Sedation and Analgesia for the Pediatric Intensivist

Pradip P. Kamat • John W. Berkenbosch
Editors

Sedation and Analgesia for the Pediatric Intensivist

A Clinical Guide

Springer

Editors
Pradip P. Kamat
Associate Professor of Pediatrics
Emory University School of Medicine
Department of Pediatrics
Division of Pediatric Critical Care Medicine
Children's Healthcare of Atlanta at Egleston
Atlanta, GA
USA

John W. Berkenbosch
Professor of Pediatrics/Pediatric Critical Care
University of Louisville
"Just For Kids" Critical Care Center
Norton Children's Hospital
Louisville, KY
USA

ISBN 978-3-030-52554-5 ISBN 978-3-030-52555-2 (eBook)
https://doi.org/10.1007/978-3-030-52555-2

This Springer imprint is published by the registered company Springer Nature Switzerland AG
The registered company address is: Gewerbestrasse 11, 6330 Cham, Switzerland

To my wife, Veronica, and my children, Seth, Mason, and Elena, who have continued to encourage me to be the best physician, husband, and father I can be, I thank you from the bottom of my heart. Your support, understanding, and love never cease to inspire and bless me.

John W. Berkenbosch, MD, FAAP, FCCM

This work is dedicated to my wife Madhavi, who embodies perseverance and dedication to the cause of humanity, my children Lily and Prem, who make me want to be a better human, and all my colleagues in Critical Care and Sedation at Children's Healthcare of Atlanta, who push me to be a better physician everyday.

Pradip P. Kamat, MD, MBA, FCCM

Foreword

Sedation and Analgesia are two of the most important topics that patients, providers, and families all think about, discuss, and worry about before, during, and after a child's intensive care experience. In this book, *Sedation and Analgesia for the Pediatric Intensivist*, the editors (Berkenbosch and Kamat) have orchestrated and conducted a thoughtful and comprehensive discussion of these important and interrelated topics. From the past, through present, to predictions for the future, they build from a basic science foundation through clinical pearls to next-generation potential solutions. Chapters are dedicated to basic and advanced principles of agent selection, monitoring, and titration. Special circumstances such as congenital heart disease, neonatal, traumatic brain injury, and neurotoxicity are comprehensively addressed. Important emerging interactions of sedative and analgesic agents and their potential role in sleep disorders, delirium, mobility, and palliative care are thoughtfully discussed. The book provides something for everyone and is a "must" for students, multidisciplinary providers, and anyone who has or is thinking about caring for critically ill children. It is gratifying to have a modern text written by experts in the field that addresses all facts and facets of this most important aspect of our care for critically ill and injured children.

Philadelphia, PA, USA Vinay Nadkarni, MD, MS, FAAP, FAHA, FERC, FCCM

Preface

In the past two decades, pediatric critical care medicine (PCCM) physicians have been at the forefront of providing care to critically ill infants and children not just within the walls of the pediatric intensive care units (PICUs) but also outside. The training of PCCM physicians in the early recognition and management of airway and hemodynamic compromise makes them uniquely positioned to provide sedation analgesia both within and outside the walls of the PICU. The performance of procedural sedation by pediatric intensivists is a cost-effective option and allows anesthesiologists to provide care for patients who demand their unique expertise, such as in the operating room. Within the PICU, patients often require sedation, anxiolysis, and/or analgesia for the tolerance of mechanical ventilation and other PICU therapies, invasive procedure performance, and management of their underlying disease or reason for PICU admission. The provision of these therapies in the PICU has become routine and increasingly occurs in critically ill patients not being managed with an invasive airway. As any PICU patient may decompensate and require placement of an invasive airway, all members of the care team (physicians, advanced practice providers, registered nurses, and respiratory therapists) are readily available, are all attuned to monitor for these decompensations, and can rapidly respond as needed should endotracheal intubation be required.

In contrast, outpatient procedural sedation, also termed as natural airway sedation, tends to be provided with more limitations in the number of personnel available (usually a physician and nurse with no respiratory therapist), and the need to escalate to endotracheal intubation for decompensation is often viewed as a failure and may even be associated with "punitive" consequences as the procedure may not end up being completed and delays in patient discharge may occur. As sedative and analgesic agents became available whose pharmacologic properties were desirable in the outpatient setting, such as short duration of action and limited potential for cardiac and/or respiratory compromise, providers quickly embraced them. While these agents (e.g., ketamine, propofol, dexmedetomidine) have ultimately become valued and even "game-changing", there is a risk that their introduction may occur without adequate education for all caregivers involved in the care of patients receiving them.

This textbook is meant for all providers administering and monitoring the use of sedative and analgesic agents to critically ill children in the PICU or those requiring them for procedural sedation. It is directed not only to medical students, residents, fellows, attendees, and general practitioners but also to allied healthcare providers such as advance practice nurses, physician assistants, and pharmacists. Our goal, therefore, has been to make this a multidisciplinary resource, with invaluable contributions from authors with varied backgrounds and expertise, and is meant to be treatise to the readers incorporating the latest knowledge on sedation and analgesia provision within both the PICU and procedural sedation environments.

Besides extensive detailed reviews on pharmaceutical agents, we have also attempted to acknowledge that sedation and analgesia do not just mean medications and that these therapies have potential adverse effects beyond the immediate. This work, therefore, also includes chapters describing the role of child life specialists within and outside of the PICU. It also includes chapters discussing the potential for neurotoxicity in the developing brain, tolerance and withdrawal, the importance of early mobility, and the more recently recognized appreciation of and understanding regarding the development, consequences, and management of delirium.

In an effort to be as comprehensive, our hope is that readers will also enjoy chapters addressing sedation prescreening as well as the approach to the sedation of high-risk patients such as patients with cardiac disease, prematurity, obstructive sleep apnea, or those receiving extracorporeal membrane oxygenation. Contributions regarding the use of regional anesthetics to decrease systemic agent requirements and inhalational agents including nitrous oxide can also expand options often available to both the critically ill patient and the child receiving elective outpatient procedural sedation. The inclusion of a chapter on simulation for sedation recognizes the importance of continuing education while that on palliative sedation therapy underscores the fact that provision of pediatric critical care includes both acute resuscitation as well as, unfortunately, palliation care.

As editors, we are grateful to the editorial team at Springer for appreciating the importance of this topic and supporting this work. We also thank all of the authors for their hard work in providing chapters balancing both theory and bedside practice. We are optimistic that readers will find this textbook useful while caring for children inside or outside the PICU.

Finally, we are thankful to our families who have supported us in both our clinical work as Intensivists and our desire to aid current and future caregivers of all children, critically ill and otherwise, by publishing this work.

Atlanta, GA, USA — Pradip P. Kamat
Louisville, KY, USA — John W. Berkenbosch

Contents

Contributors

Olutola Adu, PharmD, BCPPS Children's Healthcare of Atlanta, Atlanta, GA, USA

Jessica A. Berger, MD, MHS Anesthesiology and Critical Care Medicine, Pediatrics, Johns Hopkins Hospital, Baltimore, MD, USA

John W. Berkenbosch, MD, FAAP, FCCM University of Louisville, "Just For Kids" Critical Care Center, Norton Children's Hospital, Louisville, KY, USA

Kaitlin M. Best, PhD, RN, CCRN Center for Sleep and Circadian Neurobiology, Perelman School of Medicine, University of Pennsylvania, Philadelphia, PA, USA

Department of Nursing & Clinical Care Services, Children's Hospital of Philadelphia, Philadelphia, PA, USA

Kristina A. Betters, MD Departments of Pediatric Anesthesiology and Critical Care Medicine; Pediatrics; Physical Medicine and Rehabilitation, Johns Hopkins Hospital, Baltimore, MD, USA

Juan P. Boriosi, MD Department of Pediatrics, University of Wisconsin School of Medicine and Public Health, Madison, WI, USA

Jessica Brown, CCLS Children's Healthcare of Atlanta, Atlanta, GA, USA

Siti N. H. Buang, MB, BCh, BAO, MRCPCH Department of Paediatric Subspecialties, Children's Intensive Care Unit, KK Women's and Children's Hospital, Singapore, Singapore

Yoke Hwee Chan, MBBS MRCP(Paed) M MED(Paed) MBA Department of Paediatric Subspecialties, Children's Intensive Care Unit, KK Women's and Children's Hospital, Singapore, Singapore

Kevin G. Couloures, DO, MPH Stanford School of Medicine, Stanford, CA, USA

Pediatric Intensive Care Unit, California Pacific Medical Center, San Francisco, CA, USA

Nancy Crego, PhD, Alumnus CCRN, CHSE Duke University School of Nursing, Durham, NC, USA

Heather Damhoff, PharmD Norton Children's Hospital, Pharmacy, Louisville, KY, USA

Leslie Dervan, MD, MS Division of Pediatric Critical Care Medicine, Department of Pediatrics, University of Washington, Seattle, WA, USA

Center for Clinical and Translational Research; Seattle Children's Research Institute, Seattle, WA, USA

Girish G. Deshpande, MD, FAAP Critical Care Medicine, University of Illinois College of Medicine at Peoria, Children's Hospital of Illinois, Peoria, IL, USA

Michael Fiedorek, MD Emory + Children's Pediatric Institute, Children's Healthcare of Atlanta, Atlanta, GA, USA

James D. Fortenberry, MD, MCCM, FAAP Critical Care Medicine, Emory University School of Medicine/Children's Hospital of Atlanta, Atlanta, GA, USA

Maria Gabriela Dominguez Garcia, MD Division of Neonatal Perinatal Medicine, LAC + USC Medical Center, Keck School of Medicine, University of Southern California, Los Angeles, CA, USA

Jessie E. Gordon, M. Ed, CCLS, CIMI "Just For Kids" Critical Care Center, Norton Children's Hospital, Louisville, KY, USA

Jocelyn R. Grunwell, MD, PhD Pediatrics, Emory University School of Medicine/Children's Healthcare of Atlanta at Egleston, Atlanta, GA, USA

Sherika Haire-Kendall, PharmD Children's Healthcare of Atlanta, Atlanta, GA, USA

Kevin Havlin, MD University of Louisville, Louisville, KY, USA

Gregory A. Hollman, MD Department of Pediatrics, University of Wisconsin School of Medicine and Public Health, Madison, WI, USA

Michael Hooper, MD Yale Medicine, New Haven, CT, USA

Pradip P. Kamat, MD, MBA, FCCM Department of Pediatrics, Emory University School of Medicine, Atlanta, GA, USA

Sapna R. Kudchadkar, MD, PhD Pediatric Anesthesiology and Critical Care Medicine, Pediatrics, Physical Medicine and Rehabilitation, Johns Hopkins Hospital, Baltimore, MD, USA

Department Critical Care Medicine; Pediatrics, Vanderbilt University, Nashville, TN, USA

Cheri D. Landers, MD, FCCM Pediatrics, University of Kentucky, Kentucky Children's Hospital, Lexington, KY, USA

Mary Landrigan-Ossar, MD, PhD Department of Anesthesia, Perioperative & Pain Medicine, Boston Children's Hospital, Harvard Medical School, Boston, MA, USA

Elizabeth Laverriere, MD, MPH Anesthesiology and Critical Care Medicine, Children's Hospital of Philadelphia, Philadelphia, PA, USA

Efrat Lelkes, MD Department of Pediatrics, Division of Critical Care Medicine, Integrated Pediatric Pain and Palliative Care, University of California San Francisco, San Francisco, CA, USA

Lisa M. Lima, MD Critical Care Medicine, University School of Medicine/ Children's Hospital of Atlanta, Atlanta, GA, USA

Mohammad Tariq Malik, MD Pediatric Critical Care, Southern California Permanente Medical Group, Fontana, CA, USA

Elizabeth Sanders Martin, LPAT, ATR-BC, LPCC, CCLS Norton Children's Hospital, Louisville, KY, USA

Mudit Mathur, MD, MBA, FAAP, FCCM, CPPS Pediatric Critical Care, Southern California Permanente Medical Group, Fontana, CA, USA

Kaiser Permanente School of Medicine, Pasadena, CA, USA

Cynthia L. McCune, PharmD, MBA, BCCCP Dell Children's Medical Center, Pharmacy, Austin, TX, USA

Anuradha Menon, MBBS(Spore) M Med(Paed)(Spore) MRCPCH (Paed) Department of Paediatric Subspecialties, Children's Intensive Care Unit, KK Women's and Children's Hospital, Singapore, Singapore

Whitney Moore, PharmD Children's Healthcare of Atlanta, Atlanta, GA, USA

Wynne Morrison, MD, MBE Department of Anesthesiology and Critical Care Medicine, Pediatric Advanced Care Team, The Children's Hospital of Philadelphia and Perelman School of Medicine at the University of Pennsylvania, Philadelphia, PA, USA

Eitan Neeman, MD Yale School of Medicine, New Haven, CT, USA

Pediatric Intensive Care Unit, Soroka University Medical Center and Faculty of Health Sciences, Ben-Gurion University of the Negev, Beer-Sheva, Israel

Akira Nishisaki, MD, MSCE Anesthesiology and Critical Care Medicine, Children's Hospital of Philadelphia, Philadelphia, PA, USA

Chhaya Patel, MD Emory University School of Medicine, Emory + Children's Pediatric Institute, Satellite Blvd. Surgery Center, Division of Pediatric and Ambulatory Anesthesiology, Children's Healthcare of Atlanta, Atlanta, GA, USA

Megan E. Peters, MD Department of Pediatrics, University of Wisconsin School of Medicine and Public Health, Madison, WI, USA

Robert Pettignano, MD Emory University School of Medicine, Atlanta, GA, USA

Gregory S. Podolej, MD Emergency Medicine, OSF St Francis Medical Center, Peoria, IL, USA

Erin R. Powell, MD Pediatrics, University of Kentucky, Kentucky Children's Hospital, Lexington, KY, USA

Veronica Ramirez-Ramon, MD Department of Pediatrics, Division of Pediatric Critical Care Medicine, Weill Cornell Medical College, New York, NY, USA

Jessica Raper, PhD Yerkes National Primate Research Center, Emory University, Atlanta, GA, USA

Lindsey Rasmussen, MD Stanford University, Stanford, CA, USA

Eileen Rhee, MD, MS Department of Pediatrics, Division of Pediatric Critical Care Medicine, Division of Bioethics and Palliative Care, Seattle Children's Hospital, Seattle, WA, USA

Erin V. Rosenberg, MD Emory University School of Medicine, Emory + Children's Pediatric Institute, Pediatric Anesthesiology Fellowship Program, Children's Healthcare of Atlanta, Atlanta, GA, USA

Amanda Ruth, MD Texas Children's Hospital, Baylor College of Medicine, Pediatric Critical Care, Houston, TX, USA

Mary Sandquist, MD Department of Pediatrics, Division of Pediatric Critical Care, University of Louisville and Norton Children's Hospital, Louisville, KY, USA

Smeeta Sardesai, MD, MS Ed, FAAP Keck School of Medicine, University of Southern California, Los Angeles, CA, USA

Nadia Shaikh, MD, FAAP Pediatric Hospital Medicine, University of Illinois College of Medicine at Peoria, Children's Hospital of Illinois, Peoria, IL, USA

Anne Stormorken, MD Case Western Reserve University, Cleveland, OH, USA

Kristin A. Tiedt, MD Department of Pediatrics, University of Wisconsin School of Medicine and Public Health, Madison, WI, USA

Chani Traube, MD Department of Pediatrics, Division of Pediatric Critical Care Medicine, Weill Cornell Medical College, New York, NY, USA

Scott Watson, MD, MPH Division of Pediatric Critical Care Medicine, Department of Pediatrics, University of Washington, Seattle, WA, USA

Center for Child Health, Behavior, and Development; Seattle Children's Research Institute, Seattle, WA, USA

Michael Wolf, MD, FCCM Divisions of Cardiology and Critical Care Medicine, Department of Pediatrics, Emory University School of Medicine/Children's Healthcare of Atlanta, Atlanta, GA, USA

Judith J. M. Wong, MB BCh BAO LRCP&SI MRCPCH (Paed) Department of Paediatric Subspecialties, Children's Intensive Care Unit, KK Women's and Children's Hospital, Singapore, Singapore

Angela S. H. Yeo, MBBS, M Med (Anes) Department of Pediatric Anaesthesia, KK Women's and Children's Hospital, Singapore, Singapore

Lily Young, MD Emory University School of Medicine, Emory + Children's Pediatric Institute, Children's Healthcare of Atlanta, Atlanta, GA, USA

Part I
Sedation and Analgesia for the Critically Ill Child

Chapter 1
Introduction to Sedation and Analgesia

Mary Sandquist and John W. Berkenbosch

Brief History of Pediatric Sedation and Analgesia

The first use of operative anesthetic in a pediatric patient occurred in 1842 when Dr. Crawford Long administered sulphuric ether via inhalation to a child for removal of one of two fingers; the author noted that "he suffered from one operation and was insensible during the other" [1]. In 1857, Dr. John Snow reported that the effect of inhaled chloroform occurred "more quickly" in pediatric patients when compared with adults, the first testimonial of a difference between pediatric and adult anesthetic absorption and metabolism. Between the 1800s and the pre–World War II era, minimal distinctions were made between pediatric and adult patients in the field of anesthesia despite the successful anesthesia of countless children. However, in the 1940s–1950s, the expansion of the pediatric surgery field mandated further exploration and refinement of pediatric anesthesia techniques.

Concurrent with advances in anesthesia post–World War II, the advent of the intensive care unit (ICU) corresponded significantly with the development and dissemination of positive-pressure mechanical ventilation capabilities [2]. The first ICU was created in Denmark in 1953 and brought anesthesiology out of the operating room to care for patients requiring longer-term mechanical ventilation during the polio epidemic in the early 1950s [3]. Over the next decade, ICUs became common in larger hospitals in developed countries [4], as did specialized neonatal and

M. Sandquist · J. W. Berkenbosch (✉)
Department of Pediatrics, Division of Pediatric Critical Care, University of Louisville and Norton Children's Hospital, Louisville, KY, USA
e-mail: john.berkenbosch@louisville.edu

P. P. Kamat, J. W. Berkenbosch (eds.), *Sedation and Analgesia for the Pediatric Intensivist*, https://doi.org/10.1007/978-3-030-52555-2_1

pediatric ICUs [5], which provided the first long-term positive-pressure ventilation to children suffering from diseases such as tetanus. This was typically achieved via tracheostomy, neuromuscular relaxation with curare or mephenesin, and occasionally sedation, typically phenobarbitone [6].

The introduction of anesthesia and analgesia to children outside of the operating room and the development of technologically sophisticated support have led to an evolution in the way pediatric ICU practitioners view pain, discomfort, and the needs surrounding their management. Importantly, this evolution has been characterized by an increasing recognition of the prevalence and sources of pain, discomfort, and anxiety in critically ill children, as well as the adverse consequences of untreated or inadequately treated pain.

Goal of Sedation and Analgesia in the Critically Ill Child

At first glance, the goals of sedation and analgesia provision to the critically ill child appear simple and almost solely altruistic, specifically to ease pain and anxiety at a time the child is highly likely to be experiencing one or both of these stressors. However, additional benefits also exist which may, in the long run, be more significant. Multiple adverse effects of inadequately treated pain have been reported, including increased myocardial oxygen consumption [7, 8], ineffective cough with associated altered pulmonary secretion clearance leading to atelectasis and/or infection [8, 9], immunosuppression [10], delayed wound healing [11], impaired sleep [12, 13], and development of hyperalgesia [14]. From a sedation perspective, adequate sedation is required in many critically ill children to prevent inadvertent removal of life-sustaining devices; facilitate cooperation with therapies, such as mechanical ventilation [15–17]; decrease anxiety; and, in many cases, confer a degree of amnesia. Importantly, sedation must be seen as a balance since inadequate sedation may also be associated with excessive anxiety, post-traumatic stress development post-hospitalization, and aversion to future medical interventions and care [15, 18]. Conversely, oversedation may contribute to increased risks of extubation failure [19, 20], increased duration of pediatric ICU stay [15], development of iatrogenic tolerance and withdrawal syndromes [21, 22], and delirium [23–25].

Despite these recognitions, the literature continues to report that inadequate management of both pain [26, 27] and sedation [28, 29] are common. It is likely that an underappreciation of the adverse effects listed above are partially responsible, but it is also likely that myths regarding the ability of children to sense and process pain continue to exist across all disciplines of healthcare providers. A list of some of these myths and the evidence disputing them can be found in Table 1.1.

Table 1.1 Myths about pain in children [30]

Myth	Evidence disputing
Infants cannot feel pain due to nervous system immaturity	Pain receptors develop from 7 to 20 weeks gestation [31], and pain conduction pathways are present at 13 weeks gestation with full myelination by 30 weeks [32]. Cortical interconnections responsible for pain perception are present by 24 weeks gestation [33].
Children do not feel pain as acutely as adults	While behaviors to pain differ between children and adults, there is no evidence that pain in children is less severe than in adults [34]. As the neuroinhibitory pathways of pain develop later than propogatory mechanisms, it is conceivable that neonates may have an increased sensitivity to pain than adults [33, 35].
Children who are active are not experiencing pain	Children may remain active while in pain to (1) decrease the likelihood that they will be taken to be further examined and managed [36] or (2) use movement and activity as a distraction and/or coping mechanism for dealing with pain [30].
Children who are sleeping must not be experiencing pain	Compared with healthy controls, children with various sources of pain have disordered sleep [37]. However, children with both acute and chronic pain demonstrate sleep architecture by polysomnogram, suggesting that sleep occurs during the presence of pain [38, 39].
Children will always truthfully report their pain presence and severity	While self-report has become the gold standard for pain assessment in children aged 6 years or higher [40, 41], children may also deny pain for fear of reprisals, including parental/caregiver disapproval, cultural norms or attitudes regarding pain, and fear of needing an injection for pain management [42, 43].
Children are not capable of describing and/or localizing their pain	The validity of self-report scales for assessing pain suggests that children are capable of expressing their pain [40, 41]. While children cannot describe the characteristics of their pain in manners as sophisticated as adults, by using body outlines and pointing strategies, children can effectively localize pain sites [36, 44].
When children cry, it is usually due to reasons other than pain (i.e., restraint, anxiety, parental absence, etc.)	While children may cry for reasons other than pain (hunger, anxiety, being restrained, etc.), crying is a frequent behavior associated with pain as well. For this reason, crying is a common component of several validated pain scales, especially those used in younger children/infants or those with developmental delays in whom self-report is not feasible [45, 46].
Parents know all the answers about children's pain	Parents are generally thought to be the most reliable interpreters of their child's behavior. However, in the setting of acute pain, regardless of the cause, the reliability of parental report may be reduced due to their own stress [47]. Especially in children unable to self-report pain, parental report has been shown to vary from bedside caregivers, making true assessment difficult [48].
Opioids are unsafe for treating children's pain	Despite some age-related differences in both pharmacokinetic and pharmacodynamic responses to opioids in children compared with adults [49], an increasing body of evidence suggests that opioids can be safely used in all ages of children [50–52], including the premature neonate [53]. Opioids remain the most commonly used analgesic in critically ill children [20, 54] and should be considered part of the standard of care for managing moderate and severe pain [40, 55].

Physiology of Pain

Pain is defined as "an unpleasant sensory and emotional experience associated with actual or potential tissue damage, or described in terms of such damage" by the International Association for the Study of Pain. Nociception, on the other hand, is the unconscious activity induced by a harmful stimulus applied to sense receptors [56]. Therefore, pain should be interpreted as the emotional response to a nociceptive stimulus with the acknowledgement that the same stimulus may produce variable pain perception in different individuals.

During critical illness, children are exposed to numerous potential sources of pain. These can be broadly divided into four categories, including (a) postsurgical pain, (b) disease-related pain, (c) device-related pain, and (d) treatment-related pain. The first two sources are intuitive and should be readily apparent to caregivers, although consideration of pain related to medical disease appears to be underappreciated compared with surgical pain [57]. Due to developmental capacities and diminished patient awareness while critically ill, it may also be difficult for bedside providers to identify the presence of pain and/or understand its source which may compound inadequate treatment. While data are limited, numerous device and/or treatment sources of pain have been identified in critically ill children. Similar to data in adults [58], endotracheal tube suctioning has been found to be a significant source of procedural pain during critical illness [59, 60]. Other sources of invasive pain not routinely pretreated included venipuncture and/or capillary blood sampling [61]. Care-related sources of pain include dressing changes, skin care, and mobilization [61, 62].

The physiology and neurobiology of the pain response system is complex but can be viewed as having two basic components: the neural pathways and interactions responsible for transmitting and processing the response to a stimulus and the biochemical mediators responsible for activating and mediating those neural pathways.

Pain arises first and foremost from tissue damage. Depending on the location of the insult, the stimulus is detected by either cutaneous nociceptors which are free nerve endings in peripheral tissue or deep-tissue nociceptors (e.g., joints, bones, and viscera). Whereas cutaneous nociceptors transmit a highly localizable response, the receptive field of deep tissue receptors is significantly wider, especially for visceral insults, making the stimulus more difficult to localize. Following nociceptor stimulation, the signal is transmitted via a number of potential neurons to the central locations for processing. Somatic tissue injuries (mechanical and thermal) are transmitted via thinly myelinated A∂ fibers which respond to mechanical and thermal impulses and are considered "fast" velocity. Visceral tissues do not contain A∂ fibers and transmit via C fibers which are much slower in velocity and produce a duller pain sensation [63].

Whereas A∂ fibers utilize glutamate to communicate the immediate localizing response to pain, C fiber transmissions are mediated via both glutamate and substance P. Additionally, chemical mediators of the pain response include release of bradykinin and prostaglandins that sensitize or activate nociceptors, which release substance P and calcitonin gene-related peptide. Substance P causes the degranulation of mast cells, releasing histamine which further activates the nociceptors, and in combination with calcitonin gene-related peptide, release further bradykinin [64].

Complexities of Sedation and Analgesia in the Critically Ill Child

The "critically ill child" can encompass a complex array of heterogeneous conditions involving multiple organ systems, especially in the growing population of chronic complex systems patients being admitted to pediatric ICUs today. These acute and chronic conditions may affect the patient's metabolism and tolerance of the multitude of agents which might be utilized to achieve these previously established goals. While the body of literature is growing, there is inadequate data regarding the pharmacokinetic and pharmacodynamic effects of sedation and analgesic drugs in the critically ill pediatric population. Drug choice and dosing are further complicated by the presence of (1) multi-organ injury, specifically hepatic and renal dysfunction, due to their impacts on drug metabolism and excretion, (2) fluid shifts due to capillary leak syndrome which may alter a drug's volume of distribution and subsequent clearance, and (3) obesity which also significantly impacts drug distribution and clearance. For this population, specifically, the practitioner is encouraged to dose drugs based on ideal rather than actual body weight. It should also be considered that drug accumulation in the adipose tissue can be substantial, especially during the use of continuous infusions, which markedly prolong elimination and dissipation of clinical effects. Periodic "holidays" during which infusions are either stopped or temporarily replaced by alternative agents may be especially important in the obese population to avoid these undesired effects. All of these factors, and likely others, challenge the provider to make calculated choices in drug selection and dosing to both achieve the desired effects for the required duration while minimizing potential adverse effects.

The subsequent chapters are intended to be a guide to all providers caring for critically ill children in making informed choices regarding the provision of appropriate sedation and analgesia in the pediatric ICU, as well as the procedural sedation setting. The principles laid out in this introduction will be expanded upon and encompass choices related to agent choice(s), safety and monitoring, special populations presenting specific risks, and specific situations commonly encountered in either the pediatric ICU or procedural sedation environments.

References

1. Long CW. An account of the first use of sulphuric ether by inhalation as an anaesthetic in surgical operations. South Med Surg J. 1849;5:705–13.
2. Marshall JC, Bosco L, Adhikari NK, Connolly B, Diaz JV, Dorman T, Fowler RA, Meyfroidt G, Nakagawa S, Pelosi P, Vincent JL, Vollman K, Zimmerman J. What is an intensive care unit? A report of the task force of the World Federation of Societies of Intensive and Critical care Medicine. J Crit Care. 2017;37:270–6.
3. Reisner-Senelar L. The birth of intensive care medicine: Bjorn Ibsen's records. Intensive Care Med. 2011;37:1084–6.

4. Weil MH, Tang W. From intensive care to critical care medicine: a historical perspective. Am J Respir Crit Care Med. 2011;183:1451–3.
5. Levin DL, Downes JJ, Todres ID. History of pediatric critical care medicine. In: Fuhrman BP, Zimmerman JJ, editors. Fuhrman and Zimmermans pediatric critical care. 5th ed. Philadelphia: Elsevier Publishing; 2017. p. 3–18.
6. Smythe PM, Bull A. Treatment of tetanus neonatorum with intermittent positive-pressure respiration. Br Med J. 1959;2:107–13.
7. Ismail A. The challenges of providing effective pain management for children in the pediatric intensive care unit. Pain Manag Nurs. 2016;17:372–83.
8. Nimmo WS, Duthie DJR. Pain relief after surgery. Anaesth Crit Care. 1987;15:68–71.
9. Oakes L. Compact clinical guide to infant and child pain management. New York: Springer; 2011.
10. Eckterowocz N, Quinlan-Colwell A, Vanderveer B, et al. Acute pain management. In: St Marie B, editor. Core curriculum for pain management nursing. 2nd ed. Philadelphia: Saunders; 2010. p. 329–79.
11. American Academy of Pediatrics, American Pain Society. The assessment and management of acute pain in infants, children, and adolescents. Pediatrics. 2001;108:793–7.
12. Aitken LM, Elliott R, Mitchell M, Davis C, Macfarlane B, Ullman A, Wetzig K, Datt A, McKinley S. Sleep assessment by patients and nurses in the intensive care: an exploratory and descriptive study. Aust Crit Care. 2017;30:59–66.
13. Armour AD, Khoury JC, Kagan RJ, Gottschlich MM. Clinical assessment of sleep among pediatric burn patients does not correlate with polysomnography. J Burn Care Res. 2011;32:529–34.
14. Hermann C, Hohmeister J, Demirakc S, et al. Long-term alteration of pain sensitivity in school-aged children with early pain experiences. Pain. 2006;125:278–85.
15. Vet NJ, Ista E, de Wildt SN, van Dijk M, Tibboel D, de Hoog M. Optimal sedation in pediatric intensive care patients: a systematic review. Intensive Care Med. 2013;39:1524–34.
16. Hartman ME, McCrory DC, Schulman SR. Efficacy of sedation regimens to facilitate mechanical ventilation in the pediatric intensive care unit: a systematic review. Pediatr Crit Care Med. 2009;10:246–55.
17. Nasr VG, DiNardo JA. Sedation and analgesia in pediatric cardiac critical care. Pediatr Crit Care Med. 2016;17:S225–31.
18. Colville G, Kerry S, Pierce C. Children's factual and delusional memories of intensive care. Am J Respir Crit Care Med. 2008;177:976–82.
19. Randolph AG, Wypij D, Venkataraman ST, et al. Effect of mechanical ventilator weaning protocols on respiratory outcomes in infants and children: a randomized controlled trial. JAMA. 2002;288:2561–8.
20. Twite MD, Rashid A, Zuk J, Friesen RH. Sedation, analgesia, and neuromuscular blockade in the pediatric intensive care unit: survey of fellowship training programs. Pediatr Crit Care Med. 2004;5:521–32.
21. Fonsmark L, Rasmussen YH, Carl P. Occurrence of withdrawal in critically ill sedated children. Crit Care Med. 1999;27:196–9.
22. Ista E, van Dijk M, Gamel C, Tibboel D, de Hoog M. Withdrawal symptoms in critically ill children after long-term administration of sedatives and/or analgesics: a first evaluation. Crit Care Med. 2008;36:2427–32.
23. Silver G, Traube C, Gerber LM, et al. Pediatric delirium and associated risk factors: a single-center prospective observational study. Pediatr Crit Care Med. 2015;16:303–9.
24. Traube C, Silver G, Gerber LM, et al. Delirium and mortality in critically ill children: epidemiology and outcomes of pediatric delirium. Crit Care Med. 2017;45:891–8.
25. Patel AK, Biagas KV, Clarke EC, et al. Delirium in children after cardiac bypass surgery. Pediatr Crit Care Med. 2017;18:165–71.
26. Groenewald CB, Rabbits JA, Schroeder DR, Harrison TE. Prevalence of moderate to severe pain in hospitalized children. Pediatr Anesth. 2012;22:661–8.
27. Shoemaker K, Dutton S, Mark M. Pain prevalence and treatment patterns in a US children's hospital. Hosp Pediatr. 2015;5:363–70.

28. Marx CM, Rosenberg DI, Ambuel B, Hamlett KW, Blumer JL. Pediatric intensive care sedation: survey of fellowship programs. Pediatrics. 1993;91:369–78.
29. Curley MAQ, Wypij D, Watson RS, Grant MJC, Asaro LA, Cheifetz IM, Dodson B, Franck LS, Gedeit RG, Angus DC, Matthay MA, and Pediatric Acute Lung Injury and Sepsis Investigators (PALISI) Network for the RESTORE Study Investigators. Protocolized sedation versus usual care in pediatric patients mechanically ventilated for acute respiratory failure: a randomized clinical trial. JAMA. 2015;313:379–89.
30. Twycross A. Dispelling modern day myths about children's pain. J Child Health Care. 1998;2:31–5.
31. Humphrey T. Some correlations between the appearance of human fetal reflexes and the development of the nervous system. Prog Brain Res. 1964;4:93–135.
32. Biljani V, Rizvi TA, Wadhwa S. Development of spinal substrate for nociception in man. NIDA Res Monogr. 1988;87:167–79.
33. Scanlon JW. Appreciating neonatal pain. Adv Pediatr Infect Dis. 1991;38:317–33.
34. The Royal College of Surgeons of England and the College of Anaesthetists. Report of the working party on pain after surgery. London: The College; 1990. p. 1–36.
35. Taddio A, Katz J, Ilersich AL, Koren G. Effect of neonatal circumcision on pain response during subsequent routine vaccination. Lancet. 1997;349:599–603.
36. Eland J. The child who is hurting. Semin Oncol Nurs. 1985;1:116–22.
37. Valrie CR, Bronberg MH, Palermo T, Schanberg LE. A systematic review of sleep in pediatric pain populations. J Dev Behav Pediatr. 2013;34:120–8.
38. Roizenblatt S, Tufik S, Goldenberg J, et al. Juvenile fibromyalgia: clinical and polysomnographic aspects. J Rheumatol. 1997;24:579–85.
39. Tayag-Kier CE, Keenan GF, Scalzi LV, et al. Sleep and periodic limb movement in sleep in juvenile fibromyalgia. Pediatrics. 2000;106:E70.
40. American Academy of Pediatrics. The assessment and management of acute pain in infants, children, and adolescents. Pediatrics. 2001;108:793–7.
41. Beltramini A, Melojevic K, Pateron D. Pain assessment in newborns, infants, and children. Pediatr Ann. 2017;46:e387–95.
42. McCaffery M, Wong DL. Nursing interventions for pain control in children. In: Schechter NL, Berde CB, Yaster M, editors. Pain in infants, children and adolescents. Baltimore: Williams and Williams; 1993. p. 295–316.
43. McGrath PJ, Unrah AM, Finlay GA. Pain measurement in children. Pain Clin Update. 1995;3:1–4.
44. McGrath PA. Evaluating a child's pain. J Pain Symptom Manage. 1989;4:198–214.
45. Merkel SI, Voepel-Lewis T, Shayevitz JR, Malviya S. The FLACC: a behavioral scale for scoring postoperative pain in younger children. Pediatr Nurs. 1997;23:293–7.
46. Voepel-Lewis T, Merkel SI, Tait AR, Trzcinka A, Malviya S. The reliability and validity of the faces, legs, activity, cry, consolability observational tool as a measure of pain in children with cognitive impairment. Anesth Analg. 2002;95:1224–9.
47. Bearden DJ, Feinstein A, Cohen LL. The influence of parent preprocedural anxiety on child procedural pain: mediation by child procedural anxiety. J Pediatr Psychol. 2012;37:680–6.
48. Khin Hla T, Hegarty M, Russell P, Drake-Brockman TF, Ramgolam A, Von Ungern-Sternberg BS. Perception of pediatric pain: a comparison of postoperative pain assessments between child, parent, nurse, and independent observer. Pediatr Anesth. 2014;24:1127–31.
49. Thigpen JC, Odle BL, Harirforoosh S. Opioids: a review of pharmacokinetics and pharmacodynamics in neonates, infants, and children. Eur J Drug Metab. 2019;44:591–609.
50. Brasher C, Gafsous B, Dugue S, Thiollier A, Kinderf J, Nivoche Y, Grace R, Dahmani S. Postoperative pain management in children and infants: an update. Paediatr Drugs. 2014;16:129–40.
51. Palmer GM. Pain management in the acute care setting: updates and debates. J Paediatr Child Health. 2016;52:213–20.
52. Krauss BS, calligaris L, Green SM, Barbi E. Current concepts in management of pain in children in the emergency department. Lancet. 2016;387:83–92.

53. Carter BS, Brunkhorst J. Neonatal pain management. Semin Perinatol. 2017;41:111–6.
54. Jenkins IA, Playfor SD, Bevan C, Davies G, Wolf AR. Current UK sedation practice in pediatric intensive care. Pediatr Anesth. 2007;17:675–83.
55. World Health Organization. Cancer pain relief: with a guide to opioid availability. 2nd ed. Geneva: WHO; 1996. p. 15.
56. Pain terms: a list with definitions on notes and usage, recommended by the IASP Subcommittee on Taxonomy. Pain. 1979;6:249.
57. Taylor EM, Boyer K, Campbell FA. Pain in hospitalized children: a prospective cross-sectional survey of pain prevalence, intensity, assessment, and management in a Canadian pediatric teaching hospital. Pain Res Manage. 2008;13:25–32.
58. Rotondi AJ, Chelluri L, Sirio C, Mendelsohn A, Schulz R, Belle S, Im K, Donahoe M, Pinsky MR. Patients' recollections of stressful experiences while receiving prolonged mechanical ventilation in an intensive care unit. Crit Care Med. 2002;30:746–52.
59. Duzkaya DS, Kuguoglu S. Assessment of pain during endotracheal suction in the pediatric intensive care unit. Pain Manag Nurs. 2015;16:11–9.
60. Fisk AC. The effects of endotracheal suctioning in the pediatric population: an integrative review. Dimens Crit Care Nurs. 2018;37:44–56.
61. Stevens BJ, Abbott LK, Yamada J, Harrison D, Stinson J, Taddio A, Barwick M, Latimer M, Scott SD, Rashotte J, Campbell F, Finley GA. Epidemiology and management of painful procedures in children in Canadian hospitals. CMAJ. 2011;183:E403–10. https://doi.org/10.1503/cmaj.101341.
62. Cummings EA, Reid GJ, Finley A, McGrath PJ, Ritchie JA. Prevalence and source of pain in pediatric inpatients. Pain. 1996;68:25–31.
63. Juneja R, Jaggar SI. The physiology of pain. Semant Schol. 2008:1–16. https://www.researchgate.net/publication/237480512_1_The_Physiology_of_Pain.
64. Kim EB, William FG. Ganong's review of medical physiology. New York: McGraw-Hill Medical; 2010.

Chapter 2
Safety and Monitoring During Pediatric ICU Sedation

Kaitlin M. Best

Ensuring safe care for critically ill children necessitates, in part, effective analgesia and sedation. Yet, the use of analgesic and sedative medications also carries risks. Opioids and benzodiazepines are associated with respiratory depression, the development of tolerance, iatrogenic withdrawal syndrome, and delirium [1–7]. Ketamine can cause hypertension, increased oral secretions, emergence delirium, agitation, and severe hallucinations [6, 8]. Dexmedetomidine has cardiovascular effects, including bradycardia and hypo- or hypertension that may limit its use in select patient subpopulations. It has also been associated with withdrawal after prolonged infusions [8–12]. Several studies have reported that exposure to analgesic and sedative medications early in life has been linked to adverse neurodevelopmental outcomes [13–15]. Although these outcomes have not been reported consistently [16–18], they remain a legitimate cause of longer-term concern. Oversedation can lengthen the duration of mechanical ventilation, increase the risk of extubation failure, and increase health-care costs, in addition to increased exposure to analgesic and sedative medications, further contributing to the development of tolerance, iatrogenic withdrawal syndrome and delirium [19–21]. Meanwhile, undersedation is associated with agitation; increased risk for adverse events, such as self-extubation or dislodgement of invasive devices; and psychological distress for both patients and their parents [22–25].

Achieving adequate analgesia and sedation in the pediatric intensive care unit (PICU) is an ongoing challenge. Evidence-based guidelines have increasingly advocated for the assessment of analgesia and sedation using standardized observational assessment tools and titrating depth of sedation to a prespecified goal [26–28]. However, surveys and observational studies of critical care practice indicate that the

K. M. Best (✉)
Center for Sleep and Circadian Neurobiology, Perelman School of Medicine, University of Pennsylvania, Philadelphia, PA, USA

Department of Nursing & Clinical Care Services, Children's Hospital of Philadelphia, Philadelphia, PA, USA
e-mail: kbest@upenn.edu

P. P. Kamat, J. W. Berkenbosch (eds.), *Sedation and Analgesia for the Pediatric Intensivist*, https://doi.org/10.1007/978-3-030-52555-2_2

implementation of such practices is far from universal; in one survey, only 36% of respondents reported the use of sedation protocols [29], and in another, only 42% of units routinely set patient-specific sedation goals [30]. There is burgeoning evidence for the safety and role of daily sedation interruption and standardized, goal-directed sedation in reducing cumulative exposure to analgesic and sedative agents [31–40], thereby reducing the incidence of complications, such as withdrawal and delirium [37, 41–44]. Nevertheless, considerable variation exists in the dosing and administration of analgesic and sedative medications across institutions [2, 20, 29, 45–47], in part due to clinician biases and variable implementation of evidence-based practices [48–55]. With the goal of providing safe, developmentally appropriate analgesia and sedation to critically ill children, this chapter will discuss available assessment tools for monitoring sedation and analgesia in the PICU and their roles in the context of analgesia and sedation management, including evidence-based clinical practice guidelines.

Assessment Tools

Pain Assessment

It is increasingly understood that adequate analgesia must be achieved prior to attempting to titrate sedation in a critically ill child. Consequently, increasing sedation in the setting of ongoing pain represents a failure to recognize one key source of patient agitation and contributes to apparent sedation "failures." Painful procedures are common in the PICU environment, with one recent study finding a median of 11 painful and stressful procedures occurring per patient per day [48]. Additionally, there is an increasing recognition that routine care practices in critically ill patients, such as endotracheal tube suctioning, repositioning, and mobilization, are significant sources of pain rather than mere agitation [56–58]. Pain expression also changes across age and developmental spectrums [59]; therefore, different tools have been developed and validated for use in specific age groups and for particular types of pain among critically ill infants and children. Providers must use their clinical acumen to select the appropriate assessment tool for a given patient, based on the child's verbal and cognitive abilities, clinical status, and consideration of the applicable population and purpose of available tools. Any assessment tools that are chosen for use in a given institution should be implemented with extensive education of clinical staff on appropriate application and scoring of the tool, and procedures should be put in place for establishing and maintaining interrater reliability to ensure consistent assessment of pain across raters [60–62].

Self-Report Tools and Surrogate Reporting

Self-report of pain is widely recommended but challenging to achieve in the PICU. In addition to individual patients' developmental capacity, the impact of underlying disease, use of sedation therapies, and endotracheal intubation and mechanical ventilation may all adversely impact the child's ability to communicate regarding pain, verbally or otherwise. Despite these limitations, research suggests that children age eight and older can provide valid self-reports of pain using a numeric rating scale of 0–10 [63–65] or faces pain scale, such as the widely known Wong–Baker Faces Pain Rating Scale [66]. These scales have been shown to be valid in populations of children as young as 3 years and older who are able to engage in self-report [67]. Unfortunately, development and validation of numeric rating scales or faces pain scales specifically for use in intubated and mechanically ventilated children have received limited research. While recent studies have shown that children can safely be maintained in a more awake state during mechanical ventilation [31], which may facilitate the child's self-report of pain using appropriate augmentative and alternative communication devices [68], further evidence is needed to explore the efficacy and validity of such approaches. Therefore, it is currently recommended that the assessment of pain through self-report be limited to children with verbal abilities who can utilize either a faces pain scale (age 3 and up) or a numeric rating scale (age 8 and up).

Surrogate reporting of pain by a parent or other caregiver familiar with the child's typical pain behaviors can provide valuable information, particularly in nonverbal children or patients who may exhibit more subtle behavioral cues. However, significant discrepancies have been reported between parent, nurse, and patient (when able to self-report) ratings of pain. In a meta-analysis comparing these assessment sources, only moderate correlations between either nurse or parent ratings of pain and the child's self-report were found [69]. A recent cohort study identified only 50–68% agreement between parent and child reports of pain [70], and another reported that parents of children with cerebral palsy tended to report significantly lower pain scores compared with both their children and other observers [71]. Thus, in children unable to self-report pain, it is recommended that a multimodal approach be utilized in which surrogate reporting is combined with other observational methods of pain assessment [72].

Observational Tools

Among neonates and infants, the Crying, Requires increased oxygen, Increased vital signs, Expression, Sleeplessness (CRIES) scale [73] and the Neonatal Pain, Agitation and Sedation Scale (N-PASS) [74, 75] have been developed to evaluate acute procedural and postoperative pain. The N-PASS has additionally been found to have good reliability and validity for assessing prolonged pain, such as that associated with a critical illness [74], and has moderate correlations with nursing assessments of pain and agitation [76]. Both tools can also be used to assess premature neonates. The CRIES has been reported effective in neonates down to 32 weeks gestational age, whereas the N-PASS has been evaluated in neonates as young as 23 weeks gestational age. The CRIES tool has five domains (see above), each scored between 0 and 2, resulting in a summary score ranging from 0 (no pain) to10 (most intense pain severity). Since the N-PASS measures both pain and sedation, its scoring is slightly more complex. It also has five domains (Crying/irritability, Behavior state, Facial expression, Extremity tone, and Vital signs), which are graded 0–2 for pain/agitation and 0, −1, or −2 for sedation, resulting in scores ranging from −10 (deeply sedated) to 10 (intense pain/agitation). Scores are corrected for gestational age [74]. Older consensus statements on pain assessment in nonverbal neonates and infants have particularly recommended the CRIES [72, 77], but those documents were released prior to the development of the N-PASS. A 2016 policy statement from the American Academy of Pediatrics simply recommends routine assessment of pain in critically ill neonates and infants, without endorsing the use of one particular tool [28]. A recent study comparing five available assessment tools for pain in neonates similarly concluded that the available tools have comparable and acceptable psychometric performance, and the authors recommend that clinical utility and practicality of tool implementation be used as the basis for selection of a specific tool [78].

The Face, Legs, Activity, Cry and Consolability (FLACC) scale was designed to evaluate acute procedural pain in children that are 2 months to 7 years of age in the postanesthesia care unit [79]. Its use was subsequently extended to the assessment of preverbal patients in the PICU [80] and for procedural pain in children that are 5–16 years old [81]. A modified FLACC has been found to be valid for the measurement of acute pain in critically ill and mechanically ventilated children up to 13 years of age [82, 83]. The FLACC tool has five domains scored between 0 and 2, resulting in a summary score ranging 0–10 and higher scores reflecting increasing pain severity. It relies solely upon behavioral indicators of pain, an important consideration since physiologic parameters, such as blood pressure, respiratory rate, and heart rate, have been found to be unreliable measures of pain and poor predictors of analgesic requirements [84, 85]. Consensus recommendations for pain assessment in nonverbal infants and children have encouraged the use of the FLACC [27, 72, 86], and it has been implemented in a variety of clinical settings [29, 45, 87, 88]. For children with cognitive impairment, a revised FLACC with individualized pain behaviors added by parents has demonstrated reliability and validity for postoperative pain assessment [83, 89].

Two additional scales have been published but are more limited in that they have only been validated for use during specific procedures or in specific populations. The Hartwig scale specifically assesses pain during endotracheal tube suctioning and is, thus, limited in generalizability. The scale utilizes five criteria (motor response, facial grimace, eye movement, respiratory pattern, and reaction to endotracheal tube aspiration), each graded from 1 to 5 for a possible score range of 5–25 [90]. In critically ill patients aged newborn to 15 years, the scale has demonstrated good internal consistency and validity [90, 91]. The Cardiac Analgesia Assessment Score (CAAS) was specifically developed to evaluate postoperative pain in mechanically ventilated children following cardiac surgical procedures [92]. It includes one behavioral (motor/respiratory response) and three physiologic (HR, BP, and pupillary size) components, each scored from 0 to 2 for a score range of 0–8. While it has been validated in cardiac surgical patients aged 0–19 years, the specificity of this population makes generalizability to broader PICU populations, surgical or otherwise, unclear.

Agitation and Sedation Assessment

Once adequate analgesia is ensured, the child's level of sedation can be assessed, which typically requires providers to make subjective judgments or conclusions regarding behavioral responses to stimuli. Optimal sedation has been defined in clinical guidelines as a state in which the child is somnolent but responsive to the environment, while tolerating therapeutic procedures without excessive movements [20, 27]. Two instruments have been developed and are used in many ICUs in an attempt to standardize assessment and improve titration of sedative medications [29, 30, 45]: the State Behavioral Scale (SBS) score and the COMFORT score.

Similar to the Richmond Agitation-Sedation Scale (RASS) used in adult critical care, the SBS score describes a patient's level of sedation across a continuum of behavioral responses, from −3 (unresponsive/comatose) to +2 (severely agitated), during normal care [93]. If a child is unresponsive during the initial, pre-stimulus observation period, a progressive stimulus is used to evaluate the patient's level of sedation. The SBS has demonstrated good inter-rater reliability and constructs validity in assessing sedation and agitation among critically ill children across the age spectrum, though it was initially validated in children that are 0–6 years old. It has been incorporated into several published studies and standardized sedation protocols [31, 32, 94, 95].

The COMFORT score was originally developed as a tool with six behavioral dimensions and two physiologic dimensions, to be used for assessment during continuous analgesic and/or sedative infusions in the PICU [96, 97]. However, subsequent psychometric testing and the recognition that physiologic variables may be influenced by both common medications used in the PICU and by critical illness itself, led to the exclusion of physiologic items and development of the COMFORT-Behavioral (COMFORT-B) scale [85]. The COMFORT-B scale demonstrated improved internal consistency, is reliable and valid for the assessment of children that are 0–17 years of age, and discriminates between under- and oversedated children in the PICU, with good sensitivity to change in level of comfort following analgesic and sedative administration [85, 98, 99]. It has six domains scored between 1 and 5, with summary scores ranging 7–30 and higher scores reflecting increasing agitation. However, the tool's length and simultaneous assessment of pain and sedation/agitation has hindered its use in some clinical settings, and the quality of evidence regarding its use is mixed [100]. A recent survey suggested that the SBS score is more commonly used for sedation assessment in the USA, whereas the COMFORT and COMFORT-B scales have been widely implemented internationally [30].

As indicated above, the RASS is commonly utilized in adult critical care while only a single validation study has been performed in critically ill children aged 2 months to 21 years [101]. Scores range from −5 (unarousable) to +4 (combative) with a score of 0 representing an awake, alert, and calm state. Despite this limited evaluation in critically ill children, use of the RASS is likely to continue to grow, as it is the score which both the pediatric Confusion Assessment Method for the ICU (pCAM-ICU) and Cornell Assessment of Pediatric Delirium (CAPD) tools use for determining eligibility to perform delirium screening in children [102–104].

Objective Monitoring Tools

The subjective nature of observational assessment tools has led many clinicians to desire an objective monitoring method that can be used to titrate sedation to more precisely fit an individual patient's needs. From a safety standpoint, cardiorespiratory monitors and pulse oximetry should be considered standards of care in monitoring for sedation-induced effects on hemodynamic status and respiratory effort. For procedural sedation in non-intubated children, the use of end-tidal capnography is additionally recommended to detect hypoventilation that would not be detected by pulse oximetry [105]. Careful examination of the capnographic waveforms can additionally allow early identification of different sources of airway compromise [106]. Heart rate variability (HRV) is an emerging area of interest in analgesia and sedation monitoring. The analgesia nociception index (ANI) is a quantitative value derived from measures of HRV that may allow detection of lesser degrees of nociception during sedation or anesthesia which the above-discussed observational assessment tools are inadequately sensitive to identify [107–109]. Research in critically ill adults suggests that the ANI may be most useful for detection of pain during routine care [110]. However, to date, this tool has not been evaluated specifically in the PICU setting. Its utility may be further limited by the effects of sedative medications common in the critical care setting, such as dexmedetomidine, that affect sympathetic tone and, consequently, HRV [109].

Electroencephalography (EEG) sensitively measures electrical activity within the brain in the clinical setting. However, the complexity of the output typically requires in-depth training and experience to interpret accurately, and the volume of information gleaned generally precludes comprehensive, real-time analysis. Advanced mathematical modeling allows EEG signals to be broken down into frequency, phase, and amplitude components, which can then be interpreted using proprietary algorithms. Such processed EEG measures have been investigated for bedside neurological monitoring and sedation assessment, including the Bispectral Index score (BIS) and amplified EEG (aEEG), which will be reviewed in the sections that follow.

Processed EEG

The BIS was developed and released in the mid 1990s as a brain function monitor to assist with monitoring depth of anesthesia in the operating room, but its use has subsequently been expanded to a number of other clinical areas [111]. The BIS is a processed EEG measure that uses a proprietary and unpublished algorithm to distill cerebral electrical activity into a numeric scale with values ranging from 0 (isoelectric EEG) to 100 (fully awake) [111–113]. Those values can be further stratified into four clinically relevant categories reflecting increasing depth of sedation: from fully awake or lightly sedated with potential for recall, to very deep sedation similar to general anesthesia. Additional parameters provided along with the BIS value are the suppression ratio, representing the cumulative percentage of burst suppression corresponding to cortical silence over the previous 65 seconds; electromyographic (EMG) activity, reflecting high frequency from muscle movement; and signal quality index (SQI), a global parameter reflecting electrode impedance and artifacts, including EMG activity. Considering the BIS value alongside the suppression ratio, EMG activity and SQI is meant to help the clinician evaluate the quality of the BIS signal and determine whether it is a reliable indicator of the patient's level of sedation.

Though originally developed and tested in adults, several studies have examined the use of BIS monitoring in the pediatric critical care setting in children from neonates to 18 years old [114–124]. BIS values have demonstrated reasonable sensitivity and specificity in differentiating between inadequate and adequate levels of sedation in older children [115, 118, 125, 126], whereas the burst suppression ratio and other EEG parameters have been shown to change with increasing age as a function of cerebral maturation and should be interpreted with caution [118, 126]. In general, it appears that the BIS is more accurate in differentiating inadequate from adequate sedation than it is for differentiating adequate from excessive sedation [114, 119, 120, 125, 126], with low to moderate correlations with sedation scores, such as the COMFORT score [116, 117, 124, 125]. Given the trend towards avoiding deep sedation except when clinically necessary, this drawback is a significant hindrance to extending the use of BIS monitoring. EMG activity can lead to interference that artificially elevates BIS scores [127], which may or may not reflect inadequate analgesia and sedation depending on the source [113, 128]. Elimination of EMG interference by neuromuscular blockade may not improve the accuracy of BIS monitoring [123, 124, 128–130], and in fact reliance on BIS values seems to lead to oversedation [130, 131]. Thus, BIS monitoring may have challenges in both cases of under- and oversedation. BIS monitoring during the use of ketamine and dexmedetomidine may not accurately quantify sedation as those agents appear to affect the EEG differently than other sedatives [111–113, 126, 132], which may be a significant limitation in the context of increasing use of both medications in current sedation practice [2, 6, 133]. Finally, abnormal brain activity as a consequence of delirium, encephalopathy, trauma, or other focal neurologic processes may all be reflected in EEG changes that could be misinterpreted as sedation, depending on electrode placement [113, 116, 128].

Amplitude-integrated EEG (aEEG) filters continuous EEG output to remove both low-frequency (<2 Hz) and high-frequency (>15 Hz) signals, smoothing and reformatting the signal for display in a single time-compressed waveform. In some neonatal ICUs, aEEG has become standard for prognostication after hypoxic–ischemic injury [134], but its use for sedation monitoring is less-well studied. Sedative and antiepileptic medications lower the background EEG amplitude and alter sleep–wake cycling (SWC). However, the results across studies of aEEG use during sedation are mixed: midazolam was shown to delay onset of normal SWC and fentanyl caused continuous low voltage in newborns undergoing cardiac surgery [135], whereas in another study of neonates undergoing noncardiac surgery, neither morphine nor midazolam altered background aEEG pattern [136]. Giordano et al. (2018) reported that aEEG was able to differentiate between no sedation and either light or deep sedation in ventilated neonates, but, similar to the BIS, it could not sensitively differentiate between light and deep sedation, and it was not superior to assessment using the N-PASS tool [119]. All aEEG parameters were depressed by increasing doses of analgesics and sedatives. Therefore, there is insufficient evidence to recommend the routine use of aEEG alone for sedation monitoring in the PICU, particularly outside the neonatal population given the lack of data in this older pediatric population.

Conventional EEG

Conventional continuous EEG monitoring is currently indicated for use in the PICU for children with refractory status epilepticus, acute encephalopathy, intracranial pressure management, acute brain injury, including traumatic brain injury and hypoxic–ischemic brain injuries, and altered mental status of unknown etiology [137]. There is also evidence that children who have undergone surgery for congenital heart disease are at risk for postoperative seizures [138–140], and continuous EEG monitoring in that population is increasing. For children undergoing sedation with or without neuromuscular blockade, continuous EEG monitoring offers the advantage of identifying nonconvulsive electrographic seizures; the majority of which may not have visible clinical signs but are associated with poor outcomes [137]. Reported practice among neonatologists is to perform continuous EEG monitoring for 1–2 days if no seizures are detected [141], though it has been suggested that duration of monitoring be tailored to the patient's age, clinical status, and cause of acute encephalopathy if seizures may reasonably be expected to arise with changing clinical status (e.g., during rewarming after therapeutic hypothermia) [137]. The most common use of continuous EEG data in altering the plan of care is initiating, titrating, or discontinuing anticonvulsant medications due to seizure identification (or lack thereof).

Evaluation of continuous EEG background features, such as burst suppression, discontinuity, attenuation, reactivity, and periodic or multifocal epileptiform discharges, has been used to aid in prognostication in patients who have sustained cardiac arrest, status epilepticus, or hypoxic–ischemic injuries [142, 143]. However, the need for real-time interpretation of EEG data and limited availability of neurologists during acute changes in patient status has led to increased interest in quantitative EEG algorithms that can be interpreted by bedside clinicians [134]. While such algorithms are commercially available, their use is subject to substantial variability in correct identification of seizure activity dependent upon user experience, and to date their use in practice is infrequent [137]. Given the difficulties with implementing an easily interpreted quantitative EEG in the PICU for seizure detection, it is unlikely that continuous EEG could feasibly be used for titration of sedation in the PICU, particularly given the complexities of sedative medication impact on EEG spectra in various brain regions [132, 144–146] and significant interindividual and age-related variability in calculated EEG parameters [147].

Conclusions

There is insufficient evidence for any of the currently available objective monitoring technologies to be used as stand-alone modalities for monitoring sedation in the PICU and, when used, information from these devices should be weighed in conjunction with observational assessment tools to form a global impression of the patient's level of sedation [112, 128]. In particular, it is important to consider the effect of the chosen analgesic and sedative regimen on EEG activity [112, 113], as well as altered pharmacokinetics and pharmacodynamics of analgesic and sedative medications during critical illness that may not be reflected in EEG or other objective monitoring parameters [6]. The exception to this may be the child in whom continuous neuromuscular blockade is being utilized and in whom BIS monitoring in particular may be helpful in trending depth of sedation. More research is needed to establish the role and utility of EEG-based monitoring devices, and this work is in progress; a working group of clinical and engineering experts is currently designing a "neuroPICU" display that would support rapid review of neurologic and physiologic data in specialized visualizations which would be modifiable based on the specialty of the reviewer [148]. However, such a device will require extensive testing prior to implementation to determine its efficacy specifically for sedation monitoring, as well as its effect on relevant patient outcomes, such as sedative exposure and iatrogenic complications. Furthermore, use of objective monitoring devices should not supersede the implementation of evidence-based practices, including setting sedation targets and utilizing standardized, goal-directed sedation protocols that incorporate validated pain and sedation assessment tools.

References

1. Best KM, Wypij D, Asaro LA, Curley MAQ. Patient, process, and system predictors of iatrogenic withdrawal syndrome in critically ill children. Crit Care Med. 2017;45(1):e7–15.
2. Anand KJS, Clark AE, Willson DF, Berger J, Meert KL, Zimmerman JJ, et al. Opioid analgesia in mechanically ventilated children: results from the multicenter measuring opioid tolerance induced by fentanyl study. Pediatr Crit Care Med. 2013;14(1):27–36.
3. Ista E, van Dijk M, Gamel C, Tibboel D, de Hoog M. Withdrawal symptoms in critically ill children after long-term administration of sedatives and/or analgesics: a first evaluation. Crit Care Med. 2008;36(8):2427–32.
4. Traube C, Silver G, Gerber LM, Kaur S, Mauer EA, Kerson A, et al. Delirium and mortality in critically ill children: epidemiology and outcomes of pediatric delirium. Crit Care Med. 2017;45(5):891–8.
5. Mody K, Kaur S, Mauer EA, Gerber LM, Greenwald BM, Silver G, et al. Benzodiazepines and development of delirium in critically ill children: estimating the causal effect. Crit Care Med. 2018;46(9):1486–91.
6. Zuppa AF, Curley MAQ. Sedation analgesia and neuromuscular blockade in pediatric critical care: overview and current landscape. Pediatr Clin North Am. 2017;64(5):1103–16.
7. Smith HAB, Gangopadhyay M, Goben CM, Jacobowski NL, Chestnut MH, Thompson JL, et al. Delirium and benzodiazepines associated with prolonged ICU stay in critically ill infants and young children. Crit Care Med. 2017;45(9):1427–35.

8. Johnson PN, Miller JL, Hagemann TM. Sedation and analgesia in critically ill children. AACN Adv Crit Care. 2012;23(4):415–34.
9. Shutes BL, Gee SW, Sargel CL, Fink KA, Tobias JD. Dexmedetomidine as single continuous sedative during noninvasive ventilation. Pediatr Crit Care Med. 2018;19(4):287–97.
10. Whalen LD, Di Gennaro JL, Irby GA, Yanay O, Zimmerman JJ. Long-term dexmedetomidine use and safety profile among critically ill children and neonates. Pediatr Crit Care Med. 2014;15(8):706–14.
11. Riker RR, Fraser GL. Adverse events associated with sedatives, analgesics, and other drugs that provide patient comfort in the intensive care unit. Pharmacotherapy. 2005;25(5 Pt 2):8S–18S.
12. Gong M, Man Y, Fu Q. Incidence of bradycardia in pediatric patients receiving dexmedetomidine anesthesia: a meta-analysis. Int J Clin Pharm. 2017;39(1):139–47.
13. Duerden EG, Guo T, Dodbiba L, Chakravarty MM, Chau V, Poskitt KJ, et al. Midazolam dose correlates with abnormal hippocampal growth and neurodevelopmental outcome in preterm infants. Ann Neurol. 2016;79(4):548–59.
14. Kocek M, Wilcox R, Crank C, Patra K. Evaluation of the relationship between opioid exposure in extremely low birth weight infants in the neonatal intensive care unit and neurodevelopmental outcome at 2years. Early Hum Dev [Internet]. 2016;92:29–32. Available from: https://doi.org/10.1016/j.earlhumdev.2015.11.001.
15. van Zellem L, Utens EM, de Wildt SN, Vet NJ, Tibboel D, Buysse C. Analgesia-sedation in PICU and neurological outcome: a secondary analysis of long-term neuropsychological follow-up in meningococcal septic shock survivors. Pediatr Crit Care Med. 2014;15(3):189–96.
16. Giordano V, Deindl P, Fuiko R, Unterasinger L, Waldhoer T, Cardona F, et al. Effect of increased opiate exposure on three years neurodevelopmental outcome in extremely preterm infants. Early Hum Dev [Internet]. 2018;123(June):1–5. Available from: https://doi.org/10.1016/j.earlhumdev.2018.06.010.
17. Watson RS, Asaro LA, Hertzog JH, Sorce LR, Kachmar AG, Dervan LA, et al. Long-term outcomes after protocolized sedation versus usual care in ventilated pediatric patients. Am J Respir Crit Care Med. 2018;197(11):1457–67.
18. Larroque B, Rozé J-C, André M, Ancel P-Y, Marret S, Kaminski M, et al. Prolonged sedation and/or analgesia and 5-year neurodevelopment outcome in very preterm infants. Arch Pediatr Adolesc Med. 2008;162(8):728.
19. Anand KJS, Willson DF, Berger J, Harrison R, Meert KL, Zimmerman J, et al. Tolerance and withdrawal from prolonged opioid use in critically ill children. Pediatrics. 2010;125(5):e1208–25.
20. Vet NJ, Ista E, de Wildt SN, van Dijk M, Tibboel D, de Hoog M. Optimal sedation in pediatric intensive care patients: a systematic review. Intensive Care Med. 2013;39(9):1524–34.
21. Kollef MH, Levy NT, Ahrens TS, Schaiff R, Prentice D, Sherman G. The use of continuous IV sedation is associated with prolongation of mechanical ventilation. Chest. 1998;114(2):541–8.
22. Kachmar AG, Irving SY, Connolly CA, Curley MAQ. A systematic review of risk factors associated with cognitive impairment after pediatric critical illness*. Pediatr Crit Care Med. 2018;19(3):e164–71.
23. Lucas Da Silva PS, De Carvalho WB. Unplanned extubation in pediatric critically ill patients: a systematic review and best practice recommendations. Pediatr Crit Care Med. 2010;11(2):287–94.
24. Colville G. The psychologic impact on children of admission to intensive care. Pediatr Clin N Am. 2008;55(3):605–16.
25. Rennick JE, Rashotte J. Psychological outcomes in children following pediatric intensive care unit hospitalization: a systematic review of the research. J Child Health Care. 2009;13(2):128–49.
26. Playfor S, Jenkins I, Boyles C, Choonara I, Davies G, Haywood T, et al. Consensus guidelines on sedation and analgesia in critically ill children. Intensive Care Med. 2006;32(8):1125–36.
27. Harris J, Ramelet A-S, van Dijk M, Pokorna P, Wielenga J, Tume L, et al. Clinical recommendations for pain, sedation, withdrawal and delirium assessment in critically ill infants

and children: an ESPNIC position statement for healthcare professionals. Intensive Care Med [Internet]. 2016;42(6):972–86. Available from: https://doi.org/10.1007/s00134-016-4344-1.
28. Committee on Fetus and Newborn and Section on Anesthesiology and Pain Medicine. Prevention and management of procedural pain in the neonate: an update. Pediatrics. 2016;137(2):e20154271.
29. Guerra GG, Joffe AR, Cave D, Duff J, Duncan S, Sheppard C, et al. Survey of sedation and analgesia practice among Canadian pediatric critical care physicians. Pediatr Crit Care Med. 2016;17(9):823–30.
30. Kudchadkar SR, Yaster M, Punjabi NM. Sedation, sleep promotion, and delirium screening practices in the care of mechanically ventilated children. Crit Care Med [Internet]. 2014;42(7):1592–600. Available from: http://content.wkhealth.com/linkback/openurl?sid=WKPTLP:landingpage&an=00003246-201407000-00002.
31. Curley MAQ, Wypij D, Watson RS, Grant MJC, Asaro LA, Cheifetz IM, et al. Protocolized sedation vs usual care in pediatric patients mechanically ventilated for acute respiratory failure. JAMA. 2015;313(4):379–89.
32. Keogh SJ, Long DA, Horn DV. Practice guidelines for sedation and analgesia management of critically ill children: a pilot study evaluating guideline impact and feasibility in the PICU. BMJ Open. 2015;5(3):1–9.
33. Verlaat CWM, Heesen GP, Vet NJ, De Hoog M, Van Der Hoeven JG, Kox M, et al. Randomized controlled trial of daily interruption of sedatives in critically ill children. Paediatr Anaesth. 2014;24(2):151–6.
34. Gupta K, Gupta VK, Muralindharan J, Singhi S. Randomized controlled trial of interrupted versus continuous sedative infusions in ventilated children. Pediatr Crit Care Med. 2012;13(2):131–5.
35. Thomas M, Dhanani S. Development, dissemination and implementation of a sedation and analgesic guideline in a pediatric intensive care unit... It takes creativity and collaboration. Dynamics. 2010;21(4):16–25.
36. Deeter KH, King MA, Ridling D, Irby GL, Lynn AM, Zimmerman JJ. Successful implementation of a pediatric sedation protocol for mechanically ventilated patients. Crit Care Med. 2011;39(4):683–8.
37. Ista E, de Hoog M, Tibboel D, van Dijk M. Implementation of standard sedation management in paediatric intensive care: effective and feasible? J Clin Nurs. 2009;18(17):2511–20.
38. Randolph AG, Wypij D, Hanson JH, Gedeit RG, Meert KL, Luckett PM, et al. Effect of mechanical ventilator weaning protocols on respiratory outcomes in infants and children: a randomized controlled trial. J Am Med Assoc. 2002;288(20):2561–8.
39. Wildschut ED, Hanekamp MN, Vet NJ, Houmes RJ, Ahsman MJ, Mathot RAA, et al. Feasibility of sedation and analgesia interruption following cannulation in neonates on extracorporeal membrane oxygenation. Intensive Care Med. 2010;36(9):1587–91.
40. Larson GE, McKeever S. Nurse titrated analgesia and sedation in intensive care increases the frequency of comfort assessment and reduces midazolam use in paediatric patients following cardiac surgery. Aust Crit Care [Internet]. 2018;31(1):31–6. Available from: https://doi.org/10.1016/j.aucc.2017.02.001.
41. Sanchez-Pinto LN, Nelson LP, Lieu P, Koh JY, Rodgers JW, Larson KA, et al. Implementation of a risk-stratified opioid weaning protocol in a pediatric intensive care unit. J Crit Care [Internet]. 2018;43:214–9. Available from: https://doi.org/10.1016/j.jcrc.2017.08.049.
42. Dreyfus L, Javouhey E, Denis A, Touzet S, Bordet F. Implementation and evaluation of a paediatric nurse-driven sedation protocol in a paediatric intensive care unit. Ann Intensive Care. 2017;7(1):36.
43. Neunhoeffer F, Seitz G, Schmidt A, Renk H, Kumpf M, Fideler F, et al. Analgesia and sedation protocol for mechanically ventilated postsurgical children reduces benzodiazepines and withdrawal symptoms-but not in all patients. Eur J Pediatr Surg. 2017;27(3):255–62.
44. Neunhoeffer F, Kumpf M, Renk H, Hanelt M, Berneck N, Bosk A, et al. Nurse-driven pediatric analgesia and sedation protocol reduces withdrawal symptoms in critically ill medical pediatric patients. Paediatr Anaesth. 2015;25(8):786–94.

45. Zeilmaker-Roest GA, Wildschut ED, van Dijk M, Anderson BJ, Breatnach C, Bogers AJJC, et al. An international survey of management of pain and sedation after paediatric cardiac surgery. BMJ Paediatr Open. 2017;1(1):e000046.
46. Jenkins IA, Playfor SD, Bevan C, Davies G, Wolf AR. Current United Kingdom sedation practice in pediatric intensive care. Paediatr Anaesth. 2007;17(7):675–83.
47. Carbajal R, Eriksson M, Courtois E, Boyle E, Avila-Alvarez A, Andersen RD, et al. Sedation and analgesia practices in neonatal intensive care units (EUROPAIN): results from a prospective cohort study. Lancet Respir Med. 2015;3(10):796–812.
48. Baarslag MA, Jhingoer S, Ista E, Allegaert K, Tibboel D, van Dijk M. How often do we perform painful and stressful procedures in the paediatric intensive care unit? A prospective observational study. Aust Crit Care. 2019;32(1):4–10.
49. LaFond CM, Van Hulle Vincent C, Oosterhouse K, Wilkie DJ. Nurses' beliefs regarding pain in critically ill children: a mixed-methods study. J Pediatr Nurs. 2016;31(6):691–700.
50. Aukes DI, Roofthooft DWE, Simons SHP, Tibboel D, van Dijk M. Pain management in neonatal intensive care. Clin J Pain. 2015;31(9):830–5.
51. Burns SM. Adherence to sedation withdrawal protocols and guidelines in ventilated patients. Clin Nurse Spec. 2012;26(1):22–8.
52. Hartman ME, McCrory DC, Schulman SR. Efficacy of sedation regimens to facilitate mechanical ventilation in the pediatric intensive care unit: a systematic review. Pediatr Crit Care Med. 2009;10(2):246–55.
53. Tanios MA, de Wit M, Epstein SK, Devlin JW. Perceived barriers to the use of sedation protocols and daily sedation interruption: a multidisciplinary survey. J Crit Care. 2009;24(1): 66–73.
54. Twite MD, Rashid A, Zuk J, Friesen RH. Sedation, analgesia, and neuromuscular blockade in the pediatric intensive care unit: survey of fellowship training programs. Pediatr Crit Care Med. 2004;5(6):521–32.
55. Egerod I. Uncertain terms of sedation in ICU. How nurses and physicians manage and describe sedation for mechanically ventilated patients. J Clin Nurs. 2002;11(6):831–40.
56. Cignacco E, Hamers JP, Van Lingen RA, Zimmerman LJ, Muller R, Gessler P, Nelle M. Pain relief in ventilated preterms during endotracheal suctioning: a randomized controlled trial. Swiss Med Wkly. 2008;138:635–45.
57. Duzkaya DS, Kuguoglu S. Assessment of pain during endotracheal suction in the pediatric intensive care unit. Pain Manag Nurs. 2015;16:11–9.
58. Stevens BJ, Abbott LK, Yamada J, Harrison D, Stinson J, Taddio A, Barwick M, Latimer M, Scott SD, Rashotte J, Campbell F, Finley GA. Epidemiology and management of painful procedures in children in Canadian hospitals. CMAJ. 2011;183:E403–10. https://doi.org/10.1503/cmaj.101341.
59. Thrane SE, Wanless S, Cohen SM, Danford CA. The assessment and non-pharmacologic treatment of procedural pain from infancy to school age through a developmental lens: a synthesis of evidence with recommendations. J Pediatr Nurs. 2016;31(1):e23–32.
60. Margonary H, Hannan MS, Schlenk EA. Quality improvement initiative on pain knowledge, assessment, and documentation skills of Pediatric nurses. Pediatr Nurs [Internet]. 2017;43(2):65–70. Available from: http://www.ncbi.nlm.nih.gov/pubmed/29394479.
61. Walsh TS, Kydonaki K, Antonelli J, Stephen J, Lee RJ, Everingham K, et al. Staff education, regular sedation and analgesia quality feedback, and a sedation monitoring technology for improving sedation and analgesia quality for critically ill, mechanically ventilated patients: a cluster randomised trial. Lancet Respir Med [Internet]. 2016;4(10):807–17. Available from: https://doi.org/10.1016/S2213-2600(16)30178-3.
62. Habich M, Wilson D, Thielk D, Melles GL, Crumlett HS, Masterton J, et al. Evaluating the effectiveness of pediatric pain management guidelines. J Pediatr Nurs [Internet]. 2012;27(4):336–45. Available from: https://doi.org/10.1016/j.pedn.2011.06.002.
63. Bailey B, Daoust R, Doyon-Trottier E, Dauphin-Pierre S, Gravel J. Validation and properties of the verbal numeric scale in children with acute pain. Pain [Internet]. 2010 [cited 2013 Jun 6];149(2):216–21. Available from: http://www.ncbi.nlm.nih.gov/pubmed/20188471.

64. Voepel-Lewis T, Burke CN, Jeffreys N, Malviya S, Tait AR. Do 0-10 numeric rating scores translate into clinically meaningful pain measures for children? Anesth Analg [Internet]. 2011 [cited 2013 Jun 6];112(2):415–21. Available from: http://www.ncbi.nlm.nih.gov/pubmed/21127278.
65. von Baeyer CL, Spagrud LJ, McCormick JC, Choo E, Neville K, Connelly MA. Three new datasets supporting use of the Numerical Rating Scale (NRS-11) for children's self-reports of pain intensity. Pain. 2009;143(3):223–7.
66. Wong D, Baker C. Pain in children: comparison of assessment scales. Pediatr Nurs. 1988;14(1):9–17.
67. Tomlinson D, von Baeyer CL, Stinson JN, Sung L. A systematic review of faces scales for the self-report of pain intensity in children. Pediatrics. 2010;126(5):e1168–98.
68. Costello JM, Patak L, Pritchard J. Communication vulnerable patients in the pediatric ICU: enhancing care through augmentative and alternative communication. J Pediatr Rehabil Med [Internet]. 2010 [cited 2013 Jun 6];3(4):289–301. Available from: http://www.ncbi.nlm.nih.gov/pubmed/21791863.
69. Zhou H, Roberts P, Horgan L. Association between self-report pain ratings of child and parent, child and nurse and parent and nurse dyads: meta-analysis. J Adv Nurs. 2008;63(4):334–42.
70. Kamper SJ, Dissing KB, Hestbaek L. Whose pain is it anyway? Comparability of pain reports from children and their parents. Chiropr Man Ther. 2016;24(1):1–7.
71. Hadden KL, Lefort S, Obrien M, Coyte PC, Guerriere DN. A comparison of observers and self-report pain ratings for children with cerebral palsy. J Dev Behav Pediatr. 2015;36(1):14–23.
72. Herr K, Coyne PJ, Key T, Manworren R, McCaffery M, Merkel S, et al. Pain assessment in the nonverbal patient: position statement with clinical practice recommendations. Pain Manag Nurs [Internet]. 2006 [cited 2013 May 25];7(2):44–52. Available from: http://www.ncbi.nlm.nih.gov/pubmed/16730317
73. Krechel SW, Bildner J. CRIES: a new neonatal postoperative pain measurements score. Initial testing of validity and reliability. Paediatr Anaesth. 1995;5:53–61.
74. Hummel P, Puchalski M, Creech SD, Weiss MG. Clinical reliability and validity of the N-PASS: neonatal pain, agitation and sedation scale with prolonged pain. J Perinatol [Internet]. 2008 [cited 2013 Jun 6];28(1):55–60. Available from: http://www.ncbi.nlm.nih.gov/pubmed/18165830.
75. Hummel P, Lawlor-Klean P, Weiss MG. Validity and reliability of the N-PASS assessment tool with acute pain. J Perinatol [Internet]. 2010 [cited 2013 Jun 6];30(7):474–8. Available from: http://www.ncbi.nlm.nih.gov/pubmed/19924132.
76. Hillman BA, Tabrizi MN, Gauda EB, Carson KA, Aucott SW. The Neonatal Pain, Agitation and Sedation Scale and the bedside nurse's assessment of neonates. J Perinatol. 2015;35(2):128–31.
77. Anand KJS, International Evidence-Based Group for Neonatal Pain. Consensus statement for the prevention and management of pain in the newborn. Arch Pediatr Adolesc Med. 2001;155(2):173–80.
78. Kappesser J, Kamper-Fuhrmann E, De Laffolie J, Faas D, Ehrhardt H, Franck LS, et al. Pain-specific reactions or indicators of a general stress response? Clin J Pain. 2019;35(2):101–10.
79. Merkel SI, Voepel-Lewis T, Shayevitz JR, Malviya S. The FLACC: a behavioral scale for scoring postoperative pain in young children. Pediatr Nurs. 1997;23(3):293–7.
80. Manworren RCB, Hynan LS. Clinical validation of FLACC: preverbal patient pain scale. Pediatr Nurs. 2003;29(2):140–6.
81. Nilsson S, Finnström B, Kokinsky E. The FLACC behavioral scale for procedural pain assessment in children aged 5-16 years. Paediatr Anaesth [Internet]. 2008 [cited 2013 May 28];18(8):767–74. Available from: http://www.ncbi.nlm.nih.gov/pubmed/18613934.
82. Johansson M, Kokinsky E. The COMFORT behavioural scale and the modified FLACC scale in paediatric intensive care. Nurs Crit Care [Internet]. 2009;14(3):122–30. Available from: http://www.ncbi.nlm.nih.gov/pubmed/19366409.

83. Malviya S, Voepel-Lewis T, Burke C, Merkel S, Tait AR. The revised FLACC observational pain tool: improved reliability and validity for pain assessment in children with cognitive impairment. Paediatr Anaesth. 2006;16(3):258–65.
84. Büttner W, Finke W. Analysis of behavioural and physiological parameters for the assessment of postoperative analgesic demand in newborns, infants and young children: a comprehensive report on seven consecutive studies. Paediatr Anaesth. 2000;10(3):303–18.
85. Ista E, van Dijk M, Tibboel D, de Hoog M. Assessment of sedation levels in pediatric intensive care patients can be improved by using the COMFORT "behavior" scale. Pediatr Crit Care Med. 2005;6(1):58–63.
86. McGrath PJ, Walco GA, Turk DC, Dworkin RH, Brown MT, Davidson K, et al. Core outcome domains and measures for pediatric acute and chronic/recurrent pain clinical trials: PedIMMPACT recommendations. J Pain. 2008;9(9):771–83.
87. Crellin DJ, Harrison D, Santamaria N, Babl FE. Systematic review of the face, legs, activity, cry and consolability scale for assessing pain in infants and children: is it reliable, valid, and feasible for use? Pain. 2015;156(11):2132–51.
88. Voepel-Lewis T, Zanotti J, Dammeyer JA, Merkel S. Reliability and validity of the face, legs, activity, cry, consolability behavioral tool in assessing acute pain in critically ill patients. Am J Crit Care. 2010;19(1):55–61.
89. Malviya S, Voepel-Lewis T, Tait AR, Merkel S, Lauer A, Munro H, et al. Pain management in children with and without cognitive impairment following spine fusion surgery. Paediatr Anaesth. 2001;11(4):453–8.
90. Hunseler C, Merkt V, Gerloff M, Eifinger F, Kribs A, Roth B. Assessing pain in ventilated newborns and infants: validation of the hartwig score. Eur J Pediatr. 2011;170(7): 837–43.
91. Brunow de Carvalho W, Lucas da Silva PS, Paulo CS, Fonseca MM, Belli LA. Comparison between the comfort and hartwig sedation scales in pediatric patients undergoing mechanical lung ventilation. Sao Paulo Med J. 1999;117(5):192–6.
92. Suominen P, Caffin C, Linton S, McKinley D, Ragg P, Davie G, Eyres R. The cardiac analgesic assessment scale (CAAS): a pain assessment tool for intubated and ventilated children after cardiac surgery. Pediatr Anesth. 2004;14:336–43.
93. Curley MAQ, Harris SK, Fraser KA, Johnson RA, Arnold JH. State Behavioral Scale (SBS): a sedation assessment instrument for infants and young children supported on mechanical ventilation. Pediatr Crit Care Med. 2006;7(2):107–14.
94. Heiberger AL, Ngorsuraches S, Olgun G, Luze L, Leimbach C, Madison H, et al. Safety and utility of continuous ketamine infusion for sedation in mechanically ventilated Pediatric patients. J Pediatr Pharmacol Ther. 2019;23(6):447–54.
95. Jeffries SA, McGloin R, Pitfield AF, Carr RR. Use of methadone for prevention of opioid withdrawal in critically ill children. Can J Hosp Pharm. 2012;65(1):12–8.
96. Ambuel B, Hamlett K. Assessing distress in pediatric intensive care environments: the COMFORT scale. J Pediatr Psychol. 1992;17(1):95–109.
97. van Dijk M, de Boer JB, Koot HM, Tibboel D, Passchier J, Duivenvoorden HJ. The reliability and validity of the COMFORT scale as a postoperative pain instrument in 0 to 3-year-old infants. Pain. 2000;84(2–3):367–77.
98. Bear LA, Ward-Smith P. Interrater reliability of the COMFORT scale. Pediatr Nurs. 2006;32(5):427–34.
99. Boerlage AA, Ista E, Duivenvoorden HJ, de Wildt SN, Tibboel D, van Dijk M. The COMFORT behaviour scale detects clinically meaningful effects of analgesic and sedative treatment. Eur J Pain. 2015;19(4):473–9.
100. Maaskant J, Raymakers-Janssen P, Veldhoen E, Ista E, Lucas C, Vermeulen H. The clinimetric properties of the COMFORT scale: a systematic review. Eur J Pain (United Kingdom). 2016;20(10):1587–611.
101. Kerson AG, DeMaria R, Mauer E, et al. Validity of the Richmond agitation-sedation scale (RASS) in critically ill children. J Intensive Care. 2016;4:65-016-0189-5. eCollection 2016.

102. Smith HA, Boyd J, Fuchs DC, et al. Diagnosing delirium in critically ill children: validity and reliability of the pediatric confusion assessment method for the intensive care unit. Crit Care Med. 2011;39(1):150–7.
103. Silver G, Traube C, Kearney J, et al. Detecting pediatric delirium: development of a rapid observational assessment tool. Intensive Care Med. 2012;38(6):1025–31.
104. Traube C, Silver G, Kearney J, et al. Cornell assessment of pediatric delirium: a valid, rapid, observational tool for screening delirium in the PICU*. Crit Care Med. 2014;42(3):656–63.
105. Saunders R, Struys MMRF, Pollock RF, Mestek M, Lightdale JR. Patient safety during procedural sedation using capnography monitoring: a systematic review and meta-analysis. BMJ Open. 2017;7(6):1–10.
106. Sammartino M, Volpe B, Sbaraglia F, Garra R, D'Addessi A. Capnography and the bispectral index—their role in pediatric sedation: a brief review. Int J Pediatr. 2010;2010:1–5.
107. Avez-Couturier J, De Jonckheere J, Jeanne M, Valleé L, Cuisset JM, Logier R. Assessment of procedural pain in children using analgesia nociception index: a pilot study. Clin J Pain. 2016;32(12):1100–4.
108. Weber F, Geerts NJE, Roeleveld HG, Warmenhoven AT, Liebrand CA. The predictive value of the heart rate variability-derived analgesia nociception index in children anaesthetized with sevoflurane: an observational pilot study. Eur J Pain (United Kingdom). 2018;22(9):1597–605.
109. Gall O, Champigneulle B, Schweitzer B, Deram T, Maupain O, Montmayeur Verchere J, et al. Postoperative pain assessment in children: a pilot study of the usefulness of the analgesia nociception index † † This study was presented, in part, during the 2012 annual meeting of the French Society of Anaesthesia and Intensive Care. Br J Anaesth [Internet]. 2015;115(6):890–5. Available from: https://linkinghub.elsevier.com/retrieve/pii/S000709121731437X
110. Chanques G, Tarri T, Ride A, Prades A, De Jong A, Carr J, et al. Analgesia nociception index for the assessment of pain in critically ill patients: a diagnostic accuracy study. Br J Anaesth [Internet]. 2017;119(4):812–20. Available from: https://doi.org/10.1093/bja/aex210.
111. Johansen JW. Update on bispectral index monitoring. Best Pract Res Clin Anaesthesiol. 2006;20(1):81–99.
112. McKeever S, Johnston L, Davidson A. A review of the utility of EEG depth of anaesthesia monitors in the paediatric intensive care environment. Intensive Crit Care Nurs. 2012;28(5):294–303.
113. Fraser GL, Riker RR. Bispectral index monitoring in the intensive care unit provides more signal than noise. Pharmacotherapy. 2005;25(5 II):19S–27S.
114. Twite MD, Zuk J, Gralla J, Friesen RH. Correlation of the Bispectral Index Monitor with the COMFORT scale in the pediatric intensive care unit. Pediatr Crit Care Med. 2005;6(6):648–53.
115. Berkenbosch JW, Fichter CR, Tobias JD. The correlation of the bispectral index monitor with clinical sedation scores during mechanical ventilation in the pediatric intensive care unit. Anesth Analg. 2002;94:506–11.
116. Courtman SP, Wardurgh A, Petros AJ. Comparison of the bispectral index monitor with the comfort score in assessing level of sedation of critically ill children. Intensive Care Med. 2003;29(12):2239–46.
117. Froom SR, Malan CA, Mecklenburgh JS, Price M, Chawathe MS, Hall JE, et al. Bispectral index asymmetry and COMFORT score in paediatric intensive care patients. Br J Anaesth. 2008;100(5):690–6.
118. Lamas A, López-Herce J, Sancho L, Mencía S, Carrillo Á, Santiago MJ, et al. Assessment of the level of sedation in children after cardiac surgery. Ann Thorac Surg. 2009;88(1):144–50.
119. Giordano V, Deindl P, Goeral K, Czaba C, Weninger M, Berger A, et al. The power of N-PASS, aEEG, and BIS in detecting different levels of sedation in neonates: a preliminary study. Paediatr Anaesth. 2018;28(12):1096–104.
120. Powers KS, Nazarian EB, Tapyrik SA, Kohli SM, Yin H, van der Jagt EW, et al. Bispectral index as a guide for titration of propofol during procedural sedation among children. Pediatrics. 2005;115(6):1666–74.

121. Crain N, Slonim A, Pollack M. Assessing sedation in the pediatric intensive care unit by using BIS and the COMFORT scale. Pediatr Crit Care Med. 2002;3(1):11–4.
122. Prins SA, de Hoog M, Blok JH, Tibboel D, Visser GH. Continuous noninvasive monitoring of barbiturate coma in critically ill children using the Bispectral™ index monitor. Crit Care. 2007;11(5):1–7.
123. Lamas A, López-Herce J, Sancho L, Mencía S, Carrillo Á, Santiago MJ, et al. Responsiveness to stimuli of bispectral index, middle latency auditory evoked potentials and clinical scales in critically ill children. Anaesthesia. 2008;63(12):1296–301.
124. Lamas A, López-Herce J, Sancho L, Mencía S, Carrillo Á, Santiago MJ, et al. Analysis of bispectral index and middle latency auditory-evoked potentials parameters in critically ill children. J Clin Neurophysiol. 2009;26(3):150–4.
125. Triltsch AE, Nestmann G, Orawa H, Moshirzadeh M, Sander M, Grobe J, et al. Bispectral index versus COMFORT score to determine the level of sedation in paediatric intensive care unit patients: a prospective study. Crit Care. 2005;9(1):R9–17.
126. Malviya S, Voepel-Lewis T, Tait AR, Watcha MF, Sadhasivam S, Friesen RH. Effect of age and sedative agent on the accuracy of bispectral index in detecting depth of sedation in children. Pediatrics. 2007;120(3):e461–70.
127. Vivien B, Di Maria S, Ouatttara A, Langeron O, Coriat P, Riou B. Overestimation of bispectral index in sedated intensive care unit patients revealed by administration of muscle relaxant. Anesthesiology. 2003;99:9–17.
128. Shander A, Lobel GP, Mathews DM. Brain monitoring and the depth of anesthesia. Anesth Analg. 2017;126(2):705–9.
129. Aneja R, Heard AMB, Fletcher JE, Heard CMB. Sedation monitoring of children by the bispectral index in the pediatric intensive care unit. Pediatr Crit Care Med [Internet]. 2003 [cited 2013 Jun 19];4(1):60–4. Available from: http://www.ncbi.nlm.nih.gov/pubmed/12656545.
130. Tobias JD, Grindstaff R. Bispectral index monitoring during the administration of neuromuscular blocking agents in the pediatric intensive care unit patient. J Intensive Care Med. 2005;20(4):233–7.
131. Amigoni A, Mozzo E, Brugnaro L, Gentilomo C, Stritoni V, Michelin E, et al. Assessing sedation in a pediatric intensive care unit using comfort behavioural scale and bispectral index: these tools are different. Minerva Anestesiol. 2012;78(3):322–9.
132. Xi C, Sun S, Pan C, Ji F, Cui X, Li T. Different effects of propofol and dexmedetomidine sedation on electroencephalogram patterns: wakefulness, moderate sedation, deep sedation and recovery. PLoS One. 2018;13(6):1–15.
133. Benedetti GM, Silverstein FS, Rau SM, Lester SG, Benedetti MH, Shellhaas RA. Sedation and analgesia influence electroencephalography monitoring in pediatric neurocritical care. Pediatr Neurol. 2018;87:57–64.
134. Riviello JJ. Digital trend analysis in the pediatric and neonatal intensive care units. J Clin Neurophysiol. 2013;30(2):143–55.
135. Bernet V, Latal B, Natalucci G, Doell C, Ziegler A, Wohlrab G. Effect of sedation and analgesia on postoperative amplitude-integrated EEG in newborn cardiac patients. Pediatr Res [Internet]. 2010;67(6):650–5. Available from: http://www.embase.com/search/results?subaction=viewrecord&from=export&id=L358842921%0Ahttp://dx.doi.org/10.1203/PDR.0b013e3181da44ba.
136. Olischar M, Davidson AJ, Lee KJ, Hunt RW. Effects of morphine and midazolam on sleep-wake cycling in amplitude-integrated electroencephalography in post-surgical neonates ≥32 weeks of gestational age. Neonatology. 2012;101(4):293–300.
137. Abend NS, Chapman KE, Gallentine WB, Goldstein J, Hyslop AE, Loddenkemper T, et al. Electroencephalographic monitoring in the pediatric intensive care unit. Curr Neurol Neurosci Rep [Internet]. 2013;13(3):330. Available from: http://link.springer.com/10.1007/s11910-012-0330-3.
138. Gaynor JW, Nicolson SC, Jarvik GP, Wernovsky G, Montenegro LM, Burnham NB, et al. Increasing duration of deep hypothermic circulatory arrest is associated with an increased

incidence of postoperative electroencephalographic seizures. J Thorac Cardiovasc Surg. 2005;130(5):1278–86.
139. Naim MY, Gaynor JW, Chen J, Nicolson SC, Fuller S, Spray TL, et al. Subclinical seizures identified by postoperative electroencephalographic monitoring are common after neonatal cardiac surgery. J Thorac Cardiovasc Surg [Internet]. 2015;150(1):169–80. Available from: https://linkinghub.elsevier.com/retrieve/pii/S0022522315004961.
140. Gunn JK, Beca J, Penny DJ, Horton SB, D'Udekem YA, Brizard CP, et al. Amplitude-integrated electroencephalography and brain injury in infants undergoing Norwood-type operations. Ann Thorac Surg [Internet]. 2012;93(1):170–6. Available from: https://doi.org/10.1016/j.athoracsur.2011.08.014.
141. Abend NS, Dlugos DJ, Hahn CD, Hirsch LJ, Herman ST. Use of EEG monitoring and management of non-convulsive seizures in critically ill patients: a survey of neurologists. Neurocrit Care. 2010;12(3):382–9.
142. Nishisaki A, Sullivan J, Steger B, Bayer CR, Dlugos D, Lin R, et al. Retrospective analysis of the prognostic value of electroencephalography patterns obtained in pediatric in-hospital cardiac arrest survivors during three years. Pediatr Crit Care Med. 2007;8(1):10–7.
143. Kessler SK, Topjian AA, Gutierrez-Colina AM, Ichord RN, Donnelly M, Nadkarni VM, et al. Short-term outcome prediction by electroencephalographic features in children treated with therapeutic hypothermia after cardiac arrest. Neurocrit Care. 2011;14(1):37–43.
144. Sleigh JW, Vacas S, Flexman AM, Talke PO. Electroencephalographic arousal patterns under dexmedetomidine sedation. Anesth Analg. 2018;127(4):951–9.
145. Montandon G, Cushing SL, Campbell F, Propst EJ, Horner RL, Narang I. Distinct cortical signatures associated with sedation and respiratory rate depression by morphine in a pediatric population. Anesthesiology [Internet]. 2016;125(5):889–903. Available from: http://www.embase.com/search/results?subaction=viewrecord&from=export&id=L611774798%0Ahttp://dx.doi.org/10.1097/ALN.0000000000001303%0Ahttp://sfx.aub.aau.dk/sfxaub?sid=EMBASE&issn=15281175&id=doi:10.1097%2FALN.0000000000001303&atitle=Distinct+Cortical+Signatu.
146. Forsyth A, McMillan R, Campbell D, Malpas G, Maxwell E, Sleigh J, et al. Comparison of local spectral modulation, and temporal correlation, of simultaneously recorded EEG/fMRI signals during ketamine and midazolam sedation. Psychopharmacology. 2018;235(12):3479–93.
147. Walsh EC, Lee JM, Terzakis K, Zhou DW, Burns S, Buie TM, et al. Age-dependent changes in the propofol-induced electroencephalogram in children with autism spectrum disorder. Front Syst Neurosci. 2018;12(June):1–12.
148. Grinspan Z, Eldar Y, Gopher D, Gottlieb A, Lammfromm R, Mangat H, et al. Guiding principles for a pediatric neurology ICU (neuroPICU) bedside multimodal monitor. Appl Clin Inform. 2016;07(02):380–98.

Chapter 3
Analgesic Use in the Pediatric Intensive Care Unit

Anne Stormorken

Causes of pain in critically ill children are as varied as their admission diagnoses. Disease-related pain may derive from traumatic injuries, surgical pain, and complications/consequences of many medical diseases. Additional sources of pain include procedures commonly performed for diagnostic and therapeutic indications, device-related discomfort (lines, drains, endotracheal tube, etc.), and care-associated pain, including repositioning and endotracheal tube suctioning, among others. Consequently, the need for analgesia is almost ubiquitous and necessitates the development of an analgesic regimen for any patient admitted to the pediatric intensive care unit (PICU). The heterogeneity and large number of etiologies for acute and chronic pain may preclude all-encompassing algorithms for care, posing unique management challenges in critically ill children. Pain experienced by these children may also be as unrecognized as in other parts of the hospital [1–4]. Pain intensity and perception of pain are not continuous variables; therefore, providing continuous opioid infusions to blunt consciousness may be associated with periods of over-sedation, as well as periods of inadequate analgesia. Multimodal analgesia incorporating non-opioid analgesics is therefore an important strategy in critically ill children. Similarly, heterogeneity and ontogeny associated with pharmacodynamics in children require age-specific consideration regarding drug selection and dosing. Optimizing analgesia for children admitted to the PICU requires sound knowledge of pharmacology embedded within appropriate patient care algorithms.

In addition to being considered compassionate and to facilitate care interventions, the provision of appropriate and adequate analgesia is underscored by the variety of adverse effects associated with inadequate treatment of pain, which may include increased myocardial oxygen consumption [5, 6], ineffective cough with associated altered pulmonary secretion clearance leading to atelectasis and/or

A. Stormorken (✉)
Case Western Reserve University, Cleveland, OH, USA
e-mail: Anne.Stormorken@UHhospitals.org

P. P. Kamat, J. W. Berkenbosch (eds.), *Sedation and Analgesia for the Pediatric Intensivist*, https://doi.org/10.1007/978-3-030-52555-2_3

infection [6, 7], immunosuppression [8], delayed wound healing [9], impaired sleep [10, 11], and development of hyperalgesia [12].

Pain management strategies, regardless of etiologies, should begin with a simple focus: pain prevention. Procedural pain is often predictable in nature and timing and therefore could be easily mitigated. A point prevalence study examining patient assessment of pain severity among hospitalized children reported a high frequency of moderate to severe pain and that the most common and most severe source of pain was related to needlesticks [1]. Preventative strategies encoded within an institutional approach to procedures may improve overall pain control, not just related to needlestick pain. Subsequent to the implementation of such a system-wide protocol, the point prevalence study was repeated and highlighted that success depends on institutional commitment and patient and parent engagement. Implementation is facilitated by parent and provider education as well as protocolized care embedded within the electronic medical record (EMR) [13].

Proactive management of procedural pain will assuredly allay any associated fear and anxiety and may also mitigate sleep–wake cycle disruption, particularly if bundled with other bedside care. Unmanaged pain and sleep disruption have been identified as factors associated with the development of post-intensive care syndrome (PICS) [14–16]. To optimize sedative and analgesic administration, these elements of care can be incorporated into clinical practice guidelines serving as part of intensive care early liberation initiatives, such as PICU-Up and Wee-move. Coordinating timing of analgesic administration such that peak analgesic effect occurs with the painful component of a procedure also optimizes analgesic effect and facilitates procedural success. Needlestick pain algorithms and procedural pain clinical practice guidelines can incorporate not only analgesic dosing and route but also procedural type. EMR-embedded order sets which are activated on admission will facilitate implementation and foster institution-wide clinical adoption [13]. While merely focusing on the laudable goal of managing pain associated with traumatic injuries, perioperative states, medical conditions, and procedural pain improves pain control; additional benefits may be realized by instituting clinical practice guidelines. Inadequate analgesia for initial procedures may diminish the effect of adequate analgesia in subsequent procedures [17]. Children had greater reduction in posttraumatic stress symptoms which correlated with administration of increased doses of morphine used to treat acute injuries and burns [18, 19].

Multimodal analgesia is often viewed as opioid-sparing, however it may also be viewed as holistically incorporating non-pharmacologic strategies in pain management. Psychological interventions are effective in decreasing postoperative pain [20]. Within the lens of early liberation goals, the provision of distraction techniques, music, art therapy, and cognitive behavioral therapy is effective and, with education, also serves to involve the family in care [21]. With regards to pharmacotherapy however, multimodal analgesia is defined as concomitant use of analgesic agents with differing mechanisms of action to promote synergy of effect while mitigating additive adverse effects by reducing total doses of any individual agent. To provide a holistic and multidisciplinary approach, recent guidelines have incorporated both pharmacologic and non-pharmacologic strategies within recommendations for pediatric perioperative care [22, 23].

Non-opioids analgesics should be considered as first-line therapy in pain management, particularly in opioid-sparing strategies [22–24]. Acetaminophen and nonsteroidal anti-inflammatory drugs (NSAIDs) are widely used and share a common mechanisms of action by acting on the prostaglandin (PG) signaling pathway. PGs are implicated as pro-nociceptive agents produced by cyclooxygenase (COX)-mediated metabolism of excess arachidonic acids created during inflammation or tissue injury. PGs exert their effect through both central and peripheral receptors; however, acetaminophen blocks COX-mediated PG production centrally, whereas NSAIDs inhibit enzymatic action peripherally. Both acetaminophen and NSAIDs are commonly administered to treat mild to moderate pain and provide synergistic analgesic effect when co-administered [25–28].

Acetaminophen is available in enteral, parenteral, and rectal formulations with the bioavailability of the enteral route (90%) approximating that of parenteral administration. The primary effect is one of analgesia due to inhibition of PG synthesis at central receptors. Acetaminophen is metabolized by glucuronide conjugation in the liver except in neonates in whom sulphate conjugation is more important due to immature glucuronide enzymatic function. Enteral and parenteral dosing is equivalent: 15 mg/kg every 6 h with a maximum daily total dose of 90 mg/kg or 4 grams. In neonates, dose reduction to a total daily dose of 60 mg/kg/day administered every 4–6 h should be implemented as this takes enzymatic immaturity into consideration.

NSAIDs are available in both enteral and parenteral formulations and provide their mechanism of action via inhibition of COX-enzyme metabolism of arachidonic acid to PGs (Table 3.1). Inhibition of the constitutive COX-1 isoenzyme found on gastric mucosa, renal parenchyma, platelets, and osteoblasts results in the more common adverse effects, such as gastric ulceration, renal dysfunction, bleeding, and bony nonunion. Inhibition of the inducible COX-2 isoenzyme mitigates the increase in PG synthesis in response to trauma and is therefore the mechanism for analgesia, antipyretic and anti-inflammatory effects. Most NSAIDs are nonselective, and the newer selective COX-2 inhibitors have yet to show fewer side effects or greater efficacy. Considering this side effect profile, it is recommended to avoid

Table 3.1 Non-opioid analgesics

Drug	Route	Dose	Maximum dose	ADE
Acetaminophen	IV/ PO	10 mg/kg/dose Q 4 h 15 mg/kg/dose Q 6 h	90 mg/kg/day OR 4 grams/day	Hepatotoxicity
NSAIDs				
Ketorolac	IV	0.5 mg/kg/dose Q 6 h for 5 days (for 3 days if <2 yo)	30 mg/dose	GI bleeding, nephrotoxicity
Ibuprofen	PO	8–10 mg/kg/dose Q 6–8 h	40 mg/kg/day OR 2400 mg/day	GI bleeding, nephrotoxicity
Naproxen	PO	5–6 mg/kg/dose Q 12 h	1000 mg/day	GI bleeding, nephrotoxicity

using NSAIDs in clinical conditions with decreased renal perfusion, such as low cardiac output or hypovolemic states as well as acute or chronic renal insufficiency. In these patients, inhibition of PG production mitigates their reno-protective effects and poses increased risk of renal dysfunction. Similarly, clinical conditions with increased risk of bleeding, such as thrombocytopenia or dysfunctional platelets, as well as associated coagulopathy, should also be avoided. The role in nonunion is unclear as, despite widespread use of short-term adjunct ketorolac following pediatric spinal fusion, there is no evidence for increased reoperation [29, 30]. Therefore, inclusion of NSAIDs in clinical scenarios having other risks for nonunion should be based on assessment of the unique patient risk-benefit ratio.

Opioids are widely administered to effectively manage moderate to severe pain and are available in a variety of formulations facilitating multiple routes of administration. Opiates refer to naturally occurring compounds, such as opium, codeine, and morphine, whereas opioids refer to modified naturally occurring agents, for example, oxycodone or synthetic agents, such as fentanyl or methadone. While an increasingly important topic for practitioners, concerns raised regarding widespread prescribing practices, extended-release formulations, and opioid addiction are beyond the scope of this chapter. The reader is referred to a thorough review on this subject in a Special Topic Series on Opioid Therapeutics and Concerns in Pediatrics in the Clinical Journal of Pain [31–35].

A rational pain management strategy should involve provision of continuous analgesia with the additional ability to titrate to effect or provide additional bolus dosing for relief of incidental breakthrough pain secondary to painful procedures, including mobilization, endotracheal tube suctioning, dressing changes, and line placement, among others. Pharmacokinetic principles governing opioid delivery include route of administration, bioavailability and absorption, drug concentration at receptor, metabolism, and elimination. Opioids may be delivered intermittently (parenterally and enterally), as continuous infusions and via patient-controlled analgesia (PCA). In equipotent doses, enteral formulations have the same adverse effect profiles as parenteral formulations [36]. Analgesic drug levels will reach 90% steady state with intermittent dosing in 3.3 half-lives and 100% steady state with 5 half-lives. Commonly used opioids, such as morphine, hydromorphone, and oxycodone, have half-lives of 3–4 h, requiring total time to achieve steady state serum analgesic levels of near 24 h [36]. Therefore, delivering intermittent analgesics scheduled at intervals appropriate to the half-life may still result in inadequate initial pain relief as serum analgesic levels may fall below therapeutic range in the 1–2 h prior to the next dose (Table 3.2). Fentanyl and morphine have historically been, and remain, the most commonly utilized opioids in pediatric critical care [37, 38]. Compared with fentanyl, morphine has a longer half-life of elimination and a shorter half-life of redistribution. Consequently, administration of these agents would favor more rapid onset of analgesia with fentanyl however prolonged time to elimination with fentanyl infusion administration [36, 39].

To obviate the inherent delays associated with intermittent delivery, such as verifying the order in EMR, obtaining the drug and verifying with another nurse prior to administration, and mitigating variation in drug levels, continuous infusions with nurse-delivered breakthrough doses or PCA are commonly performed in PICU

Table 3.2 Opioid analgesics

Drug	Route	Dose <50 kg	Dose >50 kg	Frequency
Morphine	IV	0.05–0.1 mg/kg/dose	2–5 mg/dose	Q 2–4 h
	PO	0.15–0.3 mg/kg/dose	15–20 mg/dose	Q 3–4 h
Hydromorphone	IV	10–20 mcg/kg/dose	0.2–0.6 mg/dose	Q 2–4 h
	PO	50–100 mcg/kg/dose	1- 2 mg/dose	Q 4 h
Fentanyl	IV	0.5–1 mcg/kg/dose	25–50 mcg/dose	Q 30–60 min
	IN	1–2 mcg/kg/dose	25–50 mcg/dose	Q 1 h
Methadone	IV	0.1 mg/kg/dose	5–10 mg	Q 6–12 h
	PO	0.1 mg/kg/dose	5–10 mg	Q 6–12 h
Oxycodone	PO	0.05–0.1 mg/kg/dose	5–10 mg/dose	Q 4–6 h
Hydrocodone	PO	0.1–0.2 mg/kg/dose *Only available as acetaminophen combo*	5–10 mg/dose *Only available as acetaminophen combo*	Q 4–6 h

Table 3.3 Opioid PCA Dosing

Drug	Demand dose	Lockout period (minutes)	Breakthrough dose	Basal infusion rate
Morphine	0.02–0.04 mg/kg/dose	5–15	0.04–0.08 mg/kg/dose	0.02–0.04 mg/kg/h
Hydromorphone	2–5 mcg/kg/dose	5–15	4–10 mcgkg/dose	2–5 mcg/kg/h
Fentanyl	0.5–1 mcg/kg/dose	5–15	1–2 mcg/kg/dose	0.5–1 mcg/kg/h

settings. PCA devices are microprocessor pumps that provide parenteral administration of opioids via one or a combination of the following: demand dose, breakthrough dose, and basal infusion. Patient safety is ensured by limiting the dose as well as the total dose delivered per hour by proscribing the lockout period between demand and breakthrough dosing. Additional safety guards include computerized order entry and order sets constrained by provider or location (Table 3.3). Efficacy of PCA in managing moderate to severe pain in children has been demonstrated; however, contrary to adults, use of a basal infusion does not pose an increased risk [22, 23, 40–43]. The patient must be willing to interact with the PCA as well as both cognitively and physically able to use the device. Alternatively, educated proxy users in parent-controlled and nurse-controlled analgesia can be used; however, appropriate monitoring is suggested to ensure safety [23, 40, 43–46].

Specific Agents

Morphine, a naturally occurring opiate, can be administered via sublingual, enteral, rectal, parenteral, subcutaneous, intramuscular, and intrathecal and epidural routes. Intramuscular administration of analgesics should be avoided as the pain of injection is often perceived as being greater than the pain for which analgesia was initially prescribed. Enteral bioavailability of morphine is poor (30%) due to first-pass metabolism, with peak effect at 60–90 min. Hepatic metabolism of morphine via glucuronyl transferase produces metabolites in ratios that reflect specific patient metabolism; however, inactive metabolites are generally produced in greater amounts. Morphine-3-glucuronide (M3G) is an inactive metabolite that is thought to be responsible for the adverse central nervous system effects, such as dysphoria, myoclonus, and hyperalgesia. Active metabolites include morphine-6-glucuronide (M6G), normorphone, and codeine. M6G is the most potent metabolite and provides the primary analgesic effects attributed to morphine as well as adverse effects of nausea, vomiting, pruritis, and respiratory depression. Both metabolites are renally excreted and will therefore accumulate in patients with renal dysfunction [36, 39]. The most commonly experienced side effects of nausea, vomiting, and pruritis with morphine PCA infusions can be mitigated by co-administration of low-dose naloxone infusions ranging from 0.25 to 2.0 mcg/kg/h [47].

Hydromorphone is a synthetic opioid acting at the mu receptor which is five times more potent than morphine. Lack of active metabolites makes this an appealing choice in patients with decreased clearance due to renal dysfunction. Enteral and parenteral formulations are available with enteral bioavailability being low at only 20% of parenteral administration. In some patients, hydromorphone use is associated with improved analgesia and less dysphoria, nausea, and pruritis compared to other opioid agents, underscoring the influence of individual opioid receptor pharmacogenomics. Hydromorphone is commonly administered if morphine analgesia is ineffective or these side effects are intolerable.

Fentanyl is a synthetic opioid which is highly lipid soluble and roughly 100 times more potent than morphine. Time to onset of action is very short due to rapid redistribution from plasma to fatty tissues; however, its longer elimination half-life results in significant tissue accumulation with infusions. Fentanyl is primarily delivered parenterally, although in the absence of vascular access, intranasal delivery is associated with equally prompt onset of action and effective analgesia in similar dosing. The side effect profile mirrors that of morphine and hydromorphone; however, chest wall rigidity upon rapid administration is unique to fentanyl. Tolerance has been reported to occur more rapidly than with morphine infusions in equianalgesic dosing.

Remifentanil shares similar lipophilic properties with more rapid onset of action than fentanyl. However, due to its metabolism by tissue and plasma esterases, elimination is very rapid with offset of action reported within 10 min. Adverse effects include bradycardia, chest wall rigidity, and respiratory depression, and its use has also been implicated in the development of opioid-induced hyperalgesia with nominal exposure. Practically, the pharmacokinetics are insufficient to outweigh the costs of widespread PICU use as well as side effects when compared to fentanyl [36, 39].

Considerations regarding initiation of lower opioid doses in neonates reflect the unique pharmacokinetic and pharmacodynamic features of neonates and young infants of up to 6 months of age. Opioid metabolism, clearance and protein binding favor increased serum levels of opioids, therefore necessitating beginning with smaller doses. Hepatic enzyme systems involved in conjugation of opioids do not become mature until 6 months of age. Coupled with decreased glomerular filtration rate and decreased protein binding, opioid administration in neonates is associated with increased levels of parent drug as well as accumulation of active and inactive metabolites [48]. Additionally, immature respiratory reflexes to hypoxia and hypercarbia may progress to hypoventilation and apnea if not recognized and no interventions performed. Safe administration of opioids in neonates involves not only dose adjustment but appropriate monitoring commensurate with risk of adverse events.

Methadone is a multi-mechanistic synthetic opioid that exerts its analgesic effects through agonism at the mu receptor, antagonism at the N-methyl-d-aspartate (NMDA) receptor and prevents reuptake of both noradrenaline and serotonin. Consequently, methadone has been included in the treatment of acute perioperative pain for spinal fusion, opioid-induced hyperalgesia, chronic pain, and opioid dependence [22, 23]. Available in parenteral and highly bioavailable enteral formulations with a protracted elimination half-life, methadone is metabolized via cytochrome P_{450} mixed oxidase enzymes. Neonatal dosing should be decreased to reflect the relative immaturity of this enzymatic complex. Dosing equivalency in opioid-naive patients is 1:1 with enteral and parenteral formulations; however, in opioid-tolerant patients decreasing the ratio by 50–75% due to incomplete cross tolerance to avoid over-sedation and respiratory depression is recommended [36]. Methadone is associated with respiratory depression and sedation although to a lesser extent than that observed with morphine. Dose-dependent QT prolongation may be enhanced by electrolyte abnormalities, underlying cardiac dysfunction, and concomitant administration of other drugs, increasing QT interval (erythromycin and ondansetron) or CYP3A4 inhibitors (fluoxetine, fluconazole, valproate, and clarithromycin). Through NMDA-receptor antagonism, methadone could decrease the development of tolerance and opioid-induced hyperalgesia with consequent decreased opioid requirements in critically ill children receiving opioid infusions. Methadone is commonly incorporated in weaning regimens to prevent or treat iatrogenic withdrawal syndromes associated with opioid exposure in critically ill children [49–51].

Enteral opioid formulations, including oxycodone, hydrocodone, or enterally administered morphine and hydromorphone, are commonly transitioned to once patients are able to tolerate enteral medications, as analgesic needs decrease, and to facilitate tapering from parenteral infusions to avoid development of iatrogenic withdrawal syndrome. Pediatric hospital formularies should provide liquid and solid formulations of enteral opioids to facilitate administration over a wide range of ages. Avoiding acetaminophen combination formulations will minimize acetaminophen toxicity and optimize effective opioid dosing. As in adults, extended release formulations are not indicated in the treatment of acute pain; however, they do have a role in the management of chronic pain secondary to cancer and its sequelae. Dosing recommendations for opioids should include route and initial dose with dose ranges to facilitate titration to effect (Table 3.2).

Recent guidelines regarding perioperative opioid administration in children recommended postoperative patient monitoring in specific high-risk patient subgroups as well as analgesic regimens [22, 23]. An expert opinion suggests that minimal monitoring required to identify hypoventilation and apnea would include pulse oximetry, plethysmography, and cardiorespiratory monitoring. Capnography has been described; however, it is not always practical, and transcutaneous monitoring has not been fully evaluated in children receiving opioids. Pertinent quality metrics to follow include cardiorespiratory arrest events, rapid response team consultations, and opioid antagonist administration. It is pertinent to note that perceived risks associated with opioid administration to treat severe pain postoperatively should not prevent their use. Additionally, opioids after major intracranial surgery do not substantially change mental status or result in sufficient respiratory depression to withhold their use [52].

There are subgroups of children that merit increased vigilance as they are at increased risk for adverse effects upon opioid administration [23]. These include neonates, children with cognitive impairment, neuromuscular diseases, obstructive sleep apnea (OSA), concomitant administration of other sedatives, opioid-naïve patients, and those children that have received neuraxial opioids. Severity of OSA correlates with increased risk of respiratory depression with opioid administration, and patients with chronic oxygen dependency or chronic lung disease similarly are at increased risk for respiratory depression. Postoperative care of these patients may be best accomplished in the PICU setting due to availability of closer monitoring as well as increased nurse staffing ratio which should facilitate optimal drug titration. Monitoring of these patients as described above should also include use of sedation scales, such as modified Ramsey, University of Michigan Sedation Scale (UMSS) or Pasero Opioid-Induced Sedation Scale (POSS), to objectively identify sedation. However, monitoring alone may be insufficient, and initiation of lower doses which are then titrated to effect may be most prudent. Perioperatively, it is crucial that patients chronically receiving opioids should continue this regimen to avoid experiencing iatrogenic withdrawal, and additional opioids should be titrated to address acute postoperative pain. Due to receptor downregulation associated with chronic exposure, it should be recognized that increased doses may be required. In these circumstances, addition of adjunct medications, such as ketamine, dexmedetomidine, gabapentin, and, where appropriate, diazepam or baclofen for muscle spasm be considered.

There are certain clinical circumstances that merit special considerations, including management of patients with chronic or neuropathic pain and treating end-of-life symptoms, including pain [22, 23]. Perioperative care and acute pain management in children chronically receiving opioids pose unique challenges. In order to mitigate withdrawal, opioids should be administered in equianalgesic dosing to chronic exposure. Additional opioids can be titrated to address acute pain. Multimodal analgesic regimen is uniquely poised to maximize efficacy by including agents that the patient does not usually receive: regional anesthesia, systemic pharmacotherapy, including acetaminophen, NSAIDs, and adjunctive agents. If anxiety and depression are premorbid diagnoses, psychological and psychiatric interventions should be incorporated.

Treatment of neuropathic pain poses complex issues, not only due to the wide spectrum of etiologies but also due to the lack of pediatric-specific literature to provide guidance. Adult studies highlight the lack of working definition, poor understanding of underlying pathophysiology, and unclear outcome metrics, such as improved functionality, pain intensity, and therapy duration. However, differences in etiology, neurodevelopment, and comorbidities in children preclude generalizing these studies to pediatric practice. Also, use of opioids in these patients must be balanced with opioid-associated side effects and the potential for abuse. Consequently, the role of opioid medications in managing neuropathic pain in children is not clearly established. Potential roles for multi-mechanistic opioids, such as tramadol and methadone, exist; however, there is limited literature to guide their use [53]. Patients exhibiting central sensitization pathophysiology, that is increased sensitivity to painful or non-painful stimuli as found in fibromyalgia, chronic postsurgical pain, or amplified musculoskeletal pain disorders, will similarly benefit from multimodal analgesia and non-pharmacologic interventions, including psychology [22, 23]. Opioids have a clear role in end-of-life care as they are very effective in managing end-of-life symptoms, including pain, dyspnea, and anxiety. Contrary to popular opinion, their use does not hasten death. While a full description of the holistic approach to pain management in palliative care is beyond the scope of this chapter, the reader is referred to several excellent reviews [54–56] and a separate chapter in this book, addressing palliative sedation and analgesia.

Adjunctive analgesic medications are indicated when opioids are ineffective in mitigating pain at doses that incur significant side effects, or when side effects become intolerable without adequate analgesic effect. These medications include alpha-agonists, NMDA-receptor antagonists, and gabapentinoids (Table 3.4).

Table 3.4 Adjunct analgesics

Drug class	Agent	Route	Dose	Max dose	Adverse effects
Gabapentinoids	Gabapentin	PO	6 mg/kg–24 mg/kg TID (slow uptitration from 2 mg/kg/qhs necessary)	300 mg to 1200 mg TID	Dizziness, sedation, ataxia, nystagmus
	Pregabalin	PO	1.5 mg/kg–6 mg/kg BID (slow uptitration from 0.3 mg/kg qhs necessary)	75 mg to 300 mg BID	Ataxia,nystagmus, weight gain, dizziness, sedation
NMDA-agonist	Ketamine	IV	0.5–1 mg/kg/dose		Tachycardia, hypertension, dysphoria, hallucinations
α-agonist	Dexmedetomidine	IV	0.5 mcg/kg/dose		Bradycardia, hypotension
		IV gtt	0.3–2.0 mg/kg/h		
		IN	1–2 mcg/kg/dose		

Regional anesthesia is crucial to opioid-sparing analgesic strategies and is discussed in detail in a subsequent chapter. It is worthwhile to note however that regional anesthesia can be crucial in facilitating early extubation and mitigating the need for ventilatory support in select patients. In certain postoperative conditions, opioids may be unnecessary when regional anesthesia is combined with non-opioid and adjunct analgesic agents [22, 23].

α_2-adrenoreceptor agonists, dexmedetomidine, and clonidine, act at central, spinal, and peripheral sites to inhibit nerve signal propagation and provide analgesia. Clonidine is extensively used during regional anesthesia and mitigating autonomic dysregulation. Dexmedetomidine is much more selective for α-2 receptors, providing desired effects of analgesia and mild sedation with less associated bradycardia and hypotension. Additionally, it can be delivered parenterally, intranasally, and buccally with initial dosing of 0.3 micrograms/kg/h and titrated to effect. In addition to analgesia, positive attributes include provision of mild sedation which mimics natural sleep patterns as well as relative preservation of airway tone and minute ventilation. The role of dexmedetomidine infusions to mitigate opioid requirements in patients receiving dinutuximab infusions for neuroblastoma therapy has been reported [57].

NMDA antagonists, such as ketamine, provide analgesia and dissociative sedation that is dose-dependent in its effects. Chemically similar to phencyclidine, ketamine exerts its effects through competitive antagonism at the NMDA receptor preventing voltage-dependent ion flow. Inhibition of this receptor is thought to prevent central sensitization, wind-up, and formation of a pain memory creating a role for management of neuropathic and chronic pain disorders as well as a putative role in hyperalgesic states. It is the latter that may prove to be attractive for critically ill children, particularly in opioid-sparing strategies or mitigating opioid-induced hyperalgesia [22, 23, 36].

Gabapentinoids, pregabalin and gabapentin, reduce central sensitization, hyperalgesia, and allodynia, and are part of the analgesic regimen for chronic neuropathic pain. They decrease the release of excitatory neurotransmitters by inhibiting the influx of calcium ions through voltage-sensitive calcium channels. Both drugs are well absorbed and are renally eliminated intact, and neither undergo metabolism; thus, dosing should be reduced in renal failure. The most common effects are dizziness, visual disturbances, and sedation, all of which decrease with time. There is a wide therapeutic index, and up-titration to an effective dose requires gradual increase over days [53]. Gabapentin may be incorporated in the perioperative regimen of patients to increase analgesic regimen efficacy as well as to decrease opioid needs [22, 23, 36].

Critically ill children experience pain frequently and repetitively either as a consequence of their primary reason for admission to the PICU or diagnostic and therapeutic procedures needed for their care. Indiscriminate provision of sedative and analgesic infusions to blunt awareness are no longer standard of care and may contribute to the development of delirium and PICS just as easily as inadequate analgesia. These states to some degree can be discriminated by validated scales, but preventative strategies as well as non-pharmacologic approaches would optimize multimodal analgesia. Administration of acetaminophen with NSAIDs provides effective management of mild to moderate pain with addition of opioids if escalation is needed to manage moderate to severe pain. If opioids are ineffective and particularly if dose escalation is limited by side effects, then adjunctive medications, such as ketamine, dexmedetomidine, or gabapentin, may optimize pain management. Critically ill children will most likely be well monitored; however, there are high-risk populations, such as those with OSA, obesity, and cardiopulmonary disease, that pose higher risk for opioid-related adverse effects and should be monitored accordingly.

References

1. Friedrichsdorf SJ, Postier AC, Eull D, Foster L, Weidner C, Campbell F. Pain outcomes in a US children's hospital: a prospectivecross- sectional survey. Hosp Pediatr. 2015;5(1):18–26.
2. Kozlowski LJ, Kost-Byerly S, Colantuoni E, et al. Pain prevalence, intensity, assessment and management in a hospitalized pediatric population. Pain Manag Nurs. 2014;15(1):22–35.
3. Taylor EM, et al. Pain in hospitalized children: a prospective cross-sectional survey of pain prevalence, intensity, assessment and management in a Canadian pediatric teaching hospital. Pain Res Manag. 2008;13(1):25–32. http://www.ncbi.nlm.nih.gov/pmc/articles/PMC2670807/pdf/prm13025.pdf.
4. Stevens BJ, Harrison D, Rashotte Y, Yamata J, Abbott LK, Coburn G, Stinson J, LeMay S. Pain assessment and intensity in hospitalized children in Canada. J Pain. 2012;13:857–65.
5. Ismail A. The challenges of providing effective pain management for children in the pediatric intensive care unit. Pain Manag Nurs. 2016;17:372–83.
6. Nimmo WS, Duthie DJR. Pain relief after surgery. Anaesth Crit Care. 1987;15:68–71.
7. Oakes L. Compact clinical guide to infant and child pain management. New York: Springer; 2011.
8. Eckterowocz N, Quinlan-Colwell A, Vanderveer B, et al. Acute pain management. In: St Marie B, editor. Core curriculum for pain management nursing. 2nd ed. Philadelphia: Saunders; 2010. p. 329–79.
9. American Academy of Pediatrics, American Pain Society. The assessment and management of acute pain in infants, children, and adolescents. Pediatrics. 2001;108:793–7.
10. Aitken LM, Elliott R, Mitchell M, Davis C, Macfarlane B, Ullman A, Wetzig K, Datt A, McKinley S. Sleep assessment by patients and nurses in the intensive care: an exploratory and descriptive study. Aust Crit Care. 2017;30:59–66.
11. Armour AD, Khoury JC, Kagan RJ, Gottschlich MM. Clinical assessment of sleep among pediatric burn patients does not correlate with polysomnography. J Burn Care Res. 2011;32:529–34.
12. Hermann C, Hohmeister J, Demirakc S, et al. Long-term alteration of pain sensitivity in school-aged children with early pain experiences. Pain. 2006;125:278–85.
13. Postier AC, Eull D, Schulz C, Fitzgerald M, Symalla B, Watson D, Goertzen L, Friedrichsdorf SJ. Pain experience in a US children's hospital: a point prevalence survey undertaken after the implementation of a system-wide protocol to eliminate or decrease pain caused by needles. Hosp Pediatr. 2018;8(9):1–9.
14. Herrup EA, Wieczorek B, Kudchadkar SR. Characteristics of postintensive care syndrome in children after critical illness: a systematic review. World J Crit Care Med. 2017;6(2):124–34.
15. Watson RS, Choong K, Colville G, Crow S, Dervan LA, Hopkins RO, Knoester H, Pollack MM, Rennick J, Curley MAQ. Life after critical illness in children – toward and understanding of pediatric post-intensive care syndrome. J Pediatr. 2018;198:16–24.
16. Manning JC, Pinto NP, Rennick JE, Colville G, Curley MAQ. Conceptualizing post intensive care syndrome in children – the PICS-p framework. Pediatr Crit Care Med. 2018;19(4):298–300.

17. Weisman SJ, Bernstain B, Schechter NL. Consequences of inadequate analgesia during painful procedures in children. Arch Pediatr Adolesc Med. 1998;152:147–9.
18. Nixon RD, Nehmy TJ, Ellis AA, Ball SA, Menne A, McKinnon AC. Predictors of posttraumatic stress in children following injury: the influence of appraisals heart rate and morphine use. Behav Res Ther. 2010;48(8):810–5.
19. Staddard FJ Jr, Sorrentino EA, Ceranogly TA, Saxe G, Murphy JM, Drake JE, et al. Preliminary evidence of the effects of morphine on post-traumatic stress disorder symptoms in one- to 4 year olds with burns. J Burn Care Res. 2009;30(5):836–43.
20. Davidson F, Snow S, Hayden JA, Chorney J. Psychological interventions in managing postoperative pain in children: a systematic review. Pain. 2016;157(9):1872–86.
21. Esses SA, Small S, Rodemann A, Hartmann ME. Am J Crit Care. 2019;28(1):19–27.
22. Chou R, et al. Guidelines on the Management of Postoperative Pain; Management of Postoperative Pain: a clinical practice guidelines from the American Pain Society, the American Society of Regional Anesthesia and Pain Medicine, and the American Society of Anesthesiologists' Committee on Regional Anesthesia, Executive Committee and Administrative Council. J Pain. 2016;17(2):131–57.
23. Cravero JP, et al. The Society for Pediatric Anesthesiology recommendations for the use of opioids in children during the perioperative period. Pediatr Anesth. 2019;29:547–71.
24. Finnerup NB. Nonnarcotic methods of pain management. N Engl J Med. 2019;380:2440–8.
25. Wong I, St. John-Green C, Walker SM. Opioid-sparing effects of perioperative paracetamol and nonsteroidal anti-inflammatory drugs (NSAIDs) in children. Pediatr Anesth. 2013;23:475–95.
26. Walther-Larsen S, Aagaard GB, Friis SM, et al. Structured intervention for management of pain following day surgery in children. Pediatr Anesth. 2016;26:151–7.
27. Hannam J, Anderson BJ. Explaining the acetaminophen-ibuprofen analgesic interaction using a response surface model. Pediatr Anesth. 2011;21:1234–40.
28. Hannam J, Anderson BJ, Mahadevan M, et al. Postoperative analgesia using diclofenac and acetaminophen in children. Pediatr Anesth. 2014;24:953–61.
29. Vitale MG, Choe JC, Hwang MW, et al. Use of ketorolac tromethamine in children undergoing scoliosis surgery: an analysis of complications. Spine. 2003;3:55–62.
30. Rosenberg RE, Trzcinski S, Cohen M, Erickson M, Errico T, McLoed L. The association between adjuvant pain medication use and outcomes following pediatric spinal fusion. Spine (Phila Pa 1976). 2017;42(10):E602–8.
31. Krane EJ, WAlco GA. With apologies to Lennon and McCartney, all we need is data; opioid concerns in pediatrics. Clin J Pain. 2019;35(6):461–2.
32. Anderson TA. The opioid wars-CON. The risks of opioids for pain management outweigh the benefits. Clin J Pain. 2019;35(6):463–7.
33. Krane EJ. The opioid debate – PRO. Opioids have an important role in pain management in children. Clin J Pain. 2019;35(6):468–72.
34. Groenewald CB. Opioid-prescribing patterns for pediatric patients in the United States. Clin J Pain. 2019;35(6):515–20.
35. Eisdorfer S, Galinkin J. Opioid use disorder in children and adolescents; risk factors, detection and treatment. Clin J Pain. 2019;35(6):521–4.
36. Yaster M, Reid AL, Cohen MN, Monitto CL. Opioids in the management of acute pediatric pain; an update in a time of crisis. Clin J Pain. 2019;35(6):487–96.
37. Jenkins IA, Playfor SD, Bevan C, Davies G, Wolf AR. Current United Kingdom sedation practice in pediatric intensive care. Paediatr Anaesth. 2007;17(7):675–83.
38. Garcia Guerra G, Joffe AR, Cave D, et al. Survey of sedation and analgesia practice among Canadian pediatric critical care physicians. Pediatr Crit Care Med. 2016;17(9):823–30.
39. Wright JA. An update of systemic analgesics in children. Anesth Intensive Care Med. 2019;20(6):324–9.
40. Monitto CL, Greenberg RS, Kost-Byerly S, et al. The safety and efficacy of parent-/nurse-controlled analgesia in patients less than 6 years of age. Anesth Analg. 2010;91:573–9.
41. Nelson KL, Yaster M, Kost-Byerly S, et al. Current trends in pediatric acute pain management: results of a national survey of American pediatric anesthesiologists. Anesth Analg. 2010;110:754–60.

42. Yildiz K, Tercan E, Dogru K, et al. Comparison of patient – controlled analgesia with and without a background infusion after appendectomy in children. Pedatr Anesth. 2003;13:427–31.
43. Nelson KL, Yaster M, Kost-Byerly S, et al. A national survey of American Pediatric Anesthesiologists: patient-controlled analgesia and other intravenous opioid therapies in pediatric acute care management. Anesth Analg. 2010;110:754–60.
44. Anghelescu DL, Burgoyne LL, Oakes LL, et al. The safety of patient-controlled analgesia by proxy in pediatric oncology patients. Anesth Analg. 2005;101:1623–7.
45. Voepel-Lewis T, Marinkovic A, Kostrzewa A, et al. The prevalence and risk factors for adverse events in children receiving patient-controlled analgesia by proxy or patient controlled analgesia after surgery. Anesth Analg. 2008;107:70–5.
46. Howard RF, Lloyd-Thomas A, Thomas M, et al. Nurse-controlled analgesia (NCA) following major surgery in 10, 000 patients in a children's hospital. Pedatr Anesth. 2010;20:126–34.
47. Monitto CL, Kost-Bylerly S, White E, et al. The optimal dose of prophylactic intravenous naloxone in ameliorating opioid-induced side effects in children receiving intravenous patient-controlled analgesia morphine for moderate to severe pain: a dose finding study. Anesth Analg. 2011;113:834–42.
48. Kopecky EA. Opioid pharmacology; developmental effects on opioid metabolism. Clin J Pain. 2019;35(6):481–6.
49. Meyer MT, Berens RJ. Efficacy of an enteral 10-day methadone wean to prevent opioid withdrawal in fentanyl-tolerant pediatric intensive care unit patients. Pediatr Crit Care Med. 2001;2(4):329–33.
50. Steineck KJ, Skoglund AK, Carlson MK, Gupta S. Evaluation of a pharmacist-managed methadone taper. Pediatr Crit Care Med. 2014;15(3):206–10.
51. Amirnovin R, Sanchez-Pinto LN, Okuhara C, Lieu P, Koh JY, Rodgers JW, Nelson LP. Implementation of a risk-stratified opioid and benzodiazepine weaning protocol in a pediatric cardiac ICU. Pediatr Crit Care Med. 2018;19:1024–32.
52. Maxwell LG et al. Pain Management Following Major Intracranial Surgery in Pediatric Patients: A Prospective Cohort Study in Three Academic Children's Hospitals. Pediatr Anaesth 2014;24(11):1132–40.
53. Windsor RB, et al. The use of opioids for treatment of pediatric neuropathic pain: a literature review. Clin J Pain. 2019;35:509–14.
54. Friedrichsdorf SJ. From tramadol to methadone, opioids in the treatment of pain and dyspnea in pediatric palliative care. Clin J Pain. 2019;35:501–8.
55. Snaman JM, Baker JN, Ehrentraut JH, Anghelescu DL. Pediatric oncology: managing pain at the end of life. Pediatr Drugs. 2016;18(3):161–80.
56. Wiffen PJ, Cooper TE, Anderson AK, Gray AL, Gregoire MC, Ljungman G, Zernikow B. Opioids for cancer-related pain in children and adolescents. Cochrane Database Syst Rev. 2017;7:CD012564.
57. Gorges M, West N, Deyell R, Winton P, Cheung W, Lauder G. Dexmedetomidine and hydromorphone: a novel pain management strategy for the oncology ward setting during anti-GD2 immunotherapy for high-risk neuroblastoma in children. Pediatr Blood Cancer. 2015;62:29–34.

Chapter 4
Regional Analgesia and Its Role in the PICU

Mary Landrigan-Ossar

Introduction

In the past few decades, regional anesthesia has had an increasing role in the management of pain in the pediatric intensive care unit. This has been concurrent with the expansion of regional anesthesia in the pediatric operating room, but the utility of regional anesthesia in the ICU is by no means confined to postoperative patients. In this chapter we will review the history of pediatric regional anesthesia, discuss the safety of and the risks associated with these techniques, and describe some of the benefits of regional anesthesia particularly with regard to the ICU patient. The chapter will conclude with an overview of the various regional anesthesia techniques currently in use, with some of their indications.

History

While widespread adoption of peripheral regional anesthesia techniques for pediatric patients has lagged behind their use in adults, children have been the recipients of neuraxial regional techniques since their origin. In 1898, the first group of six patients in whom Augustus Bier attempted spinal anesthesia included two children. As the twentieth century progressed, case series describing the use of spinal anesthesia in children increased. Caudal anesthesia was first described for pediatric urologic surgery in the 1930s. Epidural anesthesia was described not long after, with thoracic epidurals reportedly being used in Russia as early as the 1970s; by the 1980s pediatric epidural catheters were in wide use. Progress toward the general use

M. Landrigan-Ossar (✉)
Department of Anesthesia, Perioperative & Pain Medicine, Boston Children's Hospital, Harvard Medical School, Boston, MA, USA
e-mail: mary.landrigan-ossar@childrens.harvard.edu

P. P. Kamat, J. W. Berkenbosch (eds.), *Sedation and Analgesia for the Pediatric Intensivist*, https://doi.org/10.1007/978-3-030-52555-2_4

of peripheral nerve blocks in children was slower, although case reports of their use for pediatric patients with chronic pain were published in the mid-1980s [1].

The first large-scale description of the use of pediatric regional anesthesia was published in 1996 by the French-Language Society of Pediatric Anesthesiologists (ADARPEF) [2]. At that time, the 38 participating hospitals reported an approximate 60:40 distribution of neuraxial versus peripheral regional techniques. Fifteen years later, the 2010 report from the same organization demonstrated an inversion of this distribution, with over 60% of patients receiving peripheral nerve blocks [3]. The Pediatric Regional Anesthesia Network shows a similar distribution in their 2018 review of over 100,000 blocks, with a near 50:50 distribution of central to peripheral nerve blocks [4]. The increasing incidence of peripheral nerve blocks in children is thought to be due to the increasing use of ultrasound guidance, which allows for exact localization of the needle or catheter with respect to surrounding structures, improved block success, and decreased complications [5].

Safety and Risks of Regional Anesthesia

The first case series description of spinal anesthesia resulted in 100% headaches, nausea, and vomiting for all eight patients, including the two pediatric patients in the series [1]. Fortunately, in the 120 years since then, the safety profile of regional anesthesia has improved considerably. Several large-scale studies of the complications of regional anesthesia in pediatric patients have been published; in all the large datasets published, the incidence of harm to pediatric patients with regional anesthesia has been reassuringly low. The American Society of Regional Anesthesia (ASRA) and the European Society of Regional Anesthesia (ESRA) have issued joint communications on the topic of pediatric regional anesthesia, affirming its safety and providing guidance on various controversies in block performance [6].

The French-Language Society of Pediatric Anesthesiologists (ADARPEF) published large-scale prospective studies in 1996 and again in 2010. The 2010 publication described over 31,000 blocks from over 47 reporting institutions, with a complication rate of <0.9/1000 procedures [3]. A higher complication rate was noted for infants less than 6 months and for central versus peripheral blocks. No fatalities were recorded and no long-lasting neurologic sequelae were reported in this study.

Similar results have been reported by the Pediatric Regional Anesthesia Network (PRAN), a US-based consortium of 21 institutions who have collected a database of over 100,000 pediatric regional blocks. In their 2018 publication, they report on these blocks, half of which were peripheral nerve blocks [4]. This study also showed a very low rate of complications, similar to that reported by ADARPEF, with no deaths and no sequelae lasting longer than 3 months. Table 4.1 shows the adverse events described in the consortium's 2015 study of peripheral nerve blocks [7].

A few particular areas of controversy exist when considering the use of pediatric regional anesthesia. The most contentious for many years was the placement of either neuraxial or peripheral nerve blocks in a heavily sedated or anesthetized

Table 4.1 Incidence of specific adverse events in PRAN database

Complication	Incidence
Catheter malfunction (dislodgement, occlusion)	7.3%
Abandoned or block failure	1.3%
Catheter-related infection	0.9%
Vascular (blood aspiration, hematoma)	0.9%
Excessive motor block	0.6%
Difficult catheter removal	0.1%
Others (foot swelling, muscle spasm, dizziness, burning sensation, adverse drug reaction, nausea and vomiting, contact dermatitis)	1%

Modified and used with permission from Walker et al. [7]

child. The concern from adult anesthesiologists was that children under anesthesia or sedation would not be able to report pain or paresthesias, which could arguably increase the incidence of nerve injury. Data from both APARDEF and PRAN have shown no increase in complications in anesthetized children receiving nerve blocks, and the joint ASRA/ESRA statement has confirmed that placement of blocks under general anesthesia or sedation is the standard of care for children and states that this method may in fact be safer than placing blocks on unsedated children [6].

The question of when to perform regional anesthesia on a patient who is anticoagulated is quite pertinent in the intensive care population. Bleeding complications are more problematic for neuraxial versus peripheral blocks, since the risk of neurologic catastrophe is increased with bleeding near the spinal cord. The American and European Societies of Regional Anesthesia review this topic regularly, updating their recommendations as new anticoagulant medications arise and as new data becomes available about the relative risk of bleeding complications with various regional and interventional pain procedures [8]. In general, the recommendation is to avoid neuraxial blocks in patients with altered coagulation; if anticoagulation can be briefly reversed or held to allow for placement of a block, then that can be considered.

Another question which provokes controversy is whether regional anesthesia could mask the onset of compartment syndrome in an injured extremity. Compartment syndrome develops in an injured limb after injury such as trauma, prolonged malposition during surgery, fracture with casting, and ischemia-reperfusion. These insults, if not recognized and treated within a few hours, can result in elevated pressure in a closed muscle compartment, decreased circulation, ischemia, and eventual nerve and muscle necrosis. Conventional wisdom several decades ago was that the dense sensory block achievable with regional anesthesia would mask the increasing pain which indicates the development of increased pressure in a limb compartment. The ASRA/ESRA consensus recognizes that this diagnosis is difficult to make with or without nerve block in preverbal or nonverbal children. The societies' consensus is that there is no evidence indicating that regional anesthesia masks the development of compartment syndrome. In at-risk patients, a less dense block might be used, but the most important factor in recognition of compartment syndrome is recognition of patients at risk and close monitoring [9].

One hazard of regional anesthesia safety which cannot be overlooked is that of local anesthetic systemic toxicity (LAST); it should be recognized as a possibility by anyone taking care of a child who has received a nerve block. The PRAN database reports an incidence of LAST of 0.76/10,000, with the majority of cases in infants under 6 months of age. This may be due to a combination of reduced protein binding of local anesthetics in this age group and reduced drug clearance by infants [4]. These physiologic differences in infant local anesthesia pharmacokinetics are reflected in ASRA/ESRA guidelines for local anesthesia dosing in infants [10]. LAST is more often seen in bolus administration of local anesthetic, as opposed to steady-state infusions. A study of >200,000 adult patients receiving blocks for orthopedic surgery over a 14-year period yielded a LAST incidence of 0.18% [11]. In the same study, the authors described a decreasing incidence of severe complications of LAST such as seizure and cardiac arrest, which was likely due to an increased recognition of the role of lipid therapy to treat LAST. Lipid resuscitation is now recognized as a first-line therapy for the treatment of LAST, and lipid emulsion should be stocked in any area where blocks are performed [12].

Benefits of Regional Anesthesia

The first and most important benefit of regional anesthesia is its provision of high-quality, site-specific pain control. As every PICU physician is aware, pain is one of the more distressing aspects of a patient's experience in an intensive care unit, with 50% of patients reporting moderate to severe pain during their time in the PICU. Untreated pain has detrimental effects, not only psychologically, but by causing a host of hormonal, metabolic, and inflammatory issues which can impede recovery. Additionally, up to a third of ICU patients will develop chronic pain after their ICU stay either from postsurgical pain or otherwise [13, 14]. In many of these cases, regional anesthesia has a role to play in their relief, and it is argued that regional anesthesia may still be underutilized in the ICU.

A number of meta-analyses have demonstrated the superior pain relief which can be afforded to patients with regional techniques. A 2016 Cochrane review of 15 studies reported that for patients with an epidural catheter after open abdominal surgery, their VAS pain score was reduced compared to patients receiving systemic pain medications up to postoperative day #3 [15]. A 10-year cumulative literature review by block type similarly showed an overall improvement in both pain scores and patient satisfactions with peripheral nerve blocks versus other methods of pain relief [16]. In some patient series in this review, their satisfaction with their pain control approached 100%, and they stated that they would choose that method of pain control again in the future.

One of the great advantages of regional anesthesia in contrast with systemic pain medications is the lack of systemic side effects. Opioids, nonsteroidal anti-inflammatory medications, and acetaminophen all have deleterious effects on various organ systems which are accentuated with long-term use. Opioids in particular have come under intense scrutiny recently, with many concerns raised for the potential of long-term opioid abuse arising in patients who have been exposed to them in the hospital environment. Regional anesthesia, which allows opiate-sparing pain relief, has been embraced as a possible means to reduce this problem [17].

Another area where regional anesthesia has an increasingly significant role is in the early mobilization of PICU patients. A key factor in assisting pediatric PICU patients to regain normal sleep-wake cycles and be able to participate with efforts to increase mobility is the provision of adequate analgesia with minimal sedative side effects [18]. With its lack of sedating or delirium-promoting side effects, regional anesthesia can be a valuable adjunct to these efforts.

In addition to excellent pain control, there is a growing body of evidence that the use of regional techniques can reduce perioperative complications when compared to systemic pain medication regimens. While many of the studies in this area have focused on the adult patient, the conclusions are in many cases translatable to the pediatric population. Guay's 2016 Cochrane review noted reduced time to extubation, incidence of myocardial infarction, incidence of respiratory failure, and time to ICU discharge in patients with epidurals after open abdominal aortic aneurysm repair [15]. In another review, the same authors noted reduced time to recovery of gastrointestinal function after abdominal surgery with use of epidurals [19]. A meta-analysis of 125 studies of patients with epidural after surgery found that patients with epidurals had a reduced incidence of mortality, and epidurals were associated with a beneficial effect on major pulmonary, cardiac, and gastrointestinal symptoms [20]. These myriad benefits are likely due to a combination of factors. Fewer side effects of opioids, such as sedation which can compromise efforts to extubate and constipating side effects of opioids, are certainly one factor. Another is the known reduction in the hormones associated with the perioperative stress response in patients with epidurals. The improved pain relief and decreased surgical stress response provided by regional anesthesia may also allow patients to more comfortably participate in postoperative respiratory physiotherapy, which can speed time to extubation. Together these can add up to a powerful benefit for critically ill patients.

The evidence for benefits of peripheral nerve blocks on postoperative outcomes other than pain has lagged behind the evidence for neuraxial blockade, in part because peripheral techniques have only recently become widespread. While there may be no direct effects on the success of surgical procedure, the use of regional anesthesia to promote early mobilization and physical therapy is now well-established. Several protocols detailing the use of regional anesthesia for Enhanced Recovery After Surgery (ERAS) have been published for orthopedic procedures, allowing for reduced morbidity and length of hospital stay [21].

One aspect of regional anesthesia which is of increasing utility to the physician treating critically ill children is the use of regional anesthesia for palliative purposes. While systemic analgesic therapy has been a mainstay of palliative care for many years, there is a growing recognition of the utility of regional anesthesia in this patient population. Many of the systemic side effects of pain medication, such as oversedation, pruritis, and constipation, can be relieved by the use of regional pain techniques. Additionally, regional techniques may provide good pain relief in patients for whom systemic therapies are no longer effective due to either disease progression or tolerance and tachyphylaxis [22]. In any of these cases, a thoughtful exploration of the potential methods to treat a child at the end of life will be necessary to determine if a regional procedure and its potential risk is in congruence with overall goals of care.

Some Common Blocks

Central Neuraxial Blocks

The central neuraxial blocks consist of spinal, epidural, and caudal blocks, with caudal blocks representing the largest proportion in younger children, transitioning to lumbar epidurals as the predominant neuraxial block in older children [4]. Both caudal and epidural blocks access the epidural space surrounding the spinal cord, either by access through the sacral hiatus in the case of the caudal block or percutaneously at any of the lumbar or thoracic vertebral interspaces. These blocks have traditionally been placed without image guidance, relying on the experienced operator's feel for a "pop," or loss of resistance to a saline or air-filled syringe on entry to the epidural space. Currently both fluoroscopy and ultrasound have been described to assist with block placement, and these may be invaluable in the case of patients with challenging anatomy [23, 24].

All of the central neuraxial blocks provide excellent pain relief for thoracic, abdominal, pelvic, and lower extremity pain. Figure 4.1 describes epidural catheter placement for a variety of surgical interventions. It should be noted that particularly in infants, the epidural space can be accessed by the caudal approach, and a catheter can be advanced even to the thoracic levels under fluoroscopic guidance. Infusion rates can be titrated to allow for ambulation, or even for a "band" of analgesia at an operative level, although it is quite possible with these blocks that the area affected may be greater than what is necessary. Adjuncts such as low-dose opiates or alpha-2 agonists may be added to potentiate pain relief or to increase the length of time a single-shot block may last.

Upper Extremity Blocks

There are nearly as many approaches to the brachial plexus as there are nerves coming from it (see Fig. 4.2). Axillary, infraclavicular, interscalene, and supraclavicular approaches are described, with the supraclavicular being the most commonly reported in the PRAN database [25]. Nerves all along the upper extremity from the finger to the neck can be targeted by ultrasound depending on the area which needs surgical analgesia, or vasodilation in the case of microvascular surgery [26]. Catheters can be placed for long-term pain relief, which has proven particularly helpful for pain relief and mobility after shoulder surgery [27].

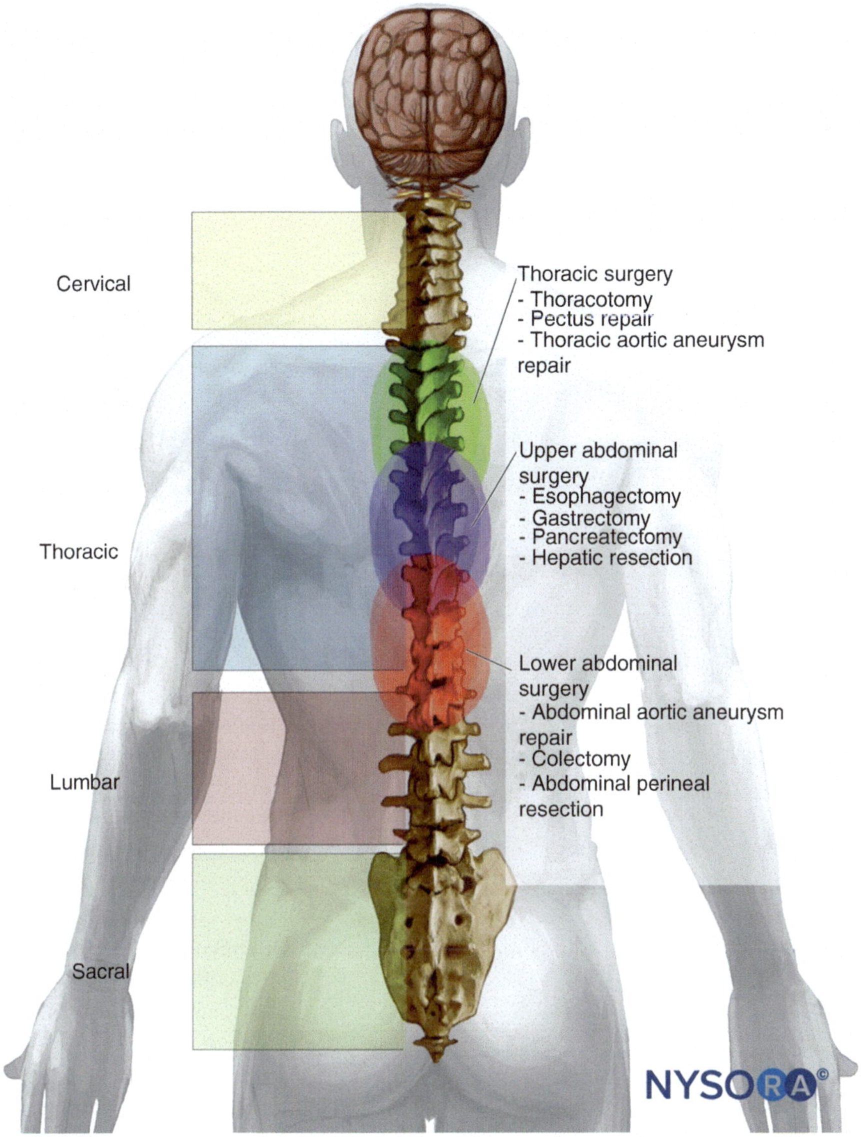

Fig. 4.1 Level of catheter placement in surgeries performed with epidural anesthesia and analgesia. (Source: nysora.com, used with permission)

A few potential complications are possible depending on the block performed, particularly for those targeting the brachial plexus. Horner's syndrome is not uncommon, and patients should be counseled that this will recede as the block wears off. More potentially concerning is hemidiaphragm paralysis, which can be potentially dangerous in patients with compromised respiratory function. Pneumothorax is a

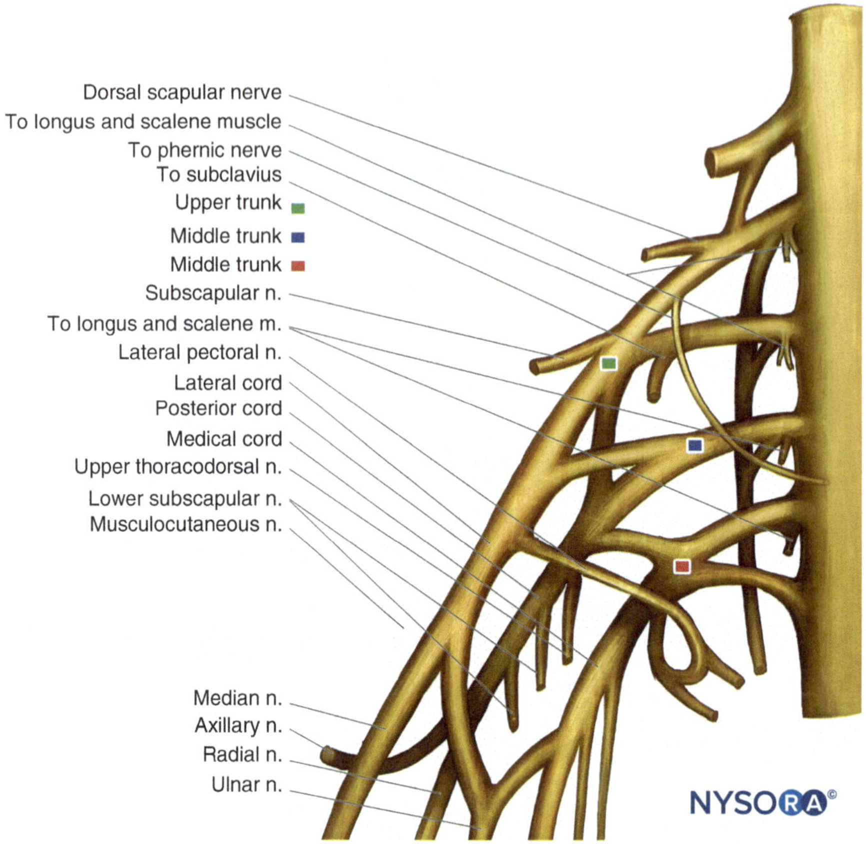

Fig. 4.2 Brachial plexus. (Source: nysora.com, used with permission)

possibility, although ultrasound guidance will hopefully minimize the chance of this complication [27].

Truncal Blocks

Truncal blocks provide analgesia to the chest, abdomen, and pelvis without the need for accessing the central neuraxis. This can be particularly useful in coagulopathic patients, in whom the risk for epidural hematoma may be unacceptably high, but is also useful when only a particular area of analgesia is desired without as high a chance of spread to nontarget areas. The most common blocks in this category include the TAP (transversus abdominis plane) block, ilioinguinal/iliohypogastric block, and rectus sheath block, with additional techniques being described on a regular basis. The paravertebral block can be thought of as transitional case between the central neuraxial block and the blocks of the abdominal and thoracic wall,

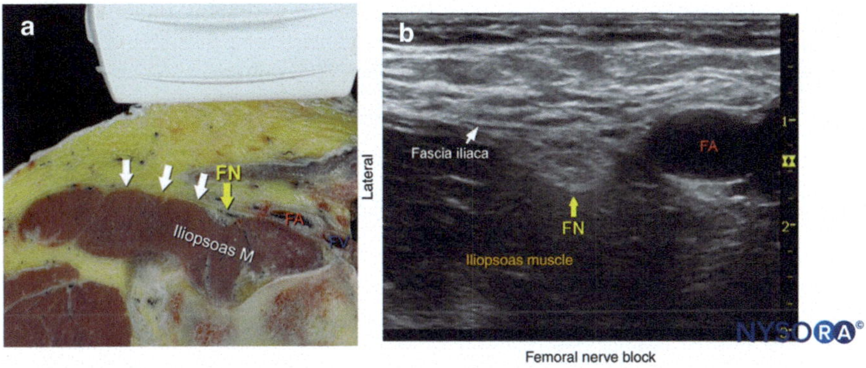

Fig. 4.3 (**a**) Cross-sectional anatomy of the femoral nerve (FN) at the level of the femoral crease. The FN is seen on the surface of the iliopsoas muscle covered by fascia iliaca (white arrows). The femoral artery (FA) and femoral vein (FV) are seen enveloped within their own vascular fascial sheath created by one of the layers of fascia lata. (**b**) Sonoanatomy of the FN at the femoral triangle. (Source: nysora.com, used with permission)

providing generally unilateral analgesia at the level of injection in the intervertebral foramen. Ultrasound guidance enhances both the rate of block success and minimizes complications such as intravascular injection, pneumothorax, and bowel perforation [25, 28].

Lower Extremity Blocks

Much like the approach to the upper extremity, there are many methods by which analgesia can be provided to the lower extremity. Blocks can range from the lumbar plexus through the femoral and sciatic nerves to the popliteal fossa and ankle. Figure 4.3 shows the cross-sectional anatomy of the femoral nerve and its surroundings, both in gross specimen and in ultrasound. Ultrasound is the most common technique for accessing nerves of the lower extremity, which ensures the greatest chance of success while minimizing complications. The most likely complication for lower extremity blocks is inadvertent vascular injection [25], although the lumbar plexus block's location does place surrounding abdominal structures at higher risk [29].

Conclusion

Regional anesthesia is a valuable analgesic technique for pediatric patients in the PICU. While the majority of patients who will benefit from nerve block are postsurgical, there are certainly opportunities for nonsurgical intensive care patients to benefit from these techniques, and these techniques are arguably underutilized in many PICUs. Close cooperation between intensive care, anesthesia, and pain service professionals will result in many benefits for PICU patients.

References

1. Brown TC. History of pediatric regional anesthesia. Paediatr Anaesth. 2012;22(1):3–9.
2. Giaufre E, Dalens B, Gombert A. Epidemiology and morbidity of regional anesthesia in children: a one-year prospective survey of the French-Language Society of Pediatric Anesthesiologists. Anesth Analg. 1996;83(5):904–12.
3. Ecoffey C, Lacroix F, Giaufre E, Orliaguet G, Courreges P. Epidemiology and morbidity of regional anesthesia in children: a follow-up one-year prospective survey of the French-Language Society of Paediatric Anaesthesiologists (ADARPEF). Paediatr Anaesth. 2010;20(12):1061–9.
4. Walker BJ, Long JB, Sathyamoorthy M, Birstler J, Wolf C, Bosenberg AT, et al. Complications in pediatric regional anesthesia: an analysis of more than 100,000 blocks from the pediatric regional anesthesia network. Anesthesiology. 2018;129(4):721–32.
5. Neal JM. Ultrasound-guided regional anesthesia and patient safety: update of an evidence-based analysis. Reg Anesth Pain Med. 2016;41(2):195–204.
6. Ivani G, Suresh S, Ecoffey C, Bosenberg A, Lonnqvist PA, Krane E, et al. The European Society of Regional Anaesthesia and Pain Therapy and the American Society of Regional Anesthesia and Pain Medicine Joint Committee Practice Advisory on Controversial Topics in Pediatric Regional Anesthesia. Reg Anesth Pain Med. 2015;40(5):526–32.
7. Walker BJ, Long JB, De Oliveira GS, Szmuk P, Setiawan C, Polaner DM, et al. Peripheral nerve catheters in children: an analysis of safety and practice patterns from the pediatric regional anesthesia network (PRAN). Br J Anaesth. 2015;115(3):457–62.
8. Narouze S, Benzon HT, Provenzano D, Buvanendran A, De Andres J, Deer T, et al. Interventional Spine and Pain Procedures in Patients on Antiplatelet and Anticoagulant Medications (Second Edition): Guidelines From the American Society of Regional Anesthesia and Pain Medicine, the European Society of Regional Anaesthesia and Pain Therapy, the American Academy of Pain Medicine, the International Neuromodulation Society, the North American Neuromodulation Society, and the World Institute of Pain. Reg Anesth Pain Med. 2018;43(3):225–62.
9. Lonnqvist PA, Ecoffey C, Bosenberg A, Suresh S, Ivani G. The European society of regional anesthesia and pain therapy and the American society of regional anesthesia and pain medicine joint committee practice advisory on controversial topics in pediatric regional anesthesia I and II: what do they tell us? Curr Opin Anaesthesiol. 2017;30(5):613–20.
10. Suresh S, Ecoffey C, Bosenberg A, Lonnqvist PA, de Oliveira GS Jr, de Leon Casasola O, et al. The European Society of Regional Anaesthesia and Pain Therapy/American Society of Regional Anesthesia and Pain Medicine Recommendations on Local Anesthetics and Adjuvants Dosage in Pediatric Regional Anesthesia. Reg Anesth Pain Med. 2018;43(2):211–6.
11. Morwald EE, Zubizarreta N, Cozowicz C, Poeran J, Memtsoudis SG. Incidence of local anesthetic systemic toxicity in orthopedic patients receiving peripheral nerve blocks. Reg Anesth Pain Med. 2017;42(4):442–5.
12. Neal JM, Woodward CM, Harrison TK. The American Society of Regional Anesthesia and Pain Medicine checklist for managing local anesthetic systemic toxicity: 2017 version. Reg Anesth Pain Med. 2018;43(2):150–3.
13. Capdevila M, Ramin S, Capdevila X. Regional anesthesia and analgesia after surgery in ICU. Curr Opin Crit Care. 2017;23(5):430–9.
14. Andreae MH, Andreae DA. Regional anaesthesia to prevent chronic pain after surgery: a Cochrane systematic review and meta-analysis. Br J Anaesth. 2013;111(5):711–20.

15. Guay J, Kopp S. Epidural pain relief versus systemic opioid-based pain relief for abdominal aortic surgery. Cochrane Database Syst Rev. 2016;1:CD005059.
16. Kessler J, Marhofer P, Hopkins PM, Hollmann MW. Peripheral regional anaesthesia and outcome: lessons learned from the last 10 years. Br J Anaesth. 2015;114(5):728–45.
17. Hah JM, Bateman BT, Ratliff J, Curtin C, Sun E. Chronic opioid use after surgery: implications for perioperative management in the face of the opioid epidemic. Anesth Analg. 2017;125(5):1733–40.
18. Wieczorek B, Ascenzi J, Kim Y, Lenker H, Potter C, Shata NJ, et al. PICU up!: impact of a quality improvement intervention to promote early mobilization in critically ill children. Pediatr Crit Care Med. 2016;17(12):e559–e66.
19. Guay J, Nishimori M, Kopp S. Epidural local anaesthetics versus opioid-based analgesic regimens for postoperative gastrointestinal paralysis, vomiting and pain after abdominal surgery. Cochrane Database Syst Rev. 2016;7:CD001893.
20. Popping DM, Elia N, Van Aken HK, Marret E, Schug SA, Kranke P, et al. Impact of epidural analgesia on mortality and morbidity after surgery: systematic review and meta-analysis of randomized controlled trials. Ann Surg. 2014;259(6):1056–67.
21. Villatte G, Mathonnet M, Villeminot J, Savary M, Theissen A, Ostermann S, et al. Interest of enhanced recovery programs in the elderly during total hip arthroplasty A systematic review. Geriatr Psychol Neuropsychiatr Vieil. 2019;17(3):234–42.
22. Rork JF, Berde CB, Goldstein RD. Regional anesthesia approaches to pain management in pediatric palliative care: a review of current knowledge. J Pain Symptom Manag. 2013;46(6):859–73.
23. Ponde VC, Bedekar VV, Desai AP, Puranik KA. Does ultrasound guidance add accuracy to continuous caudal-epidural catheter placements in neonates and infants? Paediatr Anaesth. 2017;27(10):1010–4.
24. Kao SC, Lin CS. Caudal epidural block: an updated review of anatomy and techniques. Biomed Res Int 2017;2017:9217145.
25. Shah RD, Suresh S. Applications of regional anaesthesia in paediatrics. Br J Anaesth. 2013;111(Suppl 1):i114–24.
26. Stevens GJ, Durning SJ, Stevens SD, Lowery DR. Regional anesthesia in the setting of arm replantation: a case report. A A Pract. 2018;11(2):38–40.
27. Nadeau MJ, Levesque S, Dion N. Ultrasound-guided regional anesthesia for upper limb surgery. Can J Anaesth. 2013;60(3):304–20.
28. Long JB, Birmingham PK, De Oliveira GS Jr, Schaldenbrand KM, Suresh S. Transversus abdominis plane block in children: a multicenter safety analysis of 1994 cases from the PRAN (Pediatric Regional Anesthesia Network) database. Anesth Analg. 2014;119(2):395–9.
29. Boretsky K, Hernandez MA, Eastburn E, Sullivan C. Ultrasound-guided lumbar plexus block in children and adolescents using a transverse lumbar paravertebral sonogram: initial experience. Paediatr Anaesth. 2018;28(3):291–5.

Part II
Sedative Agents

Chapter 5
Sedative Agents (Benzodiazepines)

Whitney Moore, Olutola Adu, and Sherika Haire-Kendall

Overview of Benzodiazepines and Mechanism of Action

Benzodiazepines are the most commonly used sedatives in the pediatric intensive care units [1]. In the pediatric and adult intensive care units, benzodiazepines are used for variety of indications such as anxiolysis, sedation, anterograde amnestic effects, seizures, and to treat alcohol withdrawal syndrome.

Benzodiazepines have specific action at gamma-aminobutyric acid (GABA) receptors. The mechanism of action of this sedative agonist is to improve GABAergic transmission. To better understand the mechanism of action of benzodiazepine, it helps to understand *gamma*-aminobutyric acid (GABA) neurotransmitter.

GABA is the most widely distributed inhibitory neurotransmitters in the central nervous system (CNS) and limits the excitability of neuronal activity in all areas of the brain. Increasing GABAergic activity results in sedation, amnesia, and ataxia, whereas a decrease in the GABAergic signal results in arousal, anxiety, restlessness, and insomnia [2]. The GABA receptors are widely distributed and utilized throughout the central nervous system and have two subtypes, $GABA_A$ and $GABA_B$. GABA functions as the major inhibitory neurotransmitter and controls the excitability of neurons by binding to the $GABA_A$ receptor. The $GABA_A$ receptor is the major molecular target for the action of many drugs in the brain including the benzodiazepines. The binding promotes an increased influx of chloride ions hyperpolarizing the cell membrane and preventing the generation of an action potential. This effect leads to a minor communication between neurons and, therefore, has a calming effect on many of the functions of the brain [3]. Figure 5.1 shows the $GABA_A$ receptor, which is further broken down into several subtypes two $\alpha 1$ subunits, two $\beta 2$ subunits, and one $\gamma 2$ subunit. The receptor also had a single binding site for the benzodiazepines.

W. Moore (✉) · O. Adu (✉) · S. Haire-Kendall (✉)
Children's Healthcare of Atlanta, Atlanta, GA, USA
e-mail: whitney.moore@choa.org; olutola.adu@choa.org; sherika.haire-kendall@choa.org

P. P. Kamat, J. W. Berkenbosch (eds.), *Sedation and Analgesia for the Pediatric Intensivist*, https://doi.org/10.1007/978-3-030-52555-2_5

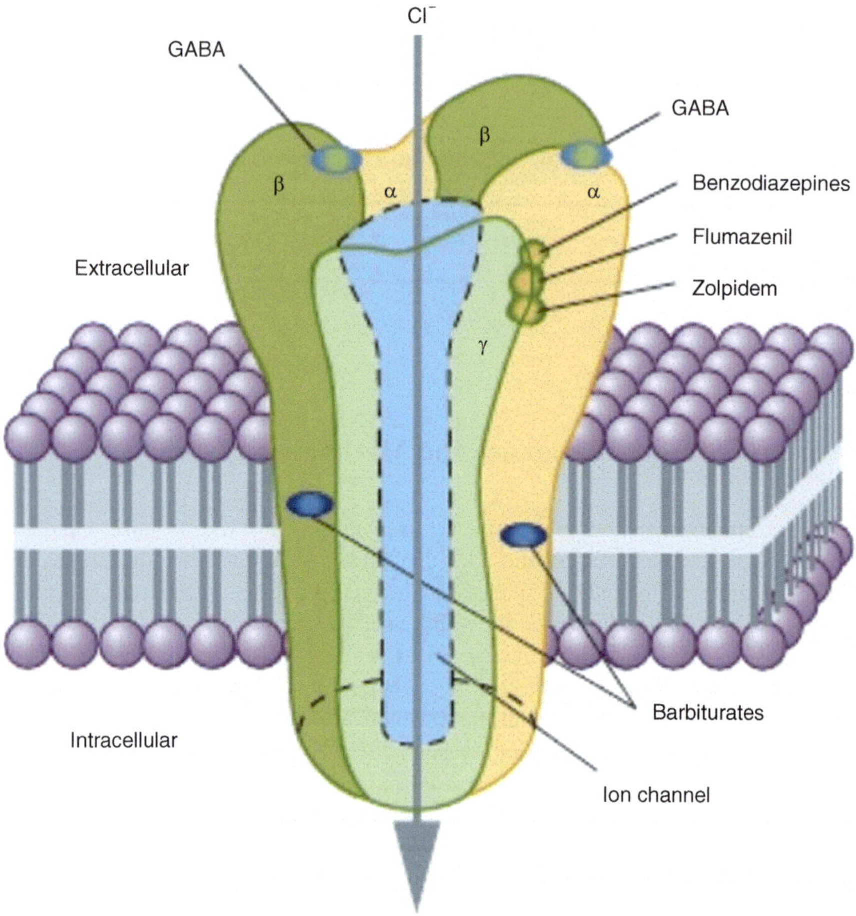

Fig. 5.1 Gamma-aminobutyric acid (GABA) receptor. (Source: Bertram G, Katzung, Anthony J. Trevor: *Basic & clinical pharmacology*, 14th ed. www.academia.edu. Copyright © McGraw-Hill Education. All rights reserved)

Benzodiazepines are allosteric modulators that require GABA to be bound to its receptor. When benzodiazepines bind to the benzodiazepine receptor on a GABA receptor, they do not stimulate it directly. Instead, it increases the frequency with which the chlorine channel opens when GABA binds its receptor resulting in an increase amount of chloride ions in the postsynaptic neuron that immediately hyperpolarizes this neuron and decreases the excitability. Benzodiazepine's advantage compared to other drugs, i.e., barbiturates, is it acts in the same receptor and decreases the activity of neurons [2–8]. Benzodiazepines are the only drugs that give GABA more affinity for its receptor and act as an allosteric modulator. They do not provide a higher activation of GABA itself. This results in less toxicity with the

Table 5.1 $GABA_A$ receptor subtypes with alpha subunit

Alpha subunit	% of CNS $GABA_A$ receptors	Know action medicated
α1	60	Sedative, amnestic, partial anticonvulsant
α2	15–20	Anxiolytic, myorelaxation
α3	10–15	Myorelaxation (only at high doses)
α4	<5	Insensitive to benzodiazepines
α5	<5	Partial myorelaxation
α6	<5	Insensitive to benzodiazepines

benzodiazepines. Sedation, anterograde amnesia, and anticonvulsant activity are promoted through $_{\alpha 1}$ receptors, whereas anxiolytic and muscle relaxation are promoted by the α_2 $GABA_A$ receptor (Table 5.1). In addition to their action on the central nervous system, benzodiazepines have a dose-dependent ventilatory depressant effect, and they also cause a modest reduction in arterial blood pressure and an increase in pulse rate as a result of a decrease of systemic peripheral resistance [1]. It is through this mechanism that sedation, hypnosis, muscle relaxation, anxiolytic, anterograde amnesia, and anticonvulsant effects occur. The most commonly used benzodiazepines for sedation in the pediatric intensive care are midazolam, lorazepam, and diazepam [4].

Pharmacokinetic and Pharmacodynamic Considerations

All benzodiazepines enhance the binding of gamma-aminobutyric acid (GABA), the major inhibitory neurotransmitter, to the GABA-A subtype of GABA receptors, resulting in GABAergic neurotransmission. All the agents in the benzodiazepine drug class have similar clinical effects. However, they differ in their pharmacokinetic profiles, such as rate of absorption, elimination half-life, and onset and duration of action. Details of benzodiazepine pharmacodynamics and pharmacokinetics are provided in Tables 5.2 and 5.3. [18].

Benzodiazepines undergo Phase I and Phase II metabolic pathways: hepatic oxidation and reduction by cytochrome P450 and glucuronide conjugation. Alprazolam, midazolam, and diazepam undergo hydroxylation, while clonazepam undergoes nitroreduction [5].

Lorazepam displays low hepatic metabolism and does not have active metabolites. Diazepam is rapidly absorbed and has the most rapid onset of action but also the greatest abuse/dependence potential. Diazepam is considered a long-acting benzodiazepine and associated with accumulation, which may result in sedation, cognitive impairment, and psychomotor retardation. Lorazepam and midazolam are considered short-acting benzodiazepine agents. The search for a water-soluble benzodiazepine with clinical properties similar to diazepam but without its potential for venous irritation led to the development of midazolam [6].

Table 5.2 Pharmacodynamic and pharmacokinetic considerations of commonly used benzodiazepines

Drug	Route of administration	Absorption	Bioavailability	Distribution	Metabolism	Active metabolite	Elimination
Clonazepam	Oral	Rapidly and completely absorbed	~90%	Children: 1.5–3 L/kg Adults: 1.5–6.4 L/kg	Hepatic Extensively via glucuronide and sulfate conjugation Nitroreduction to 7-aminoclonazepam, followed by acetylation to 7-acetamidoclonazepam	Yes	Urine (<2% as unchanged drug) Metabolites excreted as glucuronide or sulfate conjugates
Diazepam	Oral, IM, IV, rectal	Oral: Well absorbed (>90%); delayed or decreased when administered with a fatty meal Rectal: Well absorbed	IM: >90% Oral: >90% Rectal: 90%	IV: 1.2 L/kg (range 0.6–2 L/kg) Oral: 1.1 L/kg (range 0.6–1.8 L/kg) Rectal: 1 L/kg Protein binding: Oral: Neonates 84–86% Adults 98% Rectal 95–98%	Hepatic N-Demethylated by CYP3A4 and 2C19 to active metabolite N-desmethyldiazepam, and hydroxylated by CYP 3A4 to the active metabolite temazepam N-Desmethyldiazepam and temazepam are both further metabolized to oxazepam Temazepam and oxazepam are eliminated by glucuronidation	Yes	Urine (predominantly as glucuronide conjugates)

Midazolam	Oral, IM, IV, intranasal	Oral, IM, intranasal: Rapid, complete	Oral: Children ~36% Adults 40–50% IM: >90% Intranasal: IV form ~60% Nasal spray 44% Rectal: Children 40–65%	Widely distributed including CSF Vd IV: Gestation age 26–34 weeks: 1.1 L/kg (range 0.4–4.2 L/kg Infants and children 6 months to 16 years old: 1.24–2.02 L/kg Adults: 1–3.1 L/kg (increased in females, elderly, and obesity) Protein binding: ~97%, primarily albumin	Hepatic Metabolized by CYP3A4 60–70% of biotransformed midazolam is the active metabolite 1-dyroxy-midazolam (alpha-hydroxymidazolam)	Yes	Urine ~90% (predominantly as glucuronide conjugates of the hydroxylated metabolites Urine Feces ~2–10% over 5 days
Lorazepam	Oral, IM, IV	IM: Rapid and complete Oral: Readily absorbed	Oral: 90%	IV Vd: Neonates: 0.76 ± 0.37 L/kg (range 0.14–1.3 L/kg)	Hepatic Rapidly conjugated to lorazepam glucuronide (inactive)	No	Urine (~88%; predominantly as inactive metabolite) Feces (~7%)

Table 5.3 Pharmacokinetic considerations of commonly used benzodiazepines

Drug	Onset of action	Duration of action	Time to peak	Half-life (hours)
Clonazepam	~20–40 minutes	Infants and young children: 6–8 hours Adults: ≤12 hours	1–4 hours	Children: 22–33 hours Adults: 17–60 hours
Diazepam	IV: 1–5 minutes Rectal: 2–10 minutes	Sedation: 60–120 minutes Status epilepticus: 15–30 minutes	IM: 1 hour (range 0.25–2 hours) IV: ~ 1 minute Oral: 15 minutes–2.5 hours Rectal: 1.5 hours	Pediatric patients: IV: Gestation age (28–34 weeks): 54 Infants: ~30 Children 3 to 8 years old: 18 Adult patients: Oral: Parent ~44–48 Desmethyldiazepam ~100 IV: Parent 33–45 Desmethyldiazepam 87 Rectal: Parent 45–46 Desmethyldiazepam 71–99

Midazolam	Oral: 10–20 minutes IV: 3–5 minutes IM: Within 5 minutes Intranasal (nasal spray): Within 10 minutes Intranasal (IV): 5 minutes	IV: < 2 hours IM: up to 6 hours; mean 2 hours Intranasal: ~20 minutes	Children: IM: 15–30 minutes Intranasal: 10 minutes IV: 3–5 minutes Adults: IM: 30–60 minutes Intranasal: 30 minutes	Prolonged in liver failure, obesity, and renal failure In renal failure – reduced elimination of active hydroxylated metabolites leads to drug accumulation and prolonged sedation Pediatric patients: IV: Gestation age 26–34 weeks: 6.3 hours (2.6–17.7) Neonates: 4–12 hours Children: IV: 2.9–4.5 Oral: 2.2–6.8 Adults: IV: 3 (1.8–6.4) IM: 4.2 ± 1.87 Intranasal: 2.1–6.2
Lorazepam	Anticonvulsant IV: Within 10 minutes Hypnosis IM: 20 to 30 minutes Sedation IV: 2 to 3 minutes	Children: IV/IM: 3–6 hours Adults: IV/IM: 6–8 hours	Oral: ~ 2 hours IM: ≤ 3 hours	Infants/children: Full-term neonates: IV 40.2 ± 16.5 (18–73) 5 months to <3 years: 15.8 (5.9–28.4) 3 to <13 years: 16.9 (7.5–40.6) 13 to <18 years: 17.8 (8.2–42) Adults: Oral: ~12 hours IV: ~ 14 hours IM: ~ 13–18 hours ESRD: ~18 hours

Uses and Indications for benzodiazepines are listed in Table 5.4

Table 5.4 Uses and indications for benzodiazepines

Drug name	Pediatric uses/indications
Clonazepam	Neuro-irritability, agitation, seizure disorders, panic disorder
Clorazepate	Anxiety disorders, seizures
Diazepam	Seizures (acute), status epilepticus, febrile seizure, prophylaxis, spasticity/muscle spasms, sedation, anxiolysis, and amnesia prior to procedure
Midazolam	Sedation, status epilepticus, anxiolysis, acute seizures
Alprazolam	Anxiety, panic disorder, premenstrual dysphoric disorder
Lorazepam	Sedation, status epilepticus, chemotherapy-induced nausea and vomiting (anticipatory and breakthrough), insomnia due to anxiety or stress

Midazolam is the most commonly used benzodiazepine in pediatric anesthesia. It is administered orally, nasally, and rectally as well as intravenously and intramuscularly. When administered midazolam causes anterograde amnesia, sedation, and anxiolysis. Midazolam is a water-soluble benzodiazepine that has various clinical advantages over diazepam. It is not painful when administered intravenously or intramuscularly. Midazolam is FDA approved as premedication in children and is the only benzodiazepine approved by the FDA for use in neonates. Its clearance in adults (1.8–6.4 hours) is reduced compared with children (1.4–4.0 hours). Midazolam clearance is reduced even more in neonates and preterm infants compared to toddlers and older children (6–12 hours). The elimination half-life is less in preterm infants less than 32 weeks' gestational age [7, 8]. Any factor that impairs hepatic blood flow (e.g., cardiac surgery with bypass compared with cardiac surgery without bypass) may decrease elimination including hypovolemic states and patients receiving vasopressors. Midazolam has the best pharmacokinetic profile for neonates compared to other benzodiazepines because the active metabolite exhibits minimal clinical activity and has a half-life similar to the parent compound. Midazolam has been administered as a continuous infusion both in the operating room and in the intensive care unit. The depth of sedation correlates with plasma concentrations of midazolam. Prolonged use does lead to tolerance, dependency, and benzodiazepine withdrawal [9]. Long-term infusions (i.e., ≥5 days) should be tapered over days while carefully monitoring for signs of withdrawal [10]. Benzyl alcohol toxicity is a theoretical concern associated with midazolam that can cause metabolic acidosis and gasping syndrome in neonates and infants. Toxicity should not occur when midazolam is given according to the recommended dosing guidelines. Cytochrome P450 3A4 metabolizes midazolam into an active metabolite. Therefore, midazolam will interact with those drugs/foods that are CYP 3A4 inhibitors like grapefruit juice, erythromycin, calcium channel blockers, and protease inhibitors. The interaction causes prolonged duration of action of midazolam [11].

Lorazepam was approved by the FDA in September 1977 and is a benzodiazepine with sedative and antianxiety effects. It is administered orally, intramuscularly, or intravenously. Lorazepam, like diazepam, is virtually insoluble in water. Peak plasma levels of lorazepam are seen in 60–90 minutes. Lorazepam has a slower onset of action and longer duration of action compared to the other benzodiazepines. When administered IV, lorazepam produces little or no clinical effect for about 5 minutes, with its maximum effect occurring approximately 20 minutes after administration. The duration of action of lorazepam following IM administration is approximately 6–8 hours. The major side effect is excessive sleepiness and a prolonged amnesic period. Because lorazepam is dissolved in propylene glycol, it can accumulate to produce metabolic acidosis and renal dysfunction [11]. The amnesic properties of lorazepam are impressive and include both anterograde and a degree of retrograde amnesia. Lack of recall is maximal approximately 15–20 minutes after IV administration and may include events occurring throughout the treatment day [6, 12].

Diazepam has been used extensively as a premedication, adjunct to anesthesia, for sedation, amnesia, and control of seizures. It can be administered orally, intravenously, and rectally to children. Diazepam is rapidly absorbed after oral administration, with peak plasma concentrations at 30–90 minutes. In children, the absorption rate is more rapid compared to adults. IM administration is painful and results in irregular absorption and should be avoided. Rectal diazepam is used for prehospital treatment of pediatric status epilepticus [5]. IV diazepam is associated with extravasation and tissue necrosis. Administering IV lidocaine before the diazepam and administering diazepam slowly through a rapidly flowing IV catheter minimizes this pain and risk. Diazepam is highly plasma bound, with a serum half-life ranging from 20 to 80 hours. Its half-life is reduced in younger adults and children to ~18 hours. Hepatic disease may decrease the elimination of diazepam. Diazepam undergoes oxidative metabolism by demethylation (CYP 2C19) to its active metabolite, desmethyldiazepam. The active metabolite has potency similar to the parent compound and a half-life greater than the parent compound. Therefore, caution is required when using diazepam in neonates [5].

The preservative benzyl alcohol is present in many formulations of diazepam. This preservative should not be used in neonates because it is difficult to metabolize, can cause metabolic acidosis, and is associated with kernicterus. The amount of benzyl alcohol contained in a standard dose of diazepam would likely be insufficient to cause harm to a neonate [6].

Adverse Reactions, Drug-Drug Interactions, and Monitoring Parameters

Adverse reactions to benzodiazepines are usually dose dependent with more severe adverse effects occurring when doses are increased. Dose-dependent adverse reactions to benzodiazepines include CNS effects and respiratory depression. Benzodiazepine exposure has also been associated with the development and longer duration of delirium and lower likelihood of ICU discharge in critically ill infants and young children [13, 14, 17].

Table 5.5 Drug interactions with benzodiazepines

CYP family	Substrates	Inhibitors	Inducers
CYP 3A4	Midazolam	Azole antifungals Macrolides Amiodarone Diltiazem Verapamil Erythromycin Protease inhibitor	Carbamazepine Phenobarbital Phenytoin Rifampin
CYP 2C19	Diazepam	Omeprazole Oxcarbazepine Topiramate Cimetidine Fluoxetine Ketoconazole	Dexamethasone Phenobarbital Phenytoin Rifampin
UGT	Lorazepam	Probenecid Valproic acid	Lamotrigine Phenobarbital Phenytoin Rifampin

The most frequent adverse reactions reported when using benzodiazepines include sedation, dizziness, weakness, fatigue, muscle weakness, ataxia, and iatrogenic withdrawal symptoms on abrupt discontinuation or weaning [15, 17].

Other reactions to benzodiazepines include:

- Central Nervous System: confusion, depression, dysarthria, headache, slurred speech, tremor, vertigo
- Gastrointestinal System: constipation, nausea, gastrointestinal disturbances, change in appetite, jaundice, increase in bilirubin, increase in liver transaminases, increase in alkaline phosphatase
- Cardiovascular System: hypotension
- Psychiatric and Paradoxical Reactions: stimulation, restlessness, anxiety, excitation, agitation, hostility, aggression, rage, irritability, rage, hallucinations, delusions, increased muscle spasticity, nightmare, sleep disturbances or insomnia
- Urogenital System: incontinence, urinary retention, changes in libido
- Dermatological Symptoms: allergic skin reactions, alopecia

Certain medications can influence the pharmacokinetics of benzodiazepines. Medications that are known to be inhibitors may result in increased and prolonged sedation due to a decrease in plasma clearance of benzodiazepines. Medications that are known to be inducers may result in a reduced sedation due to an increase in plasma clearance of benzodiazepines. Table 5.5 shows common drug interactions with benzodiazepines. Additionally, grapefruit juice may increase serum concentrations of midazolam. It is recommended to avoid concurrent use of grapefruit juice with oral midazolam.

Contraindications to the use of benzodiazepine include:

1. Benzodiazepines are contraindicated in patients with a known hypersensitivity to the drug or to any components of the formulation.
2. Paradoxical reactions such as anxiety, agitation, hostility, aggression, excitation, sleep disturbances, insomnia, and hallucinations have been reported during benzodiazepine use. Benzodiazepine should be discontinued if the patient experiences this reaction.
3. Midazolam is not used for intrathecal or epidural administration due to presence of the preservative benzyl alcohol in the dosage form.
4. Diazepam is contraindicated in patients with severe respiratory insufficiency, sleep apnea syndrome, severe hepatic insufficiency, and myasthenia gravis.
5. Lorazepam should be used with caution with compromised respiratory function such as sleep apnea.

Benzodiazepine and Opioids

Adjuvant use of benzodiazepines and opioids increases the risk of respiratory depression due to reactions at different receptor sites in the central nervous system that control respiration [16]. Benzodiazepines interact at $GABA_A$ sites and opioids interact primarily at mu receptors. When benzodiazepines and opioids are combined, the potential for benzodiazepines to significantly increase opioid-related respiratory depression exists. Dosage and duration of concurrent use of benzodiazepines and opioids should be limited, and patients should be monitored closely for increased respiratory depression and sedation.

Administration of benzodiazepines with other central nervous system depressants such as alcohol, barbiturates, antipsychotics, sedative, hypnotics, anxiolytics, antidepressants, narcotic analgesics, sedative antihistamines, and anticonvulsants produces CNS-depressant effects.

Breastfeeding/Pregnancy Considerations

Pregnancy Considerations

Teratogenic effects have been reported with some benzodiazepines. The incidence of premature birth and low birth weights may be increased due to maternal use of benzodiazepines. Hypoglycemia and respiratory problems in the neonate may occur following exposure late in pregnancy. Neonatal withdrawal symptoms may occur within days to weeks after birth in babies exposed to some benzodiazepine in utero.

Breastfeeding Considerations

Breastfeeding is not contraindicated in women using benzodiazepines. Sedative effects of benzodiazepine exposure through breast milk appear to present minimal risk of CNS depression in infants. Infant sedation is also more likely in mothers taking a greater number of concomitant CNS depressants [2].

In Summary

Benzodiazepines are the most commonly used sedatives in the pediatric intensive care units. Recent studies have highlighted the strong association between the use of benzodiazepines and ICU-acquired delirium. Additionally, abrupt cessation of benzodiazepines will result in iatrogenic withdrawal syndrome.

References

1. Kudchadkar SR, Yaster M, Punjabi NM. Sedation, sleep promotion, and delirium screening practices in the care of mechanically ventilated children: a wake-up call for the pediatric critical care community*. Crit Care Med. 2014;42(7):1592–600.
2. Nutt D. GABAA receptors: subtypes, regional distribution, and function. J Clin Sleep Med. 2006;2(2):S7–11.
3. Griffin CE 3rd, Kaye AM, Bueno FR, Kaye AD. Benzodiazepine pharmacology and central nervous system-mediated effects. Ochsner J. 2013;13(2):214–23.
4. Vet NJ, Kleiber N, Ista E, de Hoog M, de Wildt SN. Sedation in critically ill children with respiratory failure. Front Pediatr. 2016;4:89.
5. Cote CJ, Lerman J, Ward RM, Lugo RA, Goudscouzian N. Pharmacokinetics and pharmacology of drugs used in children. In: A practice of anesthesia for infants and children. 4th ed. Philadelphia: Saunders/Elsevier; 2009. p. 89–146.
6. Malamed S. Pharmacology. In: Sedation: a guide to patient management. 6th ed. St. Louis: Elsevier, Inc; 2018. p. 319–58.
7. Gorski JC, Hall SD, Jones DR, VandenBranden M, Wrighton SA. Regioselective biotransformation of midazolam by members of the human cytochrome P450 3A (CYP3A) subfamily. Biochem Pharmacol. 1994;47(9):1643–53.
8. Kearns GL, Abdel-Rahman SM, Alander SW, Blowey DL, Leeder JS, Kauffman RE. Developmental pharmacology–drug disposition, action, and therapy in infants and children. N Engl J Med. 2003;349(12):1157–67.
9. Blumer JL. Clinical pharmacology of midazolam in infants and children. Clin Pharmacokinet. 1998;35(1):37–47.
10. Best KM, Boullata JI, Curley MA. Risk factors associated with iatrogenic opioid and benzodiazepine withdrawal in critically ill pediatric patients: a systematic review and conceptual model. Pediatr Crit Care Med. 2015;16(2):175–83.
11. Duceppe MA, Perreault MM, Frenette AJ, et al. Frequency, risk factors and symptomatology of iatrogenic withdrawal from opioids and benzodiazepines in critically ill neonates, children and adults: a systematic review of clinical studies. J Clin Pharm Ther. 2019;44(2):148–56.

12. Pentikainen PJ, Valisalmi L, Himberg JJ, Crevoisier C. Pharmacokinetics of midazolam following intravenous and oral administration in patients with chronic liver disease and in healthy subjects. J Clin Pharmacol. 1989;29(3):272–7.
13. Chicella M, Jansen P, Parthiban A, et al. Propylene glycol accumulation associated with continuous infusion of lorazepam in pediatric intensive care patients. Crit Care Med. 2002;30(12):2752–6.
14. Kraus JW, Desmond PV, Marshall JP, Johnson RF, Schenker S, Wilkinson GR. Effects of aging and liver disease on disposition of lorazepam. Clin Pharmacol Ther. 1978;24(4):411–9.
15. Traube C, Silver G, Reeder RW, et al. Delirium in critically ill children: an international point prevalence study. Crit Care Med. 2017;45(4):584–90.
16. Traube C, Greenwald BM. "The times they are a-changin": universal delirium screening in pediatric critical care. Pediatr Crit Care Med. 2017;18(6):594–5.
17. Tobias JD. Tolerance, withdrawal, and physical dependency after long-term sedation and analgesia of children in the pediatric intensive care unit. Crit Care Med. 2000;28(6):2122–32.
18. Horn E, Nesbit SA. Pharmacology and pharmacokinetics of sedatives and analgesics. Gastrointest Endosc Clin N Am. 2004;14(2):247–68.

Chapter 6
Alpha-Agonists in Pediatric Critical Care

John W. Berkenbosch

Introduction

Alpha-agonists are a class of sedatives whose unique mechanism of action in addition to advantageous non-sedative properties has led to them gaining substantial popularity among pediatric critical care providers in recent years. For many years, the only α-agonist available was clonidine, and its primary uses were for the management of a sleep or behavior disorders in children with diagnoses such as attention deficit with hyperactivity disorder, autism spectrum disorder, and Tourette's syndrome among others [1–4]. Additional uses included treatment of hypertension [5, 6] and noninvasive procedural sedation, particularly for electroencephalography [7, 8]. While available as an enteral or intravenous (IV) agent, use until recently has been primarily enteral. In the late 1990s, however, dexmedetomidine was developed and rapidly expanded the applications of α-agonists into the anesthesia and critical care environments. While it is currently only approved by the United States Food and Drug Administration (FDA) for sedation up to 24 hours in critically ill adults and for procedural sedation in non-intubated adults, uses in pediatrics and pediatric critical care have risen rapidly since the first reports of its use in the pediatric setting in 2002 [9] and for pediatric intensive care unit (PICU) sedation in 2004 [10]. It is currently a mainstay for PICU sedation in many ICUs globally; in an analysis of dexmedetomidine use among 37 PICUs contributing to the public hospital information system (PHIS) database, from 2007 to 2013 dexmedetomidine use for PICU sedation increased over sixfold [11].

J. W. Berkenbosch (✉)
University of Louisville, Norton Children's Hospital, Louisville, KY, USA
e-mail: john.berkenbosch@louisville.edu

P. P. Kamat, J. W. Berkenbosch (eds.), *Sedation and Analgesia for the Pediatric Intensivist*, https://doi.org/10.1007/978-3-030-52555-2_6

Pharmacology

The primary mechanism by which clonidine and dexmedetomidine elicit their effects is selective agonism of the α_2 receptor. Three subtypes of the α_2 receptor exist (A, B, and C), and both drugs have agonistic effects on all three subtypes, albeit in different proportions [12]. The sedative and anxiolytic effects of α-agonists are mediated via binding to central α_{2B} receptors in the locus coeruleus, whereas their most common adverse effects, bradycardia and hypotension, are mediated via both the central (bradycardia) and peripheral (hypotension) α_{2A} receptors [13]. The cardiovascular effects, especially peripherally, are dose dependent. At lower drug doses, peripheral α_{2A} binding results in vasodilation and hypotension, whereas at high doses, peripheral α_{2B} binding occurs, resulting in vasoconstriction and hypertension. This likely explains the clinical findings that, during rapid bolus dose administration of dexmedetomidine, hypertension often occurs early, presumably due to higher plasma drug levels, while hypotension is a later finding, occurring as drug levels diminish as bolus doses dissipate or drug infusions are discontinued [14, 15]. Cellular effects of agonism of all three α_2 receptor subtypes are mediated by intracellular G-proteins. In addition to their sedative and anxiolytic effects, α-agonists confer modest analgesic effects via stimulation of α_2 receptors within the spinal cord which are mediated via substance P and result in inhibition of both Aδ and C pain fibers [16]. In contrast to other sedatives, α-agonists also appear to have limited effects on the electroencephalogram (EEG) and produce a sedation that closely simulates EEG patterns seen during natural sleep [17, 18]. From a clinical perspective, children tend to rouse from this sedation more easily and with significantly less potential for post-sedation confusion, agitation, and delirium than is seen during sedation with many other agents. They also tend to be more easily rousable with stimulation during ongoing sedation and return to their sedated state upon stimulus cessation with minimal need for resedation, a pattern that some have coined "cooperative sedation" [19].

Despite many similar pharmacodynamic effects, significant differences exist in the relative potencies of these effects between clonidine and dexmedetomidine. The primary reason for this lies in the significantly greater α_2 selectivity of dexmedetomidine which has a roughly eightfold greater α_2:α_1 receptor specificity compared to clonidine at 1620:1 vs 220:1 [20]. This facilitates greater sedative effects with, theoretically, fewer cardiovascular effects.

While primarily utilized as an oral agent, in some parts of the world (Europe, Australia), clonidine is also available in IV form [21] and has recently seen increased interest for use in the sedation of PICU patients. Following IV administration, onset of action is relatively rapid (minutes). High lipid solubility leads to rapid tissue redistribution, including the central nervous system, and the potential for prolonged clinical effects with longer-term use. Metabolism is primarily via hydroxylation of the phenyl ring following splitting of the imidazoline ring [22]. While metabolites are excreted in the urine, roughly half of the drug is excreted unchanged in the urine. Dosing may be initiated with a loading dose of 3–5 mcg/kg, followed by an infusion of 1–3 mcg/kg/hr [23]. Plasma elimination $t_{1/2}$ ranges from 12 to 24 hrs [24]. Onset is slower following enteral administration, peaking at 60–90 min although bioavailability is good at 75–90% [25]. Clearance varies with age. Neonatal clearance is slow with an elimination $t_{1/2}$ of 44–72 hrs which decreases rapidly such that by 1 year of age, elimination nears the 12–16 hrs seen in adults [25]. Clinical duration of action is much shorter at 60–90 minutes [7]. Dosing for sedation is 3–5 mcg/kg, while that for treatment of withdrawal syndromes is typically lower (1–2 mcg/kg/dose) but depends on the dosages of other IV alpha-agonists being received prior to transitioning to enteral clonidine.

While enteral, intranasal, and intramuscular use have been reported for procedural sedation use with dexmedetomidine, for PICU sedation it is utilized almost exclusively as an intravenous agent. Following bolus dosing, onset of action is rapid (within minutes) although the vast majority of practitioners forego the loading dose and use the drug as an infusion only. This is likely contributed to by findings that bolus dosing may be associated with significant hemodynamic changes as well as prolonged sinus pauses if done too rapidly [15]. Like clonidine, dexmedetomidine is highly lipophilic and rapidly redistributes in tissues. In contrast to clonidine, its elimination $t_{1/2}$ is relatively short at 2–2.5 hours in both healthy volunteers [14, 26] and the critically ill [27], making titration to clinical effect easier than with clonidine. Also, unlike clonidine, dexmedetomidine undergoes almost complete metabolism in the liver via glucuronidation and cytochrome P2A6 oxidation into inactive metabolites which are renally excreted [28]. Consequently, elimination is prolonged in liver but not renal disease. Non-IV use is almost exclusively limited to procedural sedation and includes primarily intranasal and oral/buccal use. While discussed elsewhere in this book in more depth, one factor that must be considered when administering orally is that bioavailability via buccal absorption is markedly higher (82%) than it is from gastric absorption (16%, Ref. 29). This significantly limits the appeal of enteral dexmedetomidine compared to clonidine in the PICU setting. If utilized, bolus dosing in the PICU is 1–2 mcg/kg administered over no more than 10 minutes. Continuous infusion rates range from 0.2 to 2 mcg/kg/hr with recommendations being to start low and titrate up to clinical effect.

Clinical Applications

Like many other sedative/anxiolytic agents used in the PICU, α-agonists have multiple beneficial actions beyond just their sedative effects. In particular, the sympatholytic effects appear to be beneficial in reducing the incidence of clinically significant tachydysrhythmias, and the minimal respiratory-depressing effects make the class appealing for use in the non-intubated patient to facilitate cooperation with sometimes irritating therapies, especially noninvasive ventilation. Additionally, they can be used to manage symptoms of iatrogenic withdrawal associated with benzodiazepine and/or opioid use and may decrease the risk of ICU-associated delirium.

The effectiveness of both dexmedetomidine and clonidine for PICU sedation during mechanical ventilation has been well described. As a primary sedative agent, clonidine has seen relatively limited use in pediatric critical care with most early studies concentrating on use to manage iatrogenic withdrawal from opioids and/or benzodiazepines [30, 31]. These studies have reported use as both enteral [30] or as an IV infusion [21, 32] and as an adjunct to opioid and/or benzodiazepine "failure" or in an attempt to decrease opioid/benzodiazepine use several days into the PICU course. Only two studies have evaluated the addition of clonidine early in the course of PICU sedation. A retrospective review compared usual sedation with or without addition of an α-agonist (primarily clonidine) and reported slightly improved sedation efficacy but no morphine- or midazolam-sparing effects [33]. A single RCT has compared clonidine versus midazolam infusions for sedation during mechanical ventilation in critically ill children [34]. While sedation quality and time at adequate sedation was similar with each regimen, in both groups, sedation quality was suboptimal much of the time, and patients receiving clonidine required more inotropic support than those in the midazolam group. Dosing of clonidine in all the above studies included oral and IV use as well as intermittent dosing or continuous infusion. For enteral use, dosing was 3–5 mcg/kg every 6–8 hours. For intermittent IV use, dosing was 1–2 mcg/kg every 6–8 hours and continuous infusion doses ranged from 1 to 3 mcg/kg/hr.

Substantially more experience has been published regarding the use of dexmedetomidine for PICU sedation and has revealed a large, albeit likely expected, evolution in use and dosage patterns as experience increases. Initially approved in 1999 for sedation in mechanically ventilated adults, the first case reports of use in the PICU appeared in 2002 [9] followed in 2004 by the first RCT comparing two doses of dexmedetomidine infusion versus midazolam infusion in addition to intermittent morphine boluses. Time inadequately sedated and total morphine use was lower in the high dexmedetomidine dose group compared to midazolam, while no differences were observed between low-dose dexmedetomidine and midazolam groups [10]. Over the next few years, several more case series were published describing effective and apparently safe (defined as limited adverse hemodynamic effects) use of dexmedetomidine as a primary sedative agent, many describing initiation soon after arrival to the PICU. Two cohorts of postoperative cardiac surgical patients received dexmedetomidine as their primary sedative with additional analgesia via either continuous infusion or intermittent dosing of opioids [35, 36]. Sedation and analgesia were assessed as adequate in the vast majority of patients. In one cohort, compared to patients receiving midazolam sedation, dexmedetomidine use was also found to be opioid-sparing [36]. Doses required in infants were found to be slightly higher than those required in older children. Subsequently, the use of dexmedetomidine was more specifically evaluated in neonates and infants following cardiothoracic surgery to better understand safety in this population [37]. While not overtly stated as a study motivation, this question is of special interest as the sympatholytic effects of dexmedetomidine (particularly bradycardia) might, theoretically, be less well tolerated due to the greater dependence on heart rate for cardiac output in younger children. Approximately ¼ of patients in this cohort also received fentanyl infusions, although this addition did not alter either the quality of sedation/analgesia or the mean dexmedetomidine doses required to achieve adequate sedation. In more mixed PICU populations, dexmedetomidine use has been reported as either a primary sedative or adjunct to benzodiazepine and/or opioid infusions [38, 39]. Sedation quality in these populations also was reported as adequate, with dexmedetomidine use also facilitating reductions in other sedative agents. In one study this reduction was a stated goal so that the limited respiratory-suppressing effects of dexmedetomidine compared to opioids and/or benzodiazepines could be taken advantage of in order to facilitate earlier extubation. A common thread in all of these studies was that dexmedetomidine doses used were relatively low (0.1 to 0.75 mcg/kg/hr) and likely reflected both published experience in critically ill adults [40, 41] and the initial FDA label. In addition, early use tended to be time-limited, with mean infusion durations ranging from 13 to 32 hours [36, 38, 39].

Subsequent reports have described expansions in terms of both dexmedetomidine dosing and duration in multiple critically ill pediatric populations. Following burn injury, dexmedetomidine initiation after failure of opioid and benzodiazepine infusions to maintain adequate comfort was associated with improved sedation quality and maintained adequacy of sedation using doses titrated up to 2 mcg/kg/hr and infusions continued for a mean duration of 11 days [42]. In a second report following burn injury, dexmedetomidine and midazolam were both able to maintain acceptable sedation, with each drug being used for mean durations of just over 20 days. Hypotension was reported less often in patients receiving dexmedetomidine although the mean dose was relatively low at 0.44 mcg/kg/hr [43]. Similarly, safe and effective use of prolonged dexmedetomidine infusions (mean duration of 9 days) following laryngotracheal reconstruction has been reported with no differences in adverse events compared to sedation with benzodiazepines although, unlike the above reported use in burn patients, iatrogenic withdrawal was a frequent finding regardless of sedation regimen utilized [44]. In general PICU populations, prolonged (>72 hr) dexmedetomidine infusions have also been reported to be well tolerated, including hemodynamically, at doses ranging up to 2.5 mcg/kg/hr although withdrawal symptoms were, again, not uncommon and tended to correlate with rate of weaning of the infusion or failure to transition off the infusion using enteral equivalents [45–47]. In addition to withdrawal with longer-term use, the major adverse effects described in these studies were hypotension and/or bradycardia, occurring in up to 40% of patients receiving dexmedetomidine although, due to coadministration of other cardioactive medications, it is unclear what proportion of hypotension is solely attributable to dexmedetomidine (38 39, 47).

Use of dexmedetomidine for sedation of the cardiac surgical patient has been an area of special interest since its arrival. While the efficacy of sedation has been well described, the increased incidence of bradycardia and hypotension compared to many other sedative/analgesic agents used could limit usefulness in this population. However, the sympatholysis which is responsible for these adverse events could also be of benefit, particularly in reducing the risk of catecholamine-sensitive dysrhythmia development. From a sedation perspective, dexmedetomidine appears to be as well tolerated in the cardiac surgical population as in other PICU populations.

Compared to patients receiving "conventional" sedation with benzodiazepine and opioid infusions, addition of dexmedetomidine to these therapies allowed reductions in both benzodiazepine and opioid doses without any significant hemodynamic changes [48, 49]. In studies comparing sedation regimens with a dexmedetomidine/ opioid versus a midazolam/opioid-based regimen, patients receiving the dexmedetomidine-based protocol were equally well sedated compared to those receiving midazolam [50, 51]. One of these studies also reported significant reductions in the need for adjunct analgesia or sedative agents to maintain comfort but also found increased rates of hypotension and/or bradycardia development with dexmedetomidine, even though interventions for these events were rarely required [50].

As alluded to above, dexmedetomidine is of particular interest in the cardiac surgical patient with respect to postoperative dysrhythmias, particularly junctional ectopic tachycardia (JET). This is particularly malignant tachydysrhythmia that is unique to the pediatric population, occurring in up to 15% of children undergoing cardiac surgery. While decreasing, mortality rates of 8–13% have been reported in patients developing JET [52, 53]. Pathophysiologically, JET is associated with atrioventricular dissociation and progressive decreases in cardiac output as heart rates rise, making management difficult as the addition of catecholamine-based inotropic agents can exacerbate instability [54]. Treatment has focused on decreasing catecholamine levels by patient cooling, aggressively treating pain, deepening sedation, and reducing inotrope infusion rates [55]. Additional pharmacologic management focuses on reducing heart rate to enhance ventricular filling time, with amiodarone being the currently accepted standard [54]. The sympatholytic effects of dexmedetomidine are especially appealing here as, in addition to providing sedation, sympatholysis-induced catecholamine reductions may also contribute to heart rate control. In a retrospective cohort study, patients who received dexmedetomidine for postoperative sedation had a markedly reduced risk of JET development (OR 0.17) compared to non-dexmedetomidine-based sedation regimens [56]. In a subsequent trial randomizing patients to receive dexmedetomidine or placebo as an intraoperative load plus a 48-hour postoperative infusion, the incidence of JET in the dexmedetomidine group was significantly reduced (16.7% vs 3.3%) without increases in other adverse events including bradycardia and hypotension [57]. In a placebo-controlled randomized comparison of prophylactic dexmedetomidine or amiodarone following cardiac surgery, the incidence of postoperative JET was identical in the two treatment groups (6.7% each) compared to 33.3% in the placebo group [58]. All of the above studies suggest that dexmedetomidine is effective in reducing the risk of JET development. However, inadequate data exist to comment on the impact of addition of dexmedetomidine to patients who develop JET. In addition to the impacts of JET, dexmedetomidine use following cardiac surgery has been associated with reductions in other tachydysrhythmias, tachydysrhythmias requiring intervention, and ventricular tachycardia [59, 60]. In two meta-analyses of dexmedetomidine use in cardiac surgical patients, additional dexmedetomidine benefits included reductions in length of mechanical ventilation, duration of PICU and hospital stay, opioid and benzodiazepine requirements, and delirium development [61, 62]. A single study has reported that the occurrence and severity of acute kidney injury following pediatric cardiac surgery was lower in children sedated with dexmedetomidine compared to other agents, the proposed mechanisms being a combination of anti-inflammatory effects, cytoprotection via α_2-receptor-mediated cell survival signaling, and sympatholysis-mediated increased renal blood flow [63].

The absence of clinically relevant respiratory depression associated with α-agonists compared to most other sedatives available to the critical care provider has been well described and contributes largely to the basis for their use in procedural sedation. This property has also been taken advantage of in the PICU, with dexmedetomidine use described either for non-intubated patients in whom agitation control was required or as a bridge to extubation in patients deemed at higher risk of inadvertent device removal during the sedation lightening and ventilator weaning process [38, 45, 64, 65]. More recently, in correlation with the increasing use of noninvasive ventilation (NIV) for acute respiratory failure in the PICU [66], use of α-agonists has expanded to facilitate cooperation with NIV strategies, including high flow nasal cannula and continuous/bilevel positive airway pressure (CPAP/BiPAP) via nasal or full face mask. In three studies, dexmedetomidine infusions were utilized in over 600 critically ill children requiring NIV support for either primary lung disease or systemic diseases such as sepsis and septic shock [67–69]. The average doses administered to these cohorts ranged from 0.6 to 1 mcg/kg/hr with reported maximum doses of 1–1.5 mcg/kg/hr, which is similar to doses reported during use for procedural sedation. Median infusion durations ranged from 35 to 48 hrs with numerous patients requiring infusion durations of >96 hours. Two of the 3 studies provided data regarding progression of lung disease; in 242 patients initially managed with NIV and dexmedetomidine sedation, only 9 required subsequent endotracheal intubation [67, 68], and, of these, 8 were deemed to be a result of primary disease progression rather than adverse effects of dexmedetomidine use. These data suggest that, similar to its well-established respiratory safety record during procedural sedation, longer-term use of moderate-dose dexmedetomidine infusions can be safely used to facilitate cooperation with NIV therapies.

The development of tolerance and iatrogenic withdrawal syndromes following prolonged use of many sedative or analgesic agents is a well-recognized phenomenon within pediatric critical care, occurring in up to half of patients [69, 70]. To date, most literature regarding iatrogenic sedative withdrawal has focused on benzodiazepines and opioids, as they remain the most commonly utilized agents in the PICU setting. Typically, management of withdrawal is two-pronged. Firstly, prevention of symptoms is aimed for, usually by slow weaning of the sedative/analgesic agent(s) with or without transition from IV to enteral equivalents. Alongside this, a validated withdrawal scoring tool is used so that, if symptoms do develop, interventions to mitigate them such as increasing doses or reinitiation of the presumed responsible agent can be implemented. Concerns for the development of benzodiazepine and opioid withdrawal may have adverse effects on the intubated patient. In addition to potential ongoing agent-related adverse effects, endotracheal extubation may be delayed due to worries that respiratory depression may develop if infusions must be continued following extubation. Alpha-agonists, especially clonidine, have a relatively well-established history of benefit in treating withdrawal associated with substances of abuse [71–73]. More recently, these properties have been utilized to manage tolerance to, and withdrawal from, benzodiazepine and opioid infusions in PICU patients. Use of a dexmedetomidine infusion to manage iatrogenic withdrawal in the PICU setting was first described over 15 years ago [74]. Subsequent small case series describe success with IV or subcutaneous dexmedetomidine infusions [75, 76] with more rigorous data remaining limited. While it is commonly utilized, published data regarding the use of clonidine for prevention/treatment of iatrogenic withdrawal are also relatively limited, including just over 100 patients in 10 reports [77]. Both enteral and transdermal clonidine applications have been described. Regardless of which agent is used, strategies should be tailored to the unique patient situation. Dosing needs will vary depending on both the doses and duration of time the other sedative and/or analgesic agents have been administered. Unless concerns regarding hemodynamic tolerance exist, it is typically recommended that once the α-agonist is added, the benzodiazepine and opioid infusions be weaned and discontinued first so that ventilator weaning can continue with a lower likelihood of respiratory depression. It is acceptable to initiate therapy with dexmedetomidine given that it is most easily titratable. Subsequent conversion to enteral or transdermal clonidine can then occur at the practitioners discretion and patients ability to tolerate enteral intake.

Despite their value for the management of iatrogenic withdrawal, it has also been increasingly recognized that tolerance and withdrawal to α-agonists may develop. Initial descriptions of possible withdrawal occurred over 10 years ago with two case reports. In the first case, tachycardia, hypertension, and emesis developed in a 2-year-old male shortly following abrupt discontinuation of a 6-day dexmedetomidine infusion [78]. In the second, an 8-week-old female developed agitation, tachycardia, diarrhea, pupillary dilation, and seizure in the first several hours after abrupt discontinuation of a 3.5-day infusion of dexmedetomidine [79]. In both cases, symptoms resolved with reinitiation of dexmedetomidine and did not recur with a slower wean. Subsequent to these reports, several larger series have reported presumed withdrawal in patients either following abrupt discontinuation or weaning of dexmedetomidine infusions, although consensus regarding what constitutes a true withdrawal syndrome to α-agonists does not yet exist. Multiple symptoms have been described with the most common including tachycardia, hypertension, agitation, tremor, fever, and sleep disturbances [46, 48, 65, 80]. Many of these symptoms are also seen with withdrawal from either benzodiazepines or opioids. Since these medications are often coadministered with α-agonists, determination of which agent is the primary offender in terms of withdrawal development may be difficult. Use of conventional withdrawal scoring tools such as the Finnegan score for neonatal abstinence syndrome and the Modified Withdrawal Assessment Tool (M-WAT) may also be problematic as they were not specifically designed for assessing withdrawal to α-agonists and do not necessarily assess for all of the symptoms which have been described with possible α-agonist withdrawal. Thus, their use may result in an under-recognition of α-agonist-based withdrawal, which underscores the importance of practitioner being especially aware of the potential for withdrawal development during α-agonist weaning and/or termination. Similar to use for opioid and benzodiazepine withdrawal, transition from IV dexmedetomidine to enteral or transdermal clonidine is a potentially useful strategy for mitigation of withdrawal.

While initially recognized/appreciated in adult critical care, delirium in PICU patients has also come to be appreciated as a significant problem with numerous associated morbidities including prolonged ICU and hospital lengths of stay [81, 82], prolonged psychological sequelae [83], and possibly even mortality [81]. With data increasingly suggesting an association between benzodiazepine use and pediatric delirium [82, 84] and data in critically ill adults suggesting sedation that dexmedetomidine may be protective regarding delirium development [85], increased understanding of the impact of α-agonists on pediatric delirium is needed. Limited data to date have addressed this. In a small study comparing midazolam to dexmedetomidine-based sedation following scoliosis surgery, patients receiving dexmedetomidine experienced significantly less delirium [86]. In a larger meta-analysis of dexmedetomidine use in pediatric cardiac surgical patients, the odds ratio of experiencing delirium was 0.39 in patients sedated with dexmedetomidine compared to other sedatives [61]. Further study into the benefits of α-agonists for pediatric delirium remains an ongoing need and priority.

Conclusion

Alpha-agonists are increasingly utilized for pediatric ICU sedation. Useful applications include sedation efficacy, reduced risk of tachydysrhythmias following cardiac surgical procedures, treatment of withdrawal syndromes associated with benzodiazepine and opioid exposure, and possibly reductions in delirium. Their limited respiratory-suppressing properties make this class of sedatives appealing for use during noninvasive ventilation or to facilitate ventilator weaning and extubation in the otherwise potentially behavior-challenged patient. For IV sedation in the PICU, dexmedetomidine is the preferred agent due to more favorable pharmacokinetics compared to clonidine although, to facilitate termination of IV infusions, transition to enteral or transdermal clonidine is viable and useful. Significant adverse effects associated with α-agonists are limited to cardiovascular effects, particularly hypotension and bradycardia. While not uncommon, these issues usually do not require intervention other than dose reductions.

As with other sedative and analgesic agents, prolonged use can be associated with tolerance and iatrogenic withdrawal development, which can be mitigated by slow weans and/or addition of enteral α-agonist equivalents.

References

1. Willens TE, Biederman J, Spencer T. Clonidine for sleep disorders associated with attention-deficit hyperactivity disorder. J Am Acad Child Adolesc Psychiatry. 1994;33:424–6.
2. Greenhill LL. Pharmacologic treatment of attention deficit hyperactivity disorder. Psychiatr Clin North Am. 1992;15:1–27.

3. Cohen DJ, Riddle MA, Leckman JF. Pharmacotherapy of Tourette's syndrome and associated disorders. Psychiatr Clin North Am. 1992;15:109–29.
4. Goel R, Hong JS, Findling RL, Ji NY. An update on pharmacotherapy of autism spectrum disorder in children and adolescents. Int Rev Psychiatry. 2018;30:78–95.
5. Garrett BN, Kaplan NM. Clonidine in the treatment of hypertension. J Cardiovasc Pharmacol. 1980;2(Suppl 1):S61–71.
6. Falkner B, Onesti G, Lowenthal DT, Affrime MB. The use of clonidine in adolescent hypertension. Chest. 1983;83:425–7.
7. Mehta UC, Patel I, Castello FV. EEG sedation for children with autism. J Dev Behav Pediatr. 2004;25:102–4.
8. Barzegar M, Piri E, Naghavi-Behzad M, Ghasempour M. Clonidine sedation effects in children during electroencephalography. Acta Med Iran. 2017;55:568–72.
9. Tobias JD, Berkenbosch JW. Initial experience with dexmedetomidine in paediatric-aged patients. Paediatr Anaesth. 2002;12:171–5.
10. Tobias JD, Berkenbosch JW. Sedation during mechanical ventilation in infants and children: dexmedetomidine versus midazolam. South Med J. 2004;97:451–5.
11. Benneyworth BD, Downs SM, Nitu M. Retrospective evaluation of the epidemiology and practice variation of dexmedetomidine use in invasively ventilated pediatric intensive care admissions, 2007–2013. Front Pediatr. 2015;3:109. https://doi.org/10.3389/fped.2015.00109.
12. Kamibayashi T, Maze M. Clinical uses of α_2-adrenergic agonists. Anesthesiology. 2000;93:1345–9.
13. Lakhlani PP, MacMillan LB, Guo TZ, McCool BA, Lovinger DM, Maze M, Limbird LE. Substitution of a mutant a2A-adrenergic receptor via 'hit and run' gene targeting reveals the role of this subtype in sedative, analgesic, and anesthetic-sparing responses *in vivo*. Proc Natl Acad Sci U S A. 1997;94:9950–5.
14. Dyck JB, Maze M, Haack C, Vuorilehto L, Shafer SL. The pharmacokinetics and hemodynamic effects of intravenous and intramuscular dexmedetomidine hydrochloride in adult volunteers. Anesthesiology. 1993;78:813–20.
15. Bloor BC, Ward DS, Belleville JP, Maze M. Effects of intravenous dexmedetomidine in humans: II hemodynamic changes. Anesthesiology. 1992;77:1134–42.
16. Kuraishi Y, Hirota N, Sato Y, Kaneko S, Satoh M, Takagi H. Noradrenergic inhibition of the release of substance P from the primary afferents in the rabbit spinal dorsal horn. Brain Res. 1985;359:177–82.
17. Mason KP, O'Mahony E, Zurakowski D, Libenson MH. Effects of dexmedetomidine sedation on the EEG in children. Pediatr Anesth. 2009;19:1175–83.
18. Aksu R, Kumandas S, Akin A, Bicer C, Gumus H, Guler G, Per H, Bavram A, Boyaci A. The comparison of the effects of dexmedetomidine and midazolam sedation on electroencephalography in pediatric patients with febrile convulsion. Paediatr Anaesth. 2011;21:373–8.
19. Kaur M, Singh PM. Current role of dexmedetomidine in clinical anesthesia and intensive care. Anesth Essays Res. 2011;5:128–33.
20. Virtanen R, Savola JM, Saano V, Nyman L. Characterization of selectivity, specificity and potency of dexmedetomidine as alpha-2-adrenoceptor agonist. Eur J Pharmacol. 1988;150:9–14.
21. Kleiber N, van Rosmalen J, Tibboel D, de Wildt SN. Hemodynamic tolerance to IV clonidine in the PICU. Pediatr Crit Care Med. 2018;19:e409–16.
22. Lowenthal DT. Pharmacokinetics of clonidine. J Cardiovasc Pharmacol. 1980;2:529–37.
23. Wang JG, Belley-Cote E, Burry L, Duffert M, Karachi T, Perri D, Alhazzani W, D'Aragon F, Wunsch H, Rochwerg B. Clonidine for sedation in the critically ill: a systematic review and meta-analysis. Crit Care. 2017;21:75;1–11.
24. Frisk-Holmberg M, Paalzow L, Edlund PO. Clonidine kinetics in man- evidence for dose dependency and changed pharmacokinetics during chronic therapy. Br J Clin Pharmacol. 1981;12:653–8.
25. Nguyen V, Tiemann D, Park E, Salehi A. Alpha-2 agonists. Anesthesiol Clin. 2017;2:233–45.

26. Weerink MAS, Struys MMRF, Hannivoort LN, Barends CRM, Absolam AR, Colin P. Clinical pharmacokinetics and pharmacodynamics of dexmedetomidine. Clin Pharmacokinet. 2017;56:893–913.
27. Venn RM, Karol MD, Grounds RM. Pharmacokinetics of dexmedetomidine infusions for sedation of postoperative patients requiring intensive care. Br J Anaesth. 2002;88:669–75.
28. Karol MD, Maze M. Pharmacokinetics and interaction pharmacodynamics of dexmedetomidine in humans. Best Pract Res Clin Anaesthesiol. 2000;14:261–9.
29. Anttila M, Penttila¨ J, Helminen A, Vuorilehto L, Scheinin H. Bioavailability of dexmedetomidine after extravascular doses in healthy subjects. Br J Clin Pharmacol. 2003;56:691–3.
30. Arenas-Lopez S, Riphagen S, Tibby S, Durward A, Tomlin S, Davies G, Murdoch IA. Use of oral clonidine for sedation in ventilated paediatric intensive care patients. Intens Care Med. 2004;30:1625–9.
31. Duffett M, Koop A, Menon K, Meade MO, Cook DJ. Clonidine for sedation of critically ill children: a systematic review. J Pediatr Intens Care. 2012;1:5–15.
32. Hunselar C, Balling C, Rohlig C, Blickheuser R, Trieschmann U, Lieser U, Dohna-Schake C, Gebauer C, Molleer O, Hering F, Hoehn T, Schubert S, Hentschel R, Huth RG, Muller A, Muller C, Wassmer G, Hahn M, Harnischmacher U, Behr J, Roth B, For the Clonidine Study Group. Continuous infusion of clonidine in ventilated newborns and infants: a randomized clinical trial. Pediatr Crit Care Med. 2014;15:511–22.
33. Hayden JC, Doherty DR, Dawkins I, Leacy FP, Healy M, Breatnach CV, Cousins G, Gallagher PJ. The effectiveness of α2 agonists as sedatives in pediatric critical care: a propensity score-matched cohort study. Crit Care Med. 2019;47:e580–6.
34. Wolf A, McKay A, spowart C, Granvillee H, Boland A, Petrou S, Sutherland A, Gamble C. Prospective multicentre randomised, double-blind, equivalence study comparing clonidine and midazolam as intravenous sedative agents in critically ill children: the SLEEPS (Safety profiLe, Efficacy and Equivalence in Paediatric intensive care Sedation) study. Health Technol Assess. 2014;18:1–212.
35. Chrysostomou C, Di Filippo S, Manrique A-M, Schmitt CG, Orr RA, Casta A, Suchoza E, Janosky J, Davis PJ, Munoz R. Use of dexmedetomidine in children after cardiac and thoracic surgery. Pediatr Crit Care Med. 2006;7:126–31.
36. Beijan S, Valasek C, Nigro JJ, Cleveland DC, Willis BC. Prolonged use of dexmedetomidine in the pediatric cardiothoracic intensive care unit. Cardiol Young. 2009;19:98–104.
37. Chrysostomou C, Sanchez De Toledo J, Avolio T, Motoa MV, Berry D, Morrel VO, Orr RA, Munoz R. Dexmedetomidine use in a pediatric cardiac intensive care unit: can we use it in infants after cardiac surgery? Pediatr Creit Care Med. 2009;10:654–60.
38. Buck ML, Willson DF. Use of dexmedetomidine in the pediatric intensive care unit. Pharmacotherapy. 2008;28:51–7.
39. Czaja AS, Zimmerman JJ. The use of dexmedetomidine in critically ill children. Pediatr Crit Care Med. 2009;10:381–6.
40. Venn RM, Bradshaw CJ, Spencer R, Brealey D, Caudwell E, Naughton C, Vedio A, Singer M, Feneck R, Treacher D, Willatts SM, Grounds RM. Preliminary UK experience of dexmedetomidine, a novel agent for postoperative sedation in the intensive care unit. Anaesthesia. 1999;54:1136–42.
41. Martin E, Ramsay G, Mantz J, Sum-Ping ST. The role of alpha2-adrenergic agonist dexmedetomidine in postsurgical sedation in the intensive care unit. J Intens Care Med. 2003;18: 29–41.
42. Walker J, MacCallum M, Fischer C, Kopcha R, Saylors R, McCall J. Sedation using dexmedetomidine in pediatric burn patients. J Burn Care Res. 2006;27:206–10.
43. Fagin A, Palmieri T, Greenhlgh D, Sen S. A comparison of dexmedetomidine and midazolam for sedation in severe pediatric burn injury. J Burn Care Res. 2012;33:759–63.
44. McCormick ME, Johnson YJ, Pena M, Wratney AT, Pestieau SR, Zalzal GH, Preciado DA. Dexmedetomidine as a primary sedative agent after single-stage airway reconstruction. Otolaryngol Head Neck Surg. 2013;148:503–8.

45. Carroll CL, Krieger D, Campbell M, Fisher DG, Comeau LL, Zucker AR. Use of dexmedetomidine for sedation of children hospitalized in the intensive care unit. J Hosp Med. 2008;3:142–7.
46. Whalen LD, Di Gennaro JL, Irby GA, Yanay O, Zimmerman JJ. Long-term dexmedetomidine use and safety profile among critically ill children and neonates. Pediatr Crit Care Med. 2014;15:706–14.
47. Sperotto F, Mondardini MC, Vitale F, Daverio M, Campagnano E, Ferrero F, Rossetti E, Vasile B, Dusio MP, Ferrario S, Savron F, Brugnaro L, Amigoni A on behalf of the Pediatric Neurological Protection and Drugs (PeNARD) Study Group. Prolonged sedation in critically ill children: is dexmedetomidine a safe option for younger age? An off-label experience. Minerva Anestesiol. 2019;85:164–72.
48. Gupta P, Whiteside W, Sabati A, Tereso TM, Gossett JM, Tobias JD, Roth SJ. Safety and efficacy of dexmedetomidine use in critically ill children with heart disease. Pediatr Crit Care Med. 2012;13:660–6.
49. Hasegawa T, Oshima Y, Maruo A, Matsuhisa H, Tanaka A, Noda R, Matsushima S. Dexmedetomidine in combination with midazolam after pediatric cardiac surgery. Asian Cardiovasc Thorac Ann. 2015;23:802–8.
50. Hosokawa K, Shime N, Kato Y, Taniguchi A, Maeda Y, Miyazaki T, Hashimoto S. Dexmedetomidine sedation in children after cardiac surgery. Pediatr Crit Care Med. 2010;11:39–43.
51. Jiang L, Ding S, Yan H, Li Y, Zhang L, Chen X, Yin X, Liu S, Tang X, Zhang J. A retrospective comparison of dexmedetomidine versus midazolam for pediatric patients with congenital heart disease requiring postoperative sedation. Pediatr Cardiol. 2015;36:993–9.
52. Coumel P, Fidelle JE, Attuel P, Brechenmacher C, Batisse A, Bretagne J, Clementy J, Gérard R, Grolleau R, Huault G, Mouy A, Nouaille J, Kachaner J, Ribiere M, Toumieux MC. Congenital bundle-of-his focal tachycardias. Cooperative study of 7 cases. Arch Mal Coeur Vaiss. 1976;69:899–909.
53. Mildh L, Hiippala A, Rautiainen P, Pettila V, Sairanen H, Happonen JM. Junctional ectopic tachycardia after surgery for congenital heart disease: incidence, risk factors and outcome. Eur J Cardiothorac Surg. 2011;39:75–80.
54. Kylat R, Samson RA. Junctional ectopic tachycardia in infants and children. J Arrhythm. 2020;36:59–66.
55. Villain E, Vetter VL, Garcia JM, Herre J, Cifarelli A, Garson AJ. Evolving concepts in the management of congenital junctional ectopic tachycardia. A multicenter study. Circulation. 1990;81:1544–9.
56. Gautam NK, Turiy Y, Srinivasan C. Preincision initiation of dexmedetomidine maximally reduces the risk of junctional ectopic tachycardia in children undergoing ventricular septal defect repairs. J Cardiothorac Vasc Anesth. 2017;31:1960–5.
57. El Amrousy DM, El-Shmaa NS, El-Kashlan M, Hassan S, Elsanosy M, Hablas N, Elrifaey S, El-Feky W. Efficacy of prophylactic dexmedetomidine in preventing junctional ectopic tachycardia after pediatric cardiac surgery. J Am Heart Assoc. 2017;6:e004780. https://doi.org/10.1161/JAHA.116.004780.
58. El-Schmaa NS, El Amrousy D, El Feky W. The efficacy of pre-emptive dexmedetomidine versus amiodarone in preventing postoperative junctional ectopic tachycardia in pediatric cardiac surgery. Ann Card Anaesth. 2016;19:614–20.
59. Chrysostomou C, Sanchez-de-Toledo J, Wearden P, Jooste EH, Lichtenstein SE, Callahan PM, Suresh T, O'Malley E, Shiderly D, Haney J, Yoshida M, Orr R, Munoz R, Morell VO. Perioperative use of dexmedetomidine is associated with decreased incidence of ventricular and supraventricular tachyarrhythmias after congenital cardiac operations. Ann Thorac Surg. 2011;92:964–72.
60. Shuplock JM, Smith AH, Owen J, Van Driest SL, Marshall M, Saville B, Xu M, Radbill AE, Fish FA, Kannankeril PJ. The association between peri-operative dexmedetomidine and arrhythmias after surgery for congenital heart disease. Circ Arrhythm Electrophysiol. 2015;8:643–50.

61. Pan W, Wang Y, Zhou LLG, Hua X, Mo L. Outcomes of dexmedetomidine treatment in pediatric patients undergoing congenital heart disease surgery: a meta-analysis. Pediatr Anesth. 2016;26:239–48.
62. Liu Y, Bian W, Liu P, Zang X, Gu X, Chen W. Dexmedetomidine improves the outcomes in paediatric cardiac surgery: a meta-analysis of randomized clinical trials. Interact Cardiovasc Thorac Surg. 2018;26:852–8.
63. Kwiatkowski DM, Axelrod DM, Sutherland SM, Tesoro TM, Krawczeski CD. Dexmedetomidine is associated with lower incidence of acute kidney injury after congenital heart surgery. Pediatr Crit Care Med. 2016;17:128–34.
64. Tobias JD, Berkenbosch JW, Russo P. Additional experience with dexmedetomidine in pediatric patients. South Med J. 2003;96:871–5.
65. Banasch HL, Dersch-Mills DA, Boulter LL, Gilfoyle E. Dexmedetomidine use in a pediatric intensive care unit: a retrospective cohort study. Ann Pharmacother. 2018;52:133–9.
66. Marohon K, Panisello JM. Noninvasive ventilation in pediatric intensive care. Curr Opin Pediatr. 2013;25:290–6.
67. Venkatraman R, Hungerford JL, Hall MW, Moore-Clingenpeel M, Tobias JD. Dexmedetomidine for sedation during noninvasive ventilation in pediatric patients. Pediatr Crit Care Med. 2017;18:831–7.
68. Piastra M, Pizza A, Gaddi S, Luca E, Genovese O, Picconi E, De Luca D, Conti G. Dexmedetomidine is effective and safe during NIV in infants and young children with acute respiratory failure. BMC Pediatr. 2018;18:282. https://doi.org/10.1186/s12887-018-1256-y.
69. Shutes BL, Gee SW, Sargel CL, Fink KA, Tobias JD. Dexmedetomidine as single continuous sedative during noninvasive ventilation: typical usage, hemodynamic effects, and withdrawal. Pediatr Crit Care Med. 2018;19:287–97.
70. Ista E, van Dijk M, Gamel C, Tibboel D, de Hoog M. Withdrawal symptoms in children after long-term administration of sedative and/or analgesics: a literature review. "Assessment remains troublesome". Intens Care Med. 2007;33:1396–406.
71. Hoder EL, Leckman JF, Ehrenkranz R, Kleber H, Cohen DJ, Poulsen JA. Clonidine in neonatal narcotic-abstinence syndrome. N Engl J Med. 1981;305:1284–5.
72. Baumgartner GR, Rowen RC. Transdermal clonidine versus chlordiazepoxide in alcohol withdrawal: a randomized, controlled clinical trial. South Med J. 1991;84:312–21.
73. Yam PCI, Forbes A, Kox WJ. Clonidine in the treatment of alcohol withdrawal in the intensive care unit. Br J Anaesth. 1992;68:106–8.
74. Baddigam K, Russo P, Russo JA, Tobias JD. Dexmedetomidine in the treatment of withdrawal syndromes in cardiothoracic surgery patients. J Intensive Care Med. 2005;20:118–23.
75. Tobias JD. Dexmedetomidine to treat opioid withdrawal in infants following prolonged sedation in the pediatric ICU. J Opioid Manag. 2006;2:201–5.
76. Tobias JD. Subcutaneous dexmedetomidine infusions to treat or prevent drug withdrawal in infants and children. J Opioid Manag. 2008;4:187–91.
77. Capino AC, Miller JL, Johnson PN. Clonidine for sedation and analgesia and withdrawal in critically ill infants and children. Pharmacotherapy. 2016;36:1290–9.
78. Weber MD, Thammasitboon S, Rosen DA. Acute discontinuation syndrome from discontinuation from dexmedetomidine after protracted use in a pediatric patient. Pediatr Anesth. 2008;18:87–8.
79. Darnell C, Steiner J, Szmuk SP. Withdrawal from multiple sedative agent therapy in an infant: is dexmedetomidine the cause or the cure? Pediatr Crit Care Med. 2010;11:e1–3.
80. Haenecour AS, Seto W, Urbain CM, Stephens D, Laussen PC, Balit CR. Prolonged dexmedetomidine infusion and drug withdrawal in critically ill children. J Pediatr Pharmacol Ther. 2017;22:453–60.
81. Traube C, Silver G, Gerber LM, Kaur S, Mauer EA, Kerson A, Joyce C, Greenwald BM. Delirium and mortality in critically ill children: epidemiology and outcomes of pediatric delirium. Crit Care Med. 2017;45:891–8.
82. Smith HAB, Gangopadhyay M, Goben CM, Jacobowski NL, Thompson JL, Chandrasekhar R, Williams SR, Griffith K, Ely EW, Fuchs DC, Pandharipande PP. Delirium and benzodiaz-

epines associated with prolonged ICU stay in critically ill infants and young children. Crit Care Med. 2017;45:1427–35.
83. Colville G, Kerry S, Pierce C. Children's factual and delusional memories of intensive care. Am J Respir Crit Care Med. 2008;177:976–82.
84. Mody K, Kaur S, Mauer EA, Gerber LMM, Greenwald BM, Silver G, Traube C. Benzodiazepines and development of delirium in critically ill children: estimating the causal effect. Crit Care Med. 2018;46:1486–91.
85. Riker RR, Shehabi Y, Bokesch PM, Ceraso D, Wisemandle W, Koura F, Whitten P, Margolis BD, Byrne DW, Ely EW, Rocha MG, SEDCOM (Safety and Efficacy of Dexmedetomidine Compared With Midazolam) Study Group. Dexmedetomidine vs. midazolam for sedation of critically ill patients: a randomized trial. JAMA. 2009;301:489–99.
86. Aydogen MS, Korkmaz MF, Ozgul U, Erdogan MA, Yucel A, Karaman A, Togal T, Durmus M, Colak C. Pain, fentanyl consumption, and delirium in adolescents after scoliosis surgery: dexmedetomidine vs midazolam. Pediatr Anesth. 2013;23:446–52.

Chapter 7
Barbiturates in the Pediatric ICU

Heather Damhoff and Cynthia L. McCune

Introduction

Barbiturates are a class of sedative/hypnotic medications with a long history of use in pediatric critical care due to multiple potentially beneficial pharmacodynamic effects. Several options are available for the practitioner, and choices should be made based more on the agent's particular pharmacokinetic rather than pharmacodynamic properties as the latter are relatively similar between available agents. Of primary interest for the purposes of this work, barbiturates confer dose-dependent sedative and hypnotic but not analgesic effects. However, of additional interest are their anticonvulsant and intracranial pressure-modulating effects.

Pharmacology

Barbiturates exert most of their action via agonism of gamma-aminobutyric acid (GABA), the major inhibitory neurotransmitter in the central nervous system, primarily via binding of the $GABA_A$ receptor [1]. From a sedation perspective, it appears that barbiturate effects are mediated via binding to a specific site on the $GABA_A$ receptor, in essence a "barbiturate receptor" [2]. This binding results in prolongation of the downstream chloride channel and subsequent postsynaptic inhibitory effects. Additionally relevant to the critical care provider, the two most common barbiturates used in current practice, phenobarbital and pentobarbital,

H. Damhoff (✉)
Norton Children's Hospital, Pharmacy, Louisville, KY, USA
e-mail: Heather.damhoff@nortonhealthcare.org

C. L. McCune
Dell Children's Medical Center, Pharmacy, Austin, TX, USA

P. P. Kamat, J. W. Berkenbosch (eds.), *Sedation and Analgesia for the Pediatric Intensivist*, https://doi.org/10.1007/978-3-030-52555-2_7

have different properties relative to CNS depression with pentobarbital being a more potent sedative at equivalent anticonvulsant doses [1]. This difference appears to be mediated by differential potencies of $GABA_A$ binding by each agent [3] suggesting that clinical effects and potencies are mediated by more than just $GABA_A$ binding. In fact, at lower doses, the anticonvulsant effects of barbiturates are primarily mediated via GABA binding, whereas higher doses cause cell hyperpolarization via direct effects on chloride channels, independent of GABA receptor binding [4]. An additional mechanism includes inhibition of synaptic transmission via the excitatory neurotransmitter glutamate [4], an effect mediated via non-N-methyl-D-aspartate (NMDA) glutamate receptors [5] as well as high-voltage calcium channel inhibition [6]. Adverse cardiac effects appear to be mediated by inhibition of nicotinic acetylcholine receptors [7] and/or potassium and calcium channel effects [8, 9]. In animal models with dysfunctional GABA receptors, respiratory depression with barbiturates persists, suggesting this is another GABA-independent effect [10].

Barbiturates are probably most easily classified according to their duration of activity. Methohexital is an ultrashort-acting barbiturate and has more applications in the procedural sedation environment than in critical care sedation. It may be administered either intravenously (IV), intramuscularly (IM), or rectally. Pharmacokinetics when used for IV administration include a time to peak onset of about 1 minute and a dose-dependent duration of action of 4–8 minutes [11]. With IM use, onset is also rapid (3–5 minutes) with a duration of action of 45–60 minutes [12]. Onset of action with rectal administration is slightly slower [5–15] minutes but duration slightly less (25–45 min) compared to IM administration [13]. With several different routes of administration, it must be remembered that substantial route-based bioavailability exists resulting in a need to utilize route-specific dosing. Standard IV dosing is 1–2 mg/kg induction with the option of following this with an infusion of 4–6 mg/kg/hr [14]. In comparison, IM dosing is three- to fivefold greater at 6–10 mg/kg [12], whereas effective rectal use requires doses of 20–25 mg/kg with rectal use [15, 16]. Metabolism is primarily hepatic via cytochrome p450-mediated oxidation and demethylation with an elimination half-life of 3.4–4 hrs [17].

Sodium thiopental is a short-acting barbiturate which, while primarily used for anesthesia applications, continues to have a role in the critically ill, albeit relatively limited. Unlike methohexital, applications are almost exclusively IV, following which onset of anesthesia occurs within 1–2 minutes, while clinical effects last up to 30 minutes [18]. Dosing is age-dependent with infants requiring higher induction doses (5–8 mg/kg) compared to older children and adolescents (3–4 mg/kg) [19, 20]. Metabolism is via hydroxylation and oxidation within the liver, but, due to a prolonged elimination $t_{1/2}$ of up to 12 hours [21], drug accumulation can be significant and lead to a prolonged duration of clinical effect.

Pentobarbital is a medium-acting barbiturate and the most commonly used agent for PICU applications. While primarily used as an IV agent, oral and rectal use have also been described. Following IV administration, onset of sedative action is 1–5 minutes, with a peak effect at 10 minutes and duration of 45–60 min [22]. Onset of sedation following oral or rectal administration is slower at 15–30 min with a clinical duration of effect ranging from 60 to 240 min [22]. IV dosing typically starts at 1–2 mg/kg although higher doses may be utilized for specific applications (see below). As bioavailability is high following both oral and rectal administration, smaller dosing adjustments are required compared to methohexital. Age-related differences also exist with younger children requiring higher doses (3–6 mg/kg) vs older children (2–4 mg/kg). Pentobarbital undergoes hepatic metabolism via cytochrome p450-induced hydroxylation and glucuronidation. Bolus dosing of pentobarbital exhibits usual first-order elimination kinetics with an elimination $t_{1/2}$ of 12–24 hours [23]. However, following infusions of longer than 12–24-hour duration, a transition to less predictable zero-order kinetics may occur [24] due to translipid distribution and drug accumulation causing the elimination $t_{1/2}$ to be increased to as long as several days [25].

Phenobarbital is a long-acting barbiturate and can be administered via the IV or oral/enteral routes. Onset of action following IV administration is within 5 minutes, peak response is seen at 15 minutes, and duration of action is greater than 6 hours. Onset is slower with enteral administration, taking roughly 30 minutes, and clinical effects last 1–2 hours but may be as long as 6–12 hours [26]. The typical IV loading dose of phenobarbital in the setting of seizures is 20 mg/kg, while dosing for sedation is less clear as this is not a typical application. Enterally, phenobarbital is typically dosed at 3–6 mg/kg/day although adjustments to maintain either therapeutic anticonvulsant effect or sedative effect may require higher doses. All barbiturates exhibit a relatively high degree of protein binding in the plasma (35–70%), which may lead to increased free drug levels in settings of hypoalbuminemia due to either renal or hepatic disease [21, 26]. Phenobarbital is primarily metabolized by oxidation via CYP2C9 and to a lesser extent via CYP2C19 and CYP2E1. It is also a strong inducer of other hepatic drug-metabolizing enzymes, particularly CYP3A4, leading to the potential for multiple drug-drug interactions [26]. Elimination half-life is long ranging from 70 to 80 hours in adults and up to 110 hours in children [26].

Clinical Applications

Barbiturates have multiple potential applications for the pediatric intensivist, both within and outside of the critical care environment. Outside of the PICU, barbiturates are primarily used either as a sole or adjunct agent during procedural sedation, especially for radiology procedures [22]. This topic will be described in depth in another chapter of this book. Within the PICU, barbiturates have three main applications. They are potent anticonvulsants, with benefits especially in the setting of status and refractory status epilepticus. They continue to play a significant role in the management of severe intracranial hypertension following brain injury. While less well studied, they may also be useful as adjuncts for sedation of the difficult to sedate PICU patient.

Barbiturates have a long history of use for treating pediatric seizures. Due to their pharmacokinetic properties and relatively slower onset of action, barbiturates should not be considered first-line therapy for status epilepticus although they remain an effective adjunct to standard first-line therapy with benzodiazepines. As discussed above, the anticonvulsant activity of barbiturates is primarily mediated via $GABA_A$ agonism. It is significant to remember that these effects differ from the mechanism of GABA-mediated anticonvulsant effects seen with benzodiazepine use [1]. This subtle difference in pharmacology likely contributes to the potential effectiveness and even possible synergism of the two classes of drugs. This difference also probably explains the effectiveness of barbiturates for seizures otherwise refractory to benzodiazepines [27].

Despite the availability of multiple newer anticonvulsants, barbiturates, especially phenobarbital, continue to be listed as early line agents for the management of status epilepticus [28] and have been found to be as effective as other common second-line therapies including levetiracetam, phenytoin, and valproic acid. However, compared to these other agents, phenobarbital is associated with an increased incidence of adverse events including respiratory depression, prolonged sedation, and hypotension [29]. Phenobarbital continues to remain, in some authors' opinion, the agent of choice for neonatal status epilepticus [30, 31].

Relatively more evidence exists discussing the use of barbiturates for refractory status epilepticus (RSE), but pediatric data is limited to the use of phenobarbital or pentobarbital. Definitions of refractory status epilepticus still vary but generally include either status epilepticus persisting despite administration of at least two different anticonvulsant medications or status lasting longer than 1–2 hours [32–34]. Most protocols utilize intravenous pentobarbital, presumably due to its shorter duration of action and more rapid wakening following control of seizure action. A recent systematic review compared midazolam to various "anesthetic" therapies for the management of RSE [35]. While the majority of studies focused on the use of midazolam, 4 studies incorporating 95 patients utilized pentobarbital, often following failure of midazolam infusions. While most protocols utilize pentobarbital to induce a burst suppression pattern on electroencephalogram (EEG), titration to seizure control before achieving burst suppression has also been reported. In this review, seizure control was achieved in 67% of patients with a median time to seizure control of 24–48 hours. Other studies have reported up to a 90% efficacy rate [36]. However, in most available studies, pentobarbital was not initiated until RSE had persisted for >24 hours, and duration of seizure activity has been described as a contributing factor to failure of higher tier anticonvulsants [37]. In the above review, most patients received a mean pentobarbital loading dose of 5–6 mg/kg with subsequent boluses of 3–5 mg/kg as needed to achieve seizure control and/or burst suppression. While burst suppression is often able to be maintained with infusions of 1 mg/kg/hr [38], breakthrough seizures may still occur. The mean effective infusion rates required to maintain seizure control are 4–5 mg/kg/hr although rates of up to 15 mg/kg/hr were reported [35]. The average time to achieve seizure control was 24 hours, whereas maintenance of seizure control required a mean infusion duration of 6–8 days (range 1–27 days, Ref. 35).

When administering pentobarbital for RSE, it should be done, if possible, with continuous EEG monitoring in place. This both aids in appropriately identifying when a burst suppression pattern has been achieved as well as if clinical and/or electrographic seizure activity has ceased. This latter point is especially important since subclinical seizure activity has been found to be increasingly common despite the absence of clinical seizure activity in patients presenting in status epilepticus [39, 40]. Due to its pharmacokinetic properties, pentobarbital use for RSE should include a loading dose with or without a subsequent infusion. Unless significant hemodynamic instability is already present, a loading dose of 5 mg/kg with subsequent boluses of 2–3 mg/kg every 15–30 minutes is appropriate. Doses should be decreased in the setting of ongoing hypotension. Infusions should be initiated at 1–2 mg/kg/hr and titrated in 0.5–1 mg/kg/hr increments, with or without additional bolus doses, to clinical or electroencephalographic effect. Respiratory depression to the point of requiring endotracheal intubation and mechanical ventilation should be anticipated, as should the need for vasoactive agents [35].

While phenobarbital has more potent anticonvulsant properties than pentobarbital [35], its use for pediatric RSE appears to be less widespread than pentobarbital. The most likely reason for this is the long elimination half-life of phenobarbital and associated lengthier time to arousal upon cessation compared to pentobarbital. Despite this, phenobarbital remains a component of many status epilepticus algorithms, including for RSE. Crawford described a 100% success rate for control of RSE in 50 children at median phenobarbital levels 3–4 times above normal "therapeutic" levels, as well as the ability to successfully extubate many patients while phenobarbital levels were still significantly elevated [41]. A more recent report described high-dose phenobarbital use in 13 children but only after failure of at least 2 second-tier agents and attempted midazolam coma [42]. A loading dose of 10 mg/kg was used followed by an infusion of 1 mg/kg/hr which could be increased by 0.5 mg/kg/hr every 6 hours to achieve either burst suppression or a >75% reduction in epileptiform discharges on continuous EEG. Seizure control was achieved in all patients after a mean duration of 72 hours of infusion. Most patients required an infusion of >3 mg/kg/hr to achieve EEG goals. No data exist describing earlier use of high-dose phenobarbital in the RSE algorithm. However, if used earlier, it would seem prudent to use more aggressive bolus dosing including additional bolus doses at the time of infusion increases.

Barbiturates, particularly pentobarbital, have been long believed to be valuable in the management of refractory intracranial hypertension and remain a component of several intracranial hypertension management algorithms [43–45] and have, indeed, been shown to decrease intracranial pressure following traumatic brain injury [46]. The basis for this is believed to lie in a barbiturate-induced reduction in cerebral metabolic rate for oxygen which, in areas of the brain with intact autoregulatory control, leads to a reduction in cerebral blood flow, intracranial volume, and, therefore, intracranial pressure [47, 48]. Subsequent pediatric data have confirmed reduction in middle cerebral blood flow velocity in addition to significant reductions in intracranial pressure (ICP) following thiopental administration [49]. However, the reductions in both parameters did not correlate with each other, suggesting that the decreases in intracranial pressure are not solely a consequence of cerebral blood flow reductions. Pentobarbital penetrates the central nervous system rapidly and affects a relatively quick reduction in ICP without an associated reduction in cerebral perfusion pressure [50], which is believed to be important in the injured parts of the brain where autoregulatory mechanisms may be dysfunctional and cerebral blood flow is more dependent on perfusion pressure than metabolic demands. A number of studies have evaluated the impact of pentobarbital bolus plus infusion on ICP following traumatic brain injury. Use of pentobarbital was associated with normalization of ICP in 30% of 36 children with refractory intracranial hypertension although the proportion of patients with a reduction in ICP, even if not achieving normalization, was not reported [51]. In 21 severely brain-injured children with refractory intracranial hypertension, thiopental use was also associated with significant reductions in ICP although the mean overall decrease in ICP and percent of patients achieving normal ICP were not reported [52]. In 16 patients receiving 55 bolus doses of pentobarbital, the maximum decrease in ICP was 7 mmHg (30% reduction) at 120 minutes following bolus administration. Reduction in ICP was seen to start within 15 minutes of bolus initiation. However, no data regarding the impact of pentobarbital use on ICP beyond the 120-minute mark were provided. No barbiturate infusions were utilized [53]. When EEG monitoring was used, it was found that a majority of patients undergoing barbiturate therapy achieved a burst suppression pattern [51, 52]. No studies to date have been either designed for or adequately powered to assess for the impact of barbiturate therapy on survival or functional outcomes in survivors. Consequently, in the latest iteration of the Society of Critical Care Medicine's guidelines for the management of traumatic brain injury, pentobarbital received only a level III (low-grade) suggestion as an adjunct therapy for refractory intracranial hypertension in otherwise hemodynamically stable patients [54].

Dosing of barbiturates is similar to that described above for use during status epilepticus. Both pentobarbital and thiopental should be initiated via bolus dose with or without a subsequent infusion. A reasonable pentobarbital loading dose is 3–5 mg/kg in hemodynamically stable patients with lower doses if blood pressure is low or labile. Subsequent infusions should start at 1–2 mg/kg/hr and be titrated to either a burst suppression pattern on continuous EEG (if available) or ICP less than 20 mmHg. Average reported pentobarbital infusion rates to achieve these endpoints are in the 5–6 mg/kg/hr range [51]. Thiopental dosing is similar. Initial bolus dosing ranges from 3 to 5 mg/kg with infusion rates of 2–3 mg/kg/hr titrated, again, to EEG and/or ICP goals. When utilized, infusions should be maintained at the lowest possible dose required to maintain these. Once cerebral edema and/or ICP start to decrease, usually 4–5 days following injury, infusions should be weaned slowly to avoid redevelopment of intracranial hypertension or withdrawal syndromes. As with use during status epilepticus, the most common adverse event that might require additional intervention is hypotension requiring initiation or increased dosing of vasoactive medications.

While they are potent sedatives, the long duration of action makes barbiturate infusions difficult to titrate to acutely changing sedation needs in the critically ill child. Coupled with the more frequent occurrence of hypotension during infusion use compared to other agents, barbiturates tend to be reserved for the "difficult to sedate" patient in whom more conventional agents are either inadequate or have been escalated to doses where adverse effects outweigh the desired clinical goals. Few data, however, exist describing barbiturate use for PICU sedation. In a retrospective analysis of six PICU patients failing high-dose fentanyl (7–13 mcg/kg/hr) and/or midazolam (0.2–0.4 mg/kg/hr), addition of a pentobarbital infusion (1–4 mg/

kg/hr) facilitated adequate sedation as well as the ability to wean off the other agents. In four patients who required a neuromuscular blocking agent, paralysis was able to be discontinued after initiation of pentobarbital. In two patients receiving ECMO therapy, antihypertensive agents were weaned off following pentobarbital initiation. Infusions were continued for a range of 4–64 days [55]. A second series described pentobarbital infusion in eight PICU patients refractory to morphine (0.046 ± 0.03 mg/kg/hr) and lorazepam (0.054 ± 0.025 mg/kg/hr) infusions [56]. Pentobarbital was initiated using a mean loading dose of 2.1 mg/kg with infusions ranging from 1 to 4 mg/kg/hr. Mean infusion duration was just almost 11 days. In all patients, other sedatives were either reduced or discontinued and all neuromuscular blocking agents were discontinued.

It is important to note that, for ICU sedation, barbiturate doses are lower than during use for RSE or intracranial hypertension. Bolus doses of 1–2 mg/kg are often adequate to calm an agitated patient and may be added as an adjunct without subsequent infusion. When needed, infusions of 1–2 mg/kg/hr are often adequate as sedation to the point of burst suppression is not typically required. Enteral pentobarbital (4–6 mg/kg) may be alternatively utilized on a scheduled or "as needed" basis.

Regardless of the reason for initiation, adverse effects with barbiturate use are not uncommon. Hypotension occurs relatively frequently and may require volume administration and/or vasoactive agent initiation. This likely reflects the fact that mechanisms underlying hypotension development with barbiturates involve both vasodilation and negative inotropy [57, 58], whereas most other sedative/analgesic agents do so almost solely through vasodilation. Barbiturate use may lead to prolonged sedation, especially if longer-term infusions are used, due to drug accumulation and conversion from first-order to zero-order elimination kinetics. Tolerance and iatrogenic withdrawal have also been described with barbiturate use although concomitant benzodiazepine and/or opioid use makes description of a "typical" symptom constellation difficult. However, this possibility suggests that slow weaning form infusions should be practiced.

Barbiturates continue to play a key role in the management of critically ill pediatric patients, specifically as regards the management of refractory status epilepticus, intracranial hypertension, and provision of sedation when first- and/or second-line therapies have failed. While established, the paucity of high-quality evidence supporting these applications should prompt the performance of further studies to illicit their most appropriate place in therapy, particularly given the relatively high risk of associated, potentially significant, adverse events.

References

1. Loscher W, Rogawski MA. How theories evolved concerning the mechanism of action of barbiturates. Epilepsia. 2012;53:12–25.
2. Leeb-Lundberg F, Snowman A, Olsen RW. Barbiturate receptor sites are coupled to benzodiazepine receptors. Proc Natl Acad Sci U S A. 1980;77:7468–72.
3. Macdonald RL, Barker JL. Different actions of anticonvulsant and anesthetic barbiturates revealed by use of cultured mammalian neurons. Science. 1978;200:775–7.

4. Mathers DA, Barker JL. Pentobarbital opens ion channels of long duration in cultured mouse spinal neurons. Science. 1980;209:507–9.
5. Frandsen A, Quistorff B, Schousboe A. Phenobarbital protects cerebral cortex neurones against toxicity induced by kainate but not by other excitatory amino acids. Neurosci Lett. 1990;111:233–8.
6. ffrench-Mullen JM, Barker JL, Rogawski MA. Calcium current block by (−)-pentobarbital, phenobarbital, and CHEB but not (+)-pentobarbital in acutely isolated hippocampal CA1 neurons: comparison with effects on GABA-activated Cl- current. J Neurosci. 1993;13:3211–21.
7. Tonner PH, Miller KW. Molecular sites of general anaesthetic action on acetylcholine receptors. Eur J Anaesthesiol. 1995;12:21–30.
8. Gilat E, Rubinstein I, Binah O. Effect of sodium pentobarbital on the transmembrane action potential and the slow inward current of guinea pig ventricular myocytes. J Cardiovasc Pharmacol. 1987;10:485–8.
9. Bachmann A, Mueller S, Kopp K, Brueggemann A, Suessbrich H, Gerlach U, Busch AE. Inhibition of cardiac potassium currents by pentobarbital. Naunyn Schmiedeberg's Arch Pharmacol. 2002;365:29–37.
10. Zeller A, Arras M, Jurd R, Rudolph U. Identification of a molecular target mediating the general anesthetic actions of pentobarbital. Mol Pharmacol. 2007;71:852–9.
11. O'Leary J. A clinical investigation of methohexital sodium. Med J Aust. 1962;1:594–5.
12. Varner PD, Ebert JP, McKay RD, et al. Methohexital sedation of children undergoing CT scan. Anesth Analg. 1985;64:643–645.
13. Quaynor H, Corbey M, Bjorkman S. Rectal induction of anaesthesia in children with methohexitone. Br J Anaesth. 1985;57:573–7.
14. Jones NE, Kelleman MS, Simon HK, Stockwell JA, McCracken C, Mallory MD, Kamat PP. Evaluation of methohexital as an alternative to propofol in a high volume outpatient pediatric sedation service. Am J Emerg Med. 2017;35:1101–5.
15. Manuli MA, Davies L. Rectal methohexital for sedation of children during imaging procedures. Am J Roentgenol. 1993;160:577–80.
16. Pomeranz ES, Chudnofsky CR, Deegan TJ, Lozon MM, Mitchiner JC, Weber JE. Rectal methohexital sedation for computed tomography imaging of stable pediatric emergency department patients. Pediatrics. 2000;105:1110–4.
17. Hudson RJ, Stanski DR, Burch PG. Pharmacokinetics of methohexital and thiopental in surgical patients. Anesthesiology. 1983;59:215–9.
18. Wada DR, Bjorkman S, Ebling WF, et al. Computer simulation of the effects of alterations in blood flows and body composition on thiopental pharmacokinetics in humans. Anesthesiology. 1997;87:884–99.
19. Westrin P, Jonmarker C, Werner O. Thiopental requirements for induction of anesthesia in neonates and in infants one to six months of age. Anesthesiology. 1989;71:344–6.
20. Jonmarker C, Westrin P, Larsson S, et al. Thiopental requirements for induction of anesthesia in children. Anesthesiology. 1987;67:104–7.
21. Russo H, Bressolle F. Pharmacodynamics and pharmacokinetics or thiopental. Clin Pharmacokinet. 1998;35:95–134.
22. Krauss B, Green SM. Procedural sedation and analgesia in children. Lancet. 2006;367(9512):766–80.
23. Bayliff CD, Schwartz ML, Hardy BG. Pharmacokinetics of high dose pentobarbital in severe head trauma. Clin Pharmacol Ther. 1985;38:457–61.
24. Owens J. Medical management of refractory status epilepticus. Semin Pediatr Neurol. 2010;17:176–81.
25. Wermeling DP, Blouin RA, Porter WH, et al. Pentobarbital pharmacokinetics in patients with severe head injury. Drug Intell Clin Pharm. 1987;21:459–63.
26. Patsalos PN, Berry DJ, Bourgeois BFD, Cloyd JC, Glauser TA, Johannessen SI, Tomson T, Perucca E. Antiepileptic drugs – best practice guidelines for therapeutic drug monitoring: a position paper by the subcommission on therapeutic drug monitoring, ILAE Commission on Therapeutic Strategies. Epilepsia. 2008;49(7):1239–76.

27. Pittman T, Bucholz R, Williams D. Efficacy of barbiturates in the treatment of resistant intracranial hypertension in severely head-injured children. Pediatr Neurosci. 1988;14:241–9.
28. Verrotti A, Ambrosia A, Pavone P, Striano P. Pediatric status epilepticus: improved management with new drug therapies? Exp Opin Pharmacother. 2017;18:7809–798.
29. Yasiry Z, Shorvon SD. The relative effectiveness of five antiepileptic drugs in treatment of benzodiazepine-resistant convulsive status epilepticus: a meta-analysis of published studies. Seizure. 2014;23:167–74.
30. Painter MJ, Scher MS, Stein AD, Armatti S, Wang Z, Gardiner JC, Paneth N, Minnigh B, Alvin J. Phenobarbital compared with phenytoin for the treatment of neonatal seizures. N Engl J Med. 1999;341:485–9.
31. Spagnoli C, Seri S, Pavlidis E, Mazzotta S, Pelosi A, Pisani F. Phenobarbital for neonatal seizures: response rate and predictors of refractoriness. Neuropediatrics. 2016;47:318–26.
32. Bleck TP. Refractory status epilepticus. Curr Opin Crit Care. 2005;11:117–20.
33. Meierkord H, Boon P, Engelsen B, et al. EFNS guideline on the management of status epilepticus. Eur J Neurol. 2006;13:445–50.
34. Abend NS, Dlugos DJ. Treatment of refractory status epilepticus: literature review and a proposed protocol. Pediatr Neurol. 2008;38:377–90.
35. Wilkes R, Tasker RC. Treatment of uncontrolled status epilepticus. Crit Care Clin. 2013;29:239–57.
36. Tasker RC, Goodkin HP, Fernandez IS, et al. Refractory status epilepticus in children: intention-to-treat with continuous infusions of midazolam and pentobarbital. *Pediatr Crit Care Med*. 2016;17(10):968-975Wilkes R, Tasker RC. Intensive care treatment of uncontrolled status epilepticus in children: systematic literature search of midazolam and anesthetic therapies. Pediatr Crit Care Med. 2014;15:632–9.
37. DeLorenzo RJ, Garnett LK, Towne AR, Waterhouse EJ, Boggs JG, Morton L, Choudhry MA, Barnes T, Ko D. Comparison of status epilepticus with prolonged seizure episodes lasting from 10 to 29 minutes. Epilepsia. 1999;40:164–9.
38. Barberio M, Reiter PD, Kaufman J, et al. Continuous infusion pentobarbital for refractory status epilepticus in children. J Child Neurol. 2012;27:721–6.
39. Abend NS, Gutierrez-Colina AM, Topjian AA, et al. Nonconvulsive seizures are common in critically ill children. Neurology. 2011;76:1071–7.
40. Arndt DH, Lerner JT, Matsumoto JH, et al. Subclinical early posttraumatic seizures detected by continuous EEG monitoring in a consecutive pediatric cohort. Epilepsia. 2013;54:1780–8.
41. Crawford TO, Mitchell WG, Fishman LS, Snodgrass SR. Very-high-dose phenobarbital for refractory status epilepticus in children. Neurology. 1988;38:1035–40.
42. Gulati S, Sondhi V, Chakrabarty B, Jauhari P, Lodha R, Sankar J. High dose phenobarbitone coma in pediatric refractory status epilepticus; a retrospective case record analysis, a proposed protocol and review of literature. Brain Dev. 2018;40:316–24.
43. Eisenberg HM, Frankowski RF, Contant CF, et al. High-dose barbiturate control of elevated intracranial pressure in patients with severe head injury. J Neurosurg. 1988;69:15–23.
44. Adelson PD, Bratton SL, Carney NA, et al. Guidelines for the acute medical management of severe traumatic brain injury in infants, children, and adolescents. Chapter 17. Critical pathway for the treatment of established intracranial hypertension in pediatric traumatic brain injury. Pediatr Crit Care Med. 2003;4(3 Suppl):S65–7.
45. Hutchison JS, Ward RE, Lacroix J, et al. Hypothermia pediatric head injury trial investigators and the Canadian critical care trials group: hypothermia therapy after traumatic brain injury in children. N Engl J Med. 2008;358:2447–56.
46. Miller JD. Barbiturates and raised intracranial pressure. Ann Neurol. 1979;6:189–93.
47. Kassel NF, Hitchon PW, Gerk MK, Sokoll MD, Hill TR. Alterations in cerebral blood flow oxygen metabolism and electrical activity produced by high dose thiopental. Neurosurgery. 1980;7:598–603.
48. Nordstrom CK, Messeter K, Sunbarg S, Schalen W, Werner M, Ryding E. Cerebral blood flow, vaso-reactivity and oxygen consumption during barbiturate therapy in severe traumatic brain lesions. J Neurosurg. 1988;68:424–35.

49. de Bray JM, Granry JC, Monrigal JP, Leftheriotis G, Saumet JL. Effects of thiopental on middle cerebral artery blood velocities: a transcranial Doppler study in children. Childs Nerv Syst. 1993;9:220–3.
50. Cormio M, Gopinath SP, Valadka A, Robertson CS. Cerebral hemodynamic effects of pentobarbital coma in head-injured patients. J Neuro-Oncol. 1999;16(10):927.
51. Mellion SA, Bennett KS, Ellsworth GL, Moore K, Riva-Cambrin J, Metzger RR, Bratton SL. High-dose barbiturates for refractory intracranial hypertension in children with severe traumatic brain injury. Pediatr Crit Care Med. 2013;14:239–47.
52. Velle F, Lewen A, Howells T, Enblad P, Nillson P. Intracranial pressure-based barbiturate coma treatment in children with refractory intracranial hypertension due to traumatic brain injury. J Neurosurg Pediatr. 2019:1–9. https://doi.org/10.3171/2019.10.PEDS19268. [Epub ahead of print].
53. Schein SL, Ferguson NM, Kochanek PM, Bayir H, Clark RSB, Fink EL, Tyler-Kabara EC, Wisniewski SR, Tian Y, Babasbramani GK, Bell MJ. Effectiveness of pharmacological therapies for intracranial hypertension in children with severe traumatic brain injury – results from an automated data collection system time-synched to drug administration. Pediatr Crit Care Med. 2016;17:236–45.
54. Kochanek PM, Tasker R, Carney N, Totten AM, Adelson PD, Selden NR, Davis-O'Reilly C, Hart EL, Bell MJ, Bratton SL, Grant GA, Kissoon N, Reuter-Rice KE, Vavilala MS, Wainwright MS. Guidelines for the management of pediatric severe traumatic brain injury, third edition: update of the brain trauma foundation guidelines. Pediatr Crit Care Med. 2019;20:S1–S82.
55. Tobias J, Deshpande J, Pietsch J, et al. Pentobarbital sedation for patients in the pediatric intensive care unit. South Med J. 1995;88:290–4.
56. Yanay O, Brogan T, Martin L. Continuous pentobarbital infusion in children is associated with high rates of complications. J Crit Care. 2004;19:174–8.
57. Audenaert SM, Lock RL, Johnson GL, Pedigo NW Jr. Cardiovascular effects of rectal methohexital in children. J Clin Anesth. 1992;4(2):116–9.
58. Doshi AR, Malhotro MG, Balaguru D, mare D, Erikson C. Effect of intravenous phenobarbital on left ventricular myocardial contractility determined by echocardiography in children. Kans J Med. 2019;12:40–4.

Part III
Anesthetic Agents

Chapter 8
Sedation and Analgesia for the Critically Ill Child: Ketamine

Judith J. M. Wong, Angela S. H. Yeo, Siti N. H. Buang, and Yoke Hwee Chan

Introduction

Ketamine has been used as an anesthetic for decades, but its use has diversified and gained in popularity for indications in the pediatric intensive care unit (PICU) such as intensive care sedation, procedural sedation, acute and chronic pain, prevention and management of opioid withdrawal, bronchoconstriction, and seizure disorders [1]. The popularity of ketamine is due to its ability to provide analgesia, but with less respiratory depression, making it ideal for non-intubated patients undergoing painful procedures or as an analgesic to reduce postoperative pain. It is considered a dissociative agent and is closely related to phencyclidine (PCP).

Pharmacokinetics and Pharmacodynamics

Ketamine is a racemic mixture consisting of two optical enantiomers, R(−) and S(+). It is frequently administered via the intravenous (IV) or intramuscular (IM) route, which has the highest bioavailability (93%) as compared to other routes of administration such as oral (16–29%), sublingual (29%), intranasal (45–50%), rectal (25%), and epidural [2–5]. The highly lipid-soluble ketamine has a

J. J. M. Wong · S. N. H. Buang · Y. H. Chan (✉)
Department of Paediatric Subspecialties, Children's Intensive Care Unit, KK Women's and Children's Hospital, Singapore, Singapore
e-mail: Judith.Wong.JM@singhealth.com.sg; Siti.Nur.Hanim@singhealth.com.sg; Chan.Yoke.Hwee@singhealth.com.sg

A. S. H. Yeo
Department of Pediatric Anaesthesia, KK Women's and Children's Hospital, Singapore, Singapore
e-mail: Angela.Yeo.S.H@singhealth.com.sg

P. P. Kamat, J. W. Berkenbosch (eds.), *Sedation and Analgesia for the Pediatric Intensivist*, https://doi.org/10.1007/978-3-030-52555-2_8

two-compartment pharmacokinetic profile with an alpha half-life of approximately 10–16 mins and a beta half-life of 2.5–4.9 hours [2, 5–7]. Ketamine is rapidly distributed into highly perfused tissues, including the brain, and has plasma protein binding of 10–50% [7, 8]. Metabolism of ketamine occurs via demethylation by the cytochrome P450 liver enzymes – CYP2B6, CYP2C9, and CYP3A4 to predominantly biologically active norketamine and further metabolized to biologically inactive dehydronorketamine (DHNK) and hydroxynorketamine (HNK) [1, 9]. Elimination of ketamine is primarily performed by the kidneys, with low levels excreted as ketamine (2%), norketamine (2%), and DHNK (16%). Clearance is highly dependent on the liver blood flow and occurs in 2–5 hours in adults and half that time in children [1, 6, 7].

Mechanism of Action

There is a myriad of pathways by which ketamine exerts its anesthetic and analgesic effects. N-Methyl-d-aspartate receptor (NMDAR) antagonism is the predominant mechanism of action. Ketamine acts in a dose-dependent manner on the NMDAR channel, a tetrameric protein complex that forms a ligand-gated calcium ion channel. It blocks the closed NMDA channel at lower concentrations, giving rise to its analgesic properties. At higher concentrations, both open and closed channels are blocked, resulting in its dissociative, anesthetic, and amnesic properties becoming more evident [10]. Its two different mechanisms at the same receptor are the blocking of the open channels, resulting in reduction of mean open time, and the blocking of the closed channels through binding to the allosteric PCP site located within the pore, resulting in a decrease in the frequency of channel opening [11]. These receptors are highly permeable to calcium ions, which trigger the activation of intracellular pathways in neurons and glial cells. At resting state, NMDAR channels are tonically blocked by magnesium (Mg2+) and membrane depolarization is required to displace Mg2+. NMDAR binding is dependent on the differential capacity for Mg2+ binding and interactions between the drug and Mg2+ within the channel.

While NMDAR antagonism is the main mechanism for ketamine's analgesic property, other putative mechanisms through cholinergic, opioid, and serotoninergic receptors may also play a role and could explain its effect in nonneuropathic pain [12]. Binding to dopaminergic and serotoninergic receptors has also been described. Ketamine at clinically relevant doses acts as a noncompetitive antagonist of the nicotinic acetylcholine receptors [1]. Administration of ketamine also induces an increase in extracellular serotonin (5-HT) levels in the prefrontal cortex and dorsal raphe nucleus of mice and is thought to mediate its analgesic effect. Possibly contributing also to its analgesic effects is ketamine's ability to bind opioid receptors. It is likely that ketamine is an agonist to the κ opioid receptors and antagonist to the μ receptors as naloxone does not reverse its analgesic effect [13]. Interactions between ketamine and the opioid system may be more relevant in prolonged opioid use, in which ketamine reduces opioid tolerance. Ketamine's actions on δ receptors could be involved in the neuroplasticity-related effects of the drug [14, 15]. Lastly, ketamine also interacts with the hyperpolarization-activated cyclic nucleotide-gated (HCN) channels [1]. These voltage-gated cation channels are activated by membrane hyperpolarization facilitated by cyclic nucleotides, including cyclic adenosine monophosphate (cAMP), and binding mediates ketamine's anesthetic effects.

Animal studies indicate that at supratherapeutic doses, ketamine may potentiate inhibitory GABAergic postsynaptic signals in neurons [16]. This was not shown to occur at clinically relevant doses. Instead, clinically relevant concentrations of ketamine increased the activity of high-affinity extrasynaptic $GABA_A$ receptors in the hippocampus and cortex, an effect that likely contributes to ketamine's neurodepressive properties [16].

Dosing

Ketamine has a wide therapeutic index and the optimal dosage depends on the intended therapeutic effect. Ketamine has been reported to effect analgesia at plasma concentrations of 100–200 ng/ml, arousal from anesthesia at 750 ng/ml, arousal from tactile or loud verbal stimulus at 1000 ng/ml, and arousal from painful stimulus at 1500 ng/ml [2, 17]. In a population pharmacokinetics study of IM and IV ketamine in children, the recommended procedural sedation dose for IV ketamine was 2 mg/kg, and IM ketamine was 8 mg/kg (for children between 6 and 11 kg) and 6 mg/kg (for children 17–56 kg) to provide adequate sedation for up to 20 minutes [5]. The US Food and Drug Administration (FDA) prescribing information lists the anesthetic induction dose of ketamine as 1–4.5 mg/kg IV with an average dose of 2 mg/kg required for surgical anesthetic effect of 5 to 10 minutes, or 4–11 mg/kg IM with an anesthetic effect that lasts 12 to 25 minutes [18].

Subanesthetic doses of 0.15–1.0 mg/kg IV (bolus) or 0.1–2.0 mg/kg/hour IV (continuous infusion) have also been used in the pediatric population as an adjunct for postoperative pain or for sedation/analgesia in the PICU. Unfortunately, subanesthetic dosing of ketamine is not consistently defined in the literature, with one review setting the cutoff at <1.2 mg/kg/h [19]. Recent consensus guidelines on the use of IV ketamine for pain management have recommended (Grade C) that in general, ketamine boluses should not exceed 0.35 mg/kg/dose and infusions for acute pain should not exceed 1 mg/kg/h without intensive monitoring and that provider discretion and training in airway management is advisable [20].

Uses of Ketamine in the Pediatric Intensive Care Unit

Ketamine's primary benefits in PICU sedation lie in its ability to induce a dissociative state while sparing respiratory depression, its analgesic properties through its multiple actions outside of the opioid receptor, and its utility in reducing opioid tolerance, central sensitization, and opioid hyperalgesia [21]. One of the driving forces behind the resurgence in ketamine use is the push to reduce chronic opioid exposure and risk of addiction, after acute exposure [22].

In the PICU setting, the IV route is most commonly employed, but the oral, transdermal, intranasal, subcutaneous, epidural, per rectal, and IM routes may still be considered [23]. For the purposes of this chapter, these will not be expounded upon, and the authors respectfully direct the reader to other articles [23, 24]. In the hospital, it is recognized that pain originates from several sources – medical pathology, procedural interventions, and surgery, particularly in the postoperative period. In the acute postoperative setting, the patients who benefit from ketamine infusions are those expected to have severe postoperative pain, those who are non-opioid naïve and thus possibly tolerant to opioid effects, and those at risk of opioid-induced ventilatory impairment (OIVI) [20].

Ketamine for Sedation

The safety profile of ketamine in hemodynamics and respiratory function has made it an attractive option for sedation in the critically ill patients. Ketamine has been used widely as a single or combination agent for procedural sedation in children in a variety of settings. This will be discussed in further detail in the chapter on Procedural Sedation: Ketamine.

Evidence with ketamine, as a continuous infusion in the PICU for sedation, has been limited to small series or case reports [25–27]. It is often used an adjunct to benzodiazepines and opioids or used to treat opioid withdrawal. Due to its bronchodilator effects, ketamine has been used at higher infusion rates for the treatment, or as a sedative agent, in children with bronchospasm and status asthmaticus in the PICU. Its use in brain injury has been debated due to its potential to cause cerebral vasodilatation and increase intracranial pressure [28, 29]. Subsequent studies in adults and children did not demonstrate ICP increase with ketamine in both traumatic and nontraumatic brain injuries and in some cases a reduction in ICP [30–32]. While the evidence is not strong for children given the small sample size of the pediatric population in these studies, its use for sedation and analgesia in children with traumatic brain injury is no longer an absolute contraindication.

Ketamine for Acute Pain

As an analgesic, ketamine is effective either as a stand-alone, particularly in procedural pain, or as an adjuvant. In the postoperative period, it is most commonly employed at subanesthetic dose as an adjunct to opioids in view of the expected acute nociceptive stimulus, for two important reasons – to reduce both postoperative pain intensity and opioid requirements. Benefits of combination therapy of ketamine with postoperative opioids in reducing pain scores and the requirement of opioids are more established in adults [20]. In a meta-analysis of adult studies on ketamine use in spine surgeries, bolus doses ranging from 0.15 to 10 mg/kg and infusion rates ranging from 0.06 to 5.0 mg/kg/h resulted in reduced postoperative pain scores and less morphine consumption 24 h postoperatively [33]. A longitudinal cohort of children and young adults with heterogeneous medical conditions showed that ketamine doses ranging from 0.05 to 1 mg/kg/h could achieve a significant reduction in pain scores with minimal adverse effects. However, the effect was more prominent in the group with cancer-related pain and inflammatory conditions. The opioid-sparing effect in postoperative pain, however, was minimal. In a meta-analysis of 47 adult and pediatric randomized controlled trials, ketamine was shown to have an opioid-sparing effect, both in the reduction of opioid administered and prolongation of time to first analgesic [34]. The greatest benefit in opioid reduction was seen in upper abdominal and thoracic surgeries, and to lesser extent with intra- and lower abdominal and limb and spine surgeries, but not for tonsillectomies and dental and head and neck surgeries [12, 13]. However, the pediatric subgroup analysis which was highly represented by tonsillectomy studies revealed a lack of benefit in children. Similarly, a recent meta-analysis of 11 pediatric studies did not demonstrate global opioid-sparing effect at 48 hours, nor did it reduce postoperative pain intensity [35]. However, this meta-analysis was limited by the lack of power to be conclusive about the primary outcome. Thus, it seems that despite the robust data in the adult population, there remain questions about ketamine's utility in the pediatric population for postoperative analgesia.

Apart from its use as a postoperative analgesic, ketamine as an adjunct also improves analgesia in circumstances not ascribable to surgery, such as cancer and inflammatory pain associated with pancreatitis and Crohn's disease, whereas patients with functional gastrointestinal disorders had the lowest benefit [36]. Adults and children with acute on chronic exacerbations of pain such as sickle cell disease, renal colic, or central pain from Ehler-Danlos syndrome have also been reported to have improved analgesia, but there have been no randomized controlled trials thus far [37–39].

Opioid-induced ventilatory impairment (OIVI) risk is increased in patients with obstructive sleep apnea and can be exacerbated by exposure to general anesthetics for surgery [40]. While subanesthetic ketamine has been shown to reduce opioid consumption postoperatively, there have been few studies that specifically address its utility in reducing the risk of opioid-induced respiratory depression (OIRD) or OIVI [34]. Healthy volunteers subjected to remifentanil-induced respiratory depression, in a randomized double-blind placebo-controlled crossover trial of esketamine vs placebo, demonstrated that esketamine effectively countered the OIRD [41]. In their statement on the principles for identifying and preventing OIVI, the Faculty of Pain Medicine of Australia and New Zealand had endorsed low-dose ketamine as a helpful adjuvant for opioid-sparing measure in patients who are sedated but still in pain [42].

Ketamine for Chronic Pain

The nonopioid-naïve population includes the children with painful chronic medical conditions, oncological or palliative cases, or children who have been on prolonged opioid infusions for sedation and analgesia. Current data on the short-term infusions suggest that potent analgesia is produced only during administration of ketamine, while prolonged infusions of 4–14 days may result in long-term effects of up to 3 months in patients with chronic pain with neuropathic components [20, 41]. In adults with complex regional pain syndrome, there is moderate evidence to support the use of ketamine infusions [43]. The evidence for ketamine use in children with chronic pain is scant. The use of intraoperative ketamine on a group opioid-dependent children undergoing orthopedic surgeries demonstrated a reduction in 48-hour opioid usage and lower pain intensity scores, suggesting at least a mild benefit for this population [44].

Ketamine has also been touted as an opioid tolerance-protective drug [45]. In experimental models, co-administration of ketamine and opioid attenuated the development of opioid tolerance to varying degrees [46]. Neunhoeffer described a retrospective study wherein 32 mechanically ventilated children with tolerance from prolonged IV infusion of opioids received ketamine infusions as an opioid substitute on a drug rotation protocol (median ketamine dose of 4 mg/kg/h and median duration of 3 days) [47]. This resulted in a significant reduction in subsequent fentanyl requirement, suggesting that ketamine has a role in reversing or reducing tolerance development [47].

The intensive care physician should be also aware of two oft-forgotten mechanisms which may contribute to abnormal pain hypersensitivity in the critically ill pediatric patient – central sensitization and opioid-induced hyperalgesia (OIH). In poorly controlled pain states, a prolonged but reversible increase in the excitability and synaptic efficacy of neurons in nociceptive pathways results in central sensitization through what is termed the "wind-up" phenomenon. In severe cases, chronification of the pain occurs with secondary changes in brain activity, and pain becomes pathologic, manifesting as pain hypersensitivity, either through allodynia or hyperalgesia [48]. This often results in pain which is refractory to the usual analgesia cocktails and thus rapid escalation of opioid use and, hence, tolerance. Prevention of central sensitization with low-dose ketamine infusions has been seen in basic science studies but has not always held true in clinical trials [48, 49]. In a systematic review of 17 studies, the overall risk of developing persistent postsurgical pain, a result of central sensitization, was not significantly reduced in the ketamine vs placebo group, but sensitivity analysis of exclusively IV ketamine studies did demonstrate statistically significant reductions in the risk of developing persistent postsurgical pain at 3 months and 6 months [50].

Contributing to the problem of pain hypersensitivity, a growing body of evidence suggests that opioids can elicit an exaggerated nociceptive response to noxious stimulation after continuous delivery, a common PICU postoperative sedation practice [51–53]. This is attributed to activation of μ opioid receptor resulting in a sustained increase in glutamate synaptic effectiveness at the level of the NMDAR with a resultant paradoxical hypersensitivity, OIH [54]. This translates to a need for an alternative or adjunctive analgesia since the use of opioids contributes to, rather than detracts, the pain. The evidence suggests that development of OIH can be attenuated by ketamine in subanalgesic doses, thus potentially reducing opioid consumption [51, 55].

Ketamine Side Effects

Short-term ketamine use causes dose-dependent, transient, and self-resolving side effects including a decrease in mental sharpness, concentration, recall, and recognition, as well as explicit (episodic and semantic) and implicit (procedural) forms of memory [1]. Psycho-cognitive effects such as hallucinations, dreams/nightmares, and visual disturbances are dose-related and minimal at infusion rates of less than 2.5 mcg/kg/min [19]. It can lead to vestibular perturbations, including dizziness and nausea/vomiting. Sympathetic effects include tachycardia, hypertension, and palpitations. Respiratory depression is usually mild at clinically relevant doses. Other side effects include ocular effects (e.g., nystagmus, diplopia, dilation) and musculoskeletal effects (e.g., myoclonus, twitching, spasms, ataxia, fasciculation) [1]. Of note in PICU care, ketamine causes an increase in secretions which presents another problem for the caregivers to manage.

More crucial, however, is the neurodevelopmental effects of ketamine. Indeed, multiple other sedative drug options produce similar neurotoxic effects in the pediatric brain, and the pediatric intensivist needs to carefully weigh the risks and benefits of each sedative [56]. In animal and basic science studies, long-term ketamine use has been demonstrated to have potential neurotoxic effects including reversible neuronal vacuolation, necrosis, and loss of integrity within the posterior cingulate, retrosplenial, prefrontal, and frontal-thalamic-temporal cortices [57–60]. Even low doses of ketamine were shown to impair dendritic arborization [61].

It is, however, argued that unattenuated pain may also induce cell death in cortical, thalamic, hypothalamic, and hippocampal areas of the neonatal rat brain and the amygdala, and this may be followed by subsequent neurocognitive impairment, such as an impaired cognitive, emotional, and psychosocial functioning and impaired ability to form memories [62, 63]. Conversely, concurrent surgery and procedural pain has been shown to attenuate ketamine-induced neuroapoptosis, and ketamine has also been shown to inhibit pain-induced neurotoxicity in neonatal rat brains [64]. Thus, it seems that pain, in the absence of analgesia, is detrimental to neurodevelopment, while analgesia in the presence of pain may be protective.

Conclusion

Ketamine remains a useful drug in the anesthetic/sedative/analgesic armamentarium. Its ability to provide sedation and analgesia, while preserving hemodynamics and without blunting the respiratory reflexes and drive, makes it highly suitable for facilitating painful procedures in non-intubated patients or in postoperative patients. Its optimal dose, duration, and role in a multimodal regimen for acute pain will require further elucidation. Given the neurotoxic concerns of repetitive ketamine exposure to the developing brain, it is not recommended for routine use in the absence of nociceptive stimulus which in itself is neurotoxic.

References

1. Zanos P, Moaddel R, Morris PJ, Riggs LM, Highland JN, Georgiou P, et al. Ketamine and ketamine metabolite pharmacology: insights into therapeutic mechanisms. Pharmacol Rev. 2018;70(3):621–60. PubMed PMID: 29945898. Pubmed Central PMCID: PMC6020109. Epub 2018/06/28. eng.
2. Clements JA, Nimmo WS, Grant IS. Bioavailability, pharmacokinetics, and analgesic activity of ketamine in humans. J Pharm Sci. 1982;71(5):539–42. PubMed PMID: 7097501. Epub 1982/05/01. eng.
3. Rolan P, Lim S, Sunderland V, Liu Y, Molnar V. The absolute bioavailability of racemic ketamine from a novel sublingual formulation. Br J Clin Pharmacol. 2014;77(6):1011–6. PubMed PMID: 24977293. Pubmed Central PMCID: PMC4093926. Epub 2014/07/01. eng.
4. Malinovsky JM, Servin F, Cozian A, Lepage JY, Pinaud M. Ketamine and norketamine plasma concentrations after i.v., nasal and rectal administration in children. Br J Anaesth. 1996;77(2):203–7. PubMed PMID: 8881626. Epub 1996/08/01. eng.
5. Hornik CP, Gonzalez D, van den Anker J, Atz AM, Yogev R, Poindexter BB, et al. Population pharmacokinetics of intramuscular and intravenous ketamine in children. J Clin Pharmacol. 2018. PubMed PMID: 29677389. Pubmed Central PMCID: PMC6195858. Epub 2018/04/21. eng.
6. Hijazi Y, Bodonian C, Bolon M, Salord F, Boulieu R. Pharmacokinetics and haemodynamics of ketamine in intensive care patients with brain or spinal cord injury. Br J Anaesth. 2003;90(2):155–60.
7. Mion G, Villevieille T. Ketamine pharmacology: an update (pharmacodynamics and molecular aspects, recent findings). CNS Neurosci Ther. 2013;19(6):370–80.
8. Dayton PG, Stiller RL, Cook DR, Perel JM. The binding of ketamine to plasma proteins: emphasis on human plasma. Eur J Clin Pharmacol. 1983;24(6):825–31. PubMed PMID: 6884418. Epub 1983/01/01. eng.
9. Hijazi Y, Boulieu R. Contribution of CYP3A4, CYP2B6, and CYP2C9 isoforms to<em>N-</em>demethylation of ketamine in human liver microsomes. Drug Metab Dispos. 2002;30(7):853–8.
10. Orser BA, Pennefather PS, MacDonald JF. Multiple mechanisms of ketamine blockade of N-methyl-D-aspartate receptors. Anesthesiology. 1997;86(4):903–17. PubMed PMID: 9105235. Epub 1997/04/01. eng.
11. Yamamura T, Harada K, Okamura A, Kemmotsu O. Is the site of action of ketamine anesthesia the N-methyl-D-aspartate receptor? Anesthesiology. 1990;72(4):704–10. PubMed PMID: 1969718. Epub 1990/04/01. eng.
12. Persson J. Ketamine in pain management. CNS Neurosci Ther. 2013;19(6):396–402. PubMed PMID: 23663314. Epub 2013/05/15. eng.
13. Hirota K, Okawa H, Appadu BL, Grandy DK, Devi LA, Lambert DG. Stereoselective interaction of ketamine with recombinant mu, kappa, and delta opioid receptors expressed in Chinese hamster ovary cells. Anesthesiology. 1999;90(1):174–82. PubMed PMID: 9915326. Epub 1999/01/23. eng
14. Bowen WD, Hellewell SB, McGarry KA. Evidence for a multi-site model of the rat brain sigma receptor. Eur J Pharmacol. 1989;163(2–3):309–18. PubMed PMID: 2542066. Epub 1989/04/25. eng.

15. Robson MJ, Elliott M, Seminerio MJ, Matsumoto RR. Evaluation of sigma (sigma) receptors in the antidepressant-like effects of ketamine in vitro and in vivo. Eur Neuropsychopharmacol J Eur Coll Neuropsychopharmacol. 2012;22(4):308–17. PubMed PMID: 21911285. Epub 2011/09/14. eng.
16. Wang D-S, Penna A, Orser BA. Ketamine increases the function of γ-Aminobutyric acid type a receptors in hippocampal and cortical neurons. Anesthesiology J Am Soc Anesthesiol. 2017;126(4):666–77.
17. Herd DW, Anderson BJ, Keene NA, Holford NH. Investigating the pharmacodynamics of ketamine in children. Paediatr Anaesth. 2008;18(1):36–42. PubMed PMID: 18095964. Epub 2007/12/22. eng
18. Administration. UFaD. Ketalar (ketamine hydrochloride) injection. [updated October 3, 2017.]. Available from: https://www.accessdata.fda.gov/drugsatfda_docs/label/2017/016812s043lbl.pdf.
19. Schmid RL, Sandler AN, Katz J. Use and efficacy of low-dose ketamine in the management of acute postoperative pain: a review of current techniques and outcomes. Pain. 1999;82(2):111–25. PubMed PMID: 10467917. Epub 1999/09/01. eng.
20. Schwenk ES, Viscusi ER, Buvanendran A, Hurley RW, Wasan AD, Narouze S, et al. Consensus guidelines on the use of intravenous ketamine infusions for acute pain management from the American Society of Regional Anesthesia and Pain Medicine, the American Academy of Pain Medicine, and the American Society of Anesthesiologists. Reg Anesth Pain Med. 2018;43(5):456–66. PubMed PMID: 29870457. Pubmed Central PMCID: PMC6023582. Epub 2018/06/06. eng.
21. Visser E, Schug SA. The role of ketamine in pain management. Biomed Pharmacother = Biomedicine & pharmacotherapy. 2006;60(7):341–8. PubMed PMID: 16854557. Epub 2006/07/21. eng.
22. Sun EC, Darnall BD, Baker LC, Mackey S. Incidence of and risk factors for chronic opioid use among opioid-naive patients in the postoperative period. JAMA Intern Med. 2016;176(9):1286–93. PubMed PMID: 27400458. Epub 2016/07/12. eng.
23. Vadivelu N, Schermer E, Kodumudi V, Belani K, Urman RD, Kaye AD. Role of ketamine for analgesia in adults and children. J Anaesthesiol Clin Pharmacol. 2016;32(3):298–306. PubMed PMID: 27625475. Pubmed Central PMCID: PMC5009833. Epub 2016/09/15. eng
24. Kronenberg RH. Ketamine as an analgesic. J Pain Palliat Care Pharmacother. 2002;16(3):27–35.
25. Tobias JD, Martin LD, Wetzel RC. Ketamine by continuous infusion for sedation in the pediatric intensive care unit. Crit Care Med. 1990;18(8):819–21. PubMed PMID: 2379394. Epub 1990/08/01. eng.
26. Hartvig P, Larsson E, Joachimsson PO. Postoperative analgesia and sedation following pediatric cardiac surgery using a constant infusion of ketamine. J Cardiothorac Vasc Anesth. 1993;7(2):148–53. PubMed PMID: 8477017. Epub 1993/04/01. eng.
27. Barbi E, Rizzello E, Taddio A. Use of ketamine continuous infusion for pediatric sedation in septic shock. Pediatr Emerg Care. 2010;26(9):689–90. PubMed PMID: 20838196. Epub 2010/09/15. eng.
28. List WF, Crumrine RS, Cascorbi HF, Weiss MH. Increased cerebrospinal fluid pressure after ketamine. Anesthesiology. 1972;36(1):98–9. PubMed PMID: 5006995. Epub 1972/01/01. eng.
29. Wyte SR, Shapiro HM, Turner P, Harris AB. Ketamine-induced intracranial hypertension. Anesthesiology. 1972;36(2):174–6. PubMed PMID: 5059108. Epub 1972/02/01. eng.
30. Bar-Joseph G, Guilburd Y, Tamir A, Guilburd JN. Effectiveness of ketamine in decreasing intracranial pressure in children with intracranial hypertension. J Neurosurg Pediatr. 2009;4(1):40–6. PubMed PMID: 19569909. Epub 2009/07/03. eng.
31. Zeiler FA, Teitelbaum J, West M, Gillman LM. The ketamine effect on ICP in traumatic brain injury. Neurocrit Care. 2014;21(1):163–73. PubMed PMID: 24515638. Epub 2014/02/12. eng
32. Zeiler FA, Teitelbaum J, West M, Gillman LM. The ketamine effect on intracranial pressure in nontraumatic neurological illness. J Crit Care. 2014;29(6):1096–106. PubMed PMID: 24996763. Epub 2014/07/06. eng

33. Pendi A, Field R, Farhan SD, Eichler M, Bederman SS. Perioperative ketamine for analgesia in spine surgery: a meta-analysis of randomized controlled trials. Spine. 2018;43(5):E299–307. PubMed PMID: 28700455. Pubmed Central PMCID: PMC5846492. Epub 2017/07/13. eng.
34. Laskowski K, Stirling A, McKay WP, Lim HJ. A systematic review of intravenous ketamine for postoperative analgesia. Can J Anaesth Journal canadien d'anesthesie. 2011;58(10):911–23. PubMed PMID: 21773855. Epub 2011/07/21. eng.
35. Michelet D, Hilly J, Skhiri A, Abdat R, Diallo T, Brasher C, et al. Opioid-sparing effect of ketamine in children: a meta-analysis and trial sequential analysis of published studies. Pediatr Drugs. 2016;18(6):421–33.
36. Sheehy KA, Lippold C, Rice AL, Nobrega R, Finkel JC, Quezado ZM. Subanesthetic ketamine for pain management in hospitalized children, adolescents, and young adults: a single-center cohort study. J Pain Res. 2017;10:787–95. PubMed PMID: 28435316. Pubmed Central PMCID: PMC5388303. Epub 2017/04/25. eng
37. Zempsky WT, Loiselle KA, Corsi JM, Hagstrom JN. Use of low-dose ketamine infusion for pediatric patients with sickle cell disease-related pain: a case series. Clin J Pain. 2010;26(2):163–7. PubMed PMID: 20090444. Epub 2010/01/22. eng.
38. Abbasi S, Bidi N, Mahshidfar B, Hafezimoghadam P, Rezai M, Mofidi M, et al. Can low-dose of ketamine reduce the need for morphine in renal colic? A double-blind randomized clinical trial. Am J Emerg Med. 2018;36(3):376–9.
39. Lo TC, Yeung ST, Lee S, Skavinski K, Liao S. Reduction of central neuropathic pain with ketamine infusion in a patient with Ehlers-Danlos syndrome: a case report. J Pain Res. 2016;9:683–7. PubMed PMID: 27695362. Pubmed Central PMCID: PMC5029839. Epub 2016/10/04. eng
40. Mulier JP. Perioperative opioids aggravate obstructive breathing in sleep apnea syndrome: mechanisms and alternative anesthesia strategies. Curr Opin Anaesthesiol. 2016;29(1):129–33. PubMed PMID: 26595546. Epub 2015/11/26. eng.
41. Jonkman K, van Rijnsoever E, Olofsen E, Aarts L, Sarton E, van Velzen M, et al. Esketamine counters opioid-induced respiratory depression. Br J Anaesth. 2018;120(5):1117–27. PubMed PMID: 29661389. Epub 2018/04/18. eng.
42. Anaesthetists AaNZCo. Statement on principles for identifying and preventing opioid-induced ventilatory impairment (OIVI). Available from: http://www.anzca.edu.au/resources/endorsed-guidelines/oivi-statement.
43. Cohen SP, Bhatia A, Buvanendran A, Schwenk ES, Wasan AD, Hurley RW, et al. Consensus guidelines on the use of intravenous ketamine infusions for chronic pain from the American Society of Regional Anesthesia and Pain Medicine, the American Academy of Pain Medicine, and the American Society of Anesthesiologists. Reg Anesth Pain Med. 2018;43(5):521–46. PubMed PMID: 29870458. Pubmed Central PMCID: PMC6023575. Epub 2018/06/06. eng.
44. Loftus RW, Yeager MP, Clark JA, Brown JR, Abdu WA, Sengupta DK, et al. Intraoperative ketamine reduces perioperative opiate consumption in opiate-dependent patients with chronic back pain undergoing back surgery. Anesthesiology. 2010;113(3):639–46. PubMed PMID: 20693876. Epub 2010/08/10. eng
45. Raith K, Hochhaus G. Drugs used in the treatment of opioid tolerance and physical dependence: a review. Int J Clin Pharmacol Ther. 2004;42(4):191–203. PubMed PMID: 15124977. Epub 2004/05/06. eng
46. Lilius TO, Jokinen V, Neuvonen MS, Niemi M, Kalso EA, Rauhala PV. Ketamine coadministration attenuates morphine tolerance and leads to increased brain concentrations of both drugs in the rat. Br J Pharmacol. 2015;172(11):2799–813. PubMed PMID: 25297798. Pubmed Central PMCID: PMC4439876. Epub 2014/10/10. eng.
47. Neunhoeffer F, Hanser A, Esslinger M, Icheva V, Kumpf M, Gerbig I, et al. Ketamine infusion as a counter measure for opioid tolerance in mechanically ventilated children: a pilot study. Paediatr Drugs. 2017;19(3):259–65. PubMed PMID: 28299720. Epub 2017/03/17. eng.
48. Woolf CJ, Thompson SW. The induction and maintenance of central sensitization is dependent on N-methyl-D-aspartic acid receptor activation; implications for the treatment of post-injury pain hypersensitivity states. Pain. 1991;44(3):293–9. PubMed PMID: 1828878. Epub 1991/03/01. eng.

49. Hayes C, Armstrong-Brown A, Burstal R. Perioperative intravenous ketamine infusion for the prevention of persistent post-amputation pain: a randomized, controlled trial. Anaesth Intensive Care. 2004;32(3):330–8. PubMed PMID: 15264726. Epub 2004/07/22. eng.
50. McNicol ED, Schumann R, Haroutounian S. A systematic review and meta-analysis of ketamine for the prevention of persistent post-surgical pain. Acta Anaesthesiol Scand. 2014;58(10):1199–213. PubMed PMID: 25060512. Epub 2014/07/26. eng.
51. Kissin I, Brown PT, Robinson CA, Bradley EL Jr. Acute tolerance in morphine analgesia: continuous infusion and single injection in rats. Anesthesiology. 1991;74(1):166–71. PubMed PMID: 1986642. Epub 1991/01/11. eng.
52. Martin WR, Eades CG. Demonstration of tolerance and physical dependence in the dog following a short-term infusion of morphine. J Pharmacol Exp Ther. 1961;133:262–70. PubMed PMID: 13767428. Epub 1961/08/01. eng.
53. Angst MS, Koppert W, Pahl I, Clark DJ, Schmelz M. Short-term infusion of the mu-opioid agonist remifentanil in humans causes hyperalgesia during withdrawal. Pain. 2003;106(1–2):49–57. PubMed PMID: 14581110. Epub 2003/10/29. eng
54. Mao J, Price DD, Mayer DJ. Mechanisms of hyperalgesia and morphine tolerance: a current view of their possible interactions. Pain. 1995;62(3):259–74. PubMed PMID: 8657426. Epub 1995/09/01. eng.
55. Laulin JP, Maurette P, Corcuff JB, Rivat C, Chauvin M, Simonnet G. The role of ketamine in preventing fentanyl-induced hyperalgesia and subsequent acute morphine tolerance. Anesth Analg. 2002;94(5):1263–9, table of contents. PubMed PMID: 11973202. Epub 2002/04/26. eng
56. Jevtovic-Todorovic V, Hartman RE, Izumi Y, Benshoff ND, Dikranian K, Zorumski CF, et al. Early exposure to common anesthetic agents causes widespread neurodegeneration in the developing rat brain and persistent learning deficits. J Neurosci. 2003;23(3):876–82. PubMed PMID: 12574416. Epub 2003/02/08. eng.
57. Sun L, Li Q, Li Q, Zhang Y, Liu D, Jiang H, et al. Chronic ketamine exposure induces permanent impairment of brain functions in adolescent cynomolgus monkeys. Addict Biol. 2014;19(2):185–94. PubMed PMID: 23145560. Epub 2012/11/14. eng.
58. Li Q, Shi L, Lu G, Yu H-L, Yeung F-K, Wong N-K, et al. Chronic ketamine exposure causes white matter microstructural abnormalities in adolescent cynomolgus monkeys. Front Neurosci. 2017;11:285. PubMed PMID: 28579941.
59. Olney JW, Labruyere J, Price MT. Pathological changes induced in cerebrocortical neurons by phencyclidine and related drugs. Science (New York, NY). 1989;244(4910):1360–2. PubMed PMID: 2660263. Epub 1989/06/16. eng.
60. Fryer HJL, Knox RJ, Strittmatter SM, Kalb R. Excitotoxic death of a subset of embryonic rat motor neurons in vitro. J Neurochem. 1999;72(2):500–13.
61. Vutskits L, Gascon E, Potter G, Tassonyi E, Kiss JZ. Low concentrations of ketamine initiate dendritic atrophy of differentiated GABAergic neurons in culture. Toxicology. 2007;234(3):216–26. PubMed PMID: 17418473. Epub 2007/04/10. eng.
62. Goulart BK, de Lima MN, de Farias CB, Reolon GK, Almeida VR, Quevedo J, et al. Ketamine impairs recognition memory consolidation and prevents learning-induced increase in hippocampal brain-derived neurotrophic factor levels. Neuroscience. 2010;167(4):969–73. PubMed PMID: 20338225. Epub 2010/03/27. eng.
63. Anand KJ, Garg S, Rovnaghi CR, Narsinghani U, Bhutta AT, Hall RW. Ketamine reduces the cell death following inflammatory pain in newborn rat brain. Pediatr Res. 2007;62(3):283–90. PubMed PMID: 17551412. Epub 2007/06/07. eng.
64. Liu JR, Liu Q, Li J, Baek C, Han XH, Athiraman U, et al. Noxious stimulation attenuates ketamine-induced neuroapoptosis in the developing rat brain. Anesthesiology. 2012;117(1):64–71. PubMed PMID: 22617253. Epub 2012/05/24. eng

Chapter 9
Propofol for Sedation of the Critically Ill Child

Leslie A. Dervan and R. Scott Watson

Introduction

Propofol is an intravenous (IV) anesthetic medication that modulates gamma-aminobutyric acid-A ($GABA_A$) receptors and inhibits N-methyl-D-aspartate (NMDA) receptors, inhibiting postsynaptic neuronal depolarization with resulting hypnotic, sedative, and amnestic effects [1, 2] as well as dose-dependent side effects, including respiratory depression and hypotension. It is highly lipophilic, readily crossing the blood-brain barrier and diffusing into fatty tissues [2]. Its short half-life makes it a popular option for titratable sedation with over 80% of mechanically ventilated adults receiving continuous IV sedation via propofol only a decade ago [3]. Due to its rapid onset, titratable depth of anesthesia/sedation, rapid offset, and low incidence of adverse events when used by appropriately trained, experienced providers, propofol has become a very popular choice for procedural sedation and anesthesia in pediatrics, including frequent use outside the operating room by non-anesthesia providers. In a review of over 90,000 procedural sedations provided by pediatric critical care medicine physicians using propofol, serious adverse events were reported in 2.2% of encounters, while <1% required airway intervention, and no deaths occurred [4].

L. A. Dervan (✉)
Division of Pediatric Critical Care Medicine, Department of Pediatrics, University of Washington, Seattle, WA, USA

Center for Clinical and Translational Research; Seattle Children's Research Institute, Seattle, WA, USA
e-mail: leslie.dervan@seattlechildrens.org

R. S. Watson
Division of Pediatric Critical Care Medicine, Department of Pediatrics, University of Washington, Seattle, WA, USA

Center for Child Health, Behavior, and Development; Seattle Children's Research Institute, Seattle, WA, USA

P. P. Kamat, J. W. Berkenbosch (eds.), *Sedation and Analgesia for the Pediatric Intensivist*, https://doi.org/10.1007/978-3-030-52555-2_9

Despite this adult intensive care unit (ICU) and pediatric procedural experience, propofol is less commonly used for continuous sedation in the pediatric intensive care unit (PICU) setting for several reasons. The US Food and Drug Administration issued a label change in 2001 recommending against off-label use of propofol for continuous sedation in the PICU, possibly related to an unpublished industry study that observed increased mortality for children in the ICU receiving propofol vs. standard sedation [5, 6]. Despite the label recommendations, PICU patients are frequently exposed to propofol; 39% in one study received propofol during the ICU stay [7], and exposure increased from 2001 to 2007 [8]. Data on efficacy and clinical outcomes for pediatric patients receiving propofol versus other continuous sedatives in the ICU setting are lacking, and serious safety concerns persist, chiefly related to propofol-related infusion syndrome (PRIS). Acknowledging these concerns, propofol remains an important sedative option for the pediatric intensivist, as its pharmacokinetic and pharmacodynamic properties are ideally suited to certain specific sedation goals.

Pharmacology

Mechanism of Action

Propofol (2,6-diisopropylphenol) is a $GABA_A$-receptor agonist; binding to the receptor increases cellular chloride influx, resulting in hyperpolarization and inhibition of synaptic conduction in the central nervous system (CNS). It also acts on presynaptic GABA receptors, inhibiting GABA reuptake and augmenting its release in animal models. Tonic GABAergic signaling inhibits acetylcholine (ACh) release in multiple brain areas; propofol augments ACh inhibition in the frontal cortex and the hippocampus, resulting in decreased arousal and ultimately loss of consciousness. Other areas of the brain, including the substantia nigra, are also affected [9].

Pharmacokinetics

Pharmacokinetics differ for propofol infusions compared to bolus dosing. In bolus dosing, propofol has a rapid onset of action (10–50 seconds). Offset is related to rapid drug distribution into tissues (9 min) rather than metabolism, which is primarily hepatic [1, 10]. A typical anesthetic induction dose is 1.5–3 mg/kg, divided into two to three doses to allow titration to effect while minimizing dose-related hemodynamic and respiratory side effects. Maintenance of anesthesia is achieved by repeat bolus doses of 0.5–1 mg/kg, an infusion, dosed from 50 to 250 mcg/kg/min [1, 11–15], or both. Higher doses may be needed if propofol is used alone [16, 17]. Younger children may also require higher doses, due to differences in volume of distribution and clearance [1, 11].

Infusion pharmacokinetics (PK) fit a three-compartment PK model, with clearance approximated by hepatic blood flow [18]. With infusions used for maintenance of anesthesia, children require higher doses and have longer context-sensitive half-life for propofol than adults. The half-life doubles from hour 1 of propofol infusion to hour 4 and continues to increase over time due to tissue redistribution [19]. These observations likely also apply to lower-dose infusions employed for continuous sedation. One short-term PICU-based PK study observed pharmacokinetics among 28 patients receiving propofol infusions for up to 13 hours. In this study, the initial propofol bolus dose diffused rapidly into a second and third compartment, both with extremely large volume of distribution, suggesting that a prolonged infusion could result in a very long terminal half-life of the drug. At this duration, average offset time was 15 min, although there was substantial variability among patients [10]. PK modeling data suggest that the offset following prolonged infusion varies by depth of sedation and duration of infusion and could take over 3 days for infusions lasting 7–14 days [20]. Longer recovery has been observed with long-term infusions of propofol in adult patients, with offset times of up to 24 h [21].

Besides targeted depth of sedation and infusion duration, additional clinical factors may impact the clearance and offset following prolonged infusion. Critically ill adults have decreased clearance, attributed to lower hepatic blood flow from shock [22, 23]. Patients treated with therapeutic hypothermia (33–34 degrees) also have decreased propofol clearance [24]. Unlike other options for continuous pharmacologic sedation, renal dysfunction, obesity, and liver dysfunction are not associated with delayed awakening after receiving propofol [23].

Pharmacodynamics

Commonly recognized systemic effects of propofol are dose-dependent and include CNS depression, ranging from anxiolysis to anesthesia; respiratory depression, ranging from hypoventilation to apnea [25]; upper airway obstruction [1]; and hemodynamic effects including vasodilation, decreased cardiac index, and hypotension [26, 27]. Other properties include antiemetic [28, 29] and anticonvulsant effects [30, 31], which can be additionally beneficial in certain patient populations. The hemodynamic effects of propofol result in decreased cerebral blood flow (CBF); this, combined with a decrease in cerebral metabolic demand, results in decreased intracranial pressure (ICP) [32, 33]. Despite the decrease in CBF, cerebral tissue oxygenation is preserved, due to an accompanying decrease in cerebral metabolic demand [26]. Up to 60% of patients experience pain at the injection site. Propofol does not provide any analgesic effect, so it is often paired with opioids or ketamine for painful procedures, which can alter systemic side effects and decrease the dose of propofol needed to achieve adequate sedation [1, 34]. This is also true when used for continuous sedation in the ICU; using propofol alone is associated with increased agitation in ventilated adult trauma patients [35] compared to its use in combination with other agents.

Nutritionally, propofol can contribute a significant amount of calories from fat when used for continuous sedation in adult ICU patients. In one study, propofol provided an average of 46 +/− 117 kcal/d in ICU patients receiving this drug. Fat from propofol constituted an average of 17% of total energy intake, and provided up to 100% for some patients during the first ICU days, which may be disadvantageous; among survivors, proportion of calories due to fat intake was associated with prolonged ventilation time [36]. Hypertriglyceridemia occurs in 18% of adults receiving propofol for over 24 h; in one study, 10% developed pancreatitis [37]. For pediatric calculations, an infusion of 50 mcg/kg/min (3 mg/kg/hr) provides 7.9 kcal/kg/day.

With prolonged (>24 h) exposure, evidence suggests an increased risk of ICU-acquired weakness in adult patients with sepsis and respiratory failure receiving propofol compared to other sedatives (OR = 3.4) [38]. This may be a consequence of impaired mitochondrial activity, also shown to be the mechanism behind PRIS [39]. In vitro, propofol profoundly impairs fatty acid oxidation in skeletal muscle cells, even at low doses [40]. Animal model studies demonstrate impaired neutrophil chemotaxis, phagocytosis, and bacterial clearance with propofol exposure [23]. It is also associated with impaired neutrophil oxidative response in vitro, although studies have not identified this effect in vivo after short exposures [41].

Finally, prolonged infusions raise concerns regarding the potential toxicity of diluents and preservatives in the propofol formulation, which differ by manufacturer. Egg phosphatide, soybean oil, and sulfites may be present and precipitate allergy or anaphylaxis, although this is uncommon in newer formulations. Disodium EDTA can cause hypocalcemia, and the lipid emulsion can cause hypertriglyceridemia, pancreatitis, phlebitis, fat emboli (particularly in sulfite-containing formulations), and solubility and compatibility issues; it may also be associated with the development of PRIS [23]. It is unknown how frequently these complications occur in patients on prolonged propofol infusions, but they are likely dose- and duration-dependent.

Clinical Considerations for Use

Indications for Short-Term, Deep Sedation

Continuous sedation in critically ill patients should follow adequate treatment of pain, should be targeted to a prescribed goal, and should be minimized when possible. Targeting a light, rather than deep, level of sedation is associated with improved outcome in adult ICU patients, including shorter time to extubation, less frequent tracheostomy, and reduced length of stay [42]. Targeting a light level of sedation can be safe and feasible in the pediatric population [43, 44].

The pharmacologic properties of propofol are well-suited to certain specific sedation goals. For short-term use compared to dexmedetomidine, propofol achieves a greater depth of sedation with a faster offset [45]. Similarly, ventilated adult ICU patients receiving propofol for continuous sedation were more frequently able to achieve deep sedation or coma (RASS ≤-4) as a targeted depth of sedation, compared to patients receiving dexmedetomidine [46]. Therefore, propofol can be ideal for patients who require deep sedation for short periods of time (e.g., young patients who require several hours of immobility after arterial access for interventional procedures). Deep sedation or coma may benefit some patients with increased ICP. Propofol reduces cerebral metabolic demand and reduces ICP, although if hypotension occurs, this may reduce cerebral perfusion pressure, which would limit the acceptable propofol dose for that patient [26, 32, 33].

Due to its fast offset with bolus and short-term anesthetic dosing, propofol is an attractive option for patients who require sedation but who also require intermittent interruption of sedation for neurologic examination, or as a short-term bridge to allow other sedatives to be weaned for extubation. However, propofol is only a good option for these indications for a short time frame. Patients with neurologic injury have increased risk of PRIS (described in detail below,) and due to the pharmacokinetics of propofol infusion, the offset time is expected to increase with longer infusion times [20].

Propofol "Drug Washout"

Pediatric ICU patients who require prolonged analgosedation with opioids and benzodiazepines are at high risk of developing tolerance and opioid-induced hyperalgesia, resulting in ineffective symptom control despite escalating doses [47, 48]. By employing a different class of medication, an intermittent transition to propofol could theoretically allow periodic interruption of opioids and benzodiazepines to reduce tolerance and improve efficacy. It is unknown how much reduction of tolerance would be achieved within the time and dose range generally considered safe for continuous propofol infusion. To date, no clinical evidence supports the use of propofol in this role.

The Impact of Propofol on Sleep and Delirium in ICU Patients

While propofol readily achieves deep sedation, it has negative impacts on physiologic sleep. The proportion of patients achieving rapid eye movement (REM) sleep, and the amount of time spent in REM sleep, is decreased when patients are receiving propofol compared to other sedatives [49]. Patients receiving continuous propofol infusion lose normal circadian cycling [50]. Altogether, sleep in patients sedated with propofol has been evaluated in only a handful of small studies, and a recent Cochrane review [51] concluded that evidence suggests no beneficial effect. Early adult studies suggested that, compared to benzodiazepine-based sedation, propofol was associated with less delirium in ICU patients [52, 53]. However, subsequent research has found that, compared to propofol and benzodiazepines, dexmedetomidine is associated with even less delirium and coma [54–56]. The depth of sedation achieved may be partly responsible; propofol exposure, as well as hours under deep sedation, is independently associated with delirium in adults [57].

Palliative Sedation

Providing relief of pain, dyspnea, anxiety, and other symptoms at the end of life is a crucial component of critical care. Palliative sedation refers to "the use of sedative medications to relieve intolerable and refractory distress by the reduction in patient consciousness" [58]. While maintaining consciousness and the ability to interact with loved ones is often a goal at the end of life, if standard medications fail to alleviate symptoms, prioritizing the relief from suffering may outweigh the preservation of consciousness. In this setting, palliative sedation may be consistent with a patient and family's goals. Propofol has been successfully used, in addition to benzodiazepines and opiates, for palliative sedation in both children and adults. Propofol offers a rapid onset, the opportunity to titrate to a deep level of sedation if required, and some beneficial side effects including antiemetic properties. Unfortunately, its narrow therapeutic index typically requires a critical care setting for administration. In published pediatric case series, propofol for palliative sedation has been used for up to 30 days, with infusion doses ranging from 12 to 200 mcg/kg/hr, with reports of good symptom control and both family and provider satisfaction [59, 60]. For a more in-depth discussion of palliative analgesia and sedation, the reader is referred to that specific chapter (Chapter 22).

Propofol-Related Infusion Syndrome (PRIS)

In 1992, a case series was published describing a clinical syndrome of metabolic acidosis, bradyarrhythmia, progressive myocardial failure, and death among five children receiving propofol infusion (>83 mcg/kg/min for >48 h) [61]. This syndrome, PRIS, is estimated to occur in about 1% of patients receiving propofol infusion, but it can be irreversible once identified, with 18–30% mortality among those affected [62]. Other symptoms include rhabdomyolysis [63, 64], elevated cardiac enzymes, inverted T wave [65], hyperkalemia [66], elevated serum acylcarnitines [67], and Brugada-like electrocardiographic pattern (ST segment elevation in the precordial leads) [68]. Risk factors include pediatric age; concurrent vasopressor therapy; higher Acute Physiology, Age, Chronic Health Evaluation (APACHE) score (in adults); and neurologic injury including seizure and traumatic brain injury [63, 69]. The risk is primarily dose- and duration-dependent [70], but cases have been reported in patients receiving <4 mg/kg/hr (=67 mcg/kg/min). Diagnosis can be difficult and the presenting symptoms may be sudden arrhythmia development or cardiac arrest [69]. Unfortunately, biochemical monitoring does not prevent all cases; one case report describes fatality despite negative screening creatinine kinase and lactate [71]. The largest case series, examining over 1000 patients with suspected PRIS, described 10% mortality among patients deemed to be low risk; mortality for the highest-risk patients approached 90% [63].

Pathophysiology

Propofol interferes with free fatty acid metabolism and mitochondrial respiratory pathways. In multiple human cell types in vitro, propofol interferes with mitochondrial complexes I–III, resulting in a metabolic switch from oxidative phosphorylation to glycolysis, increasing the generation of reactive oxygen species, and causing apoptosis [72]. Propofol also inhibits the enzyme carnitine palmitoyltransferase I (CPT1), preventing mitochondrial metabolization of free fatty acids, resulting in structural changes and deposition of free fatty acids in cardiac and hepatic tissues [67]. Even at low-dose exposures, skeletal muscle cells demonstrate impaired fatty acid oxidation and mitochondria have reduced spare electron transfer chain capacity [40]. Decreased utilization of free fatty acids as an energy source results in myocardial fat deposition, which has been observed at autopsy in affected patients [73].

Prevention and Treatment

Consensus in the literature and across international institutional practice is that propofol infusions are generally considered safe when limited to doses <4 mg/kg/hr (= 67 mcg/kg/min) and duration <24–48 hours [74, 75]. In one study of 210 pediatric patients after introduction of an institutional policy with good adherence to these limits (98% of infusions were used for <24 h, and 87% were dosed at <4 mg/kg/hr (= 67 mcg/kg/min)), no full cases of PRIS occurred, although 8% still developed at least one symptom consistent with PRIS [76]. Additional recommendations for prevention include using dextrose infusion to suppress fat metabolism and avoiding propofol in high-risk patients, including those with neurologic injury, vasopressor requirements, or shock [23]. Screening patients for rhabdomyolysis and limiting use to those with low CK may also help [77]. In obese patients, doses should be based on predicted/ideal body weight to avoid inadvertent dose-related toxicity [78].

The cornerstone of treatment is discontinuing propofol as soon as toxicity is recognized. Case reports describe successful treatment with invasive physiologic support and drug removal, including partial exchange transfusion [79], plasma exchange [80], and hemofiltration with extracorporeal life support [81].

Consideration in Special Populations

Mitochondrial and Metabolic Disorders

Propofol exposure is associated with mitochondrial toxicity, myocyte apoptosis, and resulting muscular injury, even at low doses. Single doses of propofol have been reported to cause toxicity in patients with mitochondrial encephalopathy, lactic acidosis, and stroke-like episodes (MELAS), which may have been exacerbated by not providing a concomitant dextrose infusion [82]. Although there are also case series demonstrating some safe experiences using propofol in patients with mitochondrial disorders, patients with mitochondrial disorders are at overall increased risk of PRIS [83]. There are also reports of propofol unmasking mitochondrial disorders by causing toxicity in otherwise healthy patients who developed PRIS and were then found to have mitochondrial complex deficiencies [84]. Recommendations are that patients with known or suspected mitochondrial disorders should not receive prolonged or high-dose propofol for anesthesia or sedation [83].

Concern has also been raised whether patients with fatty acid oxidation disorders should receive propofol, due to risk that its lipid emulsion formulation could cause metabolic toxicity in these patients. For short-term (<1 hr) use in a series of patients with specific fatty acid oxidation disorders (long-chain L-3 hydroxyacyl-CoA dehydrogenase deficiency and trifunctional protein deficiency) undergoing sedated procedures, propofol accounted for only ~10% of their daily lipid intake limit and was not associated with any clinical side effects [39]. However, longer-term or higher-dose infusions will increase lipid exposure and toxicity in this patient population.

Conclusions

Propofol is an IV anesthetic drug with favorable short-term pharmacokinetics to provide rapid-onset, deep, and rapid-offset sedation. It results in dose-dependent CNS depression, hypotension, and respiratory depression; providers using propofol require experience and preparedness in airway management and advanced cardiorespiratory support. Long-term use is pharmacokinetically challenging, due to prolonged half-life with increasing infusion duration, and is not universally recognized as safe, due to the association between propofol infusion duration and mitochondrial toxicity (PRIS). In selected populations and for well-matched indications, propofol can be a useful sedation adjunct for the critically ill child.

Bibliography

1. Khurmi N, Patel P, Kraus M, Trentman T. Pharmacologic considerations for pediatric sedation and anesthesia outside the operating room: a review for anesthesia and non-anesthesia providers. Paediatr Drugs. 2017;19:435–46.
2. Devlin JW, Roberts RJ. Pharmacology of commonly used analgesics and sedatives in the ICU: benzodiazepines, propofol, and opioids. Anesthesiol Clin. 2011;29:567–85.
3. Wunsch H, Kahn JM, Kramer AA, Rubenfeld GD. Use of intravenous infusion sedation among mechanically ventilated patients in the United States. Crit Care Med. 2009;37:3031–9.
4. Kamat PP, McCracken CE, Gillespie SE, et al. Pediatric critical care physician-administered procedural sedation using propofol: a report from the Pediatric Sedation Research Consortium Database. Pediatr Crit Care Med. 2015;16:11–20.
5. Ahlen K, Buckley CJ, Goodale DB, Pulsford AH. The 'propofol infusion syndrome': the facts, their interpretation and implications for patient care. Eur J Anaesthesiol. 2006;23:990–8.
6. Diedrich DA, Brown DR. Analytic reviews: propofol infusion syndrome in the ICU. J Intensive Care Med. 2011;26:59–72.
7. Hsu B, Brazelton T. Off-label medication use in an academic hospital pediatric critical care unit. WMJ. 2009;108:343–8.
8. Heaton PC, Schuchter J, Lannon CM, Kemper AR. Impact of drug label changes on propofol use in pediatrics for moderate conscious sedation. Clin Ther. 2011;33:886–95.
9. Trapani G, Altomare C, Liso G, Sanna E, Biggio G. Propofol in anesthesia. Mechanism of action, structure-activity relationships, and drug delivery. Curr Med Chem. 2000;7:249–71.
10. Reed MD, Yamashita TS, Marx CM, Myers CM, Blumer JL. A pharmacokinetically based propofol dosing strategy for sedation of the critically ill, mechanically ventilated pediatric patient. Crit Care Med. 1996;24:1473–81.
11. Jasiak KD, Phan H, Christich AC, Edwards CJ, Skrepnek GH, Patanwala AE. Induction dose of propofol for pediatric patients undergoing procedural sedation in the emergency department. Pediatr Emerg Care. 2012;28:440–2.
12. Alletag MJ, Auerbach MA, Baum CR. Ketamine, propofol, and ketofol use for pediatric sedation. Pediatr Emerg Care. 2012;28:1391–5; quiz 6-8.
13. Patel KN, Simon HK, Stockwell CA, et al. Pediatric procedural sedation by a dedicated nonanesthesiology pediatric sedation service using propofol. Pediatr Emerg Care. 2009;25:133–8.
14. Hassan NE, Betz BW, Cole MR, et al. Randomized controlled trial for intermittent versus continuous propofol sedation for pediatric brain and spine magnetic resonance imaging studies. Pediatr Crit Care Med. 2011;12:e262–5.
15. Klein SM, Hauser GJ, Anderson BD, et al. Comparison of intermittent versus continuous infusion of propofol for elective oncology procedures in children. Pediatr Crit Care Med. 2003;4:78–82.
16. Hollman GA, Schultz MM, Eickhoff JC, Christenson DK. Propofol-fentanyl versus propofol alone for lumbar puncture sedation in children with acute hematologic malignancies: propofol dosing and adverse events. Pediatr Crit Care Med. 2008;9:616–22.
17. Milius EM, Papademetrious TR, Heitlinger LA. Retrospective review of propofol dosing for procedural sedation in pediatric patients. J Pediatr Pharmacol Ther. 2012;17:246–51.
18. Smuszkiewicz P, Wiczling P, Przybylowski K, et al. The pharmacokinetics of propofol in ICU patients undergoing long-term sedation. Biopharm Drug Dispos. 2016;37:456–66.
19. McFarlan CS, Anderson BJ, Short TG. The use of propofol infusions in paediatric anaesthesia: a practical guide. Paediatr Anaesth. 1999;9:209–16.
20. Barr J, Egan TD, Sandoval NF, et al. Propofol dosing regimens for ICU sedation based upon an integrated pharmacokinetic-pharmacodynamic model. Anesthesiology. 2001;95:324–33.
21. Bailie GR, Cockshott ID, Douglas EJ, Bowles BJ. Pharmacokinetics of propofol during and after long-term continuous infusion for maintenance of sedation in ICU patients. Br J Anaesth. 1992;68:486–91.

22. Bodenham A, Shelly MP, Park GR. The altered pharmacokinetics and pharmacodynamics of drugs commonly used in critically ill patients. Clin Pharmacokinet. 1988;14:347–73.
23. Devlin JW, Mallow-Corbett S, Riker RR. Adverse drug events associated with the use of analgesics, sedatives, and antipsychotics in the intensive care unit. Crit Care Med. 2010;38:S231–43.
24. Bjelland TW, Klepstad P, Haugen BO, Nilsen T, Dale O. Effects of hypothermia on the disposition of morphine, midazolam, fentanyl, and propofol in intensive care unit patients. Drug Metab Dispos. 2013;41:214–23.
25. Marik PE. Propofol: therapeutic indications and side-effects. Curr Pharm Des. 2004;10: 3639–49.
26. Fleck T, Schubert S, Ewert P, Stiller B, Nagdyman N, Berger F. Propofol effect on cerebral oxygenation in children with congenital heart disease. Pediatr Cardiol. 2015;36:543–9.
27. Morgan DJ, Campbell GA, Crankshaw DP. Pharmacokinetics of propofol when given by intravenous infusion. Br J Clin Pharmacol. 1990;30:144–8.
28. Sahyoun C, Krauss B. Clinical implications of pharmacokinetics and pharmacodynamics of procedural sedation agents in children. Curr Opin Pediatr. 2012;24:225–32.
29. Cravero JP, Beach ML, Blike GT, Gallagher SM, Hertzog JH, Pediatric Sedation Research C. The incidence and nature of adverse events during pediatric sedation/anesthesia with propofol for procedures outside the operating room: a report from the Pediatric Sedation Research Consortium. Anesth Analg. 2009;108:795–804.
30. Zhang Q, Yu Y, Lu Y, Yue H. Systematic review and meta-analysis of propofol versus barbiturates for controlling refractory status epilepticus. BMC Neurol. 2019;19:55.
31. Claassen J, Hirsch LJ, Emerson RG, Mayer SA. Treatment of refractory status epilepticus with pentobarbital, propofol, or midazolam: a systematic review. Epilepsia. 2002;43:146–53.
32. Kelly DF, Goodale DB, Williams J, et al. Propofol in the treatment of moderate and severe head injury: a randomized, prospective double-blinded pilot trial. J Neurosurg. 1999;90:1042–52.
33. Ravussin P, Guinard JP, Ralley F, Thorin D. Effect of propofol on cerebrospinal fluid pressure and cerebral perfusion pressure in patients undergoing craniotomy. Anaesthesia. 1988;43 Suppl:37–41.
34. Roback MG, Carlson DW, Babl FE, Kennedy RM. Update on pharmacological management of procedural sedation for children. Curr Opin Anaesthesiol. 2016;29(Suppl 1):S21–35.
35. Mahmood S, Mahmood O, El-Menyar A, Asim M, Al-Thani H. Predisposing factors, clinical assessment, management and outcomes of agitation in the trauma intensive care unit. World J Emerg Med. 2018;9:105–12.
36. Charriere M, Ridley E, Hastings J, Bianchet O, Scheinkestel C, Berger MM. Propofol sedation substantially increases the caloric and lipid intake in critically ill patients. Nutrition. 2017;42:64–8.
37. Devlin JW, Lau AK, Tanios MA. Propofol-associated hypertriglyceridemia and pancreatitis in the intensive care unit: an analysis of frequency and risk factors. Pharmacotherapy. 2005;25:1348–52.
38. Abdelmalik PA, Rakocevic G. Propofol as a risk factor for ICU-acquired weakness in septic patients with acute respiratory failure. Can J Neurol Sci. 2017;44:295–303.
39. Martin JM, Gillingham MB, Harding CO. Use of propofol for short duration procedures in children with long chain 3-hydroxyacyl-CoA dehydrogenase (LCHAD) or trifunctional protein (TFP) deficiencies. Mol Genet Metab. 2014;112:139–42.
40. Krajcova A, Lovsletten NG, Waldauf P, et al. Effects of Propofol on cellular bioenergetics in human skeletal muscle cells. Crit Care Med. 2018;46:e206–e12.
41. Frohlich D, Trabold B, Rothe G, Hoerauf K, Wittmann S. Inhibition of the neutrophil oxidative response by propofol: preserved in vivo function despite in vitro inhibition. Eur J Anaesthesiol. 2006;23:948–53.
42. Devlin JW, Skrobik Y, Gelinas C, et al. Clinical practice guidelines for the prevention and management of pain, agitation/sedation, delirium, immobility, and sleep disruption in adult patients in the ICU. Crit Care Med. 2018;46:e825–e73.

43. Deeter KH, King MA, Ridling D, Irby GL, Lynn AM, Zimmerman JJ. Successful implementation of a pediatric sedation protocol for mechanically ventilated patients. Crit Care Med. 2011;39:683–8.
44. Dreyfus L, Javouhey E, Denis A, Touzet S, Bordet F. Implementation and evaluation of a paediatric nurse-driven sedation protocol in a paediatric intensive care unit. Ann Intensive Care. 2017;7:36.
45. Wu J, Mahmoud M, Schmitt M, Hossain M, Kurth D. Comparison of propofol and dexmedetomidine techniques in children undergoing magnetic resonance imaging. Paediatr Anaesth. 2014;24:813–8.
46. Ruokonen E, Parviainen I, Jakob SM, et al. Dexmedetomidine versus propofol/midazolam for long-term sedation during mechanical ventilation. Intensive Care Med. 2009;35:282–90.
47. Best KM, Boullata JI, Curley MA. Risk factors associated with iatrogenic opioid and benzodiazepine withdrawal in critically ill pediatric patients: a systematic review and conceptual model. Pediatr Crit Care Med. 2015;16:175–83.
48. Best KM, Wypij D, Asaro LA. Curley MA and randomized evaluation of sedation titration for respiratory failure study I. Patient, process, and system predictors of iatrogenic withdrawal syndrome in critically ill children. Crit Care Med. 2017;45:e7–e15.
49. Kondili E, Alexopoulou C, Xirouchaki N, Georgopoulos D. Effects of propofol on sleep quality in mechanically ventilated critically ill patients: a physiological study. Intensive Care Med. 2012;38:1640–6.
50. Bienert A, Kusza K, Wawrzyniak K, et al. Assessing circadian rhythms in propofol PK and PD during prolonged infusion in ICU patients. J Pharmacokinet Pharmacodyn. 2010;37:289–304.
51. Lewis SR, Schofield-Robinson OJ, Alderson P, Smith AF. Propofol for the promotion of sleep in adults in the intensive care unit. Cochrane Database Syst Rev. 2018;1:CD012454.
52. Lonardo NW, Mone MC, Nirula R, et al. Propofol is associated with favorable outcomes compared with benzodiazepines in ventilated intensive care unit patients. Am J Respir Crit Care Med. 2014;189:1383–94.
53. Wang H, Wang C, Wang Y, et al. Sedative drugs used for mechanically ventilated patients in intensive care units: a systematic review and network meta-analysis. Curr Med Res Opin. 2019;35:435–46.
54. Skrobik Y, Duprey MS, Hill NS, Devlin JW. Low-dose nocturnal Dexmedetomidine prevents ICU delirium. A randomized, placebo-controlled trial. Am J Respir Crit Care Med. 2018;197:1147–56.
55. Riker RR, Shehabi Y, Bokesch PM, et al. Dexmedetomidine vs midazolam for sedation of critically ill patients: a randomized trial. JAMA. 2009;301:489–99.
56. Pandharipande PP, Pun BT, Herr DL, et al. Effect of sedation with dexmedetomidine vs lorazepam on acute brain dysfunction in mechanically ventilated patients: the MENDS randomized controlled trial. JAMA. 2007;298:2644–53.
57. Bryczkowski SB, Lopreiato MC, Yonclas PP, Sacca JJ, Mosenthal AC. Risk factors for delirium in older trauma patients admitted to the surgical intensive care unit. J Trauma Acute Care Surg. 2014;77:944–51.
58. Morita T, Akechi T, Sugawara Y, Chihara S, Uchitomi Y. Practices and attitudes of Japanese oncologists and palliative care physicians concerning terminal sedation: a nationwide survey. J Clin Oncol. 2002;20:758–64.
59. McWilliams K, Keeley PW, Waterhouse ET. Propofol for terminal sedation in palliative care: a systematic review. J Palliat Med. 2010;13:73–6.
60. Anghelescu DL, Hamilton H, Faughnan LG, Johnson LM, Baker JN. Pediatric palliative sedation therapy with propofol: recommendations based on experience in children with terminal cancer. J Palliat Med. 2012;15:1082–90.
61. Parke TJ, Stevens JE, Rice AS, et al. Metabolic acidosis and fatal myocardial failure after propofol infusion in children: five case reports. BMJ. 1992;305:613–6.
62. Roberts RJ, Barletta JF, Fong JJ, et al. Incidence of propofol-related infusion syndrome in critically ill adults: a prospective, multicenter study. Crit Care. 2009;13:R169.

63. Fong JJ, Sylvia L, Ruthazer R, Schumaker G, Kcomt M, Devlin JW. Predictors of mortality in patients with suspected propofol infusion syndrome. Crit Care Med. 2008;36:2281–7.
64. Linko R, Laukkanen A, Koljonen V, Rapola J, Varpula T. Severe heart failure and rhabdomyolysis associated with propofol infusion in a burn patient. J Burn Care Res. 2014;35:e364–7.
65. Mijzen EJ, Jacobs B, Aslan A, Rodgers MG. Propofol infusion syndrome heralded by ECG changes. Neurocrit Care. 2012;17:260–4.
66. Mali AR, Patil VP, Pramesh CS, Mistry RC. Hyperkalemia during surgery: is it an early warning of propofol infusion syndrome? J Anesth. 2009;23:421–3.
67. Vollmer JP, Haen S, Wolburg H, et al. Propofol related infusion syndrome: ultrastructural evidence for a mitochondrial disorder. Crit Care Med. 2018;46:e91–e4.
68. Riera AR, Uchida AH, Schapachnik E, Dubner S, Filho CF, Ferreira C. Propofol infusion syndrome and Brugada syndrome electrocardiographic phenocopy. Cardiol J. 2010;17:130–5.
69. Krajcova A, Waldauf P, Andel M, Duska F. Propofol infusion syndrome: a structured review of experimental studies and 153 published case reports. Crit Care. 2015;19:398.
70. Diaz JH, Prabhakar A, Urman RD, Kaye AD. Propofol infusion syndrome: a retrospective analysis at a level 1 trauma center. Crit Care Res Pract. 2014;2014:346968.
71. Veldhoen ES, Hartman BJ, van Gestel JP. Monitoring biochemical parameters as an early sign of propofol infusion syndrome: false feeling of security. Pediatr Crit Care Med. 2009;10:e19–21.
72. Sumi C, Okamoto A, Tanaka H, et al. Propofol induces a metabolic switch to glycolysis and cell death in a mitochondrial electron transport chain-dependent manner. PLoS One. 2018;13:e0192796.
73. Jorens PG, Van den Eynden GG. Propofol infusion syndrome with arrhythmia, myocardial fat accumulation and cardiac failure. Am J Cardiol. 2009;104:1160–2.
74. Kruessell MA, Udink ten Cate FE, Kraus AJ, Roth B, Trieschmann U. Use of propofol in pediatric intensive care units: a national survey in Germany. Pediatr Crit Care Med. 2012;13:e150–4.
75. Rosenfeld-Yehoshua N, Klin B, Berkovitch M, Abu-Kishk I. Propofol use in Israeli PICUs. Pediatr Crit Care Med. 2016;17:e117–20.
76. Koriyama H, Duff JP, Guerra GG, Chan AW, Sedation W, Analgesia T. Is propofol a friend or a foe of the pediatric intensivist? Description of propofol use in a PICU*. Pediatr Crit Care Med. 2014;15:e66–71.
77. Schroeppel TJ, Fabian TC, Clement LP, et al. Propofol infusion syndrome: a lethal condition in critically injured patients eliminated by a simple screening protocol. Injury. 2014;45:245–9.
78. Ramaiah R, Lollo L, Brannan D, Bhananker SM. Propofol infusion syndrome in a super morbidly obese patient (BMI = 75). Int J Crit Illn Inj Sci. 2011;1:84–6.
79. Da-Silva SS, Wong R, Coquillon P, Gavrilita C, Asuncion A. Partial-exchange blood transfusion: an effective method for preventing mortality in a child with propofol infusion syndrome. Pediatrics. 2010;125:e1493–9.
80. Levin PD, Levin V, Weissman C, Sprung CL, Rund D. Therapeutic plasma exchange as treatment for propofol infusion syndrome. J Clin Apher. 2015;30:311–3.
81. Guitton C, Gabillet L, Latour P, et al. Propofol infusion syndrome during refractory status epilepticus in a young adult: successful ECMO resuscitation. Neurocrit Care. 2011;15:139–45.
82. Mtaweh H, Bayir H, Kochanek PM, Bell MJ. Effect of a single dose of propofol and lack of dextrose administration in a child with mitochondrial disease: a case report. J Child Neurol. 2014;29:NP40–6.
83. Finsterer J, Frank M. Propofol is mitochondrion-toxic and may unmask a mitochondrial disorder. J Child Neurol. 2016;31:1489–94.
84. Savard M, Dupre N, Turgeon AF, Desbiens R, Langevin S, Brunet D. Propofol-related infusion syndrome heralding a mitochondrial disease: case report. Neurology. 2013;81:770–1.

Chapter 10
Inhalational Agents: What Volatile Inhalational Agents Are and How to Use Them in the ICU Setting

Erin V. Rosenberg, Lily Young, Michael Fiedorek, and Chhaya Patel

Introduction

Inhalational agents have played a pivotal role in anesthesia history. The first publicly demonstrated anesthetic of the modern era, diethyl ether, was an inhalational anesthetic. Volatile anesthetics play a significant role in clinical anesthesia throughout the world and are administered routinely by anesthesiologists using anesthesia machines. Technological advances have permitted volatile anesthetic administration to migrate to nontraditional areas outside of the operating room, such as the critical care unit. The development of specialized equipment such as Anesthetic Converting Device (AnaConDa; Sedana Medical, Uppsala, Sweden), which is a miniature vaporizer consisting of an antiviral and antibacterial humidifying filter, in addition to an activated charcoal membrane that allows for absorption and reuse of the anesthesia, has allowed for the use of anesthetic gases with critical care unit ventilators.

E. V. Rosenberg
Emory University School of Medicine, Emory + Children's Pediatric Institute, Pediatric Anesthesiology Fellowship Program, Children's Healthcare of Atlanta, Atlanta, GA, USA
e-mail: evrosen@emory.edu

L. Young
Emory University School of Medicine, Emory + Children's Pediatric Institute, Children's Healthcare of Atlanta, Atlanta, GA, USA
e-mail: lyoung5@emory.edu

M. Fiedorek
Emory + Children's Pediatric Institute, Children's Healthcare of Atlanta, Atlanta, GA, USA
e-mail: mfiedor@emory.edu

C. Patel (✉)
Emory University School of Medicine, Emory + Children's Pediatric Institute, Satellite Blvd. Surgery Center, Division of Pediatric and Ambulatory Anesthesiology, Children's Healthcare of Atlanta, Atlanta, GA, USA
e-mail: cpatel2@emory.edu

P. P. Kamat, J. W. Berkenbosch (eds.), *Sedation and Analgesia for the Pediatric Intensivist*, https://doi.org/10.1007/978-3-030-52555-2_10

Principles of Inhalational Agents

Inhalational anesthetic agents, which remain the principle amnestic agents used in the operating room for general anesthesia, provide unique advantages secondary to their distinctive pharmacokinetic and pharmacodynamic principles. The three volatile agents most commonly used in the USA are isoflurane, desflurane, and sevoflurane, all of which are halogenated hydrocarbons. Sevoflurane is a fluorinated methyl isopropyl ether. Isoflurane and desflurane are both methyl ethyl ethers, with desflurane differing from isoflurane by only one atom. Halogenation affords all three of these agents superior stability and less flammability compared to ether.

The inhalational mechanism of drug delivery is particularly unique. The pharmacokinetics of these agents depends upon physical properties such as partial pressure, vapor pressure, and solubility. Furthermore, uptake, distribution, and clearance are all directly dependent on alveolar ventilation and cardiac output.

The partial pressure of a gas is the fractional contribution that it makes to the overall pressure of all combined gases, which at sea level totals 760 mmHg. 1.4% isoflurane thus achieves a partial pressure of 10.64 at barometric pressure (1.4% × 760 mm Hg = 10.64 mm Hg). The partial pressure that is achieved in the alveoli (PA), which itself is dependent on inspired concentration, atmospheric pressure, and uptake into the blood, ultimately results in equilibration with arterial partial pressure (Pa) secondary to thermodynamic force that causes movement down a pressure gradient. Pa then in turn equilibrates with the central nervous system tissue (PCNS). Equilibrium results when the partial pressure gradients between PA, Pa, and PCNS equalize and achieve steady state. The goal of inhalational anesthesia is to obtain a certain partial pressure of the agent in the CNS that provides the desired effect. On account of differing solubility coefficients between tissues, at equilibrium where PA = Pa = PCNS, the actual concentration in the tissues will differ between the alveoli, arterial blood, and CNS. PA is thus an accurate and titratable measure of PCNS and thus also anesthetic plane and makes volatile anesthetics quickly and easily titratable.

The solubility of each anesthetic agent determines how readily Pa will equilibrate with PA. The blood-gas partition coefficient denotes solubility and is the ratio of the concentrations between the two states at equilibrium, i.e., an equal partial pressure. The greater the relative solubility of a volatile agent in blood as compared to the alveolar gas, the more molecules of anesthetic agent must dissolve in the blood to produce equilibration between PA and Pa. Thus, as solubility increases, uptake and time to equilibrium are both increased and induction of anesthesia slows. Likewise, as arterial blood reaches peripheral organs, tissues with high tissue-blood coefficients require more molecules (and more time) for equilibrium [1]:

$$\text{Uptake} = P\left(A - v\right) \times \text{gamma} \times \text{CO}$$

Minimum Alveolar Concentration

The minimum alveolar concentration (MAC) is used as a standard indicator of depth of anesthesia and also demonstrates the agent's relative potency [1]. 1 MAC is defined as the minimum alveolar concentration at sea level (1 atmosphere) at which 50% of patients do not move in response to a surgical incision. It is important to remember that MAC is defined by muscle immobility, which is an effect at the level of the spinal cord. This alveolar concentration corresponds to an alveolar partial pressure, which at steady state produces a partial pressure in the brain that results in immobility and amnesia. For example, 1 MAC of sevoflurane is 2.1% (2.1% × 760 = 15.96). The more potent the agent, the lower the alveolar concentration needed to achieve 1 MAC (Table 10.1). 1.14% isoflurane produces the same effect as 6% desflurane, thus indicating isoflurane is significantly more potent. MAC is highest at 6 months and then decreases with age. The duration of administration does not alter MAC [2].

Uptake and Distribution

The speed at which depth of anesthesia is achieved corresponds to the rate of rise of PA/PI (inspired partial pressure). The rate of PA rise is influenced both by anesthetic inflow into the alveoli and by anesthetic uptake into the alveolar capillary vessels. High delivery and low uptake increase this rate of rise. High PI, increased alveolar ventilation, low dead space, and low FRC all increase the rapidity of volatile anesthetic onset by increasing the rate of PA rise. Factors that increase blood uptake lower the rate of PA increase, and thus onset is slowed because the goal PA takes longer to achieve. These factors include high cardiac output, high agent solubility, and high alveolar to venous partial pressure differences [3].

There are a number of other factors that also contribute to duration of onset. Left to right shunting usually does not alter anesthetic uptake or speed of induction significantly provided cerebral perfusion is not decreased to a degree that delivery of volatile agent to the brain is decreased. Right to left shunting slows induction as less arterial blood has the opportunity to equilibrate with the PA.

Table 10.1 Properties of modern volatile anesthetics

Common anesthetics	Blood-gas partition coefficient	Minimum alveolar concentration (MAC)
Sevoflurane	0.63	2.05
Isoflurane	1.4	1.14
Desflurane	0.42	6

Concentration Effect

There are two notable pharmacokinetic principles of volatile anesthetics that also impact the speed of induction: concentration effect and second-gas effect. Concentration effect describes the impact of the inspired partial pressure on the rate of PA rise. The phenomenon describes how, after volatile absorption from the alveoli to the blood, the resulting absence of gas is replaced by an even higher (less diluted by dead space) inspired concentration of anesthetic, thus leading to higher PAs. The higher the PI, the faster the PA will rise secondary to this effect. The second-gas effect describes a unique phenomenon that occurs with the use of two agents especially with one being nitrous oxide which has a very rapid uptake. As nitrous oxide is rapidly absorbed by the blood with each breath, additional volatile agent is brought into the alveoli from the conducting airways leading to higher PA and thus faster anesthetic onset.

Delivery of the Agent

Anesthesia Machine Direct Delivery

Anesthesia machines combine the ability to mechanically ventilate and administer volatile anesthetics in a closed-loop system that reduces both the amount of anesthetic consumed and environmentally wasted. If an anesthesia machine is chosen to deliver volatile anesthetics in the ICU setting, the vaporizer attached to the machine is the mechanism by which anesthetic dose is determined. Anesthetic vapor is mixed with a combination of air, oxygen, and potentially nitrous oxide. The circle system of an anesthesia machine allows the patient's expired gas to be reused after the chemical elimination of carbon dioxide, and thus very little gas is wasted. Because at room temperature inhalational anesthetics are liquids, a vaporizer device is needed to accurately add the desired amount of anesthetic vapor to the gas flow, which is then delivered to the patient via spontaneous or mechanical ventilation. Unfortunately, anesthesia machine ventilators are generally limited in their modes and in their ability to deliver precise volumes and pressures in small children.

Alternatively, the anesthesia machine can be used to deliver the desired volatile concentration and FiO_2 to a separate, more sophisticated ventilator; however most ventilators require a higher driving pressure than this method would provide. There are special ICU ventilators that have a vaporizer in circuit with a high driving pressure gas input as well as some that utilize a circle system to reduce agent wastage. Delivery of the inhaled anesthetic drugs requires a vaporizer. A scavenging system is required to prevent environmental contamination. Continuous end-tidal concentration monitoring is utilized to monitor cerebral concentration. This can be achieved with the use of an anesthesia machine or a vaporizing device dedicated for use with an ICU ventilator such as the AnaConDa (Anesthesia Conserving Device, Sedana Medical, Sweden), MIRUS (Pall Medical, Germany), or RIVAL

(Reflector-In-line Vaporizer Anesthesia application, Thornhill Medical, Toronto, Canada) [4]. The AnaConDa system is a modified heat moisture exchanger that has been developed to allow the use of inhalational agents such as sevoflurane and isoflurane in the ICU without requiring high fresh gas flows or specialized ventilators. The device features a syringe pump that delivers isoflurane or sevoflurane to a small carbon-fiber device which goes in-line with a traditional ICU ventilator, and carbon dioxide absorbers and circle systems are not required. In many ways, this can be considered a disposable anesthetic vaporizer. The device can be used with common intensive care unit ventilators and is inserted between the Y-piece and the patient. Liquid isoflurane or sevoflurane are delivered by a syringe pump. Majority of anesthetic exhaled by the patient is absorbed by a reflector and resupplied during the next inspiration. The newer MIRUS system also uses a reflector and can deliver desflurane. RIVAL is the first commercial available in-line vaporizer in North America and Europe. RIVAL is described as an in-line vaporizer that can be placed on the inspiratory limb circuit and allows for changes of inspired concentrations of inhalational anesthetics independent of inspired gas flow or minute ventilation which may potentially lead to the higher efficiency and versatility of anesthetic delivery [5].

Necessary Equipment and Preparation

Continuous monitoring of inspired and expired volatile anesthetic concentration is vital in order to safely administer an appropriate dose of the drug. Errors may occur with the vaporizer itself whereby more or less anesthetic is actually delivered relative to what is dialed on the device. Waste gas scavenging is also important as Occupational Safety and Health Administration (OSHA) allows a maximum of 2 ppm for occupational exposure to these volatile agents. If a closed or semi-closed system is used to deliver volatile gases, expired carbon dioxide must be removed from the circuit prior to delivering the recycled gases back to the patient. This is achieved via one of several different carbon dioxide absorbents, each of which works by a similar though unique chemical reaction. Calcium hydroxide (Ca(OH)2) is the principal chemical in all available carbon dioxide (CO_2) absorbents and is combined with various catalysts. These catalysts can react with inhaled anesthetics to produce various undesirable byproducts, including carbon monoxide and compound A. Sevoflurane in particular is known to produce compound A, and thus flow rates must be at least 2 L/min per manufacturer recommendations to prevent compound A accumulation and the associated potential renal injury, though no studies have found this to be clinically significant. As these reactions are exothermic, the avoidance of thermal injury is necessary. Carbon monoxide production is most associated with desflurane and occurs most significantly when the absorbent becomes desiccated. Knowledgeable practitioners and trained staff are essential for safe delivery and quick recognition of adverse side effects such as cardiorespiratory depression. The ability to recognize and immediately treat malignant hyperthermia must also be readily available as discussed later in the chapter.

Clinical Effects of Inhalational Anesthetics

Volatile anesthetics exert dose-dependent physiological changes throughout the body, which requires an extensive understanding when used in the clinical setting.

Circulatory System

A common effect of volatile agents is relaxing vascular smooth muscle leading to a decrease in systemic vascular resistance. This will ultimately lead to a dose-related decrease in mean arterial pressure, but only minimal changes will occur to cardiac inotropy in the adult population. The neonatal myocardium is more sensitive to inhalational anesthetics and may exhibit a greater decrease in contractility.

Enflurane, isoflurane, and desflurane result in 5–10% increases in HR from baseline, while sevoflurane does not usually exhibit until doses of 1.5 MAC [2]. These increases in heart rate are likely secondary to a reflex tachycardia from noxious stimuli on the airway receptors or activation of the sympathetic nervous system. Halothane reduces the arrhythmogenic threshold for epinephrine or increases the heart's sensitivity to catecholamines and causes ventricular dysrhythmias. Sevoflurane, isoflurane, and desflurane do not demonstrate the same dysrythmogenicity [3, 6]. Inhalational agents diminish the baroreceptor reflex during general anesthesia, with halothane and enflurane more than depression of the reflex than isoflurane or sevoflurane. The baroreflex returns to normal the quickest with the use of sevoflurane.

Volatile anesthetics can decrease oxygen consumption up to 15% during general anesthesia, as well as redistribute cardiac output. Blood flow is decreased to the liver, gut, and kidneys, while flow to the brain, skin, and muscle remains essentially unchanged [2].

Nitrous oxide is frequently combined with volatile anesthetics during general anesthesia and has unique cardiovascular actions. When combined with volatile anesthetics, both systemic vascular resistance and blood pressure are greater than without the nitrous oxide. This change is thought concentration, as well as the decrease in dose of the simultaneous administration of the volatile anesthetic [2].

Cerebral

All the potent inhalational anesthetics are dose-dependent cerebral vasodilators. They reduce cerebral metabolic rate but can increase cerebral blood flow and intracranial pressure by blunting cerebral autoregulation. This occurs by the uncoupling of cerebral blood flow and metabolism. Cerebral blood flow increases more significantly at concentrations greater than one MAC, thus further increasing ICP [7].

Volatiles cause characteristic changes in EEG. As depth of anesthesia increases, periods of electrical silence become more frequent, with an isoelectric pattern occurring at a range of 1.5–2.0 MAC. All volatiles depress the amplitude and increase the latency of somatosensory evoked potentials. Increasing MAC to 1 may abolish evoked potentials [6].

Hepatic

Volatile anesthetics undergo very little hepatic metabolism and minimally effect hepatic function. The best known potentially hepatotoxic drug is halothane causing "halothane hepatitis." This hepatitis can manifest as either a mild, self-limited form with no evidence of liver failure or a more severe, fulminant hepatitis that is most likely immune-mediated. Isoflurane, desflurane, and enflurane have been associated with acute hepatic failure, but the incidences attributed to them have been very small. Risk factors for developing volatile anesthetic-associated hepatitis include female gender, obesity, age, and, most importantly, a history of prior exposure [2].

Neuromuscular

Inhalational agents induce relaxation of both skeletal and smooth muscle by blocking nicotinic acetylcholine receptors at the neuromuscular junction. They may potentiate the required dose of a neuromuscular blocking agent, though it may not be sufficient to prevent patient movement in response to all noxious stimuli.

While smooth muscle relaxation may be beneficial in certain situations, it may also prove to be detrimental in others, for instance, it can cause nausea, emesis, or ileus from gastrointestinal smooth muscle relaxation [7].

Pulmonary

All volatile anesthetics affect ventilation in a dose-dependent manner. They increase respiratory rate and decrease tidal volume with minimal effects on decreasing minute ventilation until higher inspired concentrations of the gases are reached. The net ventilatory mechanics are also impacted by inhaled anesthetics. Functional residual capacity is decreased during general anesthesia from a decrease in the intercostal muscle tone, cephalad displacement of the diaphragm position and inward displacement of the rib cage [6], and the onset of phasic expiratory activity of respiratory muscles [2]. The decrease in FRC can lead to symptomatic hypoxemia that is overcome by positive pressure ventilation.

While volatiles affect vascular smooth muscle, they have very little effect on pulmonary vascular resistance. Modern volatile agents do inhibit hypoxic pulmonary vasoconstriction at high concentrations, thereby increasing V/Q mismatch, which may result in hypoxia.

Inhaled anesthetics have been used to treat status asthmaticus when conventional treatment fails. This works as an effective treatment as volatiles relax smooth muscle in the airway by decreasing smooth muscle tone from beta$_2$ receptor activation, inhibition of acetylcholine and histamine, and blocking of hypocapnic bronchoconstriction [2, 3]. The bronchodilating effect may be lessened when the bronchial epithelium is damaged, as seen in asthmatics or patients with respiratory viruses. Isoflurane and desflurane are more irritating to the airways than sevoflurane and can produce airway irritation and, in the instance of desflurane, can increase airway resistance. This irritation may lead to coughing or laryngospasm. Sevoflurane's less noxious properties make it the volatile agent of choice for an inhalation induction of general anesthesia, though isoflurane and desflurane are used for maintenance of anesthesia without increased incidence of airway irritation [2].

Volatile anesthetics reduce ciliary movement and alter the characteristics of mucus that can result in inadequate clearing of secretions, mucus plugging, atelectasis, and hypoxemia.

Biotransformation and Toxicity of Inhalational Anesthetic Agents

Comparing currently used anesthetics, sevoflurane is prone to significant biodegradation, followed by isoflurane and desflurane (Table 10.2). The biodegradation pathways of isoflurane and desflurane are closely related. Both isoflurane and desflurane involve cytochrome P450 2E1 enzymes that insert an active oxygen atom, producing HCl (isoflurane), HF (desflurane), and an unstable product that degrades to trifluoroacetic acid, carbon dioxide, fluoride ions, and water. Sevoflurane is also metabolized via cytochrome P450 2E1 oxidative biodegradation, producing carbon dioxide, inorganic fluoride, and hexafluoroisopropanol. Biodegradation is mostly found in the liver and only insignificantly in the kidney [8].

Table 10.2 Biodegradation of modern volatile anesthetics

Common anesthetics	% of metabolism
Sevoflurane	5–8
Isoflurane	0–0.2
Desflurane	0–0.02

Isoflurane

In adult population, there has been controversy regarding the use of isoflurane in patients with coronary artery disease because of the possibility of "coronary steal," which is diversion of blood from areas of the myocardium with inadequate perfusion to the myocardium with more adequate perfusion. However, this has not been shown to be clinically significant. Isoflurane exposure has also been demonstrated to induce cognitive decline in mice. Exposure of cultured human cells to isoflurane has been reported to induce apoptosis as well as accumulation and aggregation of amyloid beta protein. However, no clear link between clinical exposure to isoflurane and cognitive decline or dementia in humans has been established. The results from observational studies of anesthetic exposure in children have been mixed, and more preclinical and clinical studies are required to determine whether anesthetics cause injury to humans.

Sevoflurane

Sevoflurane metabolites include fluoride (F−), which has the potential to cause high-output renal failure. However, because of sevoflurane's low blood-gas solubility and its rapid elimination, fluoride concentrations fall very quickly after surgery, and renal toxicity from fluoride does not occur. The interaction of sevoflurane with dry carbon dioxide absorbents produces a chemical toxic to rats called "compound A." Larger amounts of breakdown products are produced at very low fresh gas flows, as a result of increased temperature of the soda lime, and when the soda lime is desiccated. Compound A causes serious injury to kidneys in rats but is not proven to cause the same in humans [9].

Desflurane

Desflurane is minimally metabolized. The interaction of desflurane with dry CO_2 absorbents produces carbon monoxide and possibly results in increased levels of blood carboxyhemoglobin. The major clinical drawbacks of desflurane are its airway pungency and cardiovascular reactivity making it difficult to use in pediatric population.

Table 10.3 Use of volatile anesthetics outside of the operating room

Advantages	Disadvantages
Bronchodilation	Nausea, vomiting
Anticonvulsant	Specialized equipment
Potential lung and myocardial protection	Cardiorespiratory depression
Minimal drug tolerance/tachyphylaxis or withdrawal	Nephrotoxicity
Postoperative sedation	Immunomodulation
Ease of titrating depth of sedation	Neuroapoptosis
Insignificant end organ metabolism	Malignant hyperthermia

Advantages of Inhalational Anesthetic Use in the PICU

The advantages of inhalational anesthetics in the critical care setting include improved management of status epilepticus, bronchospastic airway diseases such as status asthmaticus, alternative to traditional sedation practices, and potential for myocardial and lung protection (Table 10.3).

Status Epilepticus

Status epilepticus is a potentially life-threatening medical emergency. The definition of status epilepticus historically has been variable, though its current definition is accepted as continuous seizures lasting more than 5 minutes or intermittent seizures for 30 minutes without recovery in between seizures. Approximately 10–20% of children with epilepsy will have at least one instance of status epilepticus [10]. Refractory status epilepticus is when there is clinical or EEG evidence of seizures after 60 minutes despite treatment with a first-line anticonvulsant (benzodiazepine) and second-line anticonvulsant medications (i.e., fosphenytoin, phenytoin, phenobarbital, valproate, levetiracetam). Superrefractory status epilepticus is a refractory status epilepticus that persists or recurs after 24 hours of general anesthesia [11]. General anesthesia for refractory seizures may be achieved using intravenous (IV) agents or inhalational agents with the goal of burst suppression. IV anesthetic agents include pentobarbital, midazolam, or propofol. The use of IV anesthetic agents is typically limited by side effects and complications. It should be noted that propofol, while used in the adult population, has less utility in the pediatric population due to the risk of propofol infusion syndrome [11] and is contraindicated in the setting of a ketogenic diet. While the use of inhaled volatile anesthetics is not always included in the treatment algorithm for refractory status epilepticus, its use has been described in the literature since as early as the 1960s [12], and modern-day volatiles have been reported since the 1980s [13, 14]. Volatile agents are oftentimes considered the last resort after the failure of IV anesthetic agents. Their use in the ICU is limited by the ability to safely deliver the gas with appropriately trained personnel. Inhaled anesthetic agents have a marked advantage in the ability to provide almost immediate control of seizure activity. Retrospective reports have demonstrated isoflurane was effective in almost immediately stopping long-standing superrefractory status epilepticus [14, 15]. Another distinct advantage of inhaled volatile anesthetic gases is the ease at which they are measured and titrated. The minimum alveolar concentration of isoflurane required to achieve burst suppression is between 1.5% and 2%. In conjunction with continuous EEG monitoring, inhaled anesthetics are easily titratable to maintain the minimum concentration required for burst suppression. Even in prolonged use, there do not seem to be long-standing adverse effects on hepatic or renal function [15, 16]. There is not good evidence for how long to continue burst suppression under inhalational anesthesia. The time should be used to optimize antiepileptic therapy and identify and treat underlying etiologies. Much of the evidence supporting the efficacy of volatile anesthetics in arresting refractory status epilepticus is limited to case reports or series. Ideally, larger prospective randomized controlled trials would help identify the role in which volatile anesthesia should play in the management of status epilepticus.

Bronchospastic Airway Disease and Status Asthmaticus

Status asthmaticus is a life-threatening refractory asthma exacerbation that can result in respiratory failure and death. Standard treatment of status asthmaticus includes oxygen, inhaled short-acting beta agonists, corticosteroids, anticholinergics such as ipratropium, and intravenous magnesium sulfate. Subsequent treatment may include methylxanthines, noninvasive positive pressure ventilation, heliox, ketamine, nebulized epinephrine, mechanical ventilation, or extracorporeal membrane oxygenation (ECMO) [17, 18]. Inhaled volatile anesthetics are effective bronchodilators with halothane reported in the literature to successfully treat refractory severe status asthmaticus dating as far back as the 1930s with cyclopropane [19] and 1970s and 1980s with halothane [20, 21]. Since that time, there have been several case reports noting treatment of status asthmaticus with modern-day anesthetics including isoflurane or sevoflurane when conventional therapy has failed [22]. Several larger retrospective reviews have also reported successful treatment of severe asthma with isoflurane that was refractory to traditional management in pediatric and adult patients [23, 24]. Multiple reviews report improvement of pH and PCO_2 after initiation of inhaled volatile anesthetic therapy in the setting of status asthmaticus [23, 24]. Because the patients require mechanical ventilation for long-term delivery of inhaled anesthetics, volatile anesthesia has the added benefit of providing necessary sedation, reducing or eliminating the need for intravenous sedation. To date, much of the evidence supporting the effective use of volatile anesthesia for status asthmaticus is anecdotal and limited to case reports or case series. There may be a role for volatile anesthetics in the treatment of refractory status asthmaticus that fails to respond to conventional therapy. Ideally, randomized controlled trials would help further elucidate the role that inhaled volatile anesthetics should play in the treatment of refractory status asthmaticus.

Alternative Sedation Option for ICU Sedation

Approximately 85% of ICU undergoing mechanical ventilation or invasive procedures undergo sedation [25]. The most commonly used agents are intravenous and include benzodiazepines and propofol in conjunction with opioids. Ketamine, barbiturates, and dexmedetomidine are also utilized [25]. No intravenous sedation agent is ideal. Benzodiazepines may be associated with tolerance, withdrawal, or neuropsychiatric disorders (depression, anxiety, posttraumatic stress disorder) [26, 27]. Propofol may be associated with propofol infusion syndrome (potentially fatal complication as a result of prolonged propofol infusion), resulting in metabolic acidosis, rhabdomyolysis, hyperlipidemia, cardiac and renal failure [28], hypertriglyceridemia, and pancreatitis. Along with opioids, propofol and benzodiazepines rely on the liver and kidney for elimination [29]. Certain benzodiazepines have active metabolites. Both undersedation and oversedation are problematic with IV agents. Inhaled volatile agents have been used in the operating room for surgical anesthesia for over a century. As discussed previously, over the last few decades, they have also been used on occasion in the pediatric and adult critical care setting for the treatment of refractory status asthmaticus and epilepticus when conventional therapy has failed. More recently, investigation into its use as a sedative agent outside of the operating room has increased interest. Volatile anesthetic agents have distinct advantages in that they are easily measured and titratable, have a rapid onset of action, lack tolerance or tachyphylaxis, exhibit rapid offset with pulmonary elimination, and have low hepatic metabolism and no significant metabolites [30]. The ability to measure end-tidal concentration of inhaled volatile gases helps prevent over- or undersedation. Rapid washin and washout of gases contribute to its titratability. These both contribute to faster emergence times as compared to intravenous agents. In the adult literature, several trials have demonstrated that in short-term postoperative sedation, inhaled volatile sedation has shorter times to extubation when compared to midazolam or propofol [31–33]. Similar results have been demonstrated with longer-term sedation trials [34, 35]. Mesnil et al. also demonstrated that the sevoflurane group had a reduction in morphine consumption 24 h post extubation as compared to the midazolam and propofol groups, suggesting a possible benefit of opioid sparing when inhaled volatile agents are used for sedation [35].

There may be a role for the use of inhaled volatile agents for sedation in the critical care setting. Trials are currently underway examining the use of volatile agents for long-term sedation in North America (VALTS) and Germany (IsoConDa) [4]. Prior to adopting widespread use of volatile sedation in the ICU setting, the safety, efficacy, and benefit over traditional intravenous sedation must be demonstrated. In addition to this, safe delivery with specialized devices and appropriately trained practitioners and personnel remains a large obstacle.

Potential Myocardial and Lung Protection Properties

Pharmacologic conditioning of the heart occurs when exposure to a particular drug protects the heart from ischemia or reperfusion injury. Preconditioning occurs when the protective effect follows exposure prior to the ischemic event; postconditioning occurs when the protective effect takes place when exposure occurs immediately following the ischemic event. Volatile anesthetic agents appear to be a class of drugs that demonstrate pre- and postconditioning in animal models [36, 37]. There appears to be a benefit of using volatile agents during cardiac surgery; however, there was no difference in myocardial ischemia during noncardiac surgery when comparing volatile agents to total intravenous anesthesia [38]. In one pediatric study of children undergoing ventricular septal defect repairs, preconditioning with volatiles demonstrated decreased creatinine kinase MB (CK MB) release. It showed a trend to decrease inotropic support and ventilation and intensive care unit duration; however it was not statistically significant [39].

In addition to potential cardioprotection, volatile anesthetics have demonstrated protection on other organ systems including the lungs. In rodent models, sevoflurane was shown to suppress inflammation [41], and isoflurane decreased lung injury and vascular leakage [40]. Most of the clinical data in humans regarding pulmonary protection rely on intraoperative exposure to volatile anesthetics. When compared to propofol, patients under one-lung ventilation anesthetized with volatile anesthetics had decreased markers of inflammation [41] and reduced adverse events including pneumonia, atelectasis, pleural effusion, and bronchopulmonary fistula [42]. A prospective analysis of data on 124,497 patients over an 8-year period found that higher intraoperative inhalational anesthetic dose was associated with a lower odds of postoperative respiratory complications and also with a lower 30-day mortality [43].

While preclinical evidence for the role of volatile anesthetics in cardiac conditioning and lung protection is compelling, further investigation into the role volatile agents may play in clinically relevant cardiac and pulmonary protection is necessary, especially in the pediatric population.

Disadvantages of Inhalational Anesthetic Use in the PICU

There is growing interest for the use of potent inhaled anesthetics outside the operating room especially in the ICU. The disadvantages of volatile anesthetic (Table 10.3) use in the ICU include cost, equipment needs, cardiorespiratory depression, side effect profile of the volatile anesthetics, malignant hyperthermia (MH), immunomodulatory effects, and neurocognitive dysfunction.

Specialized Equipment

The primary limitation to the use of inhalational anesthetics in the PICU setting traditionally has been related to practical difficulties associated with administration of inhaled anesthetic agents outside of the operating room. These difficulties include problems with administration, monitoring, and gas scavenging. Routine use has been limited by the requirement of vaporizers, specially adapted ventilators and high flow respiratory circuits resulting in high agent consumption, costs, and concerns about environmental contamination. Inhalational anesthetic implementation in the ICU requires engineering upgrade of a significant part of the ICU for gas-scavenging infrastructure and technical investments such as the filters, delivery pumps, and gas analyzer. The availability of miniature vaporizers, such as the Anesthesia Conserving Device (AnaConDa; Sedana Medical, Uppsala, Sweden) and the more recently introduced MIRUS system (Pall Medical, Dreieich, Germany), has attempted to simplify bedside volatile anesthetic administration [44]. AnaConDa is the most studied and widely used heat moisture exchanger in the world. Unfortunately it does add 100 ml to the dead space in the ventilator circuit, which may result in hypercapnia especially during weaning from mechanical ventilation [34]. Another potential problem is inadvertent intravenous injection as the Luer-lock anesthetic infusion line has a similar appearance to intravenous infusion lines [45]. Additionally, workplace contamination may occur during refilling of the syringes and loss of anesthetic to the environment during frequent tracheal tube suctioning. Currently, the MIRUS device and AnaConDa are available in very limited countries and have not been approved for use in the USA. The implementation of inhaled anesthetics in critical care setting requires an important educational intervention directed at the physicians, nurses, and respiratory therapists. Knowledge about agents has to be maintained round the clock across all shifts and staff rotations.

Cardiorespiratory Depression

Volatile anesthetics universally produce concentration-dependent myocardial depression. This is due primarily to altered Ca^{2+} entry and sarcoplasmic reticulum Ca^{2+} handling [46]. The negative inotropy is compounded by decreases in systemic vascular resistance (SVR) by isoflurane, desflurane, and sevoflurane to further reduce blood pressure. Reduction in SVR is most prominent with isoflurane, supporting the theory of coronary steal phenomenon in patients with coronary artery disease. All volatile anesthetics prolong the QT interval, potentially increasing the risk of torsades de pointes polymorphic ventricular tachycardia. Volatile anesthetics also cause dose-dependent respiratory depression. Inhalational anesthetics significantly affect respiration in infants and children in a dose-dependent fashion via effects on the respiratory center, chest wall muscles, and reflex responses. Isoflurane, sevoflurane, and desflurane depress ventilatory drive and response to CO_2, resulting in a dose-dependent decrease in alveolar ventilation mainly through reduction in tidal volume, while the respiratory rate is maintained or slightly increased. The increased respiratory rate during inhalational anesthesia has been attributed to sensitization of the stretch receptors within the lung as well as possible central effects. Even at subanesthetic concentrations, it blunts the hypoxic and hypercarbic ventilatory responses.

Adverse Effects of Inhalational Agents

Some of the adverse effects of inhalational anesthetics include nephrotoxicity, hepatotoxicity, and nausea and vomiting. Inhalational anesthetics affect renal function potentially due to four possible mechanisms: cardiovascular, autonomic, neuroendocrine, and metabolic. Metabolic mechanism is a serious clinical concern that has led to renal dysfunction after inhalational anesthesia. Metabolism of inhalational anesthetics releases inorganic fluoride that has been postulated to cause renal dysfunction. A second theoretical cause of sevoflurane-associated renal dysfunction is compound A, a product of alkaline hydrolysis of sevoflurane in the presence of CO_2 absorbents. In vivo, sevoflurane is metabolized by microsomal CYP IIE1 isozyme in both the liver and kidneys. The peak plasma concentration of inorganic fluoride is proportional to the duration of exposure to sevoflurane in children [8]. However, studies have failed to show any evidence of nephrotoxicity with prolonged volatile use, even in the setting of high fluoride levels.

Isoflurane, sevoflurane, and desflurane have also been associated with transient hepatic dysfunction and raised transaminase enzymes. This severe form involves massive hepatic necrosis that can lead to death. The mechanism for this severe injury is immunologic, requiring prior exposure to a volatile anesthetic. Isoflurane and desflurane all undergo oxidative metabolism by cytochrome P450 enzymes to produce trifluoroacetate. The trifluoroacetate can bind covalently to hepatocyte proteins. The trifluoroacetyl-hepatocyte moieties can act as haptens, which the body recognizes as foreign and to which the immune system forms antibodies. Subsequent exposure to any anesthetic capable of producing trifluoroacetate may provoke an immune response, leading to severe hepatic necrosis [47].

The use of volatile anesthetics is associated with a twofold increase in the risk of PONV, with risk increasing in a dose-dependent manner, and no significant difference in incidence with different volatile anesthetics [48]. The exact nature of vomiting pathways is complex and also not fully understood, but a number of pathophysiological mechanisms known to cause nausea or vomiting have been identified. The main coordinator is the vomiting center, a collection of neurons located in the medulla oblongata. Such structures include the chemoreceptor trigger zone (CRTZ), located at the caudal end of the fourth ventricle in the area postrema, and the nucleus tractus solitarius (NTS), located in the area postrema and lower pons. The CRTZ receives input from vagal afferents in the gastrointestinal tract, and it can also detect emetogenic toxins, metabolites, and drugs circulating in the blood and cerebrospinal fluid due to its lack of the blood-brain barrier. The CRTZ projects neurons to the NTS, which receives input from vagal afferents and from the vestibular and limbic systems. The NTS triggers vomiting by stimulating the rostral nucleus, the nucleus ambiguous, the ventral respiratory group, and the dorsal motor nucleus of the vagus. PONV is also linked to several other stimuli, including opioids, volatile anesthetics, anxiety, adverse drug reactions, and motion. Multiple neurotransmitter pathways are implicated in the physiology of nausea and vomiting [49]. Enterochromaffin cells in the gastrointestinal tract release serotonin, and the vagus nerve communicates with the CRTZ via 5-HT3 receptors. The CRTZ communicates with the NTS primarily via dopamine-2 (D2) receptors. The vestibular system, which detects changes in equilibrium, communicates with the NTS via histamine-1 (H1) and acetylcholine (mACh). Anticipatory or anxiety-induced nausea and vomiting appears to originate in the cerebral cortex, which communicates directly with the NTS via several types of neuroreceptors [49]. Therefore, antiemetic drugs have been developed to target these specific receptors. Given that available antiemetic drugs work on different receptor classes, multiple antiemetics can be safely and effectively combined to reduce the risk of PONV in high-risk patients.

Malignant Hyperthermia (MH)

Malignant hyperthermia (MH) is a rare (1 in 50,000 to 100,000) pharmacogenetic disorder of skeletal muscle triggered in susceptible individuals by all volatile inhalational anesthetics. In addition to volatile agents, depolarizing skeletal muscle relaxants such as succinylcholine can also trigger MH. This syndrome has been linked to mutation in the type 1 ryanodine receptor (RyR1) in more than 50% of cases studied to date. Signs of MH include tachycardia, increased expired CO_2, muscle rigidity, and increased temperature and are related to increased metabolism (hypermetabolic state). The key aspects of management include discontinuation of volatile anesthetics and succinylcholine, immediate administration of intravenous dantrolene, and treatment of potentially life-threatening electrolyte abnormalities such as hyperkalemia. The Malignant Hyperthermia Association of the United States (MHAUS) provides detailed treatment recommendations on its website http://www.mhaus.org/healthcare-professionals. MHAUS also maintains a 24-hour hotline for emergency advice (1-800-644-9737 in the USA; 001-209-417-3722 outside of the USA). Dantrolene markedly attenuates the loss of calcium from sarcoplasmic reticulum, restoring the metabolism to normal and reversing the signs of metabolic stimulation. This can be difficult to diagnose in the critically ill patient in the ICU setting due to other comorbidities [50]. Use of volatile anesthetics requires staff education, malignant hyperthermia protocol adoption, and dantrolene availability to manage this rare medical emergency.

Immunomodulatory Effects

Volatile anesthetics have long been known to moderately suppress the immune system. Numerous studies have investigated whether this suppression increased the risk of postoperative wound infection, and no correlation was ever identified.

Although specific targets of volatile anesthetics in the immune system have not been well defined, molecular and cellular events involved in immunomodulation by volatile anesthetics have been identified, including a reduction in the number of immune cells due to cell death and the suppression of immune activities. Whether this immunosuppression hinders the host's ability to kill malignant cells liberated during surgical manipulation has become a question of research interest. There have been mixed results in rat models. Theoretically, many perioperative factors potentially suppress the host immunity and augment the cancer cells, leading to the growth of minimally residual tumor cells and recurrence of cancer. Some studies have reported potentially harmful immunosuppression or cancer cell augmentation after anesthesia with volatile anesthetics [51, 52]. Other identified co-founding factors have shown intermittent association with poor outcomes, including surgical stress response, hypotension, hypothermia, hyperglycemia, blood transfusions, glucocorticoids, and NSAIDs [51]. Well-controlled randomized clinical trials are needed, although isolating effects of volatile anesthetics from other factors in a perioperative setting remains challenging. Future studies should take into consideration the surgical procedures involved, the anesthetics and other medications used, and the time dependence in immunomodulation and resolution.

Neurocognition Effects

Over the last decade, the safety of the anesthetic agents has come under scrutiny after the realization that immature animals demonstrate neurodegeneration and long-lasting neurocognitive and behavioral deficiencies and elderly animals have learning and memory impairment after exposure to general anesthesia [53]. All of the commonly used anesthetic and sedative agent classes bind either to the GABA receptor or to the N-methyl-D-aspartate receptor (NMDA – a subtype of the glutamate receptor) to produce their anesthetic and sedative effects. Evidence from animal studies suggests that most general anesthetics which block NMDA receptor or bind GABA receptors trigger neuroapoptosis or programmed cell death in the developing brain. These agents include inhalational anesthetics which bind to GABA receptors. NMDA-binding agents include nitrous oxide and ketamine.

In immature rodents and monkeys at critical developmental periods, exposure to either NMDA receptor blockers or GABAergic agents can lead to increased apoptosis [54]. The effects are dose dependent and seen over particular periods of early development. There is some evidence that rodents exposed to anesthesia during infancy have delayed neurobehavioral development. One of the proposed mechanisms for anesthetic-induced neuroapoptosis in the developing brain occurs when binding of GABA and NMDA agents blocks normal neurotransmission in the GABA and glutamate systems, resulting in synaptic deprivation [55, 56]. This in turn leads to the activation of the intrinsic neuroapoptotic cascade due to lack of neuronal stimulation. Mitochondrial disruption occurs as part of this process and can be observed in electron microscopic studies of anesthetic exposure. Caspase 9 is released from the mitochondria, resulting in increased caspase 3 concentrations, inciting the completion of the neuroapoptosis process [55, 56].

The most important human studies to assess the impact of anesthesia on the developing brain include the General Anesthesia Compared to Spinal Anesthesia (GAS) and the Pediatric Anesthesia Neurodevelopmental Assessment (PANDA). The GAS randomized infants undergoing inguinal hernia repair to either an awake-regional technique or a general anesthetic. Secondary outcomes assessed at 2 years of age showed no increased risk of adverse neurodevelopment in children exposed to a general anesthetic [57]. The PANDA study compared children who had undergone inguinal hernia repair with general anesthesia before 3 years of age with an unexposed sibling. No difference in IQ was found between exposed and unexposed siblings [58]. The results from these trials suggest that a short-duration anesthetic in otherwise-healthy children may have limited effects. Nevertheless, the concerns regarding anesthetic neurotoxicity led the US Food and Drug Administration (FDA) to issue a drug safety communication.

In 2017, the US FDA issued a drug safety communication stating that the use of general anesthetic drugs "for lengthy periods of time or over multiple surgeries or procedures may negatively affect brain development in children younger than 3 years" [59]. "Lengthy" is defined as >3 h; this warning has resulted in a labeling change to all common anesthetic drugs binding to GABA and NMDA receptors, including volatile anesthetic agents. Furthermore, US FDA warns that "…we should discuss with parents, caregivers, and pregnant women the benefits, risks, and appropriate timing of surgery or procedures requiring anesthetic and sedation drugs" [59]. The International Anesthesia Research Society, in a collaborative public-private partnership with the FDA, formed SmartTots (Smart Strategies to Reduce Anesthesia Risk in Tots; www.smarttots.org) to coordinate and fund research with the goal of ensuring safe surgery for infants and children who undergo anesthesia and/or sedation.

Conclusions

Volatile agents are a family of inhalational general anesthetics and its use in the ICU setting holds a promising potential. However, additional study and overcoming barriers to ICU adoption need to be addressed before volatiles become routinely used in critical care setting. Current evidence suggests that volatiles have beneficial properties beyond the operating room. To show that volatiles present a clear clinical benefit, larger trials are required to see whether these agents display better sedation ventilation outcomes, cytoprotective properties, and longer-term cognitive effects compared with current intravenous methods. Furthermore, introducing change to existing clinical practice and organizational behaviors and attitudes presents an additional challenge in the ICU settings. Presently, delivery of volatile agents in the ICU is a new approach for many critical care providers who have limited anesthesia training related to volatile delivery. As a result, education and training programs will be necessary to assist intensivists with the learning curve in understanding this group of agents, optimizing complex drug delivery system and avoiding pitfalls. Evolving research will continue to provide insights of whether these agents have new therapeutic indications beyond the operating room.

References

1. Quasha AL, Eger EI II, et al. Determination and application of MAC. Anesthesiology. 1980;53:315–34.
2. Barash PG, Cullen BF, Stoelting RK, Cahalan MK, Stock MC, Ortega R. Clinical anesthesia. Philadelphia: Wolters Kluwer; 2017.
3. Kaplan JA, Augoustides JG, Manecke GR, Maus T, Reich DL. Kaplan's cardiac anesthesia: for cardiac and noncardiac surgery. 7th ed. Philadelphia: Elsevier; 2017.
4. Jerath A, Parotto M, et al. Opportunity knocks? The expansion of volatile agent use in new clinical settings. J Ccardiothorac Vasc Anesth. 2018;32:1946–54.
5. Mashari A, Fisher JA, Fedorko L, et al. Technology III: in-line vaporizer with reflector. J Clin Monit Comput. 2018;32:647.
6. Pardo M, Miller RD, Miller RD. Basics of anesthesia. 6th ed. Philadelphia: Elsevier; 2018.
7. Hays SR, Joshi GP, Nussmeier NA. Inhalation anesthetic agents: Clinical Effects and uses. 2018, September 28. Retrieved March 5, 2019, from https://www.uptodate.com/home.
8. Kharasch ED, Hankins DC, Thummel KE. Human kidney methoxyflurane and sevoflurane metabolism. Intrarenal fluoride production as a possible mechanism of methoxyflurane nephrotoxicity. Anesthesiology. 1995;82:689–99.
9. Eger EI 2nd, Eisenkraft JB. In: Weiskopf RB, editor. The pharmacology of inhaled anesthetics. Chicago: Healthcare Press; 2003. p. 167–76.
10. Shinnar S, Berg AT, Moshe SL, O'Dell C, Alemany M, Newstein D, Kang H, Goldensohn ES, Hauser WASO. The risk of seizure recurrence after a first unprovoked afebrile seizure in childhood: an extended follow-up. Pediatrics. 1996;98(2 Pt 1):216.
11. Wilkes R, Tasker RC. Pediatric intensive care treatment of uncontrolled status epilepticus. Crit Care Clin. 2013;29(2):239–57. https://doi.org/10.1016/j.ccc.2012.11.007. Epub 2013 Jan 3. Review
12. Carter S, Gold AP. The critically ill child: management of status epilepticus. Pediatrics. 1969;44(5 Part I):732–3.
13. Rodney M, Soifer BE, Gelb AW. Isoflurane for the management of status epilepticus. Ann Pharmacother. 1989;23(7-8):579–81.
14. Kofke WA, Young RS, Davis P, Woelfel SK, Gray L, Johnson D, Gelb A, Meeke R, Warner DS, Pearson KS, et al. Isoflurane for refractory status epilepticus: a clinical series. Anesthesiology. 1989;71(5):653–9.
15. Mirsattari SM, Sharpe MD, Young GB. Treatment of refractory status epilepticus with inhalational anesthetic agents isoflurane and desflurane. Arch Neurol. 2004;61(8):1254–9.
16. John H, Truog RD, Rice SA. Prolonged administration of isoflurane to pediatric patients. Anesth Analg. 1993;76(3):520–6.
17. Carrie S, Anderson TA. Volatile anesthetics for status asthmaticus in pediatric patients: a comprehensive review and case series. Pediatr Anesth. 2015;25:460–7.
18. Rehder KJ. Adjunct therapies for refractory status Asthmaticus in children. Respir Care. June 2017;62(6):849–65.
19. Meyer NE, Schotz S. Relief of severe intractable bronchial asthma with cyclopropane anesthesia: report of a case. J Allergy. 1939;10:239–40.
20. Colaco CM. Halothane for status asthmaticus in the intensive care unit – a case report. Can AnaesthSoc J. 1978;25(4):329–30.
21. Schwartz SH. Treatment of status asthmaticus with halothane. JAMA. 1984;251(20):2688–9.
22. Watanabe K, et al. Prolonged sevoflurane inhalation therapy for status asthmaticus in an infant. PediatrAnesth. 2008;18(6):543–5.
23. Carrie S, Anderson TA. Volatile anesthetics for status asthmaticus in pediatric patients: a comprehensive review and case series. Pediatr Anesthes. 2015;25:460–7.
24. Schutte D, Zwitserloot AM, et al. Sevoflurane therapy for life threatening asthma in children. Br J Anaesth. 2013;111(6):967–70.
25. Weinart CR, Calvin AD. Epidemiology of sedation and sedation adequacy for mechanically ventilated patients in a medical and surgical intensive care unit. Crit Care Med. 2007;35:393–401.

26. Wade DM, et al. Investigating risk factors for psychological morbidity three months after intensive care: a prospective cohort study. Crit Care. 2012;16:R192.
27. Griffiths J, et al. The prevalence of post traumatic stress disorder in survivors of ICU treatment: a systemic review. Intensive Care Med. 2007;33:1506–18.
28. Fodale V, La Monac E. Propofol infusion syndrome: an overview of a perplexing disease. Drug Saf. 2008;31(4):293–303.
29. Barr J, Fraser GL, et al. Clinical practice guidelines for the management of pain, agitation, and delirium in adult patients in the intensive care unit. Crit Care Med. 2013;41:263–306.
30. Preckel B, Bolten J. Pharmacology of modern volatile anaesthetics. Best Pract Res Clin Anaesthesiol. 2005;19:331–48.
31. Rohm KD, Wolf MW, Schollhorn T, et al. Short term sevoflurane sedation using the anaesthetic conserving device after cardiothoracic surgery. Intensive Care Med. 2008;34:1683–9.
32. Hellstrom J, Owall A, SAckey PV. Wake-up times following sedation with sevoflurane versus propofol after cardiac surgery. Scand Cardiovasc J. 2012;46:262–8.
33. Jerath A, Ferguson ND, et al. The use of volatile anesthetic agents for long term critical care sedation (VALTS): study protocol for pilot randomized controlled trial. Trials. 2015;16:560.
34. Sackey PV, Martling CR, Granath F, et al. Prolonged isoflurane sedation of intensive care unit patients with anesthetic conserving device. Crit Care Med. 2004;32:2241–6.
35. Mesnil M, Capdevila X, Bringuier S, Trine PO, et al. Long-term sedation in intensive care unit: a randomized comparison between inhaled sevoflurane and intravenous propofol or midazolam. Intensive Care Med. 2011;37:933–41.
36. Kikuchi C, Dosenovic S, Bienengraeber M. Anesthetics as cardioprotectants: translatability and mechanism. Br J Pharmacol. 2015;172:2051–61.
37. Knapp J, Bergmann G, et al. Pre and postconditioning effect of sevoflurane on myocardial dysfunction after cardiopulmonary resuscitation in rats. Resuscitation. 2013;84:1450–5.
38. Lotz C, Kehl F. Volatile anesthetic induced cardiac protection: molecular mechanisms, clinical aspects, and interactions with non volatile agents. J Cardiothorac Vasc Anesth. 2015;29(3):749–60.
39. Singh P, Chauhan S, Jain G, et al. Comparison of cardioprotective effects of volatile anesthetics in children undergoing ventricular septal defect closure. World Pediatrcongenit Heart Surg. 2013;4:24–9.
40. Englert JA, Macias AA, Amador-Munoz D, et al. Isoflurane ameliorates acute lung injury by preserving epithelial tight junction integrity. Anesthesiology. 2015;123L:377–88.
41. Schilling T, Kozian A, Kretzschmar M, et al. Effects of propofol and desflurane anaesthesia on the alveolar inflammatory response to one-lung ventilation. Br J Anaesth. 2007;99:368–75.
42. DeConno E, Steurer MP, Wittlinger M, et al. Anesthetic-induced improvement of the inflammatory response to one-lung ventilation. Anesthesiology. 2009;110:1316–26.
43. Grabitz SD, Farhan HN, Ruscic KJ, et al. Dose dependent protective effect of inhalational anesthetics against postoperative respiratory complications: a prospective analysis of data on file from three hospitals in New England. Crit Care Med. 2017;45(1):e30–9.
44. Soukup J, Schärff K, Kubosch K, Pohl C, Bomplitz M, Kompardt J. State of the art: sedation concepts with volatile anesthetics in critically ill patients. J Crit Care. 2009;24:535–44.
45. Berton J, Sargentini C, Nguyen JL, Belii A, Beydon L. AnaConDa® reflection filter: bench and patient evaluation of safety and volatile anesthetic conservation. Anesth Analg. 2007;104:130–4.
46. Wheeler DM, Katz A, Rice RT, et al. Volatile anesthetic effects on sarcoplasmic reticulum Ca content and sarcolemmal Ca flux in isolated rat cardiac cell suspensions. Anesthesiology. 1994;80:372–82.
47. Njoku D, Laster MJ, Gong DH, et al. Biotransformation of halothane, enflurane, isoflurane and desflurane to trifluoroacetylated liver proteins: association between protein acetylation and hepatic injury. Anesth Analg. 1997;84:173–8.
48. Stern R. The psychophysiology of nausea. Acta Biol Hung. 2002;53:589–99.
49. Sclocco R, Kim J, Garcia R, Sheehan J, Beissner F, Bianchi A, et al. Brain circuitry supporting multi-organ autonomic outflow in response to nausea. Cereb Cortex. 2014;26(2):485–97.

50. Schuster F, Moegele S, Johannsen S, et al. Malignant hyperthermia in the intensive care setting. Crit Care. 2014;18:411.
51. Das J, Kumar S, Khanna S, Mehta Y. Are we causing the recurrence-impact of perioperative period on long-term cancer prognosis: review of current evidence and practice. J Anaesthesiol Clin Pharmacol. 2014;30:153–9.
52. Heaney A, Buggy DJ. Can anaesthetic and analgesic techniques affect cancer recurrence or metastasis? Br J Anaesth. 2012;109:i17–28.
53. Jevtovic-Todorovic V. Exposure of developing brain to general anesthesia: what is the animal evidence? Anesthesiology. 2018;128:832–9.
54. Jevtovic-Todorovic V. General anesthetics and neurotoxicity: how much do we know? Anesthesiol Clin. 2016;34:439–51.
55. Braun S, Gaza N, Werdehausen R, Hermanns H, Bauer K, Durieux ME, Hollman MW, Stevens MF. Ketamine induces apoptosis via the mitochondrial pathway in human lymphocytes and neuronal cells. Br J Anaesth. 2010;105:347–54.
56. Andropoulos DB. Effect of anesthesia on the developing brain: infant and fetus. Fetal Diagn Ther. 2018;43:1–11.
57. Davidson AJ, Disma N, de Graaff JC, Withington DE, Dorris L, Bell G, GAS Consortium, et al. Neurodevelopmental outcome at 2 years of age after general anaesthesia and awake-regional anaesthesia in infancy(GAS): an international multicentre, randomised controlled trial. Lancet. 2016;387:239–50.
58. Sun LS, Li G, Miller TL, Salorio C, Byrne MW, Bellinger DC, et al. Association between a single general anesthesia exposure before age 36 months and neurocognitive outcomes in later childhood. JAMA. 2016;315:231220.
59. US Food and Drug Administration Drug safety communication: FDA approves label changes for use of general anesthetic and sedation drugs in young children. https://www.fda.gov/Drugs/DrugSafety/ucm554634.htm. Date: April 27, 2017.

Chapter 11
Tolerance and Withdrawal in Critically Ill Children

Anne Stormorken

Introduction

The literature regarding sedative regimens in critically ill children is prolific. Opioids and benzodiazepines are historically the most commonly administered drugs to provide analgesia and sedation [1–3]. However, alpha-2 adrenergic agents including clonidine and dexmedetomidine are increasingly used primarily due to decreased effect on minute ventilation [4]. Historically, analgesic and sedative regimens have focused primarily on achieving physiological states that facilitated synchrony with therapy such as mechanical ventilation, bedsides care and promoted amnesia, analgesia, and hypno-sedation. Unfortunately, medications were not always administered with protocols, or their effects evaluated via consistent use of pain or sedation assessment tools. More recently, the PICU culture is shifting to focus on balancing the benefit of analgesia and sedation/hypnosis with minimizing tolerance, withdrawal, and delirium. The scope of this focus has also widened to include post-intensive care unit (PICU) impact. Acknowledging the central role of validated assessment tools in assessing pain, sedation, withdrawal, and delirium, the paradigm of care has shifted to include neurocognitive assessment as an important part of patient outcomes. Analgosedation regimens should be tailored to the individual patient to optimize analgesia and sedation and minimize tolerance, withdrawal, and delirium, while promoting mobility and intermittent periods of awareness [5]. Recent trials conducted in children to identify benefits associated with analgosedative protocols or daily sedation interruption have not provided clear paths to achieve these goals.

A. Stormorken (✉)
Case Western Reserve University, Cleveland, OH, USA
e-mail: Anne.Stormorken@UHhospitals.org

P. P. Kamat, J. W. Berkenbosch (eds.), *Sedation and Analgesia for the Pediatric Intensivist*, https://doi.org/10.1007/978-3-030-52555-2_11

Tolerance

Tolerance, dependence, and withdrawal are iatrogenic complications of critical illness in children which may be experienced during an ICU admission. Decreasing mortality through advances in critical care such as mechanical ventilation, continuous renal replacement therapy, and extracorporeal support has led to protracted exposure to analgesics and sedatives.

Tolerance is defined as escalating drug dose requirements to maintain the same clinical effect [6–8] and has been variably studied using the outcome of doubling of the dose [9] or doubling of infusion rate [10] as being clinically significant. The observation of tolerance development has been reported in both pediatric and neonatal critical care although, to date, no clear guidelines exist to mitigate its development [6, 7, 11–13]. The complete pathophysiology underlying tolerance development remains unclear although it is better understood for some agents compared to others. For opioids the mechanisms appear to include desensitization of receptor-mediated pathways involved in nociception, upregulation in expression of protein kinase C (PKC) and G protein-coupled receptor kinases (GRK) in inhibitory analgesic pathway, increased nociception via activated immune cell release of cytokines, and receptor downregulation with chronic exposure [8, 14].

Tolerance has been observed to develop earlier with continuous drug infusions [8, 10, 14], and the rate of occurrence is related to dose and duration of drug administered. Tolerance to analgesic effects of opioids occurs more rapidly than to respiratory depressive effects, requiring cautious up-titration in dosing. There have been no prospective RCTs in critically ill children which compare opioids and tolerance. Postulated mechanisms included increased affinity for opioid receptors with synthetic opioids such as fentanyl [7]. Methadone poses the least risk due to associated NMDA antagonism [13]. Anand et al. observed that in surgical patients but not medical patients, exposure to fentanyl rather than morphine infusions was associated with tolerance development. In medical and surgical patients, coadministration with benzodiazepines and increased duration of opioid delivery were both positively associated with increased risk of tolerance [9].

Preventing and minimizing the impact of tolerance may involve multiple strategies including reducing drug exposure and use of multimodal analgesic regimens including regional anesthesia as well as drug rotation. Multimodal analgesia includes delivery of non-opioids such as acetaminophen, nonsteroidal anti-inflammatory drugs, as well as adjuvants such as ketamine or gabapentin in addition to opioids. Neuraxial and peripheral regional analgesic techniques provide targeted pain relief without the adverse effects of nausea, vomiting, over-sedation, and respiratory depression encountered with the use of opioids. Switching from morphine to fentanyl may obviate increasing tolerance secondary to lack of nociceptive morphine-3-glucuronide metabolite as well as taking advantage of mu receptor subtypes [8].

Dependence and Iatrogenic Withdrawal Syndrome

Dependence is the physiologic state that occurs when drug administration must continue in order to avoid signs and symptoms of withdrawal. Iatrogenic withdrawal syndrome (IWS) refers to observed signs and symptoms experienced by patients when analgesic or sedative drug administration in a drug-dependent patient has been either abruptly discontinued or weaned too rapidly [13]. The exact constellation of signs and symptoms as well as their severity is determined by drug class and total drug exposure [13, 15–19]. The majority of the symptomatology is related to central nervous system (CNS) activation and autonomic dysfunction, presumably reflecting the location of involved receptors. Historically, IWS has been primarily described from benzodiazepine and opioid infusions as these were most frequently administered. However with increasing use of dexmedetomidine infusions, IWS from alpha-agonists has also been described. Opioid-based IWS manifests typically as irritability, agitation, inconsolability, and tremors related to CNS dysfunction. Tachycardia, hypertension, diaphoresis, and hyperpyrexia reflect autonomic dysfunction. Gastrointestinal (GI) effects occur due to mu receptors found throughout the GI tract and may manifest as feeding refusal, nausea, vomiting, and diarrhea [15]. Description of iatrogenic benzodiazepine withdrawal syndrome is not as specific as sole administration is uncommon in critically ill children. Symptoms primarily include those related to CNS and autonomic dysfunction, while GI symptoms appear to be uncommon. Additionally, delirium and seizures have been reported [20, 21]. Inclusion of alpha-2 agonists such as clonidine and dexmedetomidine in analgosedative regimens is increasing. Initial case reports revealed bradycardia and hypertension upon abrupt discontinuation of either agent. Subsequent cohort studies and reviews confirm these findings with the additional observations of irritability, agitation, sleeplessness, hypertonicity, and seizures. Similar to benzodiazepine withdrawal, it can be difficult to evaluate dexmedetomidine-related IWS as alpha-agonists are commonly employed in combination regimens, especially with opioids. Small studies of sole dexmedetomidine administration suggest this CNS and autonomic dysfunction profile comprises dexmedetomidine-related withdrawal syndrome [22–25].

Correct attribution of patient agitation to pain, under-sedation, or withdrawal is challenging enough; ascribing which agent is responsible for IWS provides additional complexity. The development of IWS-specific screening tools validated across the spectrum of ages, developmental conditions, critical illness, and patient comorbidities has contributed greatly to solving this problem [26, 27]. Initially validated in neonates born to heroin-addicted mothers, the Neonatal Abstinence Scale (NAS) defines the manifested symptomatology in these babies [28]. Subsequent development of two assessment scales more germane to the population of critically ill children, the Withdrawal Assessment Tool-1 (WAT-1) and the Sophia Observational Score (SOS), have afforded improved understanding of the prevalence of withdrawal as well as risk factors. Franck et al. derived and validated the WAT-1 in critically ill children over a representative pediatric age range as well as illness acuity. The WAT-1 is comprised of a 12-point scale that assesses the patient's vital sign changes and behavioral response to a mild stimulus such as bedside care in addition to evaluating the chart. Scores greater than or equal to 3 demonstrate specificity of 88% and sensitivity of 87% for presence of withdrawal [29, 30]. Ista et al. derived and validated the 15-item SOS in a comparable patient population, and scores greater than or equal to 4 demonstrate specificity of 95% and sensitivity of 83% for presence of withdrawal [31–33]. Systematic reviews of these assessment tools underscore the positive inter-rater reliability of both tools as well as the lack of specific attribution for opioids or benzodiazepines as study patients received both classes of drugs [27, 34]. Amigoni et al. evaluation of IWS in critically ill children found that positive values of WAT-1 and SOS were correlated in a statistically significant fashion ($p < 0.001$) [35].

To date no screening tool for alpha-agonist withdrawal has been developed. Withdrawal attributed to these agents is suspected if the clinical symptoms of tachycardia, hypertension, and CNS agitation are observed within the appropriate clinical context and lack of response is noted with administration of benzodiazepines or opioids but ameliorated with provision of dexmedetomidine or clonidine. Recognizing delirium as a clinical construct with shared symptoms in critically ill children, it must also be acknowledged that screening tools have limitations. Importantly, there is overlap in symptomatology between pain, under-sedation, iatrogenic withdrawal syndrome, and delirium. Existing assessment scoring tools must be applied within the pertinent clinical context and combined with responses to therapeutic interventions to ensure accurate diagnosis [36, 37].

Recent literature using these screening tools has revealed that the prevalence of iatrogenic withdrawal in PICU patients ranges from 34% to 87% [15, 33, 35, 38, 39]. IWS related to a specific agent or agent class is less clear. Opioid-related IWS has been reported as occurring in 29–57% of patients [6, 11, 12] and sole benzodiazepine IWS in 17–24% of recipients [20, 21]. However, these were early retrospective studies often performed without consistent use of validated screening tools. The RESTORE trial represents the largest prospective trial to date evaluating sedation in critically ill children and, following administration of the WAT-1 to all patients receiving opioids and benzodiazepines for more than 5 days, observed an IWS rate of 65% [39]. Determining the prevalence of dexmedetomidine-related IWS is hampered by lack of specific screening tool. However, in cohort studies wherein patients have received dexmedetomidine only, the reported IWS rate ranged from 27% to 83% [22, 40, 41]. In these studies, patients received lower infusion rates (less than 0.7 mcg/kg/hour) and for no longer than 5 days. In one small study, a cumulative dose of 107 mcg/kg of dexmedetomidine was associated with developing characteristic signs and symptoms of withdrawal [41]. With current practice utilizing higher dexmedetomidine infusion rates and longer infusion durations, as well as coadministration with benzodiazepines and opioids, it may be reasonably postulated that higher rates of dexmedetomidine-related IWS will occur.

There are numerous risk factors for developing iatrogenic withdrawal syndrome from any analgesic or sedative, including abrupt cessation and reported correlation with increasing dose and duration [13, 29, 42]. Current practice of coadministration of opioids, benzodiazepines, and dexmedetomidine over prolonged periods could allow estimation of total exposure so as to facilitate patient risk stratification. Duration correlation suggests a minimum of 5 days to raise the risk of IWS [12, 29, 32, 42, 43], while following greater than 9 days of exposure, the risk following abrupt drug cessation nears 100% [12]. Similar correlation of increasing IWS rate with increasing dose of opioids and benzodiazepines has also been reported [12, 19, 35]. The RESTORE trial identified that a total exposure dose of 19 mg/kg of morphine and 16 mg/kg of midazolam was associated with a statistically significant increased likelihood of developing IWS. In a secondary analysis of data from that trial, Best and colleagues identified that doubling of the opioid dose in 24 hours also increased the risk of IWS. Additional risk factors include preexisting cognitive impairment, age less than 6 years, receipt of three or more sedatives, and critical illness either of primary CNS origin or impacting CNS function [43].

Clinical practice guidelines for the prevention and treatment of iatrogenic withdrawal syndrome related to opioid, benzodiazepine, and alpha-agonist exposure in critically ill children have yet to be determined. The current literature describes protocolized care in some studies but not all instances, and many do not control for all analgesics or sedatives administered. Preventative strategies include those targeting reduction in drug exposure as this would decrease tolerance and successfully decrease dose and duration of delivery. Protocolized delivery of analgesics and sedatives and use of risk stratification in patients can optimize pain and sedation management with the added benefit of opioid and/or benzodiazepine infusion reduction [44, 45]. Similarly, Donnellan et al. optimized analgosedation delivery with near elimination of benzodiazepines in a pediatric cardiac intensive care unit using quality improvement processes [46]. However, total drug dose data is often lacking, precluding accurate a priori identification of patients at risk and generalizability of risk-dependent algorithms.

Logic would suggest that slow weaning of analgesic and sedative infusions over time would minimize IWS. However, this could substantially increase PICU length of stay and central line days and potentially increase the prevalence of delirium. Transition to intermittent administration of agents with longer half-lives would seem to be a reasonable alternative. Two approaches could be used and include replacement therapy with an agent acting at the same receptor or provision of a drug that may blunt some of the IWS symptoms. Additionally, in critically ill children, the available formulations and their delivery route are particularly important to maximize bioavailability and ensure absorption.

Prevention and treatment of opioid-related IWS studies primarily report the use of methadone due to both its long half-life and good bioavailability [47–51]. A recent systematic review suggests that, despite patient variability, provision of methadone to facilitate management of opioid-related IWS in the majority of critically ill children can be successful [52]. It is pertinent to note that weight-based dosing may be inadequate to mitigate all IWS, while formula-based equianalgesic dosing may result in over-sedation and prolonged QT interval [52, 53]. Management of benzodiazepine IWS alone has not been reported although recommendations for conversion of parenteral midazolam to enteral lorazepam have been frequently reported as part of weaning regimens to prevent IWS [44, 45, 54]. Alpha-agonist IWS management generally involves gradual weaning of dexmedetomidine infusions and transition to clonidine either in enteral or patch formulation. These studies are challenging to interpret because of small patient numbers, lack of specific alpha-agonist IWS screening tool and failure to control for opioid and/or benzodiazepine weaning and IWS management [41, 55–57]. Additionally, formulations of clonidine presently available are challenging in smaller patients, those who cannot tolerate enteral routes and the spectrum of dosing regimens. Treatment regimens not using receptor-specific therapeutic targets consist primarily of case reports or small retrospective studies. The most common are neonatal studies using benzodiazepines or alpha-agonists to treat opioid withdrawal, and this approach has not been evaluated in critically ill children.

In summary, accurate identification of pain and under-sedation using validated assessment tools will inform analgosedative agent administration. Protocols including targeted sedation levels may decrease drug exposure, a risk factor in the development of both tolerance and iatrogenic withdrawal syndrome. Evaluating individual patients for risk factors related to the development of tolerance and withdrawal as well as being cognizant of the overlap between pain, sedation, withdrawal, and delirium may facilitate management. Protocolized weaning of analgosedative agents and use of intermittent administration may prove beneficial although large-scale studies incorporating targeted sedation, weaning regimens, and primary outcomes of tolerance, withdrawal, and delirium need to be performed.

References

1. Deeter KH, King MA, Ridling D, Irby GL, Lynn AM, Zimmerman JJ. Successful implementation of a pediatric sedation protocol for mechanically ventilated patients. Crit Care Med. 2011;39(4):683–8.
2. Vet NJ, Ista E, de Wildt SN, vanDijk M, Tibboel D, de Hoog M. Optimal sedation in pediatric intensive care patients: a systematic review. Intensive Care Med. 2013;39:1524–34.
3. Poh YN, Poh PF, Buang SN, Lee JH. Sedation guidelines, protocols, and algorithms in PICUs: a systematic review. Pediatr Crit Care Med. 2014;15(9):885–92.
4. Gupta P, Whiteside W, Sabati A, Tesoro TM, Gossett JM, Tobias JD, Roth SJ. Safety and efficacy of prolonged dexmedetomidine use in critically ill children with heart disease. Pediatr Crit Care Med. 2012;13(6):660–6.
5. Saliski M, Kudchadkar SR. Optimising sedation management to promote early mobilization for critically ill children. J Pediatr Intensive Care. 2015;4:188–93.
6. Anand KJ, Arnold JH. Opioid tolerance and dependence in infants and children. Crit Care Med. 1994;22(2):334–42.
7. Tobias JD. Tolerance, withdrawal and physical dependency after long term sedation and analgesia of children in the pediatric intensive care unit. Crit Care Med. 2000;28(6):2122–32.
8. Martyn JAJ, Mao J, Bittner EA. Opioid Tolerance in Critical Illness. NEJM. 2019;380(4):365–78.
9. Anand KJ, Clark AE, Willson DF, Berger J, Meert KL, Zimmerman JJ, Harrison R, Carcillo JA, Newth CJ, Bispin S, Holubkov R, Dean JM, Nicholson CE, Eunice Kennedy Shriver National Institute of Child Health; Human Development (NICHD) Collaborative Pediatric Critical Care

Research Network (CPCCRN). Opioid analgesia in mechanically ventilated children: results from the multicenter measuring opioid tolerance induced by fentanyl study. Pediatr Crit Care Med. 2013;14(1):27–36.

10. Ibach BW, Miller JL, Woo S, Harrison D, Standifer KM, Hagemann T, Johnson PN. Characterization of tolerance in children during fentanyl continuous infusions. J Pediatr Intensive Care. 2017;6(2):83–90.
11. Arnold JH, Truog RD, Orav EJ, Scavone JM, Hershenson MB. Tolerance and dependence in neonates sedated with fentanyl during extracorporeal membrane oxygenation. Anesthesiology. 1990;73(6):1136–40.
12. Katz R, Kelly HW, Hsi A. Prospective study on the occurrence of withdrawal in critically ill children who receive fentanyl by continuous infusion. Crit Care Med. 1994;22(5):763–7.
13. Anand KJ, Willson DF, Berger J, Harrison R, Meert KL, Zimmerman J, Carcillo J, Newth C, Prodhan P, Dean JM, Nicholson C. Eunice Kennedy Shriver National Institute of Child Health and Human Development Collaborative Pediatric Critical Care Research Network. Tolerance and withdrawal from prolonged opioid use in critically ill children. Pediatrics. 2010;125(5):e1208–25.
14. Finkel JC, Pukish J. Molecular biology of opioid analgesia and its clinical considerations. Clin J Pain. 2019;35(6):473–80.
15. Franck LK, Naughton I, Winter J. Opioid and benzodiazepine withdrawal symptoms in paediatric intensive care patients. Intensive Crit Care Nurs. 2004;20(6):344–51.
16. Ista E, van Dijk M, Gamel C, Tibboel D, de Hoog M. Withdrawal symptoms in children after long-term administration of sedatives and/or analgesics: a literature review. "Assessment remains troublesome". Intensive Care Med. 2007;33(8):1396–406.
17. Ista E, van Dijk M, Gamel C, Tibboel D, de Hoog M. Withdrawal symptoms in critically ill children after long-term administration of sedatives and/or analgesics: a first evaluation. Crit Care Med. 2008;36(8):2427–32.
18. Oschman A, McCabe T, Kuhn RJ. Dexmedetomidine for opioid and benzodiazepine withdrawal in pediatric patients. Am J Health Syst Pharm. 2011;68(13):1233–8.
19. Fernandez-Carrion E, Gaboli M, Gonzalez-Celador R, Gomez de Quero-Masia P, Fernandez-de Miguel S, Murga-Herrera V, Serrano-Ayestaran O, Sanchez-Granados JM, Payo-Perez R. Withdrawal syndrome in the pediatric intensive care unit: incidence and risk factors. Med Intensiva. 2013;37(2):67–74.
20. Dominguez KD, Crowley MR, Coleman DM, Katz RW, Wilkins DG, Kelly HW. Withdrawal from lorazepam in critically ill children. Ann Pharmacother. 2006;40(6):1035–9.
21. Hughes J, Gill A, Leach HJ, Nunn AJ, Billingham I, Ratcliffe J, Thornington R, Choonara I. A prospective study of the adverse effects of midazolam on withdrawal in critically ill children. Acta Paediatr. 1994;83(11):1194–9.
22. Burbano NH, Otero AV, Berry DE, Orr RA, Munoz RA. Discontinuation of prolonged infusions of dexmedetomidine in critically ill children with heart disease. Intensive Care Med. 2012;38(2):300–7.
23. Carney L, Kendrick J, Carr R. Safety and effectiveness of dexmedetomidine in the pediatric intensive care unit (SAD-PICU). Can J Hosp Pharm. 2013;66(1):21–7.
24. Banasch HL, Dersch-Mills DA, Boulter LL, Gilfoyle E. Dexmedetomidine use in a pediatric intensive care unit: a retrospective cohort study. Ann Pharmacother. 2018;52(2):133–9.
25. Shutes BL, Gee SW, Sargel CL, Fink KA, Tobias JD. Dexmedetomidine as single continuous sedative drug in noninvasive ventilation: typical usage, hemodynamic effects, and withdrawal. Pediatr Crit Care Med. 2018;19:287–97.
26. Harris J, Ramelet AS, van Dijk M, Pokorna P, Wielenga J, Tume L, Tibboel D, Ista E. Clinical recommendations for pain, sedation, withdrawal and delirium assessment in critically ill infants and children: an ESPNIC position statement for healthcare professionals. Intensive Care Med. 2016;42(6):972–86.
27. Chiu AW, Contreras S, Mehta S, Korman J, Perreault MM, Williamson DR, Burry LD. Iatrogenic opioid withdrawal in critically ill patients: a review of assessment tools and management. Ann Pharmacother. 2017;51(12):1099–111.

28. Finnegan LP, Connaughton JF Jr, Kron RE, Emich JP. Neonatal abstinence syndrome: assessment and management. Addict Dis. 1975;2(1–2):141–58.
29. Franck LS, Harris SK, Soetenga DJ, Amling JK, Curley MA. The Withdrawal Assessment Tool-1 (WAT-1): an assessment instrument for monitoring opioid and benzodiazepine withdrawal symptoms in pediatric patients. Crit Care Med. 2008;9(6):573–80.
30. Franck LS, Scoppettuolo LA, Wypij D, Curley MA. Validity and generalizability of the Withdrawal Assessment Tool-1 (WAT-1) for monitoring iatrogenic withdrawal syndrome in pediatric patients. Pain. 2012;153(1):142–8.
31. Ista E, van der Voort E. Assessment of withdrawal symptoms in pediatric intensive care patients, a new future? Pediatr Crit Care Med. 2008;9(6):654–5.
32. Ista E, van Dijk M, de Hoog M, Tibboel D, Duivenvoorden HJ. Construction of the Sophia observation withdrawal symptoms-scale (SOS) for critically ill children. Intensive Care Med. 2009;35(6):1075–81.
33. Ista E, de Hoog M, Tibboel D, Duivenvoorden HJ, van Dijk M. Psychometric evaluation of the Sophia observation withdrawal symptoms scale in critically ill children. Pediatr Crit Care Med. 2013;14(8):761–9.
34. Lebet R, Hayakawa J, Chamblee TB, Tala JA, Singh N, Wypij D, Curley MAQ. Maintaining interrater agreement of core assessment instruments in a multisite randomized controlled clinical trial: the Randomized evaluation of sedation titration for respiratory failure (RESTORE) trial. Nurs Res. 2017;66(4):323–9.
35. Amigoni A, Mondardini MC, Vittadello I, Zaglia F, Rossetti E, Vitale F, Ferrario S, Savron F, Coffaro G, Brugnaro L, Amato R, Wolfler A, Franck LS. Network of Paediatric Intensive Care Unit Study Group (TIPNet). Withdrawal Assessment Tool-1 monitoring in PICU: a multicenter study on iatrogenic withdrawal syndrome. Pediatr Crit Care Med. 2017;18(2):e86–91.
36. Ista E, van Dijk M. We can not compartmentalize our patients! Overlapping symptoms of iatrogenic withdrawal syndrome, pediatric delirium and anticholinergic toxidrome. Pediatr Crit Care Med. 2017;18(6):603–4.
37. Madden K, Burns MM, Tasker RC. Differentiating delirium from sedative/hypnotic-related iatrogenic withdrawal syndrome lack of specificity in pediatric critical care assessment tools. Pediatr Crit Care Med. 2017;18(6):580–8.
38. DaSilva PS, Reis ME, Fonseca TS, Fonseca MS. Opioid and benzodiazepine withdrawal syndrome in PICU patients: which risk factors matter? J Addict Med. 2016;10(2):110–6.
39. Curley MA, Wypij D, Watson RS, Grant MJ, Asaro LA, Cheifetz IM, Dodson BL, Franck LS, Gedeit RG, Angus DC, Matthay MA, RESTORE Study Investigators and the Pediatric Acute Lung Injury and Sepsis Investigators Network. Protocolized sedation vs usual care in pediatric patients mechanically ventilated for acute respiratory failure: a randomized clinical trial. JAMA. 2015;313:379–89.
40. Whalen LD, DiGennaro JL, Irby GA, Yanay O, Zimmerman JJ. Long-term Dexmedetomidine use and safety profile among critically ill children and neonates. Pediatr Crit Care Med. 2014;15(8):706–14.
41. Haenecour AS, Seto W, Urbain CM, Stephens D, Laussen PC, Balit CR. Prolonged Dexmedetomidine infusion and drug withdrawal in critically ill children. J Pediatr Pharmacol Ther. 2017;22(6):453–60.
42. Best KM, Boulatta JI, Curley MA. Risk factors associated with iatrogenic opioid and benzodiazepine withdrawal in critically ill pediatric patients: s systematic review and conceptual model. Pediatr Crit Care Med. 2015;16(2):175–83.
43. Best KM, Wypij D, Asaro LA, Curley MA. Randomized Evaluation of Sedation Titration For Respiratory Failure Study Investigators. Patient, process, and system predictors of iatrogenic withdrawal syndrome in critically ill children. Crit Care Med. 2017;45(1):e7–e15.
44. Amirnovin R, Sanchez-Pinto LN, Okuhara C, Lieu P, Koh JY, Rodgers JW, et al. Implementation of a risk-stratified opioid and benzodiazepine weaning protocol in a pediatric cardiac ICU. Pediatr Crit Care Med. 2018;19(11):1024–32.

45. Sanchez-Pinto LN, Nelson LP, Lieu P, Koh JY, Rodgers JW, Larson KA, Huson JM, Amirnovin R. Implementation of a risk-stratified opioid weaning protocol in a pediatric intensive care unit. J Crit Care. 2018;43:214–9.
46. Donnellan A, Sawyer J, Peach A, Staveski S, Nelson DP, Pratap JN. Reducing exposure to opioid and benzodiazepine medications for pediatric cardiac intensive care patients; a quality improvement project. Pediatr Crit Care Med. 2019;20(4):340–9.
47. Siddappa R, Fletcher JE, Heard AM, Kielma D, Cimino M, Heard CM. Methadone dosage for prevention of opioid withdrawal in children. Paediatr Anaesth. 2003;13(9):805–10.
48. Robertson RC, Darsey E, Fortenberry JD, Pettignano R, Hartley G. Evaluation of an opiate-weaning protocol using methadone in pediatric intensive care unit patients. Pediatr Crit Care Med. 2000;1:119–23.
49. Meyer MM, Berens RJ. Efficacy of an enteral 10-day methadone wean to prevent opioid withdrawal in fentanyl-tolerant pediatric intensive care unit patients. Pediatr Crit Care Med. 2001;2(4):329–33.
50. Berens RJ, Meyer MT, Mikhailov TA, Colpaert KD, Czarnecki ML, Ghanayem NS, Hoffman GM, Soetenga DJ, Nelson TJ, Weisman SJ. A prospective evaluation of opioid weaning in opioid-dependent pediatric critical care patients. Anesth Analg. 2006;102(4):1045–50.
51. Bowens CD, Thompson JA, Thompson MT, Breitzka RL, Thompson DG, Sheeran PW. A trial of methadone tapering schedules in pediatric intensive care unit patients exposed to prolonged sedative infusions. Pediatr Crit Care Med. 2011;12(5):504–11.
52. Dervan LA, Yaghmai B, Watson RS, Wolf FM. The use of methadone to facilitate opioid weaning in pediatric critical care patients: a systemic review of the literature and meta-analysis. Paediatr Anaesth. 2017;27(3):228–39.
53. Johnson PN, Boyles KA, Miller JL. Selection of the initial methadone regimen for the management of iatrogenic opioid abstinence syndrome in critically ill children. Pharmacotherapy. 2012;32(2):148–57.
54. Warrington SE, Collier HK, Himebauch AS, Wolfe HA. Evaluation of IV to enteral benzodiazepine conversion calculations in a pediatric intensive care setting. Pediatr Crit Care Med. 2018;19:e569–75.
55. Lardieri AB, Fusco NM, Simone S, Walker LK, Morgan JA, Parbuoni KA. Effects of clonidine on withdrawal from long-term Dexmedetomidine in the pediatric patient. J Pediatr Pharmacol Ther. 2015;20(1):45–53.
56. Capino C, Miller JL, Johnson PN. Clonidine for sedation and analgesia and withdrawal in critically ill infants and children. Pharmacotherapy. 2016;36(12):1290–9.
57. Garisto C, Ricci Z, Tofani L, Benegni S, Pezzella C, Cogo P. Use of low-dose dexmedetomidine in combination with opioids and midazolam in pediatric cardiac surgical patients: randomized controlled trial. Minerva Anestesiol. 2018;84(9):1053–62.

Chapter 12
Neuromuscular Blockade for the Critically Ill Child

Amanda Ruth

Introduction

Since their introduction, neuromuscular blocking agents (NMBAs) have been frequently used in the pediatric intensive care setting. While most commonly utilized as a single dose to facilitate endotracheal intubations, prolonged administration in the form of continuous infusions is a standard practice in certain disease states and patient populations. Estimates of the use of NMBAs vary, but data have indicated that they are used in as many as 30% of mechanically ventilated pediatric patients [1], and between 10% and 16% of ventilator support-days involve the use of NMBA infusions in PICUs around the world [2].

As with all medications, NMBAs have potential adverse effects that have major clinical implications. Give the frequency of their use, pediatric intensivists should have a keen awareness of the appropriate indications for these agents. Furthermore, they should also know how to mitigate side effects that may arise.

One important point to emphasize here is NMBAs have no sedative or analgesic properties and therefore should never be administered without the concurrent use of a sedative, analgesic, or amnestic agents (e.g., opiates, benzodiazepines). It is also important to remember that patients who had received long-acting NMBAs may still remain paralyzed but aware once their sedative/amnestics have worn off.

A. Ruth (✉)
Texas Children's Hospital, Baylor College of Medicine, Pediatric Critical Care,
Houston, TX, USA
e-mail: axruth@texaschildrens.org

P. P. Kamat, J. W. Berkenbosch (eds.), *Sedation and Analgesia for the Pediatric Intensivist*, https://doi.org/10.1007/978-3-030-52555-2_12

Neuromuscular Junction

The neuromuscular junction (NMJ) is the main site of action of the NMBAs. The components of the NMJ most salient to this discussion are the presynaptic nerve terminal, the intervening gap known as the synaptic cleft, and the postsynaptic skeletal muscle membranes (Fig. 12.1). Neurotransmitters are released from the presynaptic nerve terminal across the gap to convey the excitatory impulse to the postsynaptic motor end-plates. The predominant neurotransmitter is acetylcholine (ACh). The ACh receptors are classified as muscarinic and nicotinic receptors, with the ACh receptors present in the muscle cells being nicotinic receptors. However, administration of NMBAs affects ACh action on all receptors, causing effects other than their muscle relaxation and potentially causing undesirable side effects.

Under normal physiologic conditions, ACh is stored in vesicles in the presynaptic nerve terminal. When an action potential arrives at the nerve terminal, calcium (Ca2+) binds to voltage-gated Ca2+ channels in the cell membrane, causing release of the ACh-containing vesicles into the synaptic gap. ACh then binds onto the

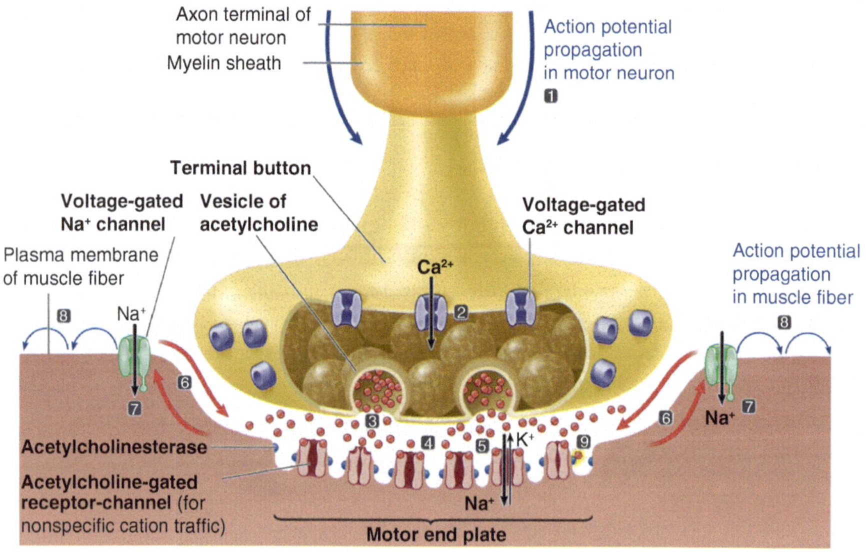

Fig. 12.1 Neuromuscular junction [3]. 1. An action potential travels along the axon membrane to a NMJ. 2. Ca2+ enters through voltage-gated Ca2+ channels. 3. Ca2+ influx triggers an increase in the exocytosis of ACh-containing vesicles. 4. ACh is released into the synaptic cleft and binds to the nicotinic receptor. 5. The binding of ACh to the receptor increases the Na+ and K+ conductance, resulting in the influx of Na+. This produces a depolarizing potential. 6. This in turn depolarizes the adjacent cell membrane. 7. More Na+ channels open, causing membrane potential to reach firing level. 8. Action potentials are generated on either side of the end-plate and are conducted along the muscle fibers. 9. These action potentials in turn initiate muscle contraction. 10. ACh is removed from the synaptic cleft by acetylcholinesterase

nicotinic ACh receptors located in the postsynaptic motor end-plates, causing depolarization. With enough ACh, this depolarization causes the activation of Na+-gated channels outside the end-plate. The opening of these in return allows for enough current to cause activation of the myocyte.

Pharmacology and Mechanism of Action

NMBAs are hydrophilic and ionized as a result, which means that they do not cross the blood-brain barrier or placental barrier between the mother and the fetus. Neonates, infants, and children have a higher proportion of extracellular water than adults, which makes their volumes of distribution of hydrophilic drugs larger. This is especially relevant in neonates and especially in premature infants. However, neonatal skeletal muscles are more sensitive to neuromuscular blockade than those of older children, likely due to the immaturity of their neuromuscular junction. Hence, despite the proportion of their extracellular water, they may be more sensitive to standard doses of NMBAs, whereas older infants and children may exhibit decreased sensitivity to the effects of NMBAs.

Dosages are commonly discussed in terms of intubating dose and maintenance dose. The intubating dose is the dosage needed to produce conditions suitable for endotracheal intubation. ED_{95} refers to the dose that produces complete flaccidity in 95% of the population, with intubating dosage usually being twice the ED_{95} although this may vary depending on other properties of the drug. Maintenance doses are generally one third or one half of the ED_{95}, but as always, titration should be based on objective monitoring. There have been numerous studies noting that onset of neuromuscular blockade in more central muscles such as the diaphragm is different compared to the onset of blockade in the peripheral muscles [4]. Blockade is achieved faster on the laryngeal muscles (vocal cord) as compared to the diaphragm. Onset and offset of neuromuscular blockade at the diaphragm are significantly shorter than the larynx. Direct monitoring of both these muscle groups (vocal cord and diaphragm) is impractical, and therefore historically, surrogate muscle groups have been utilized. Traditionally, the adductor pollicis muscle of the hand has been used [4–6], although studies show the diaphragm is more resistant to blockade than the adductor muscle. Recent studies have shown that the effect of neuromuscular blockade on the corrugator supercilii, a group of muscles around the eyes, is a more accurate reflection of the time course of neuromuscular blockade of the larynx of the diaphragm [6, 7]. Of note, these studies were mostly conducted for monitoring in the operating room. More recently, official guidelines recommend objective monitoring devices be used in critically ill patients who are receiving continuous infusions of NMBAs.

The most commonly used NMBAs in the pediatric intensive care unit (PICU) fall under two classes: depolarizing and competitive/non-depolarizing. The main site of action for both is the NMJ. Neuromuscular blocking agents and clinical properties are shown in Table 12.1.

Table 12.1 Neuromuscular blocking agents and clinical properties

Agent	Dosing	Time to onset of action	Metabolism
Depolarizing			
Succinylcholine	*Intubation*: 1 mg/kg	30–60 sec	Plasma cholinesterase
Competitive/non-depolarizing			
Aminosteroids			
Rocuronium	*Intubation*: 0.6–1.2 mg/kg *Infusion*: 3–12 mcg/kg/min	1–3 min	Hepatobiliary
Vecuronium	*Intubation*: 0.1 mg/kg *Infusion*: 10–20 mcg/kg/min	3–4 min	Biliary and renal
Pancuronium	*Intubation*: 0.1 mg/kg	3–4 min	Renal, 20% through biliary
Benzylisoquinolines			
Atracurium	*Intubation*: 0.5 mg/kg *Infusion*: 10–20 mcg/kg/min	3–5 min	Plasma esterase-mediated hydrolysis Hoffman degradation
Cisatracurium	*Intubation*: 0.1 mg/kg *Infusion*: 1–3 mcg/kg/min	4–7 min	Hoffman degradation, 15% in urine
Mivacurium	*Intubation*: 0.2 mg/kg *Infusion*: 5–8 mcg/kg/min	2–4 min	Plasma cholinesterase

Depolarizing

Currently, succinylcholine is the only depolarizing agent in clinical use. It is a quaternary ammonium compound. It acts by binding the nicotinic receptors at the postsynaptic neuromuscular junction end-plate and opening the ligand-gated channels, mimicking the action of acetylcholine. This results in depolarization and subsequent inhibition of neuromuscular transmission, producing skeletal muscle relaxation. Occasionally, the depolarization phase can manifest in older children as muscle fasciculations which may cause subsequent myalgias.

The onset of action of succinylcholine is rapid, with blockade usually seen within 30–60 seconds, making it the most rapid-acting of the commonly used NMBAs. The general effective dose for tracheal intubation is 1 mg/kg, although neonates may require up to twice the dose given their larger volume of distribution. The effect wears off within 3 minutes and is generally complete within 10–15 minutes due to its rapid distribution and degradation [8]. Succinylcholine undergoes hydrolysis by plasma cholinesterases.

Adverse Effects

Adverse effects of succinylcholine are well-known, limiting its use in certain circumstances. Some of these side effects include the following.

Cardiovascular Succinylcholine stimulates both the nicotinic and the muscarinic receptors in the sinus node of the heart. As a result, in patients with high vagal tone, administration of succinylcholine can produce bradycardia. Anticholinergic drugs (e.g., atropine) may be used to prevent or treat the resultant bradycardia.

Hyperkalemia It is known that succinylcholine produces a rise on potassium in healthy patients. However, in certain patient populations, there have been reported cases of lethal hyperkalemia after succinylcholine administration. Populations at higher risk of this event include patients with muscular dystrophy, denervation injuries, or trauma and severe burns. The underlying mechanism is thought to be excess potassium release from an upregulation of abnormal extra-junctional acetylcholine receptors (in cases of muscular dystrophy, burns, etc.). It may also trigger rhabdomyolysis in muscular dystrophy patients, similarly causing hyperkalemia.

Malignant Hyperthermia In susceptible patients, succinylcholine is a known trigger for malignant hyperthermia. While its role as the sole trigger is controversial, succinylcholine seems to enhance the potential of inhalational anesthetic agents to trigger MH.

Prolonged Paralysis In patients with inherited abnormal variant of plasma cholinesterase, succinylcholine leads to prolonged paralysis. Those with a homozygous variant produce a cholinesterase with virtually no ability to hydrolyze succinylcholine. Management of these patients includes mechanical ventilation, sedation, and supportive treatment until the drug is finally cleared by nonspecific esterases.

Others The muscle fasciculations produced in the initial phase of depolarization with succinylcholine can potentiate other side effects such as increased intraocular and intragastric pressures, rhabdomyolysis, and sustained skeletal muscle contractions.

Due to the various adverse effects of the drug and the potential of administering it to a hitherto undiagnosed muscular dystrophy patient, succinylcholine has fallen out of favor as the drug of choice for tracheal intubation in the pediatric population.

Competitive/Non-depolarizing

Non-depolarizing NMBAs act in a competitive manner in the postsynaptic nicotinic receptors. By binding to either one of both α-subunits of the receptor, these drugs prevent acetylcholine from binding to the receptor. Neuromuscular block starts becoming evident when 70–80% of the receptors are occupied. For a complete block, more than 90% of the receptors must be occupied by the NMBA [9].

The NMBAs of this class can be further subdivided into benzylisoquinolines (atracurium, mivacurium, cisatracurium) and aminosteroid compounds (pancuronium, vecuronium, rocuronium). Rocuronium and vecuronium are intermediate-acting NMBAs. Pancuronium is the only commercially available long-acting NMBA in North America.

Aminosteroid Compounds

Rocuronium

Rocuronium has the fastest onset of the depolarizing NMBAs and may be used in higher doses (1.2 mg/kg) as a substitute for succinylcholine for rapid sequence intubations. The commonly used intubating dose is 0.6–1.2 mg/kg, which achieves intubating condition in 1–3 minutes in most patients. Elimination is predominantly through a hepatobiliary route. Long-term maintenance of paralysis can be achieved through rocuronium infusion at doses of 3–12 mcg/kg/min. Rocuronium has minimal hemodynamic effects and is not vagolytic.

Vecuronium

Vecuronium has a slower onset time than rocuronium and thus is not ideal to use in rapid sequence intubations. The usual intubating dose of 0.1 mg/kg provides adequate intubating conditions in 3–4 minutes. The maintenance infusion dose is 1–2 mcg/kg/min. Its excretion is through both the biliary (50–60%) and renal (40–50%) routes. In patients with acute kidney injury or hepatic failure, the duration of vecuronium may be prolonged due to an active metabolite 3-methyldesacetylvecuronium, which has 75% of the potency of vecuronium. Like rocuronium, vecuronium has minimal hemodynamic effects.

Pancuronium

Pancuronium is the longest-acting of the steroidal NMBAs. It is rarely used due to the high incidence of postoperative residual neuromuscular weakness. An intubating dose is 0.1 mg/kg which results in maximum muscle twitch suppression in 3–4 minutes. Elimination is mostly through the renal route, although there is 20% excretion through the biliary system. Pancuronium should be avoided in patients with renal or hepatic dysfunction. It is vagolytic (blocks muscarinic receptors) and may cause tachycardia due to a weak sympathomimetic effect.

Benzylisoquinolines Compounds

Atracurium

Atracurium is an intermediate-acting NMBA. Side effects of higher doses include histamine release, which may cause flushing, hypotension, and tachycardia. The common intubating dose is 0.5 mg/kg, with intubating conditions being achieved in

3–5 minutes. Infusion may be maintained at doses of 10–20 mcg/kg/min. Atracurium is broken down by nonspecific plasma esterase-mediated hydrolysis and a pH- and temperature-dependent degradation called Hoffman elimination, which makes its metabolism essentially independent of both liver and kidney function.

Cisatracurium

Cisatracurium is a cis-isomer of atracurium. It is four times more potent and, unlike atracurium, does not produce histamine release or has any cardiovascular effect. It has a longer duration and time to onset of action. A dose of 0.1 mg/kg is used to intubate, with maximum onset of effect achieved in 4–7 minutes. Maintenance can be achieved with an infusion at 1–3 mcg/kg/min. Like atracurium, cisatracurium is also primarily metabolized through Hoffman elimination, with 15% passing unchanged in urine. Renal failure is associated with a slight reduction in the plasma clearance of the drug, but no prolonged effect is observed.

Mivacurium

Mivacurium is the shortest-acting of the benzylisoquinolinium NMBAs. It was originally developed as a non-depolarizing alternative to succinylcholine. While it has little direct cardiovascular effect, at higher doses (>0.2 mg/kg), it produces significant histamine release, which limits its uses. The intubating dose of mivacurium is 0.2 mg/kg, with intubating conditions achieved in 2–4 minutes. Infusion doses are at 5–8 mcg/kg/min. Mivacurium is mostly metabolized by butyrylcholinesterase (a plasma cholinesterase) and should not be used in patients with atypical plasma cholinesterase. Patients with hepatic and renal disease with reduced plasma cholinesterase activity may have a prolonged duration of action.

Other Adverse Effects

There have been reports of anaphylaxis with NMBA administration. The ammonium ion in many NMBAs is most likely component associated with the allergic reaction. The mechanism for severe hypersensitivity reaction to non-depolarizing NMBAs is most likely IgE mediated, with reported incidence ranging between 1:1250 and 1:13,000 anesthetic exposures. The NMBAs may be the most frequently used agents in the operating room associated with allergic reactions [10].

The NMBAs are also associated with corneal abrasions (as paralysis abolishes the blink reflex), as well as increase in deep vein thrombosis due to venous stasis from immobility [11, 12].

Table 12.2 Effects of various medications and medical conditions on the potency of non-depolarizing NMBAs

Potentiates NMBA	Diminishes NMBA
Medications	*Medications*
Inhaled anesthetics	Azathioprine
Antibiotics (aminoglycosides, clindamycin, tetracyclines, and vancomycin)	Ranitidine
Corticosteroids	Theophylline
Cyclosporine	Caffeine
Local anesthetics	Calcium
Loop diuretics	Phenytoin
Lithium	
Magnesium	
Quinidine	
Procainamide	
Conditions	*Conditions*
Hypothermia	Cerebral palsy
Hypercarbia	
Burn injuries	
Female gender	
Muscular dystrophies	

Interactions with Other Compounds

Non-depolarizing muscle relaxants can interact with other medications and medical conditions with resultant enhancement or reduction in the neuromuscular blockade. Their activity is generally enhanced by volatile anesthetics, local anesthetics, high-dose furosemide, aminoglycosides, magnesium, cyclosporine, calcium channel blockers, beta-blockers, quinidine, and lithium. Burn injuries and the female gender are also associated with increased neuromuscular blockade activity with similar doses of NMBAs. Medications such as phenytoin, ranitidine, carbamazepine, theophylline, and calcium may cause resistance to the activity of the NMBAs. Table 12.2 contains a more complete list of medications and conditions that can affect the duration of blockade.

Monitoring

As mentioned earlier, objective monitoring of patients under neuromuscular blockade, especially if the blockade is sustained, is essential [13]. The standard method employed in most PICUs is peripheral nerve stimulation (PNS), or what is more widely known as train-of-fours (TOFs). This involves a transcutaneous electrical stimulation of a peripheral nerve to assess the depth of neuromuscular blockade. Response is monitored by the twitches of either the adductor pollicis or flexor digitorum muscles, with different responses indicating the presence or absence and the degree of blockade. An alternative would be stimulation of the facial nerve, with monitoring of the contraction of the orbicularis oculi muscle for the response. The stimulator poles are placed over the nerve either at the wrist (ulnar) or cheek (facial) and current is applied, with four stimuli. As doses of NMBA are increased, the twitches decrease in force, with the fourth twitch being lost first, the third twitch being second, and so on progressively. When there are no twitches produced by the stimulator, this is referred to as a TOF of 0. As the drugs are metabolized, the twitches come back in reverse order, with the first twitch returning earliest.

Published guidelines [14] have recommended titration NMBAs to one to two of four twitches are present. For monitoring recovery from neuromuscular blockade, a TOF ratio of >0.9 is recommended. This ratio is calculated from dividing the amplitude of the fourth twitch response by that of the first twitch. Data in adults have suggested that at this ratio, vital capacity returns to normal. While no such data exists in children, this recommendation is generally extrapolated into the pediatric population.

Although PNS with TOF is the most commonly used monitoring method, it is not recommended as the sole method of monitoring the depth of neuromuscular blockade. The results of PNS using TOFs may be rendered inaccurate by patient factors such as edema, hypothermia, and monitoring site variance. Hence, the guidelines for NMBA use in critically ill adults recommend incorporating PNS with TOF into a more inclusive assessment that include clinical characteristics.

Reversal

In certain circumstances, it may be necessary to quickly achieve reversal of neuromuscular blockade. Medications that have been utilized in these clinical settings fall under two classes: acetylcholinesterase inhibitors and cyclodextrin derivatives.

Acetylcholinesterase Inhibitors

Inhibiting the enzyme acetylcholinesterase results in an increased concentration of ACh at the motor end-plate. ACh then competes with the non-depolarizing NMBA. Prolonging the time that ACh is available in the neuromuscular junction increases the chance that ACh will bind the free receptor when the NMBA dissociates from the receptors. Three commercially available medications under this class are neostigmine, edrophonium, and pyridostigmine.

These inhibitors do not act preferentially at the neuromuscular junction, and they also act at other synapses including the muscarinic receptors, leading to cholinergic side effects such as bradycardia and increased secretions. Administration of atropine prior to giving these inhibitors is recommended to counteract the potential respiratory and cardiovascular side effects.

Cyclodextrin Derivatives

Sugammadex is the only commercially available drug under this class. It works by encapsulating the steroidal NMBAs, hence blocking the NMBA from interacting with the ACh receptors. The resulting compound is inactive and is excreted by the kidneys. A recent meta-analysis found that the safety profile of sugammadex may be preferable to that of neostigmine for neuromuscular blockade reversal in adults due to lack of cholinergic side effects [15]. Hypersensitivity reactions, cardiac arrhythmias, abnormal coagulation profile, and interference with oral contraceptive pills are adverse events reported in literature [16].

Indications for Sustained Neuromuscular Blockade in Critically Ill Children

While the most common indication for the short-term use of NMBA in the PICU is facilitation of endotracheal intubation and brief procedures, there are several other situations where a sustained infusion of NMBA is deemed beneficial to patient care. The most frequent indication for the use of sustained NMBA infusions is preventing respiratory dyssynchrony in prolonged intubations. NMBAs are also used to allow patients to tolerate nonconventional ventilation mode such as high-frequency oscillatory ventilation (HFOV).

Acute Respiratory Distress Syndrome (ARDS)

Most of the available data for the use of NMBAs in patients with ARDS come from trials in the adult population. Papazian et al. [17] in 2010 conducted a randomized trial in which 340 patients were randomized to either a 48-hour infusion of cisatracurium (178 patients) or placebo (162 patients) and found that early administration of a NMBA improved the adjusted 90-day survival and increased ventilator-free time without increase in muscle weakness. A subsequent meta-analysis also found that a short-term infusion of cisatracurium reduces hospital mortality and barotrauma without increased ICU-acquired weakness in adults with ARDS [18]. Evidence for NMBA benefits in the pediatric ARDS is less vigorous, although a single-center study in 2016 found that administration of NMBA results in a short-term improvement in the oxygenation index (OI) in pediatric patients with ARDS [19]. A recent clinical trial in patients with moderate to severe ARDS (ROSE ClinicalTrials.gov number, NCT02509078), however, found no difference in 90-day mortality between patients who received early and continuous NMBA and those treated with usual care and light sedation [20].

Traumatic Brain Injury (TBI)

The evidence for the use of NMBAs in the TBI population is mixed. The most recent systematic review of 32 adult trials done in 2015 [21] found that in most studies, administration of NMBA boluses prior to stimulating procedures such as bronchoscopy helped control spikes in intracranial pressure (ICP). However, a few retrospective studies found that sustained administration of a NMBA infusion could have extracranial complications such as longer ICU stay and pneumonia. No definitive trial on the benefits or adverse effects of NMBAs in the pediatric TBI population has been performed to date.

Sepsis

Traditionally, the rationale for using sustained NMBA infusions in severe sepsis and septic shock was to facilitate mechanical ventilation and reduce metabolic demand [22]. However, evidence has been contradictory, with one placebo-controlled RCT showing the usage of NMBAs in severe sepsis did not affect oxygen delivery or oxygen consumption [23]. The most current iteration of the Surviving Sepsis Campaign [24] recommends using NMBAs <48 hours in adult patients with sepsis-induced ARDS with a Pa/FiO2 ratio of <150, although this was rated a weak recommendation. No specific recommendations were made for the pediatric population.

Others

There are a few other populations in which sustained NMBA infusions are commonly employed especially in the adult patients. These include unstable patients with pulmonary hypertension, intubated status asthmaticus patients with increased intra-abdominal hypertension critical airway, and those with recent airway surgery. A single institution's review in 2016 [25] found that in patients undergoing tracheostomy placement, those who received NMBA in the postoperative period had a longer median postoperative length of stay and were more likely to develop ileus.

No official recommendations exist regarding sustained NMBA usage in these patients, except the standard recommendation that all patients on NMBAs should have adequate sedation/analgesia and monitored appropriately.

Adverse Effects of Prolonged NMBA Administration

One of the most commonly reported side effects of prolonged NMBA use in the ICU is weakness. A potential etiology of this weakness is critical illness polyneuropathy and myopathy (CIPNM). CIPNM comprise a spectrum of conditions that manifest as general weakness and respiratory dysfunction. These are associated with high morbidity including inability to separate from the ventilator. While the true extent of these conditions is still poorly defined in children, NMBAs had been touted as a potential risk factor for the development of CIPNM.

No prospective trials have been conducted to assess the risk factors in the pediatric population. Historically, adult data have shown association between NMBA use and ICU-acquired weakness [26–28]. However, it must be noted that concomitant use of high-dose corticosteroids was also common in these trials. Recent, more high-quality literature has shown no association between the commonly used doses of NMBA with increased duration of mechanical ventilation [17, 29, 30]. There are also confounders in these studies that could contribute to muscle dysfunction, such as duration of bed rest during critical illness, the amount of sedation medication, and high-dose corticosteroids or aminoglycosides. Due to the conflicting nature of this data, no strong causation could be drawn between the use of NMBA and ICU weakness.

In 2001, a multicenter observational study by Martin et al. showed that the mortality rate among children receiving long-term NMBA was 18% [2]. However, the study also noted that children who received long-term administration of NMBA had a much higher severity of illness. Hence, it could not delineate the unique effect of NMBA on mortality rate.

A more recent retrospective cohort study in 2010 found that compared to a control group where children did not receive NMBAs, the NMBA group had a longer duration of mechanical ventilation, longer PICU stay, and an increased occurrence of ventilator-associated pneumonia [27]. Unlike Martin et al., they did not find NMBA use to be associated with a higher mortality rate or with the development of CIPNM. Of note, this study only had a small number of patients (n = 34) in the NMBA group, limiting its applicability to universal practice.

Conclusion

NMBAs remain an important adjunct in the care of critically ill children, especially those in whom prolonged mechanical ventilation is necessary. There is unfortunately sparse literature on the true effects prolonged NMBA administration may have on patients in the ICU. It is incumbent upon the pediatric critical care practitioner to be familiar with the usage and potential side effects of the different NMBAs and to be judicious in the utilization of prolonged NMBA infusions.

References

1. Jenkins IA, Playfor SD, Bevan C, Davies G, Wolf AR. Current United Kingdom sedation practice in pediatric intensive care. Paediatr Anaesth. 2007;17(7):675–83.
2. Martin LD, Bratton SL, Quint P, Mayock DE. Prospective documentation of sedative, analgesic, and neuromuscular blocking agent use in infants and children in the intensive care unit:

a multicenter perspective. Pediatr Crit Care Med J Soc Crit Care Med World Fed Pediatr Intensive Crit Care Soc. 2001;2(3):205–10.
3. ThingLink. Neuromuscular Junction by [Internet]. [cited 2019 Mar 27]. Available from: https://www.thinglink.com/scene/648196519761018880.
4. Dhonneur G, Kirov K, Slavov V, Duvaldestin P. Effects of an intubating dose of succinylcholine and rocuronium on the larynx and diaphragm: an electromyographic study in humans. Anesthesiology. 1999;90(4):951–5.
5. Cantineau JP, Porte F, d'Honneur G, Duvaldestin P. Neuromuscular effects of rocuronium on the diaphragm and adductor pollicis muscles in anesthetized patients. Anesthesiology. 1994;81(3):585–90.
6. Hemmerling TM, Donati F. Neuromuscular blockade at the larynx, the diaphragm and the corrugator supercilii muscle: a review. Can J Anaesth. 2003;50(8):779–94.
7. Plaud B, Debaene B, Donati F. The corrugator supercilii, not the orbicularis oculi, reflects rocuronium neuromuscular blockade at the laryngeal adductor muscles. Anesthesiology. 2001;95(1):96–101.
8. Neuromuscular Blockade (Anesthesia Text) [Internet]. [cited 2019 Mar 27]. Available from: https://www.openanesthesia.org/neuromuscular_blockade_anesthesia_text/.
9. Appiah-Ankam J, Hunter JM. Pharmacology of neuromuscular blocking drugs. Contin Educ Anaesth Crit Care Pain. 2004;4(1):2–7.
10. Mertes PM, Aimone-Gastin I, Guéant-Rodriguez RM, Mouton-Faivre C, Audibert G, O'Brien J, et al. Hypersensitivity reactions to neuromuscular blocking agents. Curr Pharm Des. 2008;14(27):2809–25.
11. Boddi M, Barbani F, Abbate R, Bonizzoli M, Batacchi S, Lucente E, et al. Reduction in deep vein thrombosis incidence in intensive care after a clinician education program. J Thromb Haemost. 2010;8(1):121–8.
12. Sorce LR, Hamilton SM, Gauvreau K, Mets MB, Hunter DG, Rahmani B, et al. Preventing corneal abrasions in critically ill children receiving neuromuscular blockade: a randomized, controlled trial. Pediatr Crit Care Med J Soc Crit Care Med World Fed Pediatr Intensive Crit Care Soc. 2009;10(2):171–5.
13. Playfor S, Jenkins I, Boyles C, Choonara I, Davies G, Haywood T, et al. Consensus guidelines for sustained neuromuscular blockade in critically ill children. Paediatr Anaesth. 2007;17(9):881–7.
14. Murray MJ, DeBlock H, Erstad B, Gray A, Jacobi J, Jordan C, et al. Clinical practice guidelines for sustained neuromuscular blockade in the adult critically ill patient. Crit Care Med. 2016;44(11):2079–103.
15. Hristovska A-M, Duch P, Allingstrup M, Afshari A. Efficacy and safety of sugammadex versus neostigmine in reversing neuromuscular blockade in adults. Cochrane Database Syst Rev. 2017;8:CD012763.
16. Sugammadex: a review of neuromuscular blockade reversal. - PubMed - NCBI [Internet]. [cited 2019 Sep 16]. Available from: https://www.ncbi.nlm.nih.gov/pubmed/?term=PMID+27324403+Keating+GM+2016.
17. Papazian L, Forel J-M, Gacouin A, Penot-Ragon C, Perrin G, Loundou A, et al. Neuromuscular blockers in early acute respiratory distress syndrome. N Engl J Med. 2010;363(12):1107–16.
18. Alhazzani W, Alshahrani M, Jaeschke R, Forel JM, Papazian L, Sevransky J, et al. Neuromuscular blocking agents in acute respiratory distress syndrome: a systematic review and meta-analysis of randomized controlled trials. Crit Care Lond Engl. 2013;17(2):R43.
19. Wilsterman MEF, de Jager P, Blokpoel R, Frerichs I, Dijkstra SK, Albers MJIJ, et al. Short-term effects of neuromuscular blockade on global and regional lung mechanics, oxygenation and ventilation in pediatric acute hypoxemic respiratory failure. Ann Intensive Care. 2016;6(1):103.
20. Early neuromuscular blockade in the acute respiratory distress syndrome. - PubMed - NCBI [Internet]. [cited 2019 Sep 16]. Available from: https://www.ncbi.nlm.nih.gov/pubmed/31112383.

21. Sanfilippo F, Santonocito C, Veenith T, Astuto M, Maybauer MO. The role of neuromuscular blockade in patients with traumatic brain injury: a systematic review. Neurocrit Care. 2015;22(2):325–34.
22. Hansen-Flaschen JH, Brazinsky S, Basile C, Lanken PN. Use of sedating drugs and neuromuscular blocking agents in patients requiring mechanical ventilation for respiratory failure. A national survey. JAMA. 1991;266(20):2870–5.
23. Freebairn RC, Derrick J, Gomersall CD, Young RJ, Joynt GM. Oxygen delivery, oxygen consumption, and gastric intramucosal pH are not improved by a computer-controlled, closed-loop, vecuronium infusion in severe sepsis and septic shock. Crit Care Med. 1997;25(1):72–7.
24. Rhodes A, Evans LE, Alhazzani W, Levy MM, Antonelli M, Ferrer R, et al. Surviving Sepsis campaign: international guidelines for management of sepsis and septic shock: 2016. Intensive Care Med. 2017;43(3):304–77.
25. Bauer E, Mahida JB, Boomer LA, Lutmer JE, Minneci PC, Deans KJ, et al. Outcomes following neuromuscular blockade in patients receiving tracheostomies. Int J Pediatr Otorhinolaryngol. 2016;84:101–5.
26. Behbehani NA, Al-Mane F, D'yachkova Y, Paré P, FitzGerald JM. Myopathy following mechanical ventilation for acute severe asthma: the role of muscle relaxants and corticosteroids. Chest. 1999 Jun;115(6):1627–31.
27. Adnet F, Dhissi G, Borron SW, Galinski M, Rayeh F, Cupa M, et al. Complication profiles of adult asthmatics requiring paralysis during mechanical ventilation. Intensive Care Med. 2001;27(11):1729–36.
28. Garnacho-Montero J, Madrazo-Osuna J, García-Garmendia JL, Ortiz-Leyba C, Jiménez-Jiménez FJ, Barrero-Almodóvar A, et al. Critical illness polyneuropathy: risk factors and clinical consequences. A cohort study in septic patients. Intensive Care Med. 2001;27(8):1288–96.
29. Puthucheary Z, Rawal J, Ratnayake G, Harridge S, Montgomery H, Hart N. Neuromuscular blockade and skeletal muscle weakness in critically ill patients: time to rethink the evidence? Am J Respir Crit Care Med. 2012;185(9):911–7.
30. Fan E, Dowdy DW, Colantuoni E, Mendez-Tellez PA, Sevransky JE, Shanholtz C, et al. Physical complications in acute lung injury survivors: a two-year longitudinal prospective study. Crit Care Med. 2014;42(4):849–59.

Part IV
Special Populations/Considerations

Chapter 13
Sedation Considerations for Patients with Congenital and Acquired Heart Disease

Michael Wolf

Introduction

Infants and children with congenital heart disease (CHD) often require deep sedation for procedures and imaging. The increased use of cross-sectional imaging for diagnostic purposes in congenital and acquired heart disease has also increased the need for deep sedation in this patient population. Patients with CHD and acquired heart disease are at increased risk for sedation-related complications. They often possess unique physiology as a result of their heart defects or palliative surgeries, which impacts their response to sedation. Among this group of patients, those who carry the highest risk of sedation-related complications include those younger than 2 years, single ventricle physiology, left ventricular outflow tract obstruction, impaired ventricular function, and pulmonary hypertension.

When considering sedation for the patient with heart disease it is imperative for the provider to understand anatomic variations, surgical history (if applicable), and the physiologic implications this may have on the individual patient. It is helpful to group the physiology of heart disease in children into major categories. This can assist the provider in preparing for potential consequences of providing sedation. Table 13.1 shows the preparation of a cardiac patient for procedural sedation.

The first grouping is to divide patients into congenital versus acquired heart disease. Within CHD there are several subcategories including: cyanotic versus acyanotic; repaired versus palliated; right-to-left intracardiac shunts versus left-to-right intracardiac shunts; and right and left ventricular outflow tract obstructions. The acquired heart disease category includes the cardiomyopathies (dilated, hypertrophic, restrictive), myocarditis, and arrhythmias. Understanding the general category

M. Wolf (✉)
Divisions of Cardiology and Critical Care Medicine, Department of Pediatrics, Emory University School of Medicine/Children's Healthcare of Atlanta, Atlanta, GA, USA
e-mail: wolfm@kidsheart.com

P. P. Kamat, J. W. Berkenbosch (eds.), *Sedation and Analgesia for the Pediatric Intensivist*, https://doi.org/10.1007/978-3-030-52555-2_13

Table 13.1 Preparation for sedation of the cardiac patient

Review most recent progress note from cardiology
Review most recent imaging studies including echocardiogram and ECG
Review all cardiac medications
Review baseline oxygen saturations in room air
Discuss patient with cardiology or cardiac anesthesia if any concerns arise

Table 13.1 is made by author Dr. Michael Wolf

Table 13.2 When referral to cardiac anesthesia is warranted

Unrepaired cyanotic congenital heart disease
Neonate with repaired complex congenital heart disease
Pulmonary hypertension
Single ventricle physiology
Shunt-dependent pulmonary blood flow
Left ventricular outflow tract obstruction
Cardiomyopathy with depressed systolic or diastolic ventricular function

Table 13.2 is made by author Dr. Michael Wolf

that a patient belongs to and what implications that will have on their response to sedation is the first step in preparation.

Consideration should also be given to common comorbidities associated with CHD and surgical repairs such as compromised lung compliance from congestive heart failure, genetic associations, phrenic or recurrent laryngeal nerve injury, pulmonary hypertension, or rhythm abnormalities. Table 13.2 shows patients with heart disease who should be referred to the anesthesia service.

Congenital Heart Disease

In order to simplify the grouping of patients with CHD, it is easiest to group them into three major anatomic categories: those with increased pulmonary blood flow, those with decreased pulmonary blood flow, and those with outflow tract obstruction. These anatomic subsets are not exclusive and certain patients may fit into one or more of these categories. In addition, those with single ventricle anatomy have a unique physiology that may swing from increased to decreased pulmonary blood flow with variations in their intrinsic vascular resistance.

Patients with increased pulmonary blood flow typically have CHD lesions that cause left-to-right shunting of blood and over circulation of the pulmonary vascular bed. This includes ventricular septal defects (VSD), atrial septal defects (ASD), and patent ductus arteriosus (PDA). Symptomatic patients in this category will present with symptoms of increased work of breathing, relative tachycardia, feeding intolerance, and difficulty gaining weight as a result of increased pulmonary blood flow at the expense of systemic blood flow. The balance of pulmonary and systemic circulations is influenced by the relative resistances in each circuit: pulmonary vascular resistance (PVR) and systemic vascular resistance (SVR).

Patients with decreased pulmonary blood flow typically have CHD lesions that cause right to left shunting of blood or decreased pulmonary blood flow. This includes tetralogy of Fallot, pulmonary stenosis, and Ebstein anomaly of the tricuspid valve. These patients present with cyanosis, respiratory difficulties, or exercise intolerance as a result of chronic hypoxia. Changes in lung compliance including from patient agitation can exacerbate the level of cyanosis and it can take time until saturations recover to their baseline. When an intracardiac communication is present (such as the VSD of tetralogy of Fallot) cardiac output is preserved even in the face of relative hypoxia.

Patients with left ventricular outflow tract obstructions can be in the category of CHD or acquired heart disease. This includes those with aortic stenosis (subvalvar, valvar, supravalvar), coarctation of the aorta, and hypertrophic obstructive cardiomyopathy. The downstream obstruction to outflow from the left ventricle increases the oxygen demand on that ventricle and comes at the expense of decreased cardiac output. Patients may develop symptoms related to decreased left ventricular output including respiratory difficulties from pulmonary edema, feeding intolerance from intestinal ischemia, and end-organ damage from decreased oxygen delivery. Maintaining SVR in this patient population can be an important factor in maintaining adequate cardiac output.

Patients with single ventricle physiology are generally grouped into their own physiologic category. As they move through the palliative stages of surgery, their baseline saturations, physiologic expectations, and balance of systemic and pulmonary blood flow can change drastically. Single ventricle patients with shunt-dependent pulmonary blood flow have the most tenuous physiology and their response to alterations in PVR and/or SVR can be unpredictable and dramatic. It is generally accepted that these patients, and even those who have undergone superior cavopulmonary anastomosis (Glenn operation) be referred primarily to cardiac anesthesia when sedation is needed. Following Fontan completion, there are scenarios in which these patients become acceptable candidates for deep sedation by a sedation service.

Acquired Heart Disease

Patients with cardiomyopathies are typically quite sensitive to changes in PVR and SVR and are thought to be poor sedation candidates. Dilated cardiomyopathy is usually associated with decreased left ventricular function; changes in SVR, PVR, venous return to the right side of the heart, and alterations in PVR can have devastating effects on these patients. Hypertrophic and restrictive cardiomyopathies are often present with preserved ventricular function. This should not reassure the sedation provider as both cardiomyopathies cause baseline alterations in cardiac physiology that is exquisitely sensitive to alterations in both SVR and PVR. It is generally accepted that patients with myocardial disease should be referred primarily to cardiac anesthesia when sedation is needed.

Arrhythmias are a broad category of acquired heart disease that may impact sedation candidacy. Consideration must be given to the underlying arrhythmia itself as well as to the current therapy required to treat the abnormal rhythm. Supraventricular tachyarrhythmias are controlled with medications until such time as an ablation can be performed. Ventricular arrhythmias are controlled with medication, and cause significantly more distress to providers when considering the physiologic impact of triggering the arrhythmia. Bradyarrhythmias typically require pacemaker insertion when they cause symptoms. Genetic arrhythmias such as long QT syndrome (LQTS) can also influence sedation considerations. Medication selection must be undertaken with careful consideration for potential QTc prolongation. In addition to consideration of the arrhythmia itself, many antiarrhythmic medications cause myocardial depression. Careful attention should be paid to patients' medications as well as their most recent functional evaluation by echocardiogram prior to consideration for sedation in the setting of an arrhythmia.

Pulmonary Hypertension

Pulmonary hypertension is a category of heart disease that combines the spectrum of both congenital and acquired heart disease. Congenital lesions with unrepaired left-to-right shunts can develop Eisenmenger syndrome with fixed pulmonary vascular resistance and pulmonary hypertension. Pulmonary vein obstruction, whether following CHD such as total anomalous pulmonary venous connection (TAPVC) or in former premature infants with bronchopulmonary dysplasia, causes significant pulmonary hypertension. Lesions that cause elevation in left atrial pressure such as mitral stenosis can cause pulmonary hypertension as well. In the absence of structural heart disease, patients can present with primary pulmonary hypertension from a variety of causes including etiologies such as idiopathic, chronic lung disease, or chronic thromboembolic pulmonary hypertension. Pulmonary hypertensive crises typically involve severe refractory hypoxia and decreased cardiac output; triggers are variable for different patients, but sedation is extremely high risk in this patient population out of concern for triggering a crisis.

Noncardiac Considerations

Cardiac physiology and hemodynamics in isolation is not the sole determinant of sedation candidacy; patients with both CHD and acquired heart disease can develop several noncardiac consequences of their underlying cardiac pathology. Pulmonary compliance and mechanics can be altered by increased pulmonary blood flow or chronic hypoxia. Attention should be paid to the presence of airway compression by vascular structures that may mimic tracheomalacia. Phrenic nerve injury can lead to impaired respiratory mechanics from diaphragm dysfunction, and recurrent laryngeal nerve injury may result in chronic aspiration and lung disease from vocal cord dysfunction.

Patients with chronic cyanosis will typically develop a compensatory polycythemia and resultant hyper viscosity syndrome. This can lead to neurologic sequalae including thrombotic strokes. The presence of chronic right to left shunts exposes patients to paradoxical emboli and resultant strokes or cerebral abscesses. Exposure to cardiopulmonary bypass in the neonatal period increases the risk of development of both attention deficit hyperactive disorder (ADHD), seizure disorder, and autism.

Several genetic syndromes carry strong association with CHD including: Trisomy 21, DiGeorge syndrome, William syndrome, Noonan syndrome, Mucopolysaccharidoses, Pompe disease, Alagille syndrome, to name a few. Sedation providers need to be aware that some of the genetic syndromes with CHD may have airways, which are associated with difficulty with bag-mask ventilation, laryngoscopy, and airway visualization.

Cardiac Sedation Physiology

When considering sedation for a patient with CHD there are several important hemodynamic principles to keep in mind. Patients with left-to-right intracardiac shunts (VSD, ASD, PDA) will tend to have some pulmonary edema and decreased pulmonary compliance from pulmonary vascular overload. The degree of left-to-right shunting will improve with decreased SVR; therefore, deep sedation in these patients is generally well tolerated assuming their pulmonary status is stable prior to induction of sedation.

The degree of hypoxia in patients with right to left shunts tends to improve with increased SVR; when sedated, these patients tend to have increased hypoxia as more blood flow is directed away from the pulmonary vascular bed. Supplemental oxygen and using medications that do not significantly lower SVR can be helpful in improving sedation tolerance. In addition, avoiding scenarios that increase PVR such as airway obstruction can help prevent further hypoxia. While sedation is generally well tolerated in this population, the variability in both saturations and response to supplemental oxygen tend to push them toward cardiac anesthesia referral.

Left ventricular outflow tract obstruction is exquisitely sensitive to alterations in SVR. Decreased SVR will exaggerate the gradient from the left ventricle to the systemic circulation. Intravascular volume status is equally important to maintain cardiac preload; and close attention must be paid when scheduling fasting (NPO) times prior to sedation. It is generally accepted that patients with left ventricular outflow tract obstruction require referral to cardiac anesthesia.

Contraindications to Sedation

There are no published guidelines for referral to cardiac anesthesia, but there are widely accepted principles that guide decision-making regarding sedating the cardiac patient. It is helpful to have a sedation provider who is oriented to both critical care and cardiology to review questionable cases and decide on referral necessity. Providers trained in both critical care and cardiology have a unique perspective and the ability to review echocardiographic imaging, cardiac physiology, and sedation response when formulating a plan for sedation candidacy. Residual lesions are fairly common that following pediatric cardiac surgery; having a provider who intuitively understands the physiologic impacts of those residual lesions is valuable.

Each center will have different thresholds for anesthesia referral. However, it is generally accepted that patients with the following issues are referred to cardiac anesthesia for sedation: unrepaired cyanotic CHD, neonates with repaired or unrepaired CHD, single ventricle physiology, all shunt-dependent infants, left ventricular outflow tract obstruction, cardiomyopathy with impaired systolic or diastolic ventricular function, and pulmonary hypertension. Patients with Williams syndrome (supravalvular aortic stenosis and coronary anomalies) are at inherent risk for myocardial ischemia during procedural sedation and are best referred to cardiac anesthesia. When in doubt a cardiology and/or cardiac anesthesia consult is advised to evaluate sedation candidacy.

Presedation Considerations

In addition to reviewing all medical history prior to standard sedation, there is some crucial data that should be reviewed carefully prior to sedating the pediatric patient with cardiac disease. Reviewing the most recent inpatient and/or outpatient note from a cardiologist is imperative. This should include information regarding candidacy for anesthesia and minor procedures as well as the need for endocarditis prophylaxis. The most recent echocardiogram, electrocardiogram (ECG), and cardiac catheterization (when applicable) should be reviewed. Having a cardiologist or cardiac intensivist review, this data can be extremely helpful when possible.

All medications should be reviewed with attention paid to diuretics, antihypertensives, and pulmonary vasodilators. Significant diuretic need can be a good indicator of the degree of potential respiratory compromise that may be anticipated during sedation. Lastly, reviewing the patient's baseline oxygen saturations in room air will guide the provider regarding what to expect during sedation. It is also important to understand whether oxygen may exacerbate certain conditions, such as in the presence of a left-to-right shunt.

Specific Medications

Propofol

Propofol is a potent hypnotic drug with sedative and amnestic properties. It decreases SVR while PVR remains unchanged. It can be used safely in patients with repaired CHD who have normal ventricular function. Decreasing SVR will lessen the degree of left-to-right shunting in those patients with unrepaired ASD, VSD, or PDA; this is usually well tolerated in this patient population as decreased pulmonary blood flow has the potential to decrease respiratory compromise.

Propofol has the opposite effect on those with limitation in their pulmonary blood flow such as tetralogy of Fallot or obligate right to left shunting. Decreasing SVR in this patient population will decrease pulmonary blood flow further potentiating hypoxia during sedation. Propofol's pronounce impact on SVR makes it a poor choice in patients whose pulmonary blood flow depends on balancing SVR and PVR.

Propofol is a potent myocardial depressant and should be avoided in patients with compromised ventricular function. Its effect on SVR will exacerbate left ventricular outflow tract gradients and should be avoided in any scenario that involved such obstructions including hypertrophic obstructive cardiomyopathy. It is considered safe in patients with singe right ventricles who have undergone Fontan completion and have normal systolic function. Consultation with a pediatric cardiologist is advised prior to using propofol in this population.

Propofol's effect on the QTc interval remains the subject of dispute. The literature is equivocal regarding whether QTc prolongation is an absolute contraindication for propofol use. Propofol should be avoided in patients with confirmed LQTS; and consideration should be given to avoiding its use in those with baseline prolonged QTc on ECG.

Ketamine

Ketamine is a mixed sedative and analgesic medication with a favorable hemodynamic side effect profile. It can be delivered via intramuscular injection when no intravenous line is present. It typically allows for maintenance of mean arterial pressure without meaningful changes in either SVR or PVR. It has positive effect on bronchospasm and increases upper airway tone making it an attractive choice to maintain spontaneous respiration. It is well tolerated in most patients with CHD including those with unrepaired cyanotic CHD and pulmonary hypertension. It should be used with caution in patients with airway issues because of its propensity to increase secretions.

Ketamine should be used with caution in patients with decompensated cardiogenic shock. It can potentiate circulatory collapse because of their catecholamine-depleted state; ketamine's maintenance of SVR relies on its ability to cause release of intrinsic catecholamines.

Etomidate

Etomidate is a sedative hypnotic agent with a favorable hemodynamic side effect profile. It does not cause decrease in either SVR and PVR and has no negative effect on myocardial contractility. It is an excellent choice for deep sedation in patients with impaired ventricular function. It is typically well tolerated in this population. Side effects to be aware of include laryngospasm and myoclonus. Caution is advised in patients with infectious concerns given the potential for adrenal–pituitary suppression from etomidate. Etomidate has a relatively short half-life, which should be considered when using it for longer imaging studies that may necessitate additional doses or a continuous infusion.

Fentanyl

Fentanyl is a potent opioid analgesic with sedative properties and a favorable hemodynamic profile. It is typically well tolerated even in relatively large doses in patients with repaired and unrepaired CHD. It is also well tolerated in neonates and typically does not cause appreciable changes in SVR and PVR. It is an excellent choice for invasive or painful procedures and can be used together with a sedative to provide adequate sedation and analgesia. Care should be taken regarding bolus infusion rates in neonates because of the risk of rigid chest syndrome.

Midazolam

Midazolam is a potent benzodiazepine sedative that provides both anxiolysis and sedation. It can be delivered via the oral and intranasal route when intravenous access is not available. Midazolam has pronounced effects on decreasing SVR and, therefore, its effect on left-to-right and right-to-left shunting will be similar to propofol. Although not a direct myocardial depressant, it can lead to pronounced hemodynamic compromise because of its effects on mean arterial pressure and SVR. When possible, midazolam is avoided in patients with cardiac disease because of its hemodynamic effects. The oral and intranasal routes have less impact on patient hemodynamics and can be considered safer in this patient population.

Dexmedetomidine

Dexmedetomidine has sedative, anxiolytic, and mild analgesic properties with minimal respiratory depression and variable effects on hemodynamics. By virtue of its pharmacodynamics, dexmedetomidine can cause bradycardia and hypotension that are dose dependent and not necessarily consistent from one patient to the next. It can be delivered via the intranasal route when intravenous access is not available. It is considered a safe sedation medication in patients with both repaired and unrepaired CHD and is generally well tolerated in all ages including neonates. It should be avoided in patients with bradyarrhythmias and those on digoxin because of the potential to worsen bradycardia or cause intermittent heart block.

Sedation Recovery

Sedation recovery does not differ significantly for cardiac patients. For those with hemodynamically significant cardiac disease, continuous telemetry and pulse oximetry should be monitored during the recovery period. Minimizing NPO times is crucial for certain patient populations; consideration for intravenous hydration should be given to those patients with a longer recovery time to avoid hypovolemia. Discharge from sedation is appropriate once patients have returned to their neurologic baseline with stable cardiac and respiratory status.

Summary

Infants and children with congenital and acquired heart disease are at increased risk for sedation-related complications. With increasing use of cross-sectional imaging as well as other minor procedures the demand for sedating patients with heart disease continues to increase. Careful consideration should be given to each individual patient's candidacy for sedation and consultation with a cardiac intensivist or cardiologist is recommended. A low threshold for cardiac anesthesia consultation and referral should be maintained in those patients with unrepaired, hemodynamically significant CHD, hemodynamically significant acquired heart disease, or hemodynamically significant residual lesions following cardiac surgery.

Suggested Readings

1. Williams GD, Jones TK, Hanson KA, Morray JP. The hemodynamic effects of propofol in children with congenital heart disease. Anesth Analg. 1999;87(6):1411.
2. Barton KP, Munoz R, Morell VO, Chrysostomou C. Dexmedetomidine as the primary sedative during invasive procedures in infants and toddlers with congenital heart disease. Pediatr Crit Care Med. 2008;9(6):612–5.
3. Diaz LK, Jones L. Sedating the child with congenital heart disease. Anesthesiol Clin. 2009;27(2):301–19.
4. Jain R, Petrillo-Albarano T, Parks WJ, Linzer JF, Stockwell JA. Efficacy and safety of deep sedation by non-anesthesiologists for cardiac MRI in children. Pediatr Radiol. 2013;43(5):605–11.
5. Scalese MJ, Herring HR, Rathbun RC, Skrepnek GH, Ripley TL. Propofol-associated QTc prolongation. Ther Adv Drug Safety. 2016;7(3):68–78.
6. Jayaram N, Kaine S, Divekar AA. Sedation in the pediatric and congenital catheterization laboratory: is it time we wake them up? JACC Cardiovasc Interv. 2019;12:844.

Chapter 14
Sedation Considerations for ECMO

Lisa M. Lima and James D. Fortenberry

Overview

Extracorporeal life support (ECLS) or extracorporeal membrane oxygenation (ECMO) is a form of mechanical support that can provide life sustaining respiratory and/or circulatory support when conventional measures are unsuccessful. Historically patients have been deeply sedated and paralyzed due to concern for accidental dislodgement of cannulas, interruption of flow, or self-removal of tubes or lines, and there are still populations of patients where deep sedation and neuromuscular blockade is necessary in order to sustain adequate flow, keep patients safe, and promote lung rest. Long-term utilization of ECMO while waiting for patient recovery or transplant has become common and has required clinicians to rethink sedation and neuromuscular blockade strategies due to detrimental side effects associated with long-term utilization, such as bone demineralization, muscle and strength loss, withdrawal, and delirium, among others. This has led to the trend of lightened sedation and even awake extubated patients being supported with ECMO.

Though awake ECMO may be the goal, some degree of sedation will likely still be necessary for initial cannula placement, for procedures on ECMO, or for the entire run in selected patients. Sedation strategy is highly dependent on the patient physiology-machine interactions. ECMO use poses its own set of challenges in addition to that seen in critically ill patients including: an increased volume of distribution from the increased circuit volume; drug adsorption/sequestration in the

L. M. Lima (✉)
Critical Care Medicine, University School of Medicine/Children's Hospital of Atlanta, Atlanta, GA, USA
e-mail: lisa.lima@choa.org

J. D. Fortenberry
Critical Care Medicine, Emory University School of Medicine/Children's Hospital of Atlanta, Atlanta, GA, USA
e-mail: james.fortenberry@choa.org

P. P. Kamat, J. W. Berkenbosch (eds.), *Sedation and Analgesia for the Pediatric Intensivist*, https://doi.org/10.1007/978-3-030-52555-2_14

circuit and components; and changes in drug pharmacokinetics based on charge, protein binding, and lipophilic properties. These properties all have the potential for influencing drug selection and dosing regimens.

Effect of ECMO Circuit

ECMO circuits are each unique. Circuits are assembled from constituent parts based on institutional experience and preference of components. Basic key components of the circuit include cannulas, tubing, a pump device, an oxygen exchanger (referred to as membrane oxygenator), and a heat exchanger [1]. Additional optional components include a bridge (to connect the patient side and the blood flow return side), infusion ports (useful in patients with limited venous access), a bladder (serving as a reservoir for fluctuations in circuit pressure to ensure pump function), and an arterial filter (serves as additional point to trap entrained air) [1]. Patients may also have tandem in-line plasma exchange or hemofiltration devices based on institutional practice/patient condition [2, 3].

Circuits can be primed with either blood or crystalloid solution. However, smaller pediatric/neonatal patient circuits are generally blood primed due to smaller patient blood volume relative to the volume required to maintain the circuit even in the advent of smaller ¼ inch tubing [1]. Specific priming criteria and constituents are variable based on institution, and in addition to a base of blood, they often include bicarbonate, calcium (to counter citrate from the blood), and heparin added and titrated to ensure optimal pH, calcium levels, hematocrit, as well as prevent circuit thrombosis prior to cannulation. Additionally, circuits may be pre-primed with albumin to "coat" or occupy potential binding sites from circuit-protein interactions. Circuits used for ECPR may differ in priming constituents due to time constraints. The additional circuit volume and dilutional effect lead to an increased volume of distribution [4]. There have been reports of increased need for sedation immediately following cannulation as well as throughout the entire ECMO run; conversely, some reports have demonstrated similar sedation requirements in ICU patients irrespective of ECMO utilization [5]. These reports are somewhat difficult to interpret in the light of shifting tolerance of lighter sedation and with the advent of nurse-driven sedation protocols. It is also worth mentioning that sedation may vary in different ECMO populations (i.e., an ARDS patient in the acute phase of illness with multi-organ dysfunction vs a patient with single organ dysfunction awaiting transplant) as critical illness itself leads to altered pharmacokinetics with leaky capillaries, altered renal or hepatic blood flow/clearance, and altered cardiac output [6].

The circuit plays a role affecting not just volume of distribution, but also drug adsorption and sequestration within the circuit itself. When broken down into components, each part of the circuit has potential for drug adsorption, with the worst offenders in one study being the heat exchanger and the oxygenator [7]. Other studies have found a main contributor to be the polyvinylchloride (PVC) tubing. Drugs with lipophilic properties have shown a greater tendency to sequestration, with fentanyl, dexmedetomidine, and propofol being more lipophilic than benzodiazepines and other narcotic agents. Morphine showed the lowest amount of adsorption to the circuit in several studies. Protein bound drugs may also be at risk for sequestration [8–15]. Though these studies demonstrate likely interactions between sedation agents and the ECMO circuit, the results are hard to extrapolate to a pediatric population. Studies have varied in the utilization of different circuit priming solutions and methodologies that may determine the circuits potential for protein binding and alter binding capacity based on the pH of the solution. Most studies utilized a new circuit and single bolus administration of a sedative agent with subsequent serial samples to determine drug concentration. Samples were taken at predefined time points with most studies ceasing after 24 hours. Continuous administration/bolus titration in an experimental study to determine effect on drug concentration is logistically difficult to pursue. One would also imagine that a certain binding or sequestration threshold exists and that in the setting of patient-directed sedation protocol that threshold would exceed any binding capacity of the circuit [16–18].

Propofol use in ECMO has found increasing use in adult ECMO but has demonstrated the potential for theoretical decreased membrane oxygenator lifespan due to its high lipophilicity [19–22]. Though propofol is used more cautiously in pediatric populations due to the concern of propofol-related infusion syndrome, it is a mainstay in adult sedation and has desirable properties that would lend itself to intermittent use in pediatric patients on ECMO including: fast onset of action, short duration of action, and the ability to achieve adequate sedation while maintaining spontaneous respirations [23]. It has shown to be useful in adults in bolus dosing during episodes of agitation leading to interruption of pump flow, as a benzodiazepine sparing agent in the setting of delirium, and as an opiate sparing agent [24]. Clinicians should remain thoughtful to recall potential downfalls with propofol as well due to physiologic effects including the risk of hypotension from decreased systemic vascular resistance [23]. A more recent study found no decreased length of membrane oxygenator life span and potentially an increased lifespan of oxygenators [25, 26]. Another recent, larger retrospective study supported no adverse effects on oxygenator lifespan compared to midazolam [27].

Renal replacement therapy (RRT) use has become a more common addition to the ECMO circuit with many patients having acute kidney injury or organ failure at time of cannulation, and also an increased recognition of the risk of fluid overload and its association with poor outcomes in ECMO patients [28]. A hemofilter or continuous venovenous hemofiltration device can be placed in-line with the ECMO circuit using pump pressures as a driving force for hemofiltration using an in-line hemofilter or a commercial device that has been connected to the ECMO circuit [2]. If the patient has sufficient vascular access, a third potential option is to run RRT through that access point without ever needing to connect the RRT device to the ECMO circuit. Drug clearance from in-line RRT would be expected to be similar to RRT in isolation, though most studies looking at circuit effect of drug concentration are without RRT [3, 29]. Drugs with a large volume of distribution large molecular weight, and high degree of protein binding will not have good clearance with RRT due to the membrane properties of the hemofilter. However, small, hydrophilic molecules with little protein binding will be easily filtered and circulating levels would be expected to decrease. Morphine, hydromorphone, fentanyl, midazolam, lorazepam, dexmedetomidine, and propofol all have a large volume of distribution though there is variability reported in the lower ranges seen in lorazepam and dexmedetomidine in infants and children younger than 2 years old [30, 31]. Morphine is hydrophilic with little protein binding, though has a large volume of distribution so clearance of the primary molecule would still be relatively small. Morphine does have a large number of metabolites that have been known to cause toxicity in renal insufficiency [30, 31]. Similar to the ECMO circuit, there is an expected degree of adsorption to the RRT circuit itself that may account for some degree of large molecule clearance and is partially dependent on RRT membrane selection, size of pores, and surface area [32]. Much of RRT drug dosing is extrapolated from adult data and from those with chronic renal failure; therefore, it may be difficult to apply to a pediatric population with acute kidney injury. Indication for RRT (fluid overload vs acute kidney injury) should also be taken into consideration with dose adjustments, and consultation with a pharmacist is recommended [18, 33].

Sedative Choice

No standard first-line recommendation or protocol exists for sedation of ECMO patients. An international survey of ECMO centers examining sedation practices of physicians managing adult ECMO patients found that morphine and fentanyl were the most commonly used opiates, and midazolam was the most frequently used benzodiazepine. Approximately one-third of responders used propofol routinely, and the most commonly used second-line agents were dexmedetomidine, ketamine, and clonidine, though one-third of responders stated they didn't use any second-line agents. Interestingly, only half routinely used sedation scores to monitor sedation in this particular patient population. It is unclear if this finding is secondary to ECMO patients being excluded from initial protocol inclusion or if they were targeting a deeper level of sedation as 40% of responders targeted a sluggish response to loud or physical stimuli or no response to loud or physical stimuli [34]. A more recent single-center retrospective study of pediatric PICU/CICU patients looked at their sedation practices and found opiate and benzodiazepine use in 99% and 91% respectively with 31% requiring a second-line agent. Patients requiring a second-line agent were of younger age and had higher opiate and benzodiazepine doing requirements during their time on ECMO. Median ECMO run duration was overall short 9.5 days, and there was a high incidence of additional procedures needed on ECMO (36%). The level of sedation the authors were targeting was unclear [35].

The RESTORE trial was a multicenter cluster randomized pediatric trial across 21 PICU's comparing nurse-driven sedation protocols to usual care. They performed a secondary analysis comparing sedation practices of patients on venoarterial and venovenous ECMO as well as potential factors affecting sedation. They noted a significant increase in benzodiazepine and opioid use in the first 3 days after ECMO was initiated, with an overall increase in opioid use of 108% and benzodiazepine use by 192% by the time of decannulation with lighter levels of sedation compared to pre-ECMO sedation, with a significant decrease within 3 days post decannulation. It is difficult to assess the potential for tolerance to sedation prior to cannulation as it is not clear how long patients were mechanically ventilated or required sedation prior to cannulation. By day 3, 43% of patients still required use of a neuromuscular blockade (though reasoning to continue neuromuscular blockade is not discussed) and remained heavily sedated. They also noted an increased incidence of withdrawal in patients requiring ECMO compared to those with pediatric acute respiratory distress that did not require ECMO though it is unclear if there was an overall longer period of sedation utilization between these two groups. Most frequently used second-line agents included dexmedetomidine (35%), barbiturates (32%), methadone (38%), and ketamine (17%) [5].

Approaches and Adjuncts in Difficult to Sedate Patients

Opioids and benzodiazepines are the most common first-line agents in ECMO patients reported in multiple populations. ECMO patients have been reported to have increasing sedation requirements as ECMO duration becomes longer. Adjuncts to typical sedation are, therefore, a necessary tool to have in your armamentarium though the preferred second-line agents appear to vary significantly based on population and institution [34–36].

Adult studies cite a more frequent use of quetiapine and haloperidol with some instituting inclusion as part of a standard protocol in those expecting a prolonged ECMO course as a method to combat delirium, which has been noted in up to 50% of adult ECMO patients, or in patients with agitation. Little mention of utilization of these agents is made for standard practice in pediatric ECMO patients [26, 37–39].

Ketamine has a favorable effect on hemodynamics, despite having some myocardial depressant properties, with less predisposition for hypotension which may be a concern for interruption of pump flow particularly in patients with already tenuous hemodynamics [37]. An additional benefit includes maintenance of a patient's spontaneous respiratory rate. In one study of pediatric ECMO patients, it was used in up to 17% of patients—most frequently on day of decannulation [5]. In a small retrospective study looking at ketamine use in adult ECMO patients, ketamine use was associated with decreased vasopressor dosing, though based on the study design it was hard to discern whether or not there was a meaningful change in sedation scores of patients [40].

Propofol has the benefit of having a fast onset of action and short duration of action allowing for evaluation neurologic assessment. It is generally not used continuously for a long duration in pediatric patients due to the risk of propofol infusion syndrome; however, it may be useful if deeper sedation is needed for a brief procedure [23]. An additional area of utilization in adults is as a temporary sedative measure when patient agitation causes interruption of ECMO flow, intermittent boluses can act as a physiologic "reset" or a temporizing measure until sedation adjustments can be made to address the agitation [38]. Major concerns around its utilization are related to potential interference with oxygen extraction due to its high lipid content and lipophilicity though more recent studies show no difference in oxygenator lifespan with propofol use compared to benzodiazepines [22].

Barbiturates are listed as a frequent adjunct in pediatric and neonatal patients (up to 32%) of patients. A case series of six pediatric patients with respiratory failure receiving pentobarbital for sedation (of which two required ECMO) utilized bolus dosing and then continuous infusion of 1–2 mg/kg/hr up to 4 mg/kg/hr. The patients were able to be weaned from antihypertensive agents and pentobarbital allowed discontinuation of neuromuscular blockade agents in four to six patients. It is unclear whether ability to wean antihypertensive agents were associated with improved sedation level achieved in these patients or whether it was due to a direct hemodynamic effect related to pentobarbital—though no patients were reported to need vasopressors [41]. Half of patients had withdrawal and required oral taper which was recommended in patients who required more than 7–10 days of pentobarbital, though may be seen with as little as 4 days of pentobarbital administration [42]. Pentobarbital is associated with cardiorespiratory depression and may lead to hypotension particularly in those with depressed myocardial function (has a direct negative inotropic effect as well as causes peripheral vasodilation). Hypotension may be seen more with bolus dosing compared with continuous infusion. In a retrospective review of 50 PICU patients, no excessive hypotension was seen with pentobarbital administration in these patients [42].

Inhaled anesthetics are infrequently used in PICU patients for sedation outside of life-threatening status asthmaticus due to multiple factors, though may be encountered in the operating room and in some particularly difficult to sedate patients. One of its limitations is accessibility, as it is not readily available in all PICUs. Respiratory staff may have limited training and many PICU attendings have no formal training [36]. Outside of that, there is concern in pediatric populations for neurotoxicity and the lack of long-term safety data with prolonged utilization [43]. In a recent retrospective case series looking at use of inhaled anesthetics for difficult to sedate patients in PICUs in Spain, sevoflurane showed good tolerability with the main side effects being bronchospasm in 9% (one episode potentially related to improper priming); hypotension in 30%, though none severe enough to require withdrawal of sevoflurane (all episodes hypotension observed were in cardiac patients); and withdrawal in 26% after discontinuation of sevoflurane that was responsive to dexmedetomidine, clonidine, and/or morphine [44]. An adult retrospective analysis comparing propofol and isoflurane use in ECMO patients showed no difference in ECMO duration; however, if administered via inhalation, the actual delivered anesthetic dose may be limited by the tidal volume taken by the patient. Tidal volumes of patients in this trial were not included in analysis and the patients also routinely received opiates, benzodiazepine, and delirium prophylaxis with haloperidol, clonidine, or lorazepam [45]. There have been some cases of decreased sedation noted with isoflurane during cardiac bypass cases [46]; however, in vivo studies have shown deceased uptake by the oxygenator, meaning more constant drug levels, compared to other types of sedation [9]. Some small case studies in adults have maintained sedation with isoflurane during ECMO without membrane oxygenator failure while providing adequate sedation [47].

Dexmedetomidine is a central alpha 2-adrenergic antagonist that is more potent than clonidine. It is highly lipophilic; is protein bound; and possesses several benefits such as sedation without analgesia, an opioid sparing effect, less respiratory depression, and the ability to induce sedation that mimics non-rapid eye movement sleep. The most common adverse effects are associated with the development of bradycardia, hypotension, and decreased sympathetic tone due to inhibition of the release of norepinephrine and epinephrine. It is frequently used as an adjunct for sedation in ECMO in up to 35% of patients. However, caution should be taken using this agent in patients with cardiogenic shock or those requiring pressor support [12, 37].

Neuromuscular Blockade

Concerns related to prolonged use of neuromuscular blockade (NMB) leading to myopathy have led to more conscientious use of NMB. There is little guidance for NMB use during ECMO with few papers published and large variation of utilization nationally, internationally, and institutionally within the ECMO population. Most data contributing to our knowledge of utilization comes from international and national surveys of ECMO centers as well as retrospective institutional reviews. Reported need for NMB ranges from 13% (4% in VA ECMO population) up to 64% of patients. The most common NMB agents used are cisatracurium, atracurium, vecuronium, and rocuronium, with regional and international variation appreciated [34, 48]. NMB agents are used frequently during periods of cannulation and decannulation and often accompany phases of deep sedation. In one study, when looking at the total number of days on ECMO, 54% of ECMO days were spent deeply sedated and of those 80% also included the need for NMB [48]. Data from the RESTORE trial in pediatric patients showed that 50% of patients were still using a NMB continuously 3 days prior to ECMO decannulation [5].

In an international survey of ECMO centers, NMB was utilized for >24 hours in 66–100% of patients by 21% of respondents [26, 34, 49]. It is difficult to interpret from the survey data which physician and patient characteristics contribute to the need for neuromuscular blockade and during which time of the ECMO run the NMB is needed. In a survey of pediatric ECMO centers in the United States, 70% of participants did not routinely use NMB agents, but they were administered intermittently as required for agitation and problems with pump flow and for procedures while on ECMO [49]. Additionally, variation in use may in part be accounted for by center experience, physician comfort, patient population, proportion of VV vs VA ECMO, underlying patient physiology/pathophysiology, bridge to transplantation status, and concerns for circuit function.

The use of periodic NMB has been shown to be beneficial and allow for weaning of sedation, and in addition may act as a "reset" when given in conjunction with a benzodiazepine during periods of agitation or dyspnea that cause interruption of pump flow in awake ECMO patients bridging to lung transplantation [38].

Variations in Sedation Practice and Nurse-Driven Protocols

Institution of nurse-driven protocols may increase likelihood of not only patient comfort, but also lower median doses of opioids and benzodiazepines as shown in a retrospective cohort of adult patients. This particular cohort of patients included a proportion of patients who were placed on ECMO as a bridge to transplant. It has been debated whether this population has the same sedation requirements as those with acute illness and multiorgan dysfunction. Bridge to transplant patients often have single organ dysfunction and may tolerate interruption of sedation more easily than patients with acute illness and potential for multiple organ dysfunction. There may also be a bigger push to lighten sedation in bridge to transplant patients to keep their strength and improve their transplant status [26]. However, a trend of lower sedation requirements was also noted in pediatric patients who had a decrease in dosage and length of utilization of opiates in those with a nurse-driven sedation protocol compared to those with usual care, though benzodiazepine usage remained similar between the groups [5].

Sedation holidays (or the daily interruption of sedative medications) were first noted to be of use in adult critically ill patients allowing for decreased length of mechanical ventilation and length of ICU stay as well as ability to decrease total dose of sedative infused [50]. ECMO patients have been suggested to have a higher incidence of tolerance and require higher doses of sedatives and longer duration of sedative use [10]; sedation holidays may be of particular benefit in this group. However, hesitancy over patient stability, small patient size, and potential for interruption of cannula flow have been prohibitive for instituting this in neonatal and pediatric ECMO patients. A prospective observational cohort study was performed in 20 neonates that assessed the safety and efficacy of daily sedation holidays with no adverse events such as accidental cannula displacement or self-extubation. Median time before resuming sedation was 10 hours. Numerous protocol violations were also identified with morphine not being discontinued simultaneously with midazolam, being restarted prior to patient demonstration of discomfort, or being restarted concurrently with midazolam. This may have signified nursing or physician discomfort with lighter sedation levels in the setting of ECMO, fear of potential complications, or varying interpretation of pain or distress in neonatal/pediatric patients [51].

Changing Paradigm: Transition to Awake ECMO

We are pushing the boundaries of ECMO use. Patients are now using ECMO as a bridge to transplantation, a bridge to additional therapy (i.e. a ventricular assist device), or a bridge to recovery, with the longest ECMO patient staying on ECMO for 605 days with complete recovery [52]. With those changes there is an increased push to work toward optimizing patient physical and mental condition that has led to a shift toward decreased sedation, extubation, and awake ECMO with patients undergoing physical therapy, eating regular meals, and having meaningful social interactions [24]. This has likewise added to revised strategies for sedation, physiologic considerations, and monitoring conundrums to follow respiratory status and predict need for reintubation.

Multiple physiologic changes should be taken into account when considering awake versus sedated with or without NMB physiology and intubated versus extubated physiologic effects. Physiologic processes in favor of spontaneous breathing include more optimal displacement of diaphragm for V/Q matching, improved muscular tone leading to improved FRC, improved venous return with negative pressure ventilation, and decreased risk of lung injury from mechanical ventilation. Despite potential benefits of spontaneous breathing, there is still potential risk of lung injury from high transpulmonary pressures even in the absence of mechanical ventilation; these patients would also be at risk for increased oxygen consumption and respiratory muscle fatigue [38].

In experimental settings, physiologic breathing is controlled by PCO_2 to a greater degree than PO_2 (PO_2 has to be 40–50 mm Hg prior to triggering a ventilatory response). This physiologic regulation to change minute ventilation in response to CO_2 removal has been seen experimentally while using ECMO to regulate CO_2 exchange in healthy lungs. However, this is not well studied in sick lungs, and patients with ARDS on ECMO have been observed to have a variable response suggesting other physiologic factors are also involved in this regulation [38, 53].

Another key physiologic principle to consider is the effect of intrathoracic pressure differences on blood flow through the cannula, in addition to the role of adequate preload (venous return). During physiologic breathing in healthy lungs, minimal intrathoracic pressure changes of 4–6 mm Hg occur [54]; however, in acute lung injury, large intrathoracic pressure swings (up to 20–30 mm Hg) can be seen. This large pressure swing can cause increased venous return by pulling blood from the inferior vena cava to the superior vena cava leading to collapse of the inferior vena cava around the ECMO cannula and interruption of flow, or potentially even cavitation of the vessel. This may be less frequently observed in cannulas that obtain their blood flow from both the superior vena cava and the inferior vena cava. On the opposite spectrum, increased afterload can also cause transient interruption in ECMO flow (coughing, Valsalva or bearing down with stool passage, crying).

Many nuances to management of awake ECMO patients will not be covered in this chapter. The approach to sedation in this population is unique. Some patients on ECMO as a bridge to lung transplantation have been noted to be difficult to wean from sedation partially due to exaggerated swings in intrathoracic pressure. However, there is also suspicion for an altered physiologic perception or response leading to a sensation of dyspnea that some refer to as "drowning lung". This sensation is reported to be unresponsive to opiates and can cause dangerous interruption of ECMO flow if associated with changes in intrathoracic pressure. One center has created a protocol for weaning sedation in these complex patients that involves the utilization of intermittent NMB preceded by benzodiazepines for their amnestic effect when this maladaptive response is present, eventually leading to the response being extinguished over time [39]. A stepwise approach to weaning opioid infusions is also used in conjunction with enteral methadone and eventual replacement of propofol. Dexmedetomidine is utilized to inhibit an adrenergic response, and risperidone is added for all patients to help combat agitation. Periodic NMB is continued as needed in states of hemodynamic instability or uncontrollable agitation. An alternative approach to this problem taken at some centers replaces the utilization of periodic paralysis with boluses of propofol in the setting of severe agitation or ECMO flow interruption [39].

Concluding Remarks

In conclusion, no standard approach to sedation for ECMO patients exists. Fentanyl and morphine are the most common first-line agents used for analgesia in ECMO patients, and midazolam is the most common sedative agent adjunct. The ECMO circuit has an effect on the volume of distribution and drug pharmacokinetics, as does the presence of critical illness and altered renal and hepatic perfusion. Lipophilicity, protein binding, pH, and molecular weight all play a role in circuit sequestration and may play a role in sedation levels; there is likely a threshold at which all adsorptive sites are filled though this theoretical potential has not been studied. It is difficult to extrapolate data from these studies directly to patient care as all ECMO circuits are unique with varying surface area and components individualized based on institutional practice. It is also not uncommon that some of the components or the circuit itself will need to be replaced during an ECMO run which would necessitate reaching a new steady state. The need for sedative adjuncts is common, and dexmedetomidine, quetiapine, clonidine, and ketamine are all potential adjuncts. Propofol has been safely used (though more commonly in adults) with comparable membrane oxygenator lifespan to that of benzodiazepines with no noted interference in gas exchange. Lastly, our paradigms are shifting away from heavily sedated ECMO. With the push for early mobility, the benefits of having an awake patient in long-term ECMO management necessitate new approaches to sedation to maintain safe physiologic response in these subacute patients.

References

1. Brogan TV, Lequier L, Lorusso R, MacLaren G, Peek G. The Extracorporeal Life Support Organization, Ann Arbor, Michigan, 2017.
2. Sirignano R, Patel M, Renal P-ML. Tandem therapies in extracorporeal support. In: Critical care nephrology and renal …. New York/Cham: Springer; 2018.
3. Sirignano RM, Meyer EK, Fasano R, Journal P-ML. Pediatric tandem therapeutic apheresis: a multidisciplinary approach. ASAIO J. 2018;64:382.
4. Brogan TV, Lequier L, Lorusso R, MacLaren G, Peek G. Extracorporeal life support: the ELSO red book. 5th ed: Extracorporeal Life Suport Organization; 2017.

5. Schneider JB, Sweberg T, Asaro LA, Kirby A, Wypij D, Thiagarajan RR, et al. Sedation management in children supported on extracorporeal membrane oxygenation for acute respiratory failure. Crit Care Med. 2017;45(10):e1001–e10.
6. Dzierba AL, Abrams D, Brodie D. Medicating patients during extracorporeal membrane oxygenation: the evidence is building. Crit Care. 2017;21(1):66.
7. Park J, Shin DA, Lee S, Cho YJ, Jheon S, Lee JC, et al. Investigation of key circuit constituents affecting drug sequestration during extracorporeal membrane oxygenation treatment. ASAIO J. 2017;63(3):293–8.
8. Hynynen M, Hammaren E, Rosenberg PH. Propofol sequestration within the extracorporeal circuit. Can J Anaesth. 1994;41(7):583–8.
9. Wiesenack C, Wiesner G, Keyl C, Gruber M, Philipp A, Ritzka M, et al. In vivo uptake and elimination of isoflurane by different membrane oxygenators during cardiopulmonary bypass. Anesthesiology. 2002;97(1):133–8.
10. Shekar K, Roberts JA, Mullany DV, Corley A, Fisquet S, Bull TN, et al. Increased sedation requirements in patients receiving extracorporeal membrane oxygenation for respiratory and cardiorespiratory failure. Anaesth Intensive Care. 2012;40(4):648–55.
11. Shekar K, Fraser JF, Smith MT, Roberts JA. Pharmacokinetic changes in patients receiving extracorporeal membrane oxygenation. J Crit Care. 2012;27(6):741.e9–e18.
12. Wagner D, Pasko D, Phillips K, Waldvogel J, Annich G. In vitro clearance of dexmedetomidine in extracorporeal membrane oxygenation. Perfusion. 2013;28(1):40–6.
13. Pacifici GM. Clinical pharmacology of midazolam in neonates and children: effect of disease-a review. Int J Pediatr. 2014;2014:309342.
14. Shekar K, Roberts JA, McDonald CI, Ghassabian S, Anstey C, Wallis SC, et al. Protein-bound drugs are prone to sequestration in the extracorporeal membrane oxygenation circuit: results from an ex vivo study. Crit Care. 2015;19:164.
15. Raffaeli G, Allegaert K, Koch B, Cavallaro G, Mosca F, Tibboel D, et al. In vitro adsorption of analgosedative drugs in new extracorporeal membrane oxygenation circuits. Pediatr Crit Care Med. 2018;19(5):e251–e8.
16. Mulla H, Lawson G, von Anrep C, Burke MD, Upton DU, Firmin RK, et al. In vitro evaluation of sedative drug losses during extracorporeal membrane oxygenation. Perfusion. 2000;15(1):21–6.
17. Nasr VG, Meserve J, Pereira LM, Faraoni D, Brediger S, Goobie S, et al. Sedative and analgesic drug sequestration after a single bolus injection in an ex vivo extracorporeal membrane oxygenation infant circuit. ASAIO J. 2018;65:187.
18. Bhatt-Mehta V, Annich G. Sedative clearance during extracorporeal membrane oxygenation. Perfusion. 2005;20(6):309–15.
19. Harthan AA, Buckley KW, Heger ML, Fortuna RS, Mays K. Medication adsorption into contemporary extracorporeal membrane oxygenator circuits. J Pediatr Pharmacol Ther. 2014;19(4):288–95.
20. Lemaitre F, Hasni N, Leprince P, Corvol E, Belhabib G, Fillâtre P, et al. Propofol, midazolam, vancomycin and cyclosporine therapeutic drug monitoring in extracorporeal membrane oxygenation circuits primed with whole human blood. Crit Care. 2015;19(1):40.
21. Harthan AA, Buckley KW, Heger ML, of Pediatric … F-RS. Medication adsorption into contemporary extracorporeal membrane oxygenator circuits. J Pediatr Pharmacol Ther. 2014;19:288.
22. Myers GJ, Voorhees C, Eke B, Johnstone R. The effect of Diprivan (propofol) on phosphorylcholine surfaces during cardiopulmonary bypass -- an in vitro investigation. Perfusion. 2009;24(5):349–55.
23. Chidambaran V, Costandi A, drugs DM-A. Propofol: a review of its role in pediatric anesthesia and sedation. CNS Drugs. 2015;29:573.
24. Mohite PN, Sabashnikov A, Reed A, Saez DG, Patil NP, Popov AF, et al. Extracorporeal life support in "awake" patients as a bridge to lung transplant. Thorac Cardiovasc Surg. 2015;63(8):699–705.

25. Hohlfelder B, Szumita PM, Lagambina S, Weinhouse G, Degrado JR. Safety of propofol for oxygenator exchange in extracorporeal membrane oxygenation. ASAIO J. 2017;63(2):179–84.
26. DeGrado JR, Hohlfelder B, Ritchie BM, Anger KE, Reardon DP, Weinhouse GL. Evaluation of sedatives, analgesics, and neuromuscular blocking agents in adults receiving extracorporeal membrane oxygenation. J Crit Care. 2017;37:1–6.
27. Lamm W, Nagler B, Hermann A, Robak O, Schellongowski P, Buchtele N, et al. Propofol-based sedation does not negatively influence oxygenator running time compared to midazolam in patients with extracorporeal membrane oxygenation. Int J Artif Organs. 2019;42:233. 039139881983337.
28. Selewski DT. Nephrology G-SL. The role of fluid overload in the prediction of outcome in acute kidney injury. Pediatr Nephrol. 2018;33:13.
29. Kleiber N, Mathôt RAA, Ahsman MJ, Wildschut ED, Tibboel D, de Wildt SN. Population pharmacokinetics of intravenous clonidine for sedation during paediatric extracorporeal membrane oxygenation and continuous venovenous hemofiltration. Br J Clin Pharmacol. 2017;83:1227.
30. Ghannoum M, Roberts DM, Hoffman RS, Ouellet G, Roy L, Decker BS, et al. A stepwise approach for the management of poisoning with extracorporeal treatments. Semin Dial. 2014;27(4):362–70.
31. Wolters Kluwer Clinical Drug Information, Inc. (Lexi-Drugs) [Internet]. Wolters Kluwer Clinical Drug Information, Inc.
32. Menon S, Replacement S-JM. CRRT: technology and basic concepts. In: Critical care nephrology and renal replacement .... New York/Cham: Springer; 2018.
33. Shekar K, Fraser JF, Taccone FS, Welch S, Wallis SC, Mullany DV, et al. The combined effects of extracorporeal membrane oxygenation and renal replacement therapy on meropenem pharmacokinetics: a matched cohort study. Crit Care. 2014;18(6):565.
34. Buscher H, Vaidiyanathan S, Al-Soufi S, Nguyen DN, Breeding J, Rycus P, et al. Sedation practice in veno-venous extracorporeal membrane oxygenation: an international survey. ASAIO J (American Society for Artificial Internal Organs : 1992). 2013;59(6):636–41.
35. Anton-Martin P, Modem V, Taylor D, Potter D, Darnell-Bowens C. A retrospective study of sedation and analgesic requirements of pediatric patients on extracorporeal membrane oxygenation (ECMO) from a single-center experience. Perfusion. 2016;32:183.
36. Adkins KL. Sedation strategies for extracorporeal membrane oxygenation support. ASAIO J. 2017;63(2):113–4.
37. Burcham PK, Rozycki AJ, Abel EE. Considerations for analgosedation and antithrombotic management during extracorporeal life support. Ann Transl Med. 2017;5(4):69.
38. Langer T, Santini A, Bottino N, Crotti S, Batchinsky AI, Pesenti A, et al. "Awake" Extracorporeal membrane oxygenation (ECMO):sedation and analgesia: pathophysiology, technical considerations, and clinical pioneering. Crit Care. 2016;20(1):150.
39. Timofte I, Terrin M, Barr E, Kim J, Rinaldi J, Ladikos N, et al. Adaptive periodic paralysis allows weaning deep sedation overcoming the drowning syndrome in ECMO patients bridged for lung transplantation: a case series. J Crit Care. 2017;42:157–61.
40. Tellor B, Shin N, Graetz TJ, Avidan MS. Ketamine infusion for patients receiving extracorporeal membrane oxygenation support: a case series. F1000Res. 2015;4:16.
41. Tobias JD, Deshpande JK, Pietsch JB, Wheeler TJ, Gregory DF. Pentobarbital sedation for patients in the pediatric intensive care unit. South Med J. 1995;88(3):290–4.
42. Tobias JD. Pentobarbital for sedation during mechanical ventilation in the pediatric ICU patient. J Intensive Care Med. 2000;15:115.
43. Andropoulos DB, of Medicine G-MF. Anesthesia and developing brains—implications of the FDA warning. N Engl J Med. 2017;376:905.
44. Mencia S, Palacios A, Garcia M, Llorente AM, Ordonez O, Toledo B, et al. An exploratory study of sevoflurane as an alternative for difficult sedation in critically ill children. Pediatr Crit Care Med. 2018;19(7):e335–e41.

45. Verkoyen K, Schildhauer TA, Strauch JT, Swol J. The effects of propofol and isoflurane sedation on the outcomes of surgical patients receiving extracorporeal membrane oxygenation. ASAIO J (American Society for Artificial Internal Organs : 1992). 2017;63(2):174–8.
46. Phillips AA, McLean RF, Devitt JH, Harrington EM. Recall of intraoperative events after general anaesthesia and cardiopulmonary bypass. Can J Anaesth. 1993;40(10):922–6.
47. Rand A, Zahn PK, Schildhauer TA, Waydhas C, Hamsen U. Correction to: Inhalative sedation with small tidal volumes under venovenous ECMO. J Artif Organs. 2018;21(2):206.
48. deBacker J, Tamberg E, Munshi L, Burry L, Fan E, Mehta S. Sedation practice in extracorporeal membrane oxygenation-treated patients with acute respiratory distress syndrome: a retrospective study. ASAIO J. 2018;64(4):544–51.
49. DeBerry BB, Lynch JE, Chernin JM, Zwischenberger JB, Chung DH. A survey for pain and sedation medications in pediatric patients during extracorporeal membrane oxygenation. Perfusion. 2005;20(3):139–43.
50. Kress JP, Pohlman AS, O'Connor MF, Hall JB. Daily interruption of sedative infusions in critically ill patients undergoing mechanical ventilation. N Engl J Med. 2000;342(20):1471–7.
51. Wildschut ED, Hanekamp MN, Vet NJ, Houmes RJ, Ahsman MJ, Mathot RAA, et al. Feasibility of sedation and analgesia interruption following cannulation in neonates on extracorporeal membrane oxygenation. Intensive Care Med. 2010;36(9):1587–91.
52. Nelson-McMillan K, Vricella LA, Stewart D, Young J, Shah AS, Hibino N, et al. Recovery from total acute lung failure after 20 months of extracorporeal life support. ASAIO J. 2020;66:e11. 9000;Online First.
53. Kolobow T, Gattinoni L, Tomlinson T, Pierce J. Control of breathing using an extracorporeal membrane lung. Anesthesiology. 1977;46:138–41.
54. Barnard M, Shukla A, Lovell T, Goldstone J. Esophageal-directed pressure support ventilation in normal volunteers. Chest. 1999;115(2):482–9.

Chapter 15
Analgesia and Sedation in the Neonate

Maria Gabriela Dominguez Garcia and Smeeta Sardesai

Introduction

In the past it was believed that neonates did not feel pain. In the twenty-first century there is enough evidence that newborns have developed pain receptors and have physiologic responses to stress and pain regardless of gestational age or corrected gestational age and vulnerable to both its short- and long-term effects.

Many investigations have supported the effectiveness of analgesia and comfort measures in attenuating acute pain responses and promoting long-term physiological, behavioral, and cognitive development. Infants born preterm and sick neonates during their hospital stay undergo hundreds of painful diagnostic and therapeutic procedures that are necessary for their improved survival. Pain or discomfort may occur during routine patient care procedures such as gavage tube placement, bladder catheterization, or physical examination [1].

Pain in the neonate can produce increased catecholamines, lactate and cortisol levels [2], glucose instability, respiratory instability, and changes in cerebral blood flow [3]. Chronic pain can affect the immune system, growth, and morbidity/mortality.

Procedural pain and sedation are frequently managed together, often by using the same intervention. Therefore, it is not always possible to separate sedation from pain control.

M. G. D. Garcia
Division of Neonatal Perinatal Medicine, LAC + USC Medical Center, Keck School of Medicine, University of Southern California, Los Angeles, CA, USA

S. Sardesai (✉)
Keck School of Medicine, University of Southern California,
Los Angeles, CA, USA
e-mail: sardesai@usc.edu

P. P. Kamat, J. W. Berkenbosch (eds.), *Sedation and Analgesia for the Pediatric Intensivist*, https://doi.org/10.1007/978-3-030-52555-2_15

Sedation is defined as the reduction of irritability or agitation by use of sedative medications. Sedatives are used to decrease both pain and pain response in the neonate in the NICUs and operating rooms to limit movement/agitation [4].

The American Academy of Pediatrics (AAP) and the Canadian Pediatric Society (CPS) recommend that each health care facility that treats newborns should establish a neonatal pain control program that includes routine assessment of pain, reduction in the number of painful procedures, and also reduction and prevention of acute pain from invasive procedures [5].

Neonatal Pain and Sedation Assessment

Self-reporting of pain is considered as the gold standard of pain assessment, which cannot be done in the neonates, and which means clinicians have to measure pain indirectly. In neonates, behaviors associated with pain may be similar to those associated with discomfort and currently there is no validated tool to differentiate pain from stress or agitation in neonates.

In current practice, pain assessment has been termed the fifth vital sign by the Joint Commission for the Accreditation of Hospitals and every nursing staff is required to apply validated pain scoring tool in their assessment of the neonates regularly throughout the entire hospitalization.

In their recently published update on pediatric sedation both the AAP and the AAP Dentistry recommend the use of a carefully staged process to plan for and carry out sedation for diagnostic and therapeutic procedures in neonates [6].

Currently there are several neonatal assessment tools available in clinical practice (Table 15.1). These tools are either unidimensional, dependent on either physiologic or behavioral parameters, or multidimensional, dependent on physiologic, behavioral, and contextual parameters such as gestational age [7–13].

These pain scales should be used by the nursing staff as often required for the assessment of the pain and to assess adequacy of analgesia/sedation, even though they were not developed for this purpose. It is important that the medical provider gets familiar with the tool to be used for the assessment of pain.

Sedation definition is arbitrary and there is no clear demarcation between the different levels of sedation. Assessment of level of sedation by response to verbal commands is not helpful in neonates. Assessment by gentle touch and vigorous tactile stimulation may rouse the child and interfere with the procedure. In infants sedation can progress from conscious sedation to deep sedation to general anesthesia without any demarcation.

It is important to recognize the fact that different levels of sedation require different levels of expertise in the management of the airway and physiological function for a patient [15] (Table 15.2).

Table 15.1 The pain assessment tools most commonly used in the NICU for acute pain

Tool	Indicators physiological	Behavioral	Gestational age	Nature of pain
PIPP [7]	Heart rate, oxygen saturation	Brow bulge, eyes squeezed shut, nasolabial furrow	28–49 weeks	Procedural and postoperative pain
N-PASS [8]	Heart rate, respiratory rate, blood pressure, oxygen saturation	Crying, irritability, facial expressions, tone	23–40 weeks	Acute prolonged pain in ventilated neonates, procedural and postoperative pain
NIPS [9]	Respiratory pattern	Facial expressions, crying, arm and leg movements, arousal state	24–40 weeks	Procedural pain
CRIES [10]	Oxygen saturation, heart rate, blood pressure	Crying, facial expression, sleeplessness	>32 weeks	Postoperative pain
NFCS [11]	None	Facial muscle group involvement	Preterm and full-term infants up to 18 months	Procedural pain
DAN (Douleur Aiguë du Nouveau-né) [12]		Facial expression, limb movements, vocal expression		Procedural
COMFORT-neo [13]	Respiratory rate, heart rate, blood pressure	Movements, calmness, facial tension, alertness, muscle tone	24–40 weeks	Acute procedural pain

Table modified from Witt et al. [14] (Springer publication)

Table 15.2 Levels of sedation and anticipated responses

Level of sedation	Anticipated response	Airway patency	Ventilation	Domain for assessment
3	Awake and responding	Affected	Affected	Consciousness, agitation, respirations, and pain
2	Sedated, but responds to normal voice	Affected	Affected	Consciousness, agitation, respirations, and pain
1	Sedated, but responds to loud voice or movement	Unaffected	Unaffected	Consciousness, agitation, respirations, and pain
0	Deeply sedated, unable to respond	Unaffected	Unaffected	Consciousness, agitation, respirations, and pain

Compiled from Analgesia and Sedation in Hospitalized Children, by Elizabeth J. Beckman. Ped SAP 2017 Book 3 Sedation and Analgesia

The approach to pain/sedation in the NICU should start with avoidance of painful procedures, to minimize the pain and discomfort associated with procedures, followed by nonpharmacologic methods and then pharmacologic methods for pain relief [16–18].

Analgesia and Sedation for Neonatal Procedures

Endotracheal Intubation

Endotracheal intubation is a common, painful procedure for critically ill neonates. At birth or in the life-threatening situations, intubation without premedication is warranted. Pain, discomfort traumatic injury to the airway, and physiologic instability (e.g., bradycardia, hypotension/hypertension, decreased oxygen saturation) associated with elective endotracheal intubation can be reduced by premedication. Since intubation is made more difficult by an active neonate, sedation is particularly relevant for these infants. In 2010, the AAP recommended that premedication be used for all neonates requiring elective intubations [19]. Infants are now frequently intubated for the purpose of administering surfactant only, with a plan to extubate as soon as possible to minimize chronic lung disease from mechanical ventilation, and the incidence of air leak syndromes [20].

For extubation to take place within several minutes after surfactant administration, an ultra-short-acting premedication that provides rapid, safe, and adequate analgesia to neonates while improving intubation conditions is ideal.

Opioids

Opioids produce analgesia by acting at μ receptors in the central nervous system, mimicking endogenous opioid peptides and endorphins.

Opioids have been used for treating moderate to severe pain in preterm and full-term infants in the setting of NICU, for mechanical ventilation, during and/or after surgery and before some painful procedures [21]. Opioid dosing in neonates depends on body composition, drug absorption, distribution, metabolism, and elimination which is different from the rest of the pediatric population [21]. Infants receiving opioids should be closely monitored for side effects.

Morphine, the most commonly used analgesic in the NICU, has some limitations when used in infants who need semi-urgent intubation and quick extubation. Due to its delayed onset of action after injection, it is unsuitable for this purpose [7, 22].

Fentanyl, an opiate with more rapid onset of action, can provide rapid analgesia with minimal hemodynamic effects in neonates.

Recently, remifentanil, a highly potent synthetic opioid with a rapid onset of action and a very short half-life, has been used as a premedication in neonates. Welzing et al. [23] in their study of 21 preterm infants of 29–32 weeks gestation receiving remifentanil as induction agent found that remifentanil provided good intubating conditions with 16.9 min (1–45 min) average time to extubation. In the study by Choong et al. [24], the mean time to return of spontaneous respiration in patients who received only remifentanil was 3.5 min. They found good intubation conditions (using a seven-point Likert scale) and fewer intubation attempts.

Other opioid that has been used successfully for tracheal intubation is Alfentanil, with approximately one-third the potency of fentanyl and duration of action of 20–30 min [25, 26].

For analgesia during non-emergency intubation fentanyl and remifentanil are superior to Morphine. Remifentanil, due to its rapid onset of action, may be an acceptable or even a superior alternative to fentanyl.

There are some concerns regarding chest wall rigidity with synthetic opioid use; however, this can be reversed by naloxone use or more appropriately minimized by slow administration, and co-administration of a rapid acting muscle relaxant.

Sedatives/Hyponotics

Midazolam

Midazolam is the most commonly used sedative in the NICU for the ventilated neonates. It has been shown to provide better sedation when administered with morphine [27]. In the NOPAIN trial [28], when compared to morphine, midazolam was associated with worse short-term adverse effects (death, severe IVH, or PVL) and significant oxygen desaturations when used for premedication for endotracheal intubation [29]. Midazolam has also been associated with benzyl alcohol exposure [30].

Midazolam has a long half-life, which can delay the recovery of spontaneous breathing [31].

Combining midazolam with opioids is a common practice in many NICUs despite limited data to support this practice.

Propofol

Propofol, a hypnotic agent, is growing popularity as a pre-intubation sedative, although the evidence on optimal dosing and safety is limited. The success rate of first attempt intubation with use of Propofol was 58% in study by Smits et al. [32], 49% in study by Simons et al. [33], and Welzing et al. [34] reported a success rate of 69%. The success on first attempt intubation was 85% when Propofol was used in combination with atropine in two observational studies [34, 35].

Propofol, when compared to morphine, atropine, and succinylcholine for intubation of newborns, was noted for faster intubation, better oxygen saturations, and shorter recovery time [36].

Some studies have reported hypotensive effects of Propofol [33, 34, 37, 38], while others, absence of a profound impact on mean arterial blood pressure [35, 36].

Propofol clearance and neurotoxicity are inversely related to neonatal and postmenstrual age, and data regarding optimal dosing, effects, and side effects are limited.

Propofol in theory is the most suitable premedication, but it has no analgesic effect and therefore may need to be combined with an analgesic such as an opioid.

Propofol should be used with caution in young infants and preterm neonates as its use can lead to severe hypotension, with transient decreases in heart rate and oxygen saturations.

Barbiturate

Thiopental, a short-acting oxybarbiturate, is frequently used for anesthetic induction in neonates and older children. In placebo-controlled, unblinded RCT in full-term neonates undergoing nasotracheal intubation, thiopental group had shorter time to intubation but had increased heart rate and decreased blood pressure compared to the placebo group [39] but there were no significant between-group differences in oxygen saturation during or after intubation. However, there is a clinical concern about myocardial depression and hemodynamic changes associated with thiopental in preterm neonates, although no RCTs have been reported. Thiopental is not available for use in the United States.

For preterm and term neonates, Propofol and thiopental are acceptable hypnotic agents; however, midazolam is an acceptable sedative for term infants when combined with analgesia as per the AAP recommendations [19].

Sedatives such as benzodiazepines, barbiturates, or Propofol are not recommended for non-emergency intubation, particularly in the context of surfactant administration and extubation because of high incidence of respiratory depression and hypotension [19].

Vagolytic Agents

Vagolytic agents help prevent reflex bradycardia during intubation due to an exaggerated vagal response [40]. The most commonly used vagolytic agents are glycopyrrolate and atropine. Both agents are effective and have not been directly compared to a placebo group or to each other.

Atropine has not been associated with significant adverse effects when given once in the correct dosage. Atropine is preferred to glycopyrrolate as a vagolytic agent during neonatal intubation due to its rapid onset and shorter duration of action [19].

Neuromuscular Blocking Agents

Neuromuscular blocking agents block the transmission of neurotransmitters between neurons with resultant paralysis [41].

The optimal muscle relaxant for intubation should have a rapid onset, short duration of action, and few side effects.

The paralytic agents administered for premedication in clinical trials were succinylcholine (suxamethonium) and rocuronium. Most studies administered paralytic agent in combination with analgesia and/or sedation. Only study [42] that compared administration of a paralytic to no paralytic compared atropine + fentanyl to atropine + fentanyl + rocuronium. There was greater first attempt success for intubation in the group that received rocuronium compared to no rocuronium.

Succinylcholine has rare serious side effects and causes increase in blood pressure after its use. Bronchospasm, tachycardia, and bradycardia have also been reported with use of succinylcholine [42].

Succinylcholine is contraindicated in patients with hyperkalemia and those with a family history of malignant hyperthermia [43]. The side effects Neuromuscular blocking agents block endotracheal intubation and contraindications of succinylcholine have led to the use of paralytic agents such as vecuronium and rocuronium, but the duration of muscle relaxation is too long (of up to 1 h) and therefore are not suitable premedication for intubation. Succinylcholine, which has the most rapid onset of action, would be the appropriate agent to reverse the chest wall rigidity when using potent opiate as a premedication for intubation [44].

The optimal protocol for intubation is to administer a vagolytic, an analgesic, and a muscle relaxant [44].

A summary of drugs for premedication for elective endotracheal intubation is given in Table 15.3 and a list of preferred drug combination and dosage for elective endotracheal intubation is given in Table 15.4.

Mechanical Ventilation

Mechanical ventilation is one of the most common sources of chronic pain in modern NICUs for the sickest and most premature neonates, especially when utilized for prolonged periods of time may lead to alterations in physiologic responses, neuroendocrine parameters, and pain scores [46, 47].

Improved ventilator synchrony, pulmonary function, and decreased neuroendocrine responses such as cortisol, beta-endorphin, and catecholamines have been noted in neonates treated with opiates during mechanical ventilation [48, 49].

Table 15.3 Drugs for premedication for elective endotracheal intubation

Medication	Acceptable alternative	Comments
Vagolytic		
Atropine 0.02 mg/kg intravenously (IV) bolus	*Glycopyrrolate* 4–10 g/kg IV Limited experience in newborns Contains benzyl alcohol as preservative	Dilution not recommended for Atropine Side effects: Tachycardia, dry hot skin
Analgesic		
Fentanyl 2 micrograms/kg (Range 1–4 micrograms/kg) IV slowly over 1–2 min followed by a slow 0.9% sodium chloride flush Repeat dose of 3 micrograms/kg can be given if required	*Remifentanil* 1–3 g/kg IV 2 micrograms/kg (Range 1–3 micrograms/kg) IV slowly over 1–2 min followed by a slow 0.9% sodium chloride flush Repeat dose of 3 micrograms/kg can be given if required *Morphine* 0.05–0.1 mg/kg IV or IM Use only if other opioids are not available Delayed onset and prolonged period of action	Side effects: Chest wall rigidity, seizure-like activity, respiratory depression, bradycardia Infuse slowly over 3–5 min to avoid chest wall rigidity Effects reversible with Naloxone or muscle relaxant
Muscle relaxant		
Succinylcholine 1–2 mg/kg IV bolus	*Vecuronium* 0.1 mg/kg IV bolus *Rocuronium* 0.6–1.2 mg/kg IV *Pancuronium* 0.05–0.10 mg/kg IV	Bradycardia, especially after second dose of Succinylcholine Side effects: Transient hyperkalemia, malignant hyperthermia Effects reversible with atropine and Neostigmine
Hypnotic/sedatives		
Midazolam 0.05–0.1 mg /kg IV or IM Effects can be reversed with Flumazenil	*Thiopental* 3–4 mg/kg IV When used in combination with fentanyl and/or midazolam, it may cause hypotension	Commonly used sedative for ventilated neonates and for procedural pain Better sedation when administered with morphine Hypotension may occur when used in combination with fentanyl
Propofol 2.5 mg/kg IV		Not studied extensively in neonates

Opioids

Morphine

The NEOPAIN trial [50] which evaluated the outcomes of 898 ventilated preterm infants (GA $\leq$ 32 weeks) who were randomly assigned to continuous infusion of either morphine or placebo found that the morphine group had lower pain scores on

Table 15.4 Preferred drug combination and dosage for elective endotracheal intubation

1. Atropine 20 mcg/kg over 1 min + fentanyl 2 mcg/kg over 5 min + mivacurium 200 mcg/kg in rapid infusion
2. Atropine 20 mcg/kg over 1 min + fentanyl 3–4 mcg/kg over 5 min + succinylcholine 2 mg/kg in rapid infusion
3. Morphine 100 mcg/kg + atropine 10 mcg/kg + succinylcholine 1 mg/kg
4. Propofol 2.5 mg/kg i.v. in a rapid bolus (max two doses)
5. Thiopental 6 mg/kg (2.5% solution) i.v. bolus over 1 min
6. Remifentanil 1 mcg/kg over 1 min + midazolam 200 mcg/kg

Modified from Lago et al. [45]

the PIPP scale compared to the control group, but a higher proportion of control infants received open-label morphine. Other studies have also noted that infants treated with morphine were more likely to develop hypotension, require longer duration of mechanical ventilation, and longer time to tolerate full-volume nasogastric feeds [51, 52].

In pooled data from four high-quality studies in a systematic review of 13 studies [53] on the use of opioids (primarily morphine) in ventilated infants, reduced pain scores were noted in the morphine group compared with controls (weighted mean difference −1.71, 95% CI −3.18 to −0.24) and there was no differences in the rates of mortality (five trials), duration of mechanical ventilation (10 trials), and neurodevelopment outcomes evaluated at 5–6 years of age (two trials) and secondary outcomes (rates of NEC, BPD, IVH, PVL, and hypotension). Although morphine analgesia may not alter the long-term cognitive or behavioral outcomes, it is associated with significant side effects in preterm infants and hence the routine use of morphine infusions is not recommended for ventilated preterm neonates [54–59].

A retrospective study comparing fentanyl and morphine for retinopathy of prematurity (ROP) therapy found worsening ventilation status, temperature instability (outside the 36.5–37.4 °C range), apnea and bradycardia events in the morphine group [60]. In the ventilated term neonates, morphine analgesia may not be associated with the same risks as in preterm infants but may cause increased duration of ventilation. Postoperative morphine infusions also prolonged the need for mechanical ventilation in term newborns but was not associated with apnea, hypotension, or other complications [61].

Fentanyl

A highly lipophilic drug is popular analgesic in neonates as it provides rapid analgesia with minimal hemodynamic effects in term and preterm newborns.

A multicenter randomized trial of mechanically ventilated preterm infants (GA $\leq$ 32 weeks, $n = 131$) reported lower pain scores for both ongoing pain and episodic pain for the fentanyl group compared to placebo [53]. However, fentanyl group had more respiratory depression with prolongation of the initial ventilation course versus controls (152 vs 110 hrs), with more infants in fentanyl group remaining on the ventilator at 1 week after birth (42% vs 25%) although there was no difference in the duration of mechanical ventilation between the two groups (10 versus 7 days). They also noted delayed meconium passage (55 versus 41.5 hrs) in fentanyl group.

Other smaller randomized controlled trials of ventilated infants treated with fentanyl have reported lower stress hormone levels (e.g., catecholamines and glucocorticoids), fewer episodes of hypoxia, and lower behavioral stress scores with no differences in clinical outcomes between the fentanyl- and placebo-treated groups [47, 62, 63].

Fentanyl analgesia is associated with less sedative or hypotensive effects, reduced effects on gastrointestinal motility and urinary retention, but greater opioid tolerance and withdrawal when compared to morphine [64–66].

Saarenmaa et al. [64] reported similar pain scores, catecholamine responses, and vital signs in the ventilated neonates receiving fentanyl (1.5 mcg/kg/hr) and morphine (20 mcg/kg/hr) infusions. There were no adverse respiratory effects or difficulties in weaning from ventilation in either group, but beta-endorphin levels and gastrointestinal dysmotility were lower in the fentanyl group.

Methadone

The analgesic efficacy of methadone can be explained by its p-opioid-agonist activity (L-methadone only) and its noncompetitive blockade of L-methyl-I>-aspartate (NMDA) receptors (both enantiomers, I>- and L-methadone). Methadone has high enteral bioavailability [67] and is often used in patients with opioid tolerance and withdrawal because of its safety and prolonged duration of action [68, 69] despite very little data on its efficacy, safety, or pharmacokinetics in children. One study, reported only in abstract form on methadone pharmacokinetics in children aged 1–18 years, found a prolonged elimination half-life with a range of 3.8–62 hours [70]. In the study by Rosen and Pippenger [71], the plasma half-life of methadone was 16–25 hours in neonates with gestational age 34–43 weeks showing different degrees of opioid withdrawal. Study by Mack et al. [72] also reported lower plasma clearance for methadone in the infants born to methadone addicted mothers.

In a study of children on mechanical ventilation, methadone produced significantly greater respiratory depression than morphine or pethidine, although the risk of clinically significant hypoventilation was small [73].

Methadone side effects include CNS depression, constipation, hypotension, QT prolongation, respiratory depression, and serotonin syndrome.

Benzodiazepines

Benzodiazepines (BZDs) activate gamma aminobutyric acid A ($GABA_A$) receptors and potentiate the function of endogenous GABA resulting in sedative, hypnotic, anxiolytic, anticonvulsant, and muscle-relaxant properties. BZDs do not provide analgesia and may even mask the clinical signs of pain in some neonates.

Midazolam

Midazolam is a common agent used to facilitate sedation for mechanically ventilated infants. Although a short-acting BZD, it causes prolonged sedative effects in sick preterm neonates. In NEOPAIN trial [50], relative to controls and the morphine-only group, infants treated with midazolam had low pain scores, prolonged hospital stays, and increased rates of poor neurologic outcomes (severe intraventricular hemorrhage [IVH], periventricular leukomalacia, or death). Similar results were reported in the most recent Cochrane review as well [31].

Data from newborn animal models [74, 75] suggest that midazolam induces apoptosis and/or necrosis of neurons and other brain cells, thereby raising concerns regarding the long-term effects of using midazolam for sedation in term and preterm newborns in the NICU.

However, midazolam has resulted to be a safe and effective sedation of neonates undergoing mechanical ventilation in the studies by Jacqz-Aigrain et al. [76], Anand et al. [28], and Arya and Ramji [27].

Lorazepam

Lorazepam, a highly lipophilic BZD, has serum half-life of 24–56 hours and a duration of action of 8–12 hours in critically ill neonates compared to midazolam. Continuous infusion of lorazepam in adults and older children has been shown to cause metabolic acidosis secondary to accumulation of propylene glycol, an agent used to increase the solubility of lorazepam in currently available formulations. Lorazepam's neuro-toxicity has also been reported in preterm infants [77]; therefore, lorazepam cannot be recommended for administration as a continuous infusion in neonates [78].

Although prolonged sedation can be achieved with intermittent dosing due to its longer duration of action to achieve sedation in mechanically ventilated infants, the long-term effects of BZDs on neurodevelopment remain unknown.

Alpha-Adrenergic Agonists

Dexmedetomidine

A selective alpha-adrenergic agonist with great affinity for alpha 2-receptors has hypnotic, analgesic, and anxiolytic properties. Studies in adult populations have shown easy arousal without respiratory depression, less delirium, less tachycardia, and hypertension when dexmedetomidine is used for sedation and analgesia [79].

Dexmedetomidine is used in critically ill neonates and infants with congenital heart disease because of its minimal effects on respiratory function at sedative doses, facilitating early postoperative extubation [80].

Decreased plasma clearance and prolonged half-life have been reported in neonates and preterm infants [81]. Decreased glucuronidation in the neonatal period is speculated to contribute to decreased elimination and an increase in adverse events from dexmedetomidine in this population.

Dexmedetomidine for sedation in mechanically ventilated neonates is used as a continuous infusion at doses ranging from 0.05 to 0.2 μg/kg/hr. Side effects of dexmedetomidine include bradycardia hypotension and transient hypertension, dry mouth and arrest with rapid IV or bolus administration [79].

The ideal method of analgesia for mechanical ventilation in preterm neonates remains unknown despite several well-conducted studies. There is no clear-cut advantage for any preemptive treatment. Preemptive treatment may lead to adverse effects such as tolerance, dependence, and withdrawal without improvement in death and IVH. Analgesia and sedation in mechanically ventilated patients should be based on an individual assessment of their analgesic requirements.

Intercostal Drain Placement and Removal

Intercostal drain placement and removal is a painful procedure. If the procedure is not urgent, EMLA cream (0.5–1 g) can be applied 60 min before the procedure to the puncture site. If it is urgent, then subcutaneous 1% lidocaine infiltration at a dosage of 2–4 mg/kg buffered with sodium bicarbonate ($NaCHO_3$ 8.4%) in 1:10 dilution can be used. The buffered solution can reduce the pain of the local infiltration [82].

In intubated and ventilated neonates, administer a slow intravenous bolus of opiates before the procedure, as necessary [83, 84]. In non-intubated neonates, ketamine bolus in a dose of 0.5–2 mg/kg IV can be considered, except for VLBWI. The need for intubation and ventilation in neonates breathing spontaneously should be anticipated. After the procedure, bolus or continuous intravenous infusions of opiates may be used. Monitor the pain with pain assessment tools.

No single analgesic strategy has been shown to satisfactorily alleviate pain associated with intercostal drain removal and it is likely that the optimum effects will be achieved using a combination of two or more strategies [85].

Suggested pain management approach for neonatal intercostal drain insertion:

- Non-nutritive sucking
- Oral sucrose 24%
- +/– Subcutaneous lidocaine (0.5% and/ or buffered)
- Fentanyl (if ventilated: 1–2 mcg/kg; if not ventilated: 0.5–1 mcg /kg) or ketamine (0.5–2 mg/kg IV)

Suggested pain management approach for neonatal for intercostal drain removal:

- Two or more of the following:
  - Non-nutritive sucking
  - Oral sucrose 24%
  - Fentanyl (if ventilated: 1–2 mcg/kg; if not ventilated: 0.5–1 mcg /kg) or ketamine (0.5–2 mg/kg)

Endotracheal Suction

Endotracheal suctioning (ETS), an uncomfortable and painful procedure, is commonly carried out in the NICU as routine care of ventilated neonates. There are not many studies evaluating management of pain during routine ETS. In the study by Ward-Larson et al., containment and/or use of sucrose reduced pain and the associated adverse effects experienced by neonates during ETT suctioning [86]. Another study showed that facilitated tucking position can reduce pain during ETS in premature neonates [87].

ETS should not be considered a routine procedure. Assessment of the infant's respiratory disease and clinical condition should be made to determine the need for suction.

Suggested pain management approach for neonatal ETS:

- Use non-pharmacological interventions (non-nutritive sucking, holding/swaddling). Consider oral sucrose 24%
- Consider opioid dose (such as fentanyl 1–2 mcg/kg, IV bolus 2–4 minutes prior to procedure)

Lumbar Puncture

Lumbar puncture (LP) is an invasive procedure frequently used to sample cerebrospinal fluid (CSF) in septic neonates. LP in the newborn may be associated with significant hypoxia, especially in those with prolonged duration of the procedure [88]. Sedation has been shown to reduce the likelihood of an unsuccessful LP ($p = 0.002$; RR 0.5 (95% CI 0.34–0.78)) [89]. In the same study [89], sedation was also noted to be beneficial in reducing traumatic LPs but the number of infants aged <3 months receiving sedation was very small.

In double-blind randomized study by Kaur et al. [90], in 60 consecutive newborns (Gestational Age ≥ 34 weeks) undergoing diagnostic LP, eutectic mixture of local anesthetics was efficacious in reducing the pain associated with needle insertion and withdrawal during LP.

Local anesthesia with lidocaine has been shown to decrease the degree of struggle during LP in neonates [84, 91, 92].

Suggested pain management approach for neonatal LP:

- Non-nutritive sucking
- Oral 24% sucrose 0.5–1.0 mL in 0.25 mL aliquots, commencing 2 minutes before the procedure
- +/− EMLA (≥37w) 0.5–1 g, 60–90 min prior
- +/− Subcutaneous lidocaine 0.5% and/or buffered
- +/− Fentanyl if ventilated: 1–2 mcg/kg; if not ventilated: 0.5–1 mcg /kg

Peripherally Inserted Central Catheter (PICC)

The PICC consists of a long, flexible catheter inserted in the small veins of the upper or lower extremities and aimed toward a central vein. It is a painful procedure for the neonate. During the preparatory phase of PICC insertion, sucrose and non-nutritive suck (NNS) or human milk may be used if possible. The use of systemic opiate-based analgesia with low-dose fentanyl or morphine before the procedure, as necessary is recommended. Topical analgesia is also helpful and can be achieved with EMLA.

When PICC lines are unsuccessful and surgical cut-down procedure is needed, apply EMLA 60 min before the procedure and start non-pharmacological measures as well (non-nutritive sucking, breastfeeding/human milk if possible, sucrose). If EMLA is not an option due to time, use a subcutaneous infiltration of 1% lidocaine (2–4 mg/kg). For systemic sedation/analgesia, use fentanyl (0.5–3 mcg/kg) bolus and/or midazolam, Morphine 50–100 mcg/kg can also be used before the procedure [45].

Suggested pain management approach for neonatal PICC:

- Non-nutritive sucking
- Oral sucrose 24%
- Swaddling
- Multisensory stimulation
- Fentanyl (if ventilated: 1–2 mcg/kg; if not ventilated: 0.5–1 mcg /kg)
- +/– Subcutaneous lidocaine (0.5% and/ or buffered)

Intramuscular or Subcutaneous Injection

Evidence from randomized controlled trials supports breastfeeding and sucking on sucrose solution during injections to reduce injection pain in newborns [93]. Other interventions applicable to newborns include skin to skin care, pressure, and lidocaine–prilocaine topical agents [94, 95]. Also, combining two or more analgesic interventions give superior pain relief as compared to the use of a single method [96]. In that respect, breastfeeding creates a superior response as it involves holding the baby, skin-to-skin contact, sweet-tasting milk, and the act of sucking [93]. If breastfeeding is not possible, then combined analgesia strategy can be achieved by holding the baby skin to skin and administering sucrose solution.

Screening for Retinopathy of Prematurity

Retinopathy of prematurity (ROP) examinations are medically indicated painful procedures that preterm neonates born 30 weeks' gestational age or less, or weighing 1500 g or less endures until their retina is fully matured.

ROP screening should be performed away from the feeding time [92]. Routinely, phenylephrine 2.5% (dose: 1 drop every 3–5 minutes, maximum of 3 drops per eye) and cyclopentolate 0.5% eye drops (dose: 1 drop to each eye) are applied before the examination. Currently, AAP's recommendation for pain relief during ROP screening is to use proparacaine HCl 0.5%, although randomized trials show minimal or no effects of topical anesthetic on pain during ROP screen. Sucrose and NNS or human milk have been found to be beneficial in reducing pain during ROP screening in neonates [97, 98].

Suggested pain management approach for neonatal ROP screening:

- Non-nutritive sucking
- Holding and swaddling
- Oral sucrose 24% 1–2 minutes before, and throughout procedure
- Proparacaine HCl 0.5% or tetracaine, one drop repeated as needed during the exam

Laser for ROP

Retinal surgery should be considered a major surgery. A study from Sammartino et al. in 2003 suggested remifentanil infusion for the control of pain related to laser for ROP [99] although ketamine (1–2 mg/kg per dose intravenously) can be used for neonates [100].

Circumcision

Analgesia is routinely provided when neonatal circumcision is performed. A combination of oral sucrose and dorsal penile nerve block has been found to be effective analgesic option for neonatal circumcision [101].

Local topical anesthetics commonly used for circumcision include lidocaine 4% cream (LMX4) and EMLA cream. No difference in pain control with LMX4, EMLA cream and dorsal penile nerve block (DPNB) [102, 103]. Ease of use and lack of need for specialized training are the two advantages of local topical anesthetics. The main disadvantage is skin irritation and blistering, more so in low-birth-weight infants [104].

Topical anesthetics should be applied generously to the foreskin (1–2 g) with recommended dwell times of at least 60 minutes for EMLA cream and 30 minutes for LMX4 [102].

Most commonly used agents to induce DPNB are 0.4 mL of 1% lidocaine without epinephrine and 0.25% of bupivacaine without epinephrine. Lidocaine is often preferred over bupivacaine for its shorter onset of action, although the duration of effect is shorter for lidocaine compared with bupivacaine (2–3 hrs vs. 4–8 hrs for bupivacaine) [105].

It should be noted that epinephrine-containing solutions can lead to severe vasoconstriction and varying degrees of penile loss; hence, they should never be used on the external genitalia.

Suggested pain management approach for neonatal circumcision:

- Subcutaneous ring block or dorsal penile nerve block
- EMLA 1 g 60–90 min prior to circumcision
- Oral sucrose 24% 1–2 minutes before and throughout procedure

Therapeutic Hypothermia

Therapeutic hypothermia (TH) is currently the standard of care for term neonates with hypoxic ischemic encephalopathy [106]. In the total body hypothermia trial, distressed infants were sedated with morphine infusions or with chloral hydrate [107]. In the neo.nEURO.network hypothermia randomized controlled trial, all infants were treated with morphine (0.1 mg/kg) or an equivalent dose of fentanyl every 4 hours or by continuous infusion [108]. Animal data and studies from children show decrease in the systemic clearance of cytochrome P450-metabolized drugs when body temperature is less than 37 °C. In one small study in neonates undergoing TH, serum morphine concentrations were higher and clearance was lower compared with normothermia at similar morphine infusion rates and cumulative doses [109]. Sedation, analgesia, and neuromuscular blockade during TH may alter neurologic exam and seizure detection. At present the long-term effects of sedation, analgesia, and neuromuscular blockade during TH are unclear. Currently, administration of sedation, analgesia, and neuromuscular blockade during TH is determined by center and clinician preferences, and may be dependent on the severity of illness.

Pre- and Post-Operative Sedation and Analgesia

Neonate will develop a stress response during surgery and adequate sedation and analgesia should be achieved. Fentanyl and morphine have been widely used to achieve appropriate sedation. Some studies have shown that neonates may need less morphine after cardiac surgery versus non-cardiac surgery [21]. It is very important that neonates receive perioperative pain control and that doses of opioids be modified post-operatively according to each individual case and needs [21].

Skin Breaking Procedures

Skin breaking procedures such as heel lancing, venipuncture, and arterial puncture are other common painful procedure performed in preterm and full-term neonates in the NICU. Numerous studies have documented effectiveness of

Table 15.5 Suggested pain management approach for neonatal skin breaking procedures

Heel lancing	Automated lancet for blood sampling Breastfeeding (or NNS if breastfeeding not possible) Skin-to-skin care (ideal) or holding and swaddling Oral sucrose 24%
I.M. injections *Except, routine Vitamin K	Breastfeeding (or NNS if breastfeeding not possible) Skin-to-skin care (ideal) or holding and swaddling Oral sucrose 24% +/− EMLA (≥37w) (0.5–1 g, 60–90 min prior)
Venipuncture or arterial puncture, peripheral IV insertion/removal	Breastfeeding or NNS Skin-to-skin care Oral sucrose 24% Swaddling +/− EMLA (0.5–1 g, 60–90 min prior) +/− Fentanyl if ventilated
PICC, peripheral arterial line or venous cut-down	NNS Oral sucrose 24% Swaddling Fentanyl (if ventilated: 1–2 mcg/kg; if not ventilated: 0.5–1 mcg /kg) +/− Subcutaneous lidocaine (0.5% and/or buffered)

nonpharmacologic methods of pain prevention and relief for neonates undergoing routine skin breaking procedures (Table 15.5).

Nonpharmacologic Methods of Pain Relief and Prevention in Neonates

Oral Sucrose or Glucose

Sucrose produces changes in the endogenous opioid and non-opioid mechanisms. Sucrose can decrease and improve the physiological and behavioral signs of pain [17].

Oral sucrose administration has been extensively studied in both preterm and term neonates and has been found to reduce neonatal pain responses to routine procedures [98, 110].

Optimal dose for oral sucrose has not been established in neonates. Dosing to treat neonatal pain ranges from 0.012 to 0.12 g (0.05–0.5 mL of a 24% sucrose solution) [111, 112]. Sucrose can be administered orally via a syringe or by allowing the infant to suck on a pacifier dipped in 24% sucrose solution. Multiple studies and reviews recommended an interval of 2 minutes after sucrose therapy prior to procedure, although one randomized trial found that it is unnecessary to wait after sucrose administration [113].

Non-nutritive sucking induced by sucrose has also been shown to accentuated analgesic effects [114].

Nonnutritive Sucking

Nonnutritive Suck (NNS) has been reported as a valuable analgesic for acute painful procedures and has synergistic effect when combined with oral sucrose [114].

Breastfeeding/Breast Milk

Breastfeeding is another effective method of pain reduction for term neonates. Several studies have reported breastfeeding to be a superior analgesic for term neonates undergoing heel lance procedures compared to sucrose [115–117].

In intubated or very preterm infants, in whom breastfeeding may not be possible, supplemental breast milk is a reasonable option for providing neonatal analgesia [115, 116], but is less effective than breastfeeding or sucrose/glucose [114].

Swaddling and Skin-to-Skin Care

Swaddling in both term and preterm infants has been shown to be effective at reducing pain in infants experiencing heel lance procedure [118–120].

Local Analgesia for Skin Breaking Procedures

Lidocaine–Prilocaine Mixture (EMLA)

A cream base mixture of lidocaine 2.5% and prilocaine 2.5% known as EMLA is widely used local anesthetic. It is the most extensively studied, and is the topical anesthetic of choice in many NICUs. It has long onset of action (60 min). Several studies have shown that EMLA alone or in combination with oral sucrose reduces pain for skin breaking procedures but is not effective in reducing pain related to heel lancing [121–123].

Common side effects of EMLA include mild transient skin irritation and methemoglobinemia, probably related to its prilocaine component.

Methemoglobinemia is a serious side effect and is more likely following its use on inflamed skin or inappropriately excessive doses and in patients with a predisposing condition, such as glucose-6-phosphate dehydrogenase (G6PD) deficiency.

Tetracaine Gel (Amethocaine)

Tetracaine 4%, in a cream or gel base also known as amethocaine, produces anesthesia within 30 minutes of its application with a maximum duration of 4–6 hours. Although some studies have reported greater efficacy, shorter onset of action, and longer duration of action than EMLA, most studies report similar efficacy to EMLA [124].

Transient local erythema of the skin with local edema and itching are the commonly reported adverse effects.

In clinical practice, to reduce pain associated with skin breaking procedures, amethocaine or EMLA in addition to oral sucrose can be used. It is always important to remember the non-pharmacological strategies to reduce pain with any procedure.

Other Options for Analgesia in the Neonate

Nonsteroidal Anti-inflammatory Drugs (NSAIDs)

NSAIDs are sparingly used in neonates because of their well-known adverse effects such as gastrointestinal bleeding, platelet dysfunction, and decreased glomerular filtration rate in newborn infants.

NSAIDs are not routinely recommended for neonatal analgesia because effective and safer agents are available [125, 126].

Acetaminophen

Acetaminophen (paracetamol) inhibits the COX-2 enzymes in the brain and has been well studied in newborns. Acetaminophen however has been used in the management of mild to moderate procedural and postoperative pain in neonates, but it is not effective enough when used by itself [127, 128]. However, it could be used as adjunct analgesic (combined with topical anesthetics or opioid therapy) as data suggest that IV or oral or rectal acetaminophen in combination with other analgesic agents may be useful to reduce the overall amount of administered opioid [129]. It has week anti-inflammatory effects [130].

Clearance of acetaminophen is slow in preterm and term infants. Acetaminophen has to be used carefully in neonates with liver dysfunction, but it does not cause respiratory depression or tolerance like opioids. It can be given PO, PR, and/or IV. Doses can vary from 10–20 mg/kg/dose PO to 20–40 mg/kg/dose PR 81. These doses are primarily based upon antipyretic response studies and may not apply for pain control [16].

Adverse Effects of Medications Used for Analgesia and Sedation of the Neonate

A. Withdrawal

Of all the analgesics and sedatives used in the NICU, two commonly associated with withdrawal symptoms are opioids and BZDs. Other agents associated with withdrawal include clonidine, dexmedetomidine, and barbiturates.

Withdrawal is manifestation of physical signs and symptoms when opioids/ BDZs are stopped abruptly or weaned too rapidly [131]. It is clinically difficult to distinguish between signs of opioid and benzodiazepine withdrawal. Withdrawal symptoms vary from loose, watery stools, vomiting, wretching, gagging, increased temperature, increased respiratory rate, increased secretions, tremors, sweating, yawning, sneezing, startling to touch, increased muscle tone, etc. [131]. In order to avoid signs and symptoms of opioid withdrawal, it is important to develop weaning protocols and to taper doses as slow as possible [68]. Optimal therapy for treatment of pediatric iatrogenic withdrawal is not established due to insufficient evidence. AAP recommends that each NICU should develop a protocol that provides evaluation and treatment for infants at risk of or showing signs of withdrawal [132].

There are tools available to evaluate withdrawal in neonates. Tools such as Withdrawal Assessment Tool-1 (WAT-1) [131] should be started the day before starting weaning opioids +/− benzodiazepines to obtain baseline scores and continue at least twice daily until 72 hours after the last dose. The WAT-1 scoring system consists of a review of patient's records for the past 12 hours, direct observation of the patient for 2 minutes, then evaluating patient after stimulation, level of consciousness. It consists of 11 items in a 12-point system [133].

B. Tolerance and dependence

Tolerance is described as a decreasing clinical effect of a drug after prolonged exposure to it or where increase in dosage of the drug is required to produce the same analgesic or sedative effect.

Tolerance can be innate, which is present from the first dose or acquired, and which happens over time. However, dependence is the need for continued administration of the drug to prevent precipitation of withdrawal or an abstinence syndrome [134].

Tolerance can occur in a patient, but patients who received opioids for more than 3 days and required increase in their initial dose are at a higher risk of developing tolerance [131]. Studies have shown that continuous administration of opioids produces tolerance more rapidly than intermittent doses [132, 135].

There are several weaning protocols on neonatal drug withdrawal. Protocol mostly utilized when weaning patients from opioid or benzodiazepine therapy is the one described by Hudak et al. [132].

If infants are below the threshold for prolonged exposure, a rapid taper of opioid or benzodiazepine therapy can be done within 24–48 hours.

If infants are above the threshold or withdrawal symptoms are observed during the rapid taper, they may be converted to an equivalent opioid or benzodiazepine regimen.

These therapies can then be gradually weaned by 10–20% of the initial dose every1–2 days based upon clinical response and withdrawal assessment.

There are no clear guidelines on how to wean if patient is on multiple medications for analgesia and sedation, and it seems reasonable to wean one medication at a time in order to clearly differentiate signs of withdrawal. It may be more important to wean the sedative first if there is an ongoing requirement for analgesia. Finally, the infant's pain status should be assessed and adequately managed with behavioral interventions or medications prior to and during weaning.

Summary

Every NICU should develop standardized approach to assessing and managing pain in neonates. Optimizing pain management in the neonatal population should include avoiding unnecessary painful procedures and use of noninvasive monitoring when clinically relevant and when resources are available. Nonpharmacologic measures (breastfeeding, NNS, swaddling or facilitated tucking, and skin-to-skin contact) and pharmacologic agents should be provided pre-emptively for any painful procedure. One can escalate therapy based on the degree of anticipated procedural pain, advancing through the appropriate tiers of therapy (Fig. 15.1) [136] to achieve optimal analgesia.

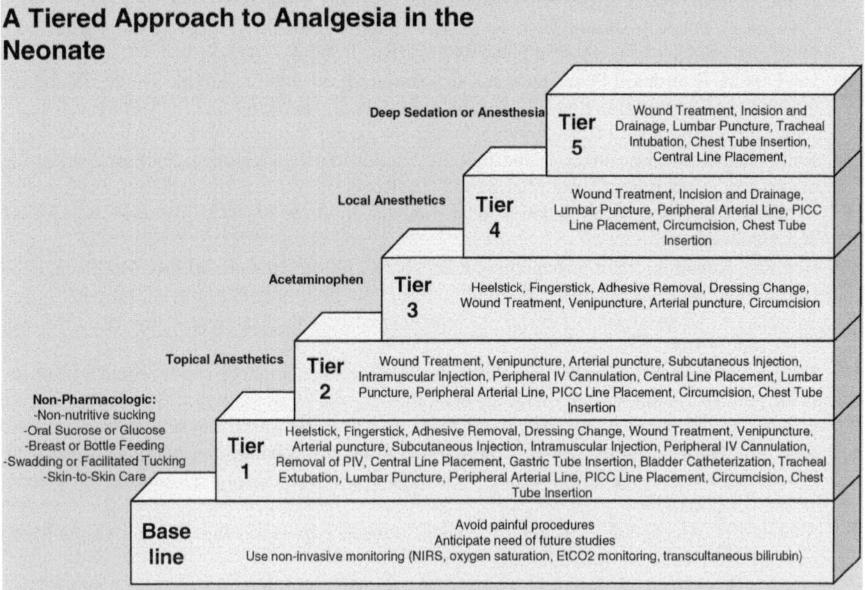

Fig. 15.1 A tiered approach to analgesia in neonates. (Ref. [14] https://doi.org/10.1007/s40138-016-0089-y)

References

1. Pereira-Da-Silva L, Bergmans KI, van Kerkhoven LA, Leal F, Virella D, Videira-Amaral JM. Reducing discomfort while measuring crown-heel length in neonates. Acta Paediatr. 2006;95(6):742–6.
2. Spitzer AR. Intensive care of the fetus and neonate. 2nd ed. Philadelphia: Elsevier-Mosby; 2005. xxii, 1440 pp
3. Taeusch HW, Ballard RA, Gleason CA. Avery's diseases of the newborn. 8th ed. Philadelphia: Elsevier Saunders; 2005. p. 1633.
4. Clark SM, Basraon SK, Hankins GDV. Intrapartum asphyxia, neonatal encephalopathy, cerebral palsy, and obstetric interventions in the term and near-term infant. NeoReviews. 2013;14(1):e13–21.

5. Prevention and management of pain in the neonate: an update. Pediatrics. 2006;118(5):2231–41.
6. Coté CJ, Wilson S. Guidelines for monitoring and management of pediatric patients before, during, and after sedation for diagnostic and therapeutic procedures: update 2016. Pediatrics. 2016;138(1):e20161212.
7. Stevens B, Johnston C, Petryshen P, Taddio A. Premature infant pain profile: development and initial validation. Clin J Pain. 1996;12(1):13–22.
8. Hummel P, van Dijk M. Pain assessment: current status and challenges. Semin Fetal Neonatal Med. 2006;11(4):237–45.
9. Lawrence J, Alcock D, McGrath P, Kay J, MacMurray SB, Dulberg C. The development of a tool to assess neonatal pain. Neonatal Netw. 1993;12(6):59–66.
10. Krechel SW, Bildner J. CRIES: a new neonatal postoperative pain measurement score. Initial testing of validity and reliability. Paediatr Anaesth. 1995;5(1):53–61.
11. Grunau RE, Oberlander T, Holsti L, Whitfield MF. Bedside application of the neonatal facial coding system in pain assessment of premature neonates. Pain. 1998;76(3):277–86.
12. Carbajal R, Paupe A, Hoenn E, Lenclen R, Olivier-Martin M. APN: evaluation behavioral scale of acute pain in newborn infants. Arch Pediatr. 1997;4(7):623–8.
13. van Dijk M, Roofthooft DW, Anand KJ, Guldemond F, de Graaf J, Simons S, et al. Taking up the challenge of measuring prolonged pain in (premature) neonates: the COMFORTneo scale seems promising. Clin J Pain. 2009;25(7):607–16.
14. Witt N, Coynor S, Edwards C, Bradshaw H. A guide to pain assessment and management in the neonate. Curr Emerg Hosp Med Rep. 2016;4:1–10.
15. Beckman EJ. Analgesia and sedation in hospitalized children. Ped SAP 2017 Book 3 Sedation and Analgesia.
16. Hall RW, Anand KJ. Pain management in newborns. Clin Perinatol. 2014;41(4):895–924.
17. Hall RW. Anesthesia and analgesia in the NICU. Clin Perinatol. 2012;39(1):239–54.
18. Allegaert K, Veyckemans F, Tibboel D. Clinical practice: analgesia in neonates. Eur J Pediatr. 2009;168(7):765–70.
19. Kumar P, Denson SE, Mancuso TJ. Premedication for nonemergency endotracheal intubation in the neonate. Pediatrics. 2010;125(3):608–15.
20. Stevens TP, Harrington EW, Blennow M, Soll RF. Early surfactant administration with brief ventilation vs. selective surfactant and continued mechanical ventilation for preterm infants with or at risk for respiratory distress syndrome. Cochrane Database Syst Rev. 2007;(4):Cd003063.
21. Simons SH, Anand KJ. Pain control: opioid dosing, population kinetics and side-effects. Semin Fetal Neonatal Med. 2006;11(4):260–7.
22. Lemyre B, Doucette J, Kalyn A, Gray S, Marrin ML. Morphine for elective endotracheal intubation in neonates: a randomized trial [ISRCTN43546373]. BMC Pediatr. 2004;4:20.
23. Welzing L, Kribs A, Huenseler C, Eifinger F, Mehler K, Roth B. Remifentanil for INSURE in preterm infants: a pilot study for evaluation of efficacy and safety aspects. Acta Paediatr. 2009;98(9):1416–20.
24. Choong K, AlFaleh K, Doucette J, Gray S, Rich B, Verhey L, et al. Remifentanil for endotracheal intubation in neonates: a randomised controlled trial. Arch Dis Child Fetal Neonatal Ed. 2010;95(2):F80–4.
25. Pereira e Silva Y, Gomez RS, Marcatto Jde O, Maximo TA, Barbosa RF, Simoes e Silva AC. Morphine versus remifentanil for intubating preterm neonates. Arch Dis Child Fetal Neonatal Ed. 2007;92(4):F293–4.
26. Saarenmaa E, Huttunen P, Leppaluoto J, Fellman V. Alfentanil as procedural pain relief in newborn infants. Arch Dis Child Fetal Neonatal Ed. 1996;75(2):F103–7.
27. Arya V, Ramji S. Midazolam sedation in mechanically ventilated newborns: a double blind randomized placebo controlled trial. Indian Pediatr. 2001;38(9):967–72.
28. Anand KJ, Barton BA, McIntosh N, Lagercrantz H, Pelausa E, Young TE, et al. Analgesia and sedation in preterm neonates who require ventilatory support: results from the NOPAIN trial. Neonatal outcome and prolonged analgesia in neonates. Arch Pediatr Adolesc Med. 1999;153(4):331–8.

29. Attardi DM, Paul DA, Tuttle DJ, Greenspan JS. Premedication for intubation in neonates. Arch Dis Child Fetal Neonatal Ed. 2000;83(2):F161.
30. Shehab N, Lewis CL, Streetman DD, Donn SM. Exposure to the pharmaceutical excipients benzyl alcohol and propylene glycol among critically ill neonates. Pediatr Crit Care Med. 2009;10:256–9.
31. Ng E, Taddio A, Ohlsson A. Intravenous midazolam infusion for sedation of infants in the neonatal intensive care unit. Cochrane Database Syst Rev. 2017;1:Cd002052.
32. Smits A, Thewissen L, Caicedo A, Naulaers G, Allegaert K. Propofol dose-finding to reach optimal effect for (semi-)elective intubation in neonates. J Pediatr. 2016;179:54–60.e9.
33. Simons SH, van der Lee R, Reiss IK, van Weissenbruch MM. Clinical evaluation of propofol as sedative for endotracheal intubation in neonates. Acta Paediatr. 2013;102(11):e487–92.
34. Welzing L, Kribs A, Eifinger F, Huenseler C, Oberthuer A, Roth B. Propofol as an induction agent for endotracheal intubation can cause significant arterial hypotension in preterm neonates. Paediatr Anaesth. 2010;20(7):605–11.
35. Nauta M, Onland W, De Jaegere A. Propofol as an induction agent for endotracheal intubation can cause significant arterial hypotension in preterm infants. Paediatr Anaesth. 2011;21(6):711–2.
36. Ghanta S, Abdel-Latif ME, Lui K, Ravindranathan H, Awad J, Oei J. Propofol compared with the morphine, atropine, and suxamethonium regimen as induction agents for neonatal endotracheal intubation: a randomized, controlled trial. Pediatrics. 2007;119(6):e1248–55.
37. Veyckemans F. Propofol for intubation of the newborn? Paediatr Anaesth. 11 France 2001. 630–1.
38. Papoff P, Mancuso M, Caresta E, Moretti C. Effectiveness and safety of propofol in newborn infants. Pediatrics. 2008;121. United States:448; author reply –9.
39. Bhutada A, Sahni R, Rastogi S, Wung JT. Randomised controlled trial of thiopental for intubation in neonates. Arch Dis Child Fetal Neonatal Ed. 2000;82(1):F34–7.
40. Bottor LT. Rapid sequence intubation in the neonate. Adv Neonatal Care. 2009;9(3):111–7; quiz 8-9.
41. Rubin MA, Sadovnikoff N. Neuromuscular blocking agents in the emergency department. J Emerg Med. 1996;14(2):193–9.
42. Feltman DM, Weiss MG, Nicoski P, Sinacore J. Rocuronium for nonemergent intubation of term and preterm infants. J Perinatol. 2011;31(1):38–43.
43. Lönnqvist P-A. Smith's anesthesia for infants and children. Br J Anaesth. 2011;107(3):479.
44. Barrington K. Premedication for endotracheal intubation in the newborn infant. Paediatr Child Health. 2011;16(3):159–71.
45. Lago P, Garetti E, Merazzi D, Pieragostini L, Ancora G, Pirelli A, et al. Guidelines for procedural pain in the newborn. Acta Paediatr. 2009;98(6):932–9.
46. Aretz S, Licht C, Roth B. Endogenous distress in ventilated full-term newborns with acute respiratory failure. Biol Neonate. 2004;85(4):243–8.
47. Guinsburg R, Kopelman BI, Anand KJ, de Almeida MF, Peres Cde A, Miyoshi MH. Physiological, hormonal, and behavioral responses to a single fentanyl dose in intubated and ventilated preterm neonates. J Pediatr. 1998;132(6):954–9.
48. Hall RW, Boyle E, Young T. Do ventilated neonates require pain management? Semin Perinatol. 2007;31(5):289–97.
49. Boyle EM, Freer Y, Wong CM, McIntosh N, Anand KJ. Assessment of persistent pain or distress and adequacy of analgesia in preterm ventilated infants. Pain. 2006;124(1–2):87–91.
50. Anand KJ, Hall RW, Desai N, Shephard B, Bergqvist LL, Young TE, et al. Effects of morphine analgesia in ventilated preterm neonates: primary outcomes from the NEOPAIN randomised trial. Lancet. 2004;363(9422):1673–82.
51. Menon G, Boyle EM, Bergqvist LL, McIntosh N, Barton BA, Anand KJ. Morphine analgesia and gastrointestinal morbidity in preterm infants: secondary results from the NEOPAIN trial. Arch Dis Child Fetal Neonatal Ed. 2008;93(5):F362–7.

52. Hall RW, Kronsberg SS, Barton BA, Kaiser JR, Anand KJ. Morphine, hypotension, and adverse outcomes among preterm neonates: who's to blame? Secondary results from the NEOPAIN trial. Pediatrics. 2005;115(5):1351–9.
53. Mitra S, Florez ID, Tamayo ME, Mbuagbaw L, Vanniyasingam T, Veroniki AA, et al. Association of Placebo, indomethacin, ibuprofen, and acetaminophen with closure of hemodynamically significant patent ductus arteriosus in preterm infants: A systematic review and meta-analysis. JAMA. 2018;319(12):1221–38.
54. Ferguson SA, Ward WL, Paule MG, Hall RW, Anand KJ. A pilot study of preemptive morphine analgesia in preterm neonates: effects on head circumference, social behavior, and response latencies in early childhood. Neurotoxicol Teratol. 2012;34(1):47–55.
55. Bellu R, de Waal K, Zanini R. Opioids for neonates receiving mechanical ventilation: a systematic review and meta-analysis. Arch Dis Child Fetal Neonatal Ed. 2010;95(4):F241–51.
56. de Graaf J, van Lingen RA, Valkenburg AJ, Weisglas-Kuperus N, Groot Jebbink L, Wijnberg-Williams B, et al. Does neonatal morphine use affect neuropsychological outcomes at 8 to 9 years of age? Pain. 2013;154(3):449–58.
57. de Graaf J, van Lingen RA, Simons SH, Anand KJ, Duivenvoorden HJ, Weisglas-Kuperus N, et al. Long-term effects of routine morphine infusion in mechanically ventilated neonates on children's functioning: five-year follow-up of a randomized controlled trial. Pain. 2011;152(6):1391–7.
58. Grunau RE, Holsti L, Peters JW. Long-term consequences of pain in human neonates. Semin Fetal Neonatal Med. 2006;11(4):268–75.
59. Anand KJ, Palmer FB, Papanicolaou AC. Repetitive neonatal pain and neurocognitive abilities in ex-preterm children. Pain. 2013;154(10):1899–901.
60. Orge FH, Lee TJ, Walsh M, Gordon K. Comparison of fentanyl and morphine in laser surgery for retinopathy of prematurity. J AAPOS. 2013;17(2):135–9.
61. El Sayed MF, Taddio A, Fallah S, De Silva N, Moore AM. Safety profile of morphine following surgery in neonates. J Perinatol. 2007;27(7):444–7.
62. Orsini AJ, Leef KH, Costarino A, Dettorre MD, Stefano JL. Routine use of fentanyl infusions for pain and stress reduction in infants with respiratory distress syndrome. J Pediatr. 1996;129(1):140–5.
63. Lago P, Benini F, Agosto C, Zacchello F. Randomised controlled trial of low dose fentanyl infusion in preterm infants with hyaline membrane disease. Arch Dis Child Fetal Neonatal Ed. 1998;79(3):F194–7.
64. Saarenmaa E, Huttunen P, Leppaluoto J, Meretoja O, Fellman V. Advantages of fentanyl over morphine in analgesia for ventilated newborn infants after birth: A randomized trial. J Pediatr. 1999;134(2):144–50.
65. Ionides SP, Weiss MG, Angelopoulos M, Myers TF, Handa RJ. Plasma beta-endorphin concentrations and analgesia-muscle relaxation in the newborn infant supported by mechanical ventilation. J Pediatr. 1994;125(1):113–6.
66. Franck LS, Vilardi J, Durand D, Powers R. Opioid withdrawal in neonates after continuous infusions of morphine or fentanyl during extracorporeal membrane oxygenation. Am J Crit Care. 1998;7(5):364–9.
67. Hall RW, Shbarou RM. Drugs of choice for sedation and analgesia in the neonatal ICU. Clin Perinatol. 2009;36(1):15–26.
68. Suresh S, Anand KJ. Opioid tolerance in neonates: mechanisms, diagnosis, assessment, and management. Semin Perinatol. 1998;22(5):425–33.
69. Tobias JD. Tolerance, withdrawal, and physical dependency after long-term sedation and analgesia of children in the pediatric intensive care unit. Crit Care Med. 2000;28(6):2122–32.
70. Berde CB, Sethna HF, Holzman RS, Reidy P, Gondek EJ. Pharmacokinetics of methadone in children and adolescents in the perioperative period. Anesthesiology. 1987;67(3):A519.
71. Rosen TS, Pippenger CE. Pharmacologic observations on the neonatal withdrawal syndrome. J Pediatr. 1976;88(6):1044–8.
72. Mack G, Thomas D, Giles W, Buchanan N. Methadone levels and neonatal withdrawal. J Paediatr Child Health. 1991;27(2):96–100.

73. Hamunen K. Ventilatory effects of morphine, pethidine and methadone in children. Br J Anaesth. 1993;70(4):414–8.
74. Bittigau P, Sifringer M, Genz K, Reith E, Pospischil D, Govindarajalu S, et al. Antiepileptic drugs and apoptotic neurodegeneration in the developing brain. Proc Natl Acad Sci U S A. 2002;99(23):15089–94.
75. Fredriksson A, Archer T, Alm H, Gordh T, Eriksson P. Neurofunctional deficits and potentiated apoptosis by neonatal NMDA antagonist administration. Behav Brain Res. 2004;153(2):367–76.
76. Jacqz-Aigrain E, Burtin P, Daoud P, Desplanques L, Beaufils F. Placebo-controlled trial of midazolam sedation in mechanically ventilated newborn babies. Lancet. 1994;344(8923):646–50.
77. Reiter PD, Stiles AD. Lorazepam toxicity in a premature infant. Ann Pharmacother. 1993;27(6):727–9.
78. Goldsmith JP, Karotkin EH, Keszler M, Suresh GK. Assisted ventilation of the neonate : evidence-based approach to newborn respiratory care. 6th ed. Philadelphia: Elsevier; 2017. p. 640.
79. Ibrahim M, Jones LJ, Lai NM, Tan K. Dexmedetomidine for analgesia and sedation in newborn infants receiving mechanical ventilation. Cochrane Database Syst Rev. 2016;2016(9):CD012361.
80. Su F, Gastonguay MR, Nicolson SC, DiLiberto M, Ocampo-Pelland A, Zuppa AF. Dexmedetomidine pharmacology in neonates and infants after open heart surgery. Anesth Analg. 2016;122(5):1556–66.
81. Chrysostomou C, Schulman SR, Herrera Castellanos M, Cofer BE, Mitra S, da Rocha MG, et al. A phase II/III, multicenter, safety, efficacy, and pharmacokinetic study of dexmedetomidine in preterm and term neonates. J Pediatr. 2014;164(2):276–82.e1-3.
82. Guideline statement: management of procedure-related pain in neonates. J Paediatr Child Health. 2006;42(Suppl 1):S31–9. PMID: 16626313.
83. Anand KJ. Consensus statement for the prevention and management of pain in the newborn. Arch Pediatr Adolesc Med. 2001;155(2):173–80.
84. Menon G, Anand KJ, McIntosh N. Practical approach to analgesia and sedation in the neonatal intensive care unit. Semin Perinatol. 1998;22(5):417–24.
85. Rosen DA, Morris JL, Rosen KR, Valenzuela RC, Vidulich MG, Steelman RJ, et al. Analgesia for pediatric thoracostomy tube removal. Anesth Analg. 2000;90(5):1025–8.
86. Ward-Larson C, A Horn R, Gosnell F. The efficacy of facilitated tucking for relieving procedural pain of endotracheal suctioning in very low Birthweight infants. MCN Am J Matern Child Nurs. 2004;29:151–6.
87. Alinejad-Naeini M, Mohagheghi P, Peyrovi H, Mehran A. The effect of facilitated tucking during endotracheal suctioning on procedural pain in preterm neonates: a randomized controlled crossover study. Glob J Health Sci. 2014;6(4):278–84.
88. Duru C, Ederiane O, Allen-Ameri D, Ibrahim Z, Pondei K, Aliyu I. Does hypoxemia occur before, during or after lumbar puncture procedure in ill newborns? Our experience in a tertiary health center. J Clin Neonatol. 2017;6(3):173–8.
89. Procter C, Buys H, Carrara H, Thomas J. Risk factors for unsuccessful lumbar puncture in children. S Afr Med J. 2016;106(12):1230–5.
90. Kaur G, Gupta P, Kumar A. A randomized trial of eutectic mixture of local anesthetics during lumbar puncture in newborns. Arch Pediatr Adolesc Med. 2003;157(11):1065–70.
91. Pinheiro JM, Furdon S, Ochoa LF. Role of local anesthesia during lumbar puncture in neonates. Pediatrics. 1993;91(2):379–82.
92. Gradin M, Eriksson M, Holmqvist G, Holstein A, Schollin J. Pain reduction at venipuncture in newborns: oral glucose compared with local anesthetic cream. Pediatrics. 2002;110(6):1053–7.
93. Taddio A, Appleton M, Bortolussi R, Chambers C, Dubey V, Halperin S, et al. Reducing the pain of childhood vaccination: an evidence-based clinical practice guideline (summary). CMAJ. 2010;182(18):1989–95.

94. Dilli D, Kucuk IG, Dallar Y. Interventions to reduce pain during vaccination in infancy. J Pediatr. 2009;154(3):385–90.
95. Kashaninia Z, Sajedi F, Rahgozar M, Noghabi FA. The effect of Kangaroo Care on behavioral responses to pain of an intramuscular injection in neonates. J Spec Pediatr Nurs. 2008;13(4):275–80.
96. Shah V, Taddio A, Rieder MJ. Effectiveness and tolerability of pharmacologic and combined interventions for reducing injection pain during routine childhood immunizations: systematic review and meta-analyses. Clin Ther. 2009;31(Suppl 2):S104–51.
97. Nesargi SV, Nithyanandam S, Rao S, Nimbalkar S, Bhat S. Topical anesthesia or oral dextrose for the relief of pain in screening for retinopathy of prematurity: a randomized controlled double-blinded trial. J Trop Pediatr. 2015;61(1):20–4.
98. Stevens B, Yamada J, Ohlsson A, Haliburton S, Shorkey A. Sucrose for analgesia in newborn infants undergoing painful procedures. Cochrane Database of Systematic Reviews 2016, Issue 7. Art. No.: CD001069. https://doi.org/10.1002/14651858.CD001069.pub5.
99. Sammartino M, Bocci MG, Ferro G, Mercurio G, Papacci P, Conti G, et al. Efficacy and safety of continuous intravenous infusion of remifentanil in preterm infants undergoing laser therapy in retinopathy of prematurity: clinical experience. Paediatr Anaesth. 2003;13(7):596–602.
100. Betremieux P, Carre P, Pladys P, Roze O, Lefrancois C, Malledant Y. Doppler ultrasound assessment of the effects of ketamine on neonatal cerebral circulation. Dev Pharmacol Ther. 1993;20(1–2):9–13.
101. Kassab M, Foster JP, Foureur M, Fowler C. Sweet-tasting solutions for needle-related procedural pain in infants one month to one year of age. Cochrane Database Syst Rev. 2012;12:Cd008411.
102. Lehr VT, Cepeda E, Frattarelli DA, Thomas R, LaMothe J, Aranda JV. Lidocaine 4% cream compared with lidocaine 2.5% and prilocaine 2.5% or dorsal penile block for circumcision. Am J Perinatol. 2005;22(5):231–7.
103. Holliday MA, Pinckert TL, Kiernan SC, Kunos I, Angelus P, Keszler M. Dorsal penile nerve block vs topical placebo for circumcision in low-birth-weight neonates. Arch Pediatr Adolesc Med. 1999;153(5):476–80.
104. American Academy of Pediatrics Task Force on Circumcision. Male Circumcision. Pediatrics. 2012;130(3):e756–e85.
105. Stolik-Dollberg OC, Dollberg S. Bupivacaine versus lidocaine analgesia for neonatal circumcision. BMC Pediatr. 2005;5(1):12.
106. Jacobs SE, Berg M, Hunt R, et al. Cooling for newborns with hypoxic ischaemic encephalopathy. Cochrane Database Syst Rev. 2013;2013(1):CD003311.
107. Azzopardi DV, Strohm B, Edwards AD, et al. Moderate hypothermia to treat perinatal asphyxial encephalopathy. N Engl J Med. 2009;361:1349–58.
108. Simbruner G, Mittal RA, Rohlmann F, et al. Systemic hypothermia after neonatal encephalopathy: outcomes of neo.nEURO.network RCT. Pediatrics. 2010;126:e771–8.
109. Tortorici MA, Kochanek PM, Poloyac SM. Effects of hypothermia on drug disposition, metabolism, and response: a focus of hypothermia-mediated alterations on the cytochrome P450 enzyme system. Crit Care Med. 2007;35:2196–204.
110. Greenberg CS. A sugar-coated pacifier reduces procedural pain in newborns. Pediatr Nurs. 2002;28(3):271–7.
111. Johnston CC, Stremler R, Horton L, Friedman A. Effect of repeated doses of sucrose during heel stick procedure in preterm neonates. Biol Neonate. 1999;75(3):160–6.
112. Johnston CC, Filion F, Snider L, Majnemer A, Limperopoulos C, Walker CD, et al. Routine sucrose analgesia during the first week of life in neonates younger than 31 weeks' postconceptional age. Pediatrics. 2002;110(3):523–8.
113. Meesters N, Simons S, van Rosmalen J, Reiss I, van den Anker J, van Dijk M. Waiting 2 minutes after sucrose administration—unnecessary? Arch Dis Child Fetal Neonatal Ed. 2017;102(2):F167–F9.

114. Thakkar P, Arora K, Goyal K, Das RR, Javadekar B, Aiyer S, et al. To evaluate and compare the efficacy of combined sucrose and non-nutritive sucking for analgesia in newborns undergoing minor painful procedure: a randomized controlled trial. J Perinatol. 2016;36(1):67–70.
115. Carbajal R, Veerapen S, Couderc S, Jugie M, Ville Y. Analgesic effect of breast feeding in term neonates: randomised controlled trial. BMJ. 2003;326(7379):13.
116. Codipietro L, Ceccarelli M, Ponzone A. Breastfeeding or oral sucrose solution in term neonates receiving heel lance: a randomized, controlled trial. Pediatrics. 2008;122(3):e716–21.
117. Shah PS, Herbozo C, Aliwalas LL, Shah VS. Breastfeeding or breast milk for procedural pain in neonates. Cochrane Database Syst Rev. 2012;12:Cd004950.
118. Weissman A, Aranovitch M, Blazer S, Zimmer EZ. Heel-lancing in newborns: behavioral and spectral analysis assessment of pain control methods. Pediatrics. 2009;124(5):e921–6.
119. Shendurnikar N, Gandhi K. Analgesic effects of breastfeeding on heel lancing. Indian Pediatr. 2005;42(7):730–2.
120. Yamada J, Stinson J, Lamba J, Dickson A, McGrath PJ, Stevens B. A review of systematic reviews on pain interventions in hospitalized infants. Pain Res Manag. 2008;13(5):413–20.
121. Prasopkittikun T, Tilokskulchai F. Management of pain from heel stick in neonates: an analysis of research conducted in Thailand. J Perinat Neonatal Nurs. 2003;17(4):304–12.
122. Huang CM, Tung WS, Kuo LL, Ying-Ju C. Comparison of pain responses of premature infants to the heelstick between containment and swaddling. J Nurs Res. 2004;12(1):31–40.
123. Foster JP, Taylor C, Spence K. Topical anaesthesia for needle-related pain in newborn infants. Cochrane Database Syst Rev. 2017;2:Cd010331.
124. Biran V, Gourrier E, Cimerman P, Walter-Nicolet E, Mitanchez D, Carbajal R. Analgesic effects of EMLA cream and oral sucrose during venipuncture in preterm infants. Pediatrics. 2011;128(1):e63–70.
125. Aldrink JH, Ma M, Wang W, Caniano DA, Wispe J, Puthoff T. Safety of ketorolac in surgical neonates and infants 0 to 3 months old. J Pediatr Surg. 2011;46(6):1081–5.
126. Anderson BJ, Holford NH, Armishaw JC, Aicken R. Predicting concentrations in children presenting with acetaminophen overdose. J Pediatr. 1999;135(3):290–5.
127. Ohlsson A, Shah PS. Paracetamol (acetaminophen) for prevention or treatment of pain in newborns. Cochrane Database Syst Rev. 2016;10:Cd011219.
128. Howard CR, Howard FM, Weitzman ML. Acetaminophen analgesia in neonatal circumcision: the effect on pain. Pediatrics. 1994;93(4):641–6.
129. Rana D, Bellflower B, Sahni J, Kaplan AJ, Owens NT, Arrindell EL Jr, et al. Reduced narcotic and sedative utilization in a NICU after implementation of pain management guidelines. J Perinatol. 2017;37(9):1038–42.
130. Haidon J, Cunliffe M. Analgesia for neonates. Continuing education in anaesthesia. Crit Care Pain. 2010;10(4):123–7.
131. Franck LS, Harris SK, Soetenga DJ, Amling JK, Curley MAQ. The Withdrawal Assessment Tool-1 (WAT-1): an assessment instrument for monitoring opioid and benzodiazepine withdrawal symptoms in pediatric patients. Pediatr Crit Care Med. 2008;9(6):573–80.
132. Hudak ML, Tan RC. Neonatal drug withdrawal. Pediatrics. 2012;129(2):e540–60.
133. Franck LS, Scoppettuolo LA, Wypij D, Curley MA. Validity and generalizability of the Withdrawal Assessment Tool-1 (WAT-1) for monitoring iatrogenic withdrawal syndrome in pediatric patients. Pain. 2012;153(1):142–8.
134. Benyamin R, Trescot AM, Datta S, Buenaventura R, Adlaka R, Sehgal N, et al. Opioid complications and side effects. Pain Physician. 2008;11(2 Suppl):S105–20.
135. Anand KJS, Clark AE, Willson DF, Berger J, Meert KL, Zimmerman JJ, et al. Opioid analgesia in mechanically ventilated children: results from the multicenter Measuring Opioid Tolerance Induced by Fentanyl study. Pediatr Crit Care Med. 2013;14(1):27–36.
136. Witt N, Coynor S, Edwards C, Bradshaw H. A guide to pain assessment and management in the neonate. Curr Emerg Hosp Med Rep. 2016;4:1–10.

Chapter 16
Sedation and Analgesia in Brain-Injured Children

Kevin Havlin and Lindsey Rasmussen

Traumatic brain injury (TBI), whether accidental or inflicted, is the leading cause of death and disability in children in the United States. Per the CDC, from 2007 to 2013, the overall age-adjusted combined rates of TBI-related ED visits, hospitalizations, and deaths have risen from 639.9 per 100,000 to 889.6 per 100,000. Much of this increase is driven by an increase in ED visits as overall age-adjusted hospitalization rates have remained stable and mortality rates have decreased slightly [1]. While the trend of increased ED visits holds true for all pediatric age groups, rates of both pediatric hospitalization and mortality have decreased over the same time period [1]. Increased public awareness of TBI, especially sports related, probably accounts for much of the increase in ED visits in recent years, and implementation of evidence-based guidelines for the management of children with severe traumatic brain injury, first published in 2003 and most recently updated in 2019 [2], likely contribute to the decrease in mortality.

Recent studies have shown that the population served by pediatric neurocritical care programs carries a higher illness severity, morbidity, and mortality when compared to the average patient in a pediatric intensive care unit [3]. Management of the brain-injured child in the pediatric intensive care unit (PICU) can be distilled to a single unifying principle, prevention of secondary injury. This secondary injury can occur through both endogenous (excitotoxicity, oxidative stress, inflammation, and delayed cell death) and exogenous (hypotension, hypoxia and impaired substrate delivery) mechanisms [4]. In clinical terms, the above processes lead to changes in cerebral blood flow/volume (CBF/CBV), and cerebral metabolic rates for oxygen ($CMRO_2$) and glucose (CMRg) that often manifest as changes in intracranial

K. Havlin (✉)
University of Louisville, Louisville, KY, USA
e-mail: kevin.havlin@louisville.edu

L. Rasmussen (✉)
Stanford University, Stanford, CA, USA
e-mail: lkrasmus@stanford.edu

P. P. Kamat, J. W. Berkenbosch (eds.), *Sedation and Analgesia for the Pediatric Intensivist*, https://doi.org/10.1007/978-3-030-52555-2_16

pressure (ICP) and cerebral perfusion pressure (CPP). It is these factors, ICP and CPP, that are most commonly monitored, targeted by intervention, and associated with good or poor outcomes in the setting of brain injury [2]. In the noninjured brain, homeostatic mechanisms exist for the coupling of CBF with $CMRO_2$/CMRG as well as autoregulation of a consistent CBF across a wide range of CPPs. These mechanisms are often impaired in TBI, making the injured brain more vulnerable to secondary insult. [4, 5]

A unique consideration in the management of the neurologically injured child is the use and inclusion of sedation as a component of the disease treatment itself rather than simply to facilitate the monitoring and treatment of the patient. Anxiety and pain can result in undesired effects, such as increased cerebral metabolic demand for oxygen and, consequently, increased ICP, whereas treatment of stress, including pain and anxiety, can impart neuroprotective effects. Similarly, inadequate or poorly chosen sedation can contribute to secondary injury, potentially worsening patient outcomes.

Role for Neuromonitoring During Sedation

The role of monitoring in the neurocritical care population has long been of interest and focus. As it is high risk and without proven benefit to place an invasive ICP monitor in every brain-injured patient, noninvasive modes of monitoring neurologic status during sedation are needed [6, 7, 18]. Despite advances in technology and medical technique, the clinical neurologic exam remains a gold standard for patient assessments.

Interruption of Sedation Trials

A reassuring neurologic exam has excellent diagnostic and prognostic value. Sedation, though often necessary, can limit or obscure the neurologic exam. As such, the practice of *Interruption of Sedation* (IS trials), sometimes referred to as *Neurologic Wake-up tests* (NWT), is frequently utilized in sedated, neurologically injured patients [8] There have been challenges to the practice of pausing sedation to allow a patient to awaken and perform neurologic functions; questioning the true benefit of these exams, the risks of abrupt cessation of any benefit from sedation medications, and the overall ratio of risk to benefit. One trial of 87 patients in an adult neurocritical care unit prospectively studied IS trials throughout the course of their intubation and sedation to identify frequency with which neurologic deficits were detected during an IS trial. This study found only one case of detection of a new deficit, and additionally found half of the IS trials to be aborted due to concerning vital sign changes [9] This brings into question the risk of awakening a neurologically injured patient, even for a short time. The same study found that patients in the aborted trials had significantly lower brain tissue oxygen tension values, with 67% of the values critically less than 20 mm Hg [9]. Another study, specifically investigating traumatic brain injury patients over 10 days following injury, showed significant decreases in CPP and increases in ICP during IS trials, although there were no associated significant alterations in microdialysis measurement of glucose, lactate, partial pressure oxygen tension, or jugular venous oxygen saturation [10]. On the other side of the argument, many promote non-neurologic benefits of IS trials such as decreased time on the ventilator [11]. As additional and multimodal options in neuromonitoring emerge, the role for sedation pauses will require continued attention and study.

End-Tidal Carbon Dioxide

As discussed in other chapters, invasive or noninvasive monitoring of carbon dioxide in a sedated child is of paramount importance. In no patient population is this more evident than in the neurocritical care cohort. As a potent vasodilator, carbon dioxide will rapidly increase CBF and cause hyperemia in the injured brain. As such, guidelines for pediatric traumatic brain injury recommend avoiding hypercarbia and maintaining normal pCO_2 levels between 35 and 45 mm Hg [2].

Hypocarbia similarly poses great danger to an already vulnerable brain. Vasoconstriction and decreased CBF, caused by hypocarbia, can lead to cerebral ischemia [12, 13]. Excessive hyperventilation and hypocarbia have been linked with worsened neurologic outcomes in TBI and in subarachnoid hemorrhage [14, 15]. Therefore, the monitoring of, and attention to, end tidal carbon dioxide to avoid both hyper- and hypocapnia, is extremely important when administering sedation, which may lead to blunting of airway protection reflexes, limitation of the neurologic exam, and decreased respiratory drive.

Near-Infrared Spectroscopy

Near-infrared spectroscopy (NIRS) is shown in the literature to correspond with cerebral venous oxygenation saturation when compared to jugular venous saturations in patients following cardiac bypass, cardiac arrest, intracranial hemorrhage, and in critically ill patients [6, 16–18]. The ease of use and noninvasive nature makes NIRS an attractive monitoring option in the neurologically injured patient. One can imagine NIRS monitoring could be useful in a patient population with concern for increased cerebral oxygen demand and potential decreased oxygen delivery due to sedation [19]. However, the application of this association during sedation is yet to be delineated. There is a growing body of literature in anesthesia, using NIRS to detect pain sensation during moderate and deep sedation in the operating room. In a study of colonoscopy patients, a consistent and reproducible change in NIRS was associated with insufflation of the colon, a procedure known to be painful [20]. In neurologically fragile patients, where a clinical pain response may not be present, but pain and stress sensation may be injurious, there may be a role for investigation of NIRS monitoring during sedation [12].

Pupillometer

The pupillometer is a device that provides a quantitative measure of pupillary size and a standardized score called the neurological pupillary index (NPi) [21, 22]. The device has become increasingly common in its use in the neurocritical care arena, as the subjectivity and reliability of the traditional bedside pupillary exam have been called increasingly into question. The ability to quantitatively detect subtle changes in pupillary reactivity, as opposed to the otherwise subjective dichotomous characterization as reactive or nonreactive, proposes new insight into the dynamic neurologic status of neurocritical care patients [22, 23]. The device is, thus far, largely utilized in detection and monitoring of increased ICP. Studies have found significantly higher ICP values, with means greater than 20 mm Hg, in patients with abnormal NPi values compared to patients with normal NPi values [21, 24]. Furthermore, abnormalities detected on pupillometer are found an average of 15.9 h prior to the actual change in the measured ICP [21]. There are no current studies in the literature specifically surrounding pupillometers as a monitoring modality during sedation. However, given the relatively low utilization of intracranial pressure monitors in children with critical neurologic illness, this technology holds promise as a noninvasive modality for obtaining more objective and vital data regarding dynamic changes in ICP in a patient whose clinical exam is less reliable due to sedation.

Drug-Specific Considerations

The choice of medication, dosing, and frequency of dosing are all important considerations when sedating the neurologically injured child. Each child should be considered individually in terms of their specific hemodynamics, the etiology of their injury, the length of their sedation, and the potential for presence of pain. In broad terms, ideal sedating drugs for the neurocritical care patient do not alter cardiovascular tone, reduce CBF and $CMRO_2$, maintain autoregulation, are easily titratable, and have clinical effects that can be turned quickly on or off.

Propofol

Propofol is a widely used medication in total intravenous anesthesia (TIVA) for neurosurgical patients. The lipid formulation penetrates the blood–brain barrier quickly [8]. Propofol causes a decrease in CBF, CMRO2, and ICP, with a dose-dependent effect on CBF and $CMRO_2$. The potential for vasodilation and hypotension in patients receiving propofol adds the caveat of careful attention to blood pressure to maintain CPP, continuous blood pressure monitoring, and quick treatment of hypotension when using propofol in this population. Its decreased incidence of vomiting, and smooth emergence without coughing, are desirable effects, which can blunt spikes in ICP when waking up. The rapid dissipation of sedating effects when discontinuing propofol is also attractive in neurologically injured patients in whom frequent neurologic exams may be warranted or desired. Furthermore, it is a potent anticonvulsant agent [8].

Propofol may have neuroprotective effects beyond those directly related to sedation. These include targeting neuroinflammation as well as ischemia-reperfusion injury, a component of the "second hit" phenomenon after brain injury. In rat studies, propofol alleviated mitochondrial-induced oxidative stress in ischemia-reperfusion by preventing accumulation of succinate in injured areas and therefore oxidation of succinate within the mitochondria. Additionally, in the same injured rats, propofol was found to prevent calcium-induced mitochondrial swelling [25]. Inflammation resulting in activated microglia in the brain may also be alleviated by use of propofol. Studies of rats with lipopolysaccharide (LPS)-activated microglia showed a significant decrease in proinflammatory mediators in the brain after receiving propofol [26]. Similar results were found in other animal studies, crediting mechanisms involving intracellular calcium homeostasis associated with propofol [27]. Further studies to corroborate these benefits in human TBI patients are needed.

Benzodiazepines

The benzodiazepine agents can all decrease CBF, $CMRO_2$, and ICP through their action on GABA type A receptors [8]. This can be desirable in the patients with intracranial hypertension or neurologic injury. Through this same mechanism, benzodiazepines are excellent agents in seizure management. With increasing literature surrounding intensive care delirium, this class of medication has arisen as independently associated with the development of delirium. Delirium in the neurocritical care population is itself associated with worse outcomes such as slower ICU progress and worse cognitive evaluations; calling for new consideration of the amount and frequency of exposure to benzodiazepines in this at-risk population [28–30].

Opioids

The opioid class has less well-defined effects on the cerebral measurements that are of concern in the brain-injured patients. CBF and ICP may be unchanged or increased with administration of opioids [8]. A commonly cited study of 2000 randomized adults with severe brain injury demonstrated an increase in ICP in both patients with intact and nonintact cerebral autoregulation, following fentanyl or morphine bolus administration. Other measures such as CBF, arteriovenous O_2 content differences, and mean flow velocity of the middle cerebral artery by transcranial doppler were unchanged. This leaves the significance of transient ICP increases associated with opioid administration uncertain [31, 32]. Similarly, a met-analysis of TBI patients demonstrated a significant increase in ICP measurements when bolus doses of opioids were administered, but failed to show changes in clinical outcomes such as mortality and length of stay [33]. Thus, the need for additional, larger randomized trials on this topic remains.

What is well known, however, is the propensity for opioids to cause respiratory depression. As the magnitude of this effect differs for each patient and is dose dependent, the opportunity for respiratory depression and hypercarbia with opioid sedation is significant in the brain-injured patient. Administration should be judicious and by a skilled clinician to avoid the known negative effects of hypercarbia in neurologically fragile children [8]. Appropriate monitoring to assess respiratory depression should also be routinely employed.

Remifentanil is an opioid often specifically utilized in the sedation of children in neurocritical care because of its extremely short half-life. The medication must be used as an infusion due to its rapid break down by plasma esterases. The short duration allows for brief pauses in sedation in order to rapidly perform neurologic examination, and it avoids accumulation of medication that may confuse the clinical picture [31]. The medication is overall felt to cause decreases in $CMRO_2$ and ICP without significant changes in the CPP or CBF [8, 31]. Remifentanil has additionally been shown to exhibit synergism with propofol, requiring a lower concentration of each to achieve the same sedation effect. This can be advantageous in a child with special concern for the adverse effects from either individual medication. However, attention should always be given to the potential for synergism in adverse effect profile as well, underscoring the importance of monitoring for earlier respiratory depression and/or hypotension when using two drugs in combination [8].

Barbiturates

Barbiturates have a long history of use in brain injury secondary to the popularity of sodium thiopental, which has fast induction action due to high lipid solubility. However, this medication is no longer available in the United States [40]. The class of barbiturates continues to be known, through its action on GABA receptors, to cause a marked decrease in CBF with some decrease in $CMRO_2$ and ICP [8]. The most commonly used barbiturates, phenobarbital and pentobarbital, can cause significant and prolonged sedation, making them less attractive options in children where frequent neurologic examinations are desired. Additionally, their negative inotropic effects can lead to decreased blood pressures, and subsequently decreased cerebral perfusion pressure. Therefore, pharmacologic hemodynamic support should be immediately available when using this class of medication in the neurocritical care population. While a separate indication than sedation alone, barbiturates are also very effective in treatment of malignant intracranial hypertension and refractory status epilepticus [8, 40].

Dexmedetomidine

Dexmedetomidine, through agonistic effects on central alpha-2 receptors, acts quickly to enact inhibitory effects in the CNS, both by sedation and analgesia [34]. The medication also has minimal respiratory depressant effects, making control of carbon dioxide less worrisome in the neurocritical care patient being sedated with a natural airway. Bradycardia is a side effect that should be acknowledged as it must be differentiated from bradycardia that may arise from intracranial hypertension [8]. Dexmedetomidine is thought to have largely neutral effects on intracranial dynamics. While it has been shown to sometimes decrease CBF, it does not cause a significant change in $CMRO_2$ or in ICP [8].

Dexmetetomidine has been shown to be neuroprotective in many animal models of brain injury via reduction of oxidative stress, decrease in inflammation, and mitigation of apoptosis [35–37]. Studies on this topic in clinical practice are sparse and, in pediatrics, are even further limited. One trial randomizing adult patients to dexmedetomidine versus placebo during epilepsy surgery found a significant reduction in the brain injury biomarker S100b, suggesting a potential neuroprotective effect of this sedation agent [38]. Further clinical studies in this area, however, are warranted.

Ketamine

An *N*-methyl-D-aspartate (NMDA) receptor antagonist, ketamine is a dissociative anesthetic with quick onset and relatively short duration of action that has potent analgesic and sedative properties. As a sympathomimetic agent, it also maintains hemodynamics in patients with replete catecholamine stores [39, 40]. These qualities, in addition to ketamine's ability to prevent spreading depolarizations in brain injury [41, 42], would appear to make it an attractive option for sedation in the neurologically injured patients. Historically, though, ketamine has been avoided in this population due to concerns related to elevated intracranial pressure [43–45]. More recent studies, however, have shown encouraging results that could lead to increased use of ketamine in brain injury. Burgoin et al. showed ketamine in combination with midazolam compared to sufentanil with midazolam caused no significant change in ICP or CPP [46]. Furthermore, Bar-Joseph showed, in children with intracranial hypertension, that ketamine alone mitigated acute spikes in ICP with noxious interventions and was capable of decreasing ICP by up to 1/3 when administered during an episode of refractory intracranial hypertension [47]. Despite the results of the latter study above, a recommendation on ketamine use was not made in the most recent pediatric severe TBI management guidelines, citing that the study did not indicate patient GCS scores and, therefore, could not meet inclusion criteria set forth by the guideline writers [2]. Main drawbacks of ketamine use include potentially dangerous increases in blood pressure, negative inotropy causing profound hypotension with decreased CPP in catecholamine-depleted patients, and concerns about upregulation of neuronal apoptotic pathways through blockage of NMDA receptors in developing brains.

Neuromuscular Blockade

At the time of publication of the 2019 update to the *Guidelines for the Management of Pediatric Severe Traumatic Brain Injury*, there remained insufficient evidence to make any recommendation regarding neuromuscular blockade (NMB) use [2]. Ideally, NMB is used sparingly in the management of severely neurologically injured patients due to the inability to follow a clinical neurologic exam beyond pupillary light response, along with the inability to detect seizures in the absence of continuous EEG monitoring. Nevertheless, most neurocritical care patients receive at least one dose of NMB at the time of endotracheal intubation for airway protection, with further use dependent on clinician judgement and clinical trajectory. Reasons for continued use of NMB include [1] facilitation of optimal mechanical ventilation through improved ventilator synchrony; [2] prevention of shivering in patients undergoing external temperature control or active cooling for neuroprotection; [3] elimination of cough reflex resulting in ICP spikes during endotracheal tube suctioning; and [4] overall decrease in metabolic demand. In a recent systematic review on the topic of NMB in TBI [48], several small and outdated studies, involving a mixed group of neuromuscular blocking agents (depolarizing and non-depolarizing), showed a potpourri of results with regard to effects on ICP and other hemodynamic parameters in the short term. Conclusions were even harder to draw regarding long-term outcomes due to lack of studies and limitations of the available studies. However, two retrospective studies found continuous infusion of NMB to be associated with prolonged ICU stay, increased frequency of pneumonia, and longer time spent with ICP > 20 mm Hg [48].

Succinylcholine, a depolarizing neuromuscular blocker, showed undesirable elevation in ICP after bolus administration in two studies, with a third study showing no effect on CBF velocity, EEG, or ICP [48]. These results, combined with concerns for potentially significant hyperkalemia in the setting of diffuse muscle breakdown (muscular dystrophy or denervation from spinal injury) or significant tissue injury (i.e., crush injury or burn) make succinylcholine a specifically unattractive choice for patients with brain injury requiring NMB. On the other hand, nondepolarizing NMB (cis/atracurium, rocuronium, vecuronium, etc.) appear to be neutral with regard to ICP, CPP, and MAP. Only one study showed significant decreases in all three after bolus of atracurium, with the remainder of the studies failing to show any significant changes in these measurements [48]. In the absence of more robust data, nondepolarizing NMB agents are preferred over succinylcholine in the setting of brain injury.

References

1. Taylor CA, Bell JM, Breiding MJ, Xu L. Traumatic brain injury-related emergency department visits, hospitalizations, and deaths – United States, 2007 and 2013. MMWR Surveill Summ. 2017;66(SS-9):1–16.
2. Kochanek PM, Tasker RC, Carney N, Totten AM, Adelson PD, Selden NR, Davis-O'Reilly C, Hart EL, Bell MJ, Bratton SL, Grant GA, Kissoon N, Reuter-Rice KE, Vavilala MS, Wainwright MS. Guidelines for the Management of Pediatric Severe Traumatic Brain Injury, Third Edition: update of the brain trauma foundation guidelines. Pediatr Crit Care Med. 2019;20:S1–S82.
3. LaRovere K, Graham R, Tasker R. Pediatric neurocritical care: a neurology consultation model and implication for education and training. Pediatr Neurol. 2013;48:206–11.
4. Kochanek PM, Bayir H, Jenkins LW, Clark RSB. Ch. 52 molecular biology of brain injury. In: Rogers' textbook of pediatric intensive care. 4th ed; Lippincott, Williams and Wilkins, Philadelphia, PA 2008. p. 826–43.
5. Jenkins LW, Kochanek PM. Ch. 51 developmental neurobiology, neurophysiology and the PICU. Rogers' textbook of pediatric intensive care . 4th Ed: Lippincott, Williams and Wilkins, Philadelphia, PA 2008. p. 810–25.
6. Balakrishnan B, Zhang L, Simpson PM, Hanson SJ. Impact of the timing of placement of an intracranial pressure monitor on outcomes in children with severe traumatic brain injury. Pediatr Neurosurg. 2018a;53(6):379–86.
7. Adams CA, Stein DM, Morrison JJ, Scalea TM. Does intracranial pressure management hurt more than it helps in traumatic brain injury? Trauma Surg Acute Care Open. 2018;3(1):e000142.
8. Badenes R, De Fez M. Sedation in neurocritical units. In: Khan Z, editor. Challenging topics in neuroanesthesia and neurocritical care. Cham: Springer; 2017. First Online24 May 2017.
9. Helbok R, Kurtz P, Schmidt MJ, Stuart MR, Fernandez L, Connolly SE, Lee K, Schmutzhard E, Mayer SA, Claassen J, Badjatia N. Effects of the neurological wake up test on clinical examination, intracranial pressure, brain metabolism and brain tissue oxygenation in severely brain-injured patients. Crit Care. 2012;16(6):R226.
10. Skoglund K, Hillered L, Purins K, Tsitsopoulos PP, Flygt J, Engquist H, Lewén A, Enblad P, Marklund N. The neurological wake-up test does not alter cerebral energy metabolism and oxygenation in patients with severe traumatic brain injury. Neurocrit Care. 2014;20(3):413–26.
11. Marklund N. The neurological wake-up test-a role in neurocritical care monitoring of traumatic brain injury patients? Front Neurol. 2017;8:540.
12. Go SL, Singh JM. Pro/con debate: should PaCO2 be tightly controlled in all patients with acute brain injuries? Crit Care. 2013;17(1):202.
13. Davis DP, Dunford JV, Poste JC, Ochs M, Holbrook T, Fortlage D, Size MJ, Kennedy F, Hoyt DB. The impact of hypoxia and hyperventilation on outcome after paramedic rapid sequence intubation of severely head-injured patients. J Trauma. 2004;57:1–8.
14. Warner KJ, Cuschieri J, Copass MK, Jurkovich GJ, Bulger EM. The impact of prehospital ventilation on outcome after severe traumatic brain injury. J Trauma. 2007;62:1330–6. discussion 1336–8
15. Von Helden A, Schneider GH, Unterberg A, Lanksch WR. Monitoring of jugular venous oxygen saturation in comatose patients with subarachnoid haemorrhage and intracerebral haematomas. Acta Neurochir Suppl (Wien). 1993;59:102–6.
16. Salonia R, Bell MJ, Kochanek PM, Berger RP. The utility of near infrared spectroscopy in detecting intracranial hemorrhage in children. J Neurotrauma. 2012;29(6):1047–53.
17. Blohm ME, Obrecht D, Hartwich J, Singer D. Effect of cerebral circulatory arrest on cerebral near-infrared spectroscopy in pediatric patients. Paediatr Anaesth. 2014;24(4):393–9.
18. Balakrishnan B, Dasgupta M, Gajewski K, Hoffmann RG, Simpson PM, Havens PL, Hanson SJ. Low near infrared spectroscopic somatic oxygen saturation at admission is associated with

need for lifesaving interventions among unplanned admissions to the pediatric intensive care unit. J Clin Monit Comput. 2018b;32(1):89–96.
19. Weiss M, Dullenkopf A, Kolarova A, Schulz G, Frey B, Baenziger O. Near-infrared spectroscopic cerebral oxygenation reading in neonates and infants is associated with central venous oxygen saturation. Paediatr Anaesth. 2005;15(2):102–9.
20. Becerra L, Aasted CM, Boas DA, George E, Yücel MA, Kussman BD, Kelsey P, Borsook D. Brain measures of nociception using near-infrared spectroscopy in patients undergoing routine screening colonoscopy. Pain. 2016;157(4):840–8.
21. Chen JW, Gombart ZJ, Rogers S, Gardiner SK, Cecil S, Bullock RM. Pupillary reactivity as an early indicator of increased intracranial pressure: the introduction of the neurological pupil index. Surg Neurol Int. 2011;2:82.
22. Clark A, Clarke TN, Gregson B, Hooker PN, Chambers IR. Variability in pupil size estimation. Emerg Med J. 2006;23(6):440–1.
23. Meeker M, Du R, Bacchetti P, et al. Pupil examination: validity and clinical utility of an automated pupillometer. J Neurosci Nurs. 2005;37(1):34–40.
24. McNett M, Moran C, Janki C, Gianakis A. Correlations between hourly Pupillometer readings and intracranial pressure values. J Neurosci Nurs. 2017;49(4):229–34.
25. Yu W, Gao D, Jin W, Liu S, Qi S. Propofol prevents oxidative stress by decreasing the ischemic accumulation of succinate in focal cerebral ischemia-reperfusion injury. Neurochem Res. 2018;43(2):420–9.
26. Zheng X, Huang H, Liu J, Lim LM, Luo T. Propofol attenuates inflammatory response in LPS-activated microglia by regulating the miR-155/SOCS1 pathway. Inflammation. 2018;41(1):11–9.
27. Lu Y, Gu Y, Ding X, Wang J, Chen J, Miao C. Intracellular Ca2+ homeostasis and JAK1/STAT3 pathway are involved in the protective effect of propofol on BV2 microglia against hypoxia-induced inflammation and apoptosis. PLoS One. 2017;12(5):e0178098.
28. Patel MB, Bednarik J, Lee P, Shehabi Y, Salluh JI, Slooter AJ, Klein KE, et al. Delirium monitoring in neurocritically ill patients: a systematic review. Crit Care Med. 2018;46(11):1832–41.
29. Mody K, Kaur S, Mauer EA, Gerber LM, Greenwald BM, Silver G, Traube C. Benzodiazepines and development of delirium in critically ill children: estimating the causal effect. Crit Care Med. 2018;46(9):1486–91.
30. Smith HAB, Gangopadhyay M, Goben CM, Jacobowski NL, Chestnut MH, Thompson JL, Chandrasekhar R, Williams SR, Griffith K, Ely EW, Fuchs DC, Pandharipande PP. Delirium and benzodiazepines associated with prolonged ICU stay in critically ill infants and young children. Crit Care Med. 2017;45(9):1427–35.
31. Jellish WS, Edelstein S. Neuroanesthesia. Handb Clin Neurol. 2014;121:1623–33.
32. De Nadal M, Munar F, Poca MA, Sahuquillo J, Garnacho A, Rosselló J. Cerebral hemodynamic effects of morphine and fentanyl in patients with severe head injury: absence of correlation to cerebral autoregulation. Anesthesiology. 2000;92(1):11–9.
33. Roberts DJ, Hall RI, Kramer AH, Robertson HL, Gallagher CN, Zygun DA. Sedation for critically ill adults with severe traumatic brain injury: a systematic review of randomized controlled trials. Crit Care Med. 2011;39(12):2743–51.
34. Carr ZJ, Cios TJ, Potter KF, Swick JT. Does Dexmedetomidine ameliorate postoperative cognitive dysfunction? A brief review of the recent literature. Curr Neurol Neurosci Rep. 2018;18(10):64.
35. Liu C, Fu Q, Mu R, Wang F, Zhou C, Zhang L, Yu B, Zhang Y, Fang T, Tian F. Dexmedetomidine alleviates cerebral ischemia-reperfusion injury by inhibiting endoplasmic reticulum stress dependent apoptosis through the PERK-CHOP-Caspase-11 pathway. Brain Res. 2018;1701:246–54.
36. Li F, Wang X, Deng Z, Zhang X, Gao P, Liu H. Dexmedetomidine reduces oxidative stress and provides neuroprotection in a model of traumatic brain injury via the PGC-1α signaling pathway. Neuropeptides. 2018;72:58–64.
37. Wang YQ, Tang YF, Yang MK, Huang XZ. Dexmedetomidine alleviates cerebral ischemia-reperfusion injury in rats via inhibition of hypoxia-inducible factor-1α. J Cell Biochem. 2019;120:7834–44.

38. Bindra A, Kaushal A, Prabhakar H, Chaturvedi A, Chandra PS, Tripathi M, Subbiah V, Sathianathan S, Banerjee J, Prakash C. Neuroprotective role of dexmedetomidine in epilepsy surgery: a preliminary study. Neurol India. 2019;67(1):163–8.
39. Ketharanathan N, Yamamoto Y, Rohlwink U, Wildschut ED, Hunfeld M, de Lange ECM, Tibboel D. Analgosedation in paediatric severe traumatic brain injury (TBI): practice, pitfalls and possibilities. Childs Nerv Syst. 2017;33(10):1703–10.
40. Mtaweh H, Bell MJ. Management of pediatric traumatic brain injury. Curr Treat Options Neurol. 2015;17(5):348.
41. Hertle DN, Dreier JP, Woitzik J, Hartings JA, Bullock R, Okonkwo DO, Shutter LA, Vidgeon S, Strong AJ, Kowoll C, Dohmen C, Diedler J, Veltkamp R, Bruckner T, Unterberg AW, Sakowitz OW, Cooperative Study of Brain Injury Depolarizations (COSBID). Effect of analgesics and sedatives on the occurrence of spreading depolarizations accompanying acute brain injury. Brain. 2012;135(Pt 8):2390–8.
42. Carlson AP, Abbas M, Alunday RL, Qeadan F, Shuttleworth CW. Spreading depolarization in acute brain injury inhibited by ketamine: a prospective, randomized, multiple crossover trial. J Neurosurg. 2018;1:1–7.
43. Gibbs JM. The effect of intravenous ketamine on cerebrospinal fluid pressure. Br J Anaesth. 1972;44(12):1298–302.
44. Ben Yehuda Y, Watemberg N. Ketamine increases opening cerebrospinal pressure in children undergoing lumbar puncture. J Child Neurol. 2006;21(6):441–3.
45. Wyte SR, Shapiro HM, Turner P, Harris AB. Ketamine-induced intracranial hypertension. Anesthesiology. 1972;36(2):174–6.
46. Burgoin A, Albanèse J, Léone M, Sampol-Manos E, Viviand X, Martin C. Effects of sufentanil or ketamine administered in target-controlled infusion on the cerebral hemodynamics of severely brain-injured patients. Crit Care Med. 2005;33(5):1109–13.
47. Bar-Joseph G, Guilburd Y, Tamir A, Guilburd JN. Effectiveness of ketamine in decreasing intracranial pressure in children with intracranial hypertension. J Neurosurg Pediatr. 2009;4(1):40–6.
48. Sanfilippo F, Santonocito C, Veenith T, Astuto M, Maybauer MO. The role of neuromuscular blockade in patients with traumatic brain injury: a systematic review. Neurocrit Care. 2015;22(2):325–34.

Chapter 17
Pediatric Anesthetic and Sedation Neurotoxicity in the Developing Brain

Jessica Raper and Pradip P. Kamat

Background

In 2012, the Food and Drug Administration (FDA), American Academy of Pediatrics, and International Anesthesia Research Society (IARS) released a consensus statement acknowledging the growing evidence that general anesthetic (GA) exposure in children aged 3 years and younger poses an increased risk for developing learning disabilities and called for research to better understand these risks [1, 2]. Then in December 2016, the FDA issued a warning about the safety of anesthesia and sedation for pediatric patients [3].

The FDA 2016 warning issued in December 2016 stated that: Repeated or lengthy use of general anesthetic and sedation drugs during surgeries or procedures in children younger than 3 years or in pregnant women during their third trimester may affect the development of children's brains.

Both preclinical animal studies and human clinical studies have shown that single short exposures to anesthesia are relatively safe for the developing brain. Thus, the FDA's warning statement focused on the most compelling preclinical and human studies (some of which are still ongoing) that demonstrate prolonged or repeated exposures to general anesthesia can have a deleterious effect on neurodevelopmental and cognitive outcomes. The FDA 2016 warning included the children younger than 3 years due to the assumption that peak synaptogenesis in most human brain regions is completed by age 3 years although brain development starts in the embryonic period and continues till adolescence. Lengthy was defined as greater than 3 hours. Although repeated was not specified, based on some clinical studies, there

J. Raper (✉)
Yerkes National Primate Research Center, Emory University, Atlanta, GA, USA
e-mail: jraper@emory.edu

P. P. Kamat
Emory University School of Medicine, Atlanta, GA, USA

P. P. Kamat, J. W. Berkenbosch (eds.), *Sedation and Analgesia for the Pediatric Intensivist*, https://doi.org/10.1007/978-3-030-52555-2_17

Table 17.1 List of general anesthetic and sedation drugs affected by the FDA label change

Generic name
Desflurane
Etomidate
Halothane
Isoflurane
Ketamine
Lorazepam injection
Methohexital
Midazolam injection, syrup
Pentobarbital
Propofol
Sevoflurane

https://www.fda.gov/Drugs/DrugSafety/ucm532356.htm

is a stepwise increase in the risk of learning disabilities with each repeated exposure [4]. The FDA also required warnings to be added to the labels of general anesthetic and sedation drugs commonly used in the operating room as well as in the pediatric intensive care units and the outpatient sedation arena (Table 17.1). The FDA's warning for potential neurotoxicity is alarming, given that almost three million children under the age of 3 years and 1.5 million infants younger than 12 months undergo procedures requiring anesthesia in the United States. This does not take into account exposure to sedation outside the operating room or the prolonged exposures in neonatal or pediatric intensive care units.

Due to controversial nature of the above warning, the FDA, in a response, published a communication (April 2017) stating that surgeries or procedures in children younger than 3 years or pregnant women should not be delayed or avoided when medically necessary. Consideration should be given to delaying potentially elective surgery in young children where medically appropriate [5].

Although previously deemed as a problem primarily-affecting patients undergoing general anesthesia in the operating room, recent focus is shifting toward patients exposed to the drugs listed in Table 17.1 outside the operating room [6–9].

Preclinical Studies

A seminal paper from John Olney's lab described the widespread apoptosis that occurs after later prenatal or early neonatal exposure to alcohol and attributed this phenomenon to alcohols' actions on neurotransmitter systems [10, 11]. Alcohol not only blocks *N*-methyl-D-aspartate (NMDA) receptors but also modulates gamma-aminobutyric acid (GABA) transmission [12, 13]. Considering that anesthetic agents act on either GABA or NMDA receptors (or both), many began to question whether similar neurotoxic effects would be found after exposure to sedative and anesthetic agents. In fact, most anesthetics and sedatives act by two principal mechanisms: (1) decreasing excitation through NMDA receptors (e.g., ketamine, nitrous oxide, and xenon) and (2) increasing inhibition through GABAA receptors (e.g., benzodiazepines, barbiturates, propofol, etomidate, isoflurane, and sevoflurane) [14]. Thus, this finding in the fetal alcohol field sparked two decades of preclinical research in animal models to investigate the potential consequences of anesthesia exposure during early brain development.

How do sedative and anesthetic medications impact the developing brain? Appropriate brain growth during the later stages of gestation is dependent on coordinated systems of programmed cell death (neuronal apoptosis) and synaptic pruning. The former process removes unused or faulty neurons from the brain, while the latter removes unnecessary neuronal structures from the brain as it matures. The main difference between the two processes is that in neuronal apoptosis, the neuron itself is killed, whereas in pruning the neuron itself is preserved and only functionally inappropriate synaptic connections are destroyed [15, 16]. These two elegantly coordinated processes in the central nervous system are dependent on neuronal activation and neurotransmitters [17]. Therefore, drugs that change GABA and/or NMDA activity, such as anesthetics, can lead to neurotoxicity by a process called drug-induced neurodevelopmental apoptosis (DIDNA), resulting in cognitive and behavioral impairment of the developing brain [18, 19]. To date, all anesthetics and sedatives have been found to produce DIDNA, depending on the length and developmental timing of exposure. For example, 5 hours of isoflurane is sufficient to induce extensive apoptosis in neonatal macaque neocortex, as is 9 h (but not 3 h) of continuous ketamine infusion [18, 20]. Also, the brain appears to be most vulnerable during peak synaptogenesis, such that apoptosis is found after anesthesia exposure at postnatal day (PND) 5–7, 20 and becomes less severe at PND 35 and 40 in infant monkeys [18–21]. Given the above preclinical data, it is of potential concern that the most commonly used agents in the pediatric intensive care unit include isoflurane, benzodiazepines, barbiturates, etomidate, propofol, and ketamine, which have all been shown to cause DIDNA [22, 23]. All the above agents are also commonly used in acute care settings and sedation services.

While many studies have focused on neural- and glial-apoptosis after anesthesia exposure, this may not be the primary or only mechanism underlying the long-term neurodevelopmental consequences. Although the exact mechanism is not conclusively known, animal studies have suggested that a neuroinflammatory response to general anesthesia exposure leads to oxidative damage, caused explicitly by microglial activation and production of interleukin-6 (IL-6), tumor necrosis factor alpha (TNF-α), and interleukin-1β (IL-1β) pro-inflammatory cytokines [24–26]. These pro-inflammatory cytokines can influence neuronal functioning via several mechanisms, including changes in neuroapoptosis, mitochondrial and oxidative damage, altered synaptogenesis by impaired neuronal branching, and ultrastructure damage [27, 28]. Importantly, general anesthesia exposure causes increased inflammation, depending on the anesthesia type and length of exposure. Elevated cytokines have been detected in plasma of human adults and animal studies have also shown increased neuroinflammation in brain tissue after anesthesia exposure [24, 25, 29]. In addition, neuroinflammation is associated with cognitive impairment in humans and animals, suggesting that anesthetic-induced neuroinflammation could be one potential mechanism of cognitive impairment after early anesthesia exposure [30–32].

What Are the Long-Term Consequences of Early Exposure to Anesthetic Agents?

Retrospective studies in humans have identified cognitive changes and increased risk of learning disability later in childhood and adolescence that are associated with early life exposure to anesthesia [4, 33, 34]. Both rodent and nonhuman primate studies have demonstrated that general anesthetics (including ketamine, nitrous oxide, propofol, isoflurane, and sevoflurane) cause persistent brain damage and learning deficits when administered during early postnatal development [18, 19, 22]. Specifically, rodent models have shown slower learning curves and impaired performance on probe trials during memory tasks. Nonhuman primate studies have found motor abnormalities, impaired retention on visual recognition memory tasks, decreased motivation, and learning on operant task [35–37]. These results from animal studies confirm that cognitive changes can result from exposure to anesthesia alone in the absence of a disease state or complications arising from surgery. Overall, the preclinical animal models data suggest that early prolonged or repeated anesthesia exposure impairs specific aspects of cognition, which may explain the increased risk of learning disabilities and attention-deficit/hyperactivity disorder (ADHD) found in clinical studies [4, 38].

Greater risk for learning disabilities and ADHD are not the only findings from clinical studies; increased internalizing behaviors have also been reported [39]. In addition, studies have shown that up to 50% of children exhibit immediate negative behavioral changes after anesthesia exposure, which does not correlate with age, gender, or length of time under anesthesia [40, 41]. Evidence from both clinical and preclinical animal studies suggests that early anesthesia exposure produces negative behavior changes, such as increased anxiety, impulsivity, aggression toward authorities, and difficulty with decision making [42, 43]. These changes in emotional behavior can persist from 1 to 6 months after anesthesia exposure and cause distress for the child and parents [41, 44]. This not only makes postoperative recovery difficult but also may have a broader negative influence on behavioral development. Nonhuman primates have similar brain morphology, genetics, and endocrine systems, live in complex social groups, and use visual cues to extract socioemotional information from their environment, perhaps making them an ideal animal model to examine emotional changes after early exposure to anesthesia [45]. Recent findings from nonhuman primate studies have shown increased anxiety behaviors after repeated (but not single) anesthesia exposure [43, 46, 47]. This increased anxiety was detected as early as 6 months of age and persisted until 2 years of age. Based on the correspondence between human and rhesus monkey lifespan, this would correspond to approximately 1- and 6-year-old human child. These findings parallel those recently found in clinical studies with increased parental reports of internalizing behavior [48].

Human Studies

Interpretation of the effect of anesthesia exposure from human studies has not been as clear-cut as preclinical studies. While some early studies have reported an association between anesthesia exposure and neurocognitive defects, others have failed to do so.

Unlike preclinical studies, human studies are limited by confounding factors such as inflammation of illness, the stress of surgery, hemodynamic fluctuations, and postoperative emotional changes. Due to ethical concerns, it is challenging to perform blinded, randomized controlled trials in humans. More recently, the International Anesthesia Research Society (IARS) formed a collaborative partnership with the FDA to form SmartTots (Smart Strategies to Reduce Anesthesia Risk in Tots; www.smarttots.org) to coordinate and fund research on neurotoxicity from sedation and anesthesia exposure in infants and children. The SmartTots investigators have highlighted the need to identify key research priorities such as preclinical studies examining dose–response relations of neurotoxicity, head-to-head comparisons of drugs or combinations of drugs that mitigate anesthetic neurotoxicity, and the search for "translatable" biomarkers [49].

Several large epidemiological studies have been performed or are ongoing evaluating risk of exposure to anesthesia in children under 3 years of age. Some relevant studies are mentioned below.

1. General Anesthesia compared to Spinal Anesthesia (GAS) trial [50]. An international multisite randomized controlled trial was designed to study cognitive outcomes at 2 and 5 years of age in more than 700 neonates randomized to either general or spinal anesthesia for hernia surgery. A recent analysis of the secondary outcome (cognitive score of the Bayley Scales of Infant and Toddler development III at age 2 years) found no evidence of adverse neurodevelopment at 2 years of age in infants receiving less than 1 hour of general anesthesia with sevoflurane compared with awake-regional anesthesia with bupivacaine. Although 20% of the patients in the spinal group crossed over to the general anesthesia group due to suboptimal operating conditions, there was no difference between the two groups. The primary outcome of the study is full-scale intelligence quotient (IQ) at age 5 years also and was not different between the two cohorts leading to the conclusion that slightly less than 1 h of general anesthesia in early infancy does not alter neurodevelopmental outcome at age 5 years compared with awake-regional anesthesia in a predominantly male study population.
2. Pediatric Anesthesia Neurodevelopmental Assessment (PANDA) [48]. This study evaluated 105 sibling pairs in which one sibling under 3 years of age underwent general anesthesia for inguinal hernia repair. The other sibling who was not exposed to general anesthesia was also under 3 years of age. Neurodevelopmental outcomes were assessed at 8–15 years of age. The primary

outcome was the full-scale, verbal, and performance intelligence quotient. Scores between groups in these outcomes were virtually identical. Secondary tests of memory, language, attention, and executive function were also not different. The ambidirectional sibling matched design minimized genetic and socioeconomic differences between groups.

3. The Mayo Anesthesia Safety in Kids (MASK) [39]. This study used a propensity-guided strategy to recruit unexposed, singly exposed, and multiply exposed children who were similar in health status and factors potentially relevant to neurodevelopment born to mothers residing in Olmsted County, Minnesota. The primary outcome was the Full-Scale intelligence quotient standard score of the Wechsler Abbreviated Scale of Intelligence. The secondary outcomes included individual domains from a comprehensive neuropsychological assessment and parent reports. The investigators in this cohort study hypothesized that exposure to multiple but not single procedures requiring anesthesia before 3 years of age is associated with adverse neurodevelopmental outcomes. The primary outcome of IQ did not differ significantly according to exposure status; however, multiple exposures were found to be associated with modest decreases in processing speed and fine motor coordination. In addition, parents reported that children who were exposed to multiple procedures had more difficulties reading and increased internalizing behaviors.
4. Neurodevelopmental Outcome After Standard Dose Sevoflurane Versus Low-Dose Sevoflurane/Dexmedetomidine/Remifentanil Anaesthesia in Young Children (TREX Trial) [49]. ClinicalTrials.gov Identifier: NCT03089905. This ongoing randomized trial will compare children after a low dose of sevoflurane (given with remifentanil and dexmedetomidine) with children administered only higher dose sevoflurane anesthesia. Neurodevelopmental outcomes will be tested in those undergoing surgery ≥2.5 hours using the full-scale IQ score of the Wechsler Preschool and Primary School Intelligence Scale.

Graham et al., in a large cohort study from Canada, used the Early Developmental Index (EDI) measuring school readiness to gauge the impact of anesthesia exposure in children <4 years of age. After controlling for gestational age, age of exposure, and socioeconomic factors, the investigators found only a weak association between EDI and anesthesia exposure [51]. Furthermore, in another large cohort study from Sweden, Glatz et al. reported small but statistically significant differences in school grades at 16 years of age as well as a lower intelligence cohort at 18 years in those exposed to anesthesia in the first 4 years of life [52]. Other factors such as maternal level of education, the month of birth had a more pronounced effect on IQ, thus confounding the association with anesthesia exposure. Both the aforementioned studies did not find any worsening of scores tested and multiple anesthesia exposures.

Though much of the definitive data demonstrating anesthesia-induced neurotoxicity has come from studies in young animals, showing that prolonged or repeated exposures result in neurodevelopmental consequences. However, preclinical studies have also shown that single, short exposures are safe, which support the recent prospective clinical studies. While some clinical studies are still ongoing examining the role of anesthesia exposure in the vulnerable cohort, especially multiple exposures, it is unlikely that a single exposure results in neurotoxicity [53]. Surgeons and anesthesiologists should be upfront with families and other stakeholders about the concern for the association between neurotoxicity and anesthesia exposure in children younger than 3 years (though not proven in human studies) and delay elective procedures, utilize regional anesthetics (whenever possible) in order to minimize exposure during the vulnerable period of brain development in this cohort.

Several other observational studies evaluating cognitive outcomes after anesthesia exposure in children have also demonstrated varying associations between anesthesia exposure and neurotoxicity as assessed by behavioral tests or academic indicators. Backeljauw et al. reported that children exposed to general anesthesia for surgical procedures before 4 years of age had problems with language and cognition, as well as volumetric alterations in brain structure [54]. Similarly, Flick et al. reported in a large, matched cohort that repeated exposure to multiple but not single anesthetics and surgeries before age 2 was a significant risk factor for later development of learning disabilities [9]. Conversely, Bartels et al. reported that there is no evidence for a causal relationship between anesthesia administration and later learning-related outcomes in twins exposed to anesthesia vs. those not exposed to anesthesia before 4 years of age [55]. New evidence appears to be emerging from preclinical nonhuman primate models, which suggests an anxious phenotype after early repeated (but not single) anesthesia exposure [43, 47]. These preclinical data echo findings from a recent ambidirectional study from the Mayo Clinic, demonstrating increased internalizing behaviors in children who experienced multiple anesthesia exposures. Therefore, new prospective clinical studies are needed to examine the potential link between multiple or prolonged anesthesia exposure and risk of anxious phenotype later in life.

Anesthesia/Sedation Exposures Outside the Operating Room

Although most research in anesthesia-induced neurotoxicity has focused on anesthesia exposures in the operating room, some recent publications have shed light on similar exposures in the neonatal, pediatric intensive care units and outpatient sedation areas. Infants and children in these locations receive prolonged sedatives, analgesics, and even inhalational anesthetics for asthma, intractable status epileptics, and prolonged deep sedation for radiological procedures such as magnetic resonance imaging. Several factors can place the neonate (especially the premature neonate) at a higher risk than older children: an immature control of cerebral blood flow and its autoregulation, immature liver enzyme activity, and poorly developed glomerular filtration with resulting drug metabolism and excretion that is not optimal. All these factors can result in potential neurotoxicity after exposure to anesthetic/sedation agents. Conservative estimates from the PICU suggest that more than 100,000 critically ill infants and children are exposed to mechanical ventilation [56]. Advancements in technology in the PICU over the years have led to an increased number of survivors who were exposed to prolonged duration of sedation or analgesia during their critical illness. Volatile anesthetics such as isoflurane are used in the PICU for refractory bronchospasm in status asthmaticus, or for burst suppression for difficult-to-treat epilepsies such as febrile infection-related epilepsy syndrome (FIRES) [57]. One recent study reported the use of inhaled sevoflurane to treat difficult-to-sedate children undergoing mechanical ventilation. Unlike the operating room, the exposure of critically ill patients in the PICU to inhaled anesthetics can be prolonged.

In the pediatric emergency department (ED), most procedural sedation is usually short; however, due to nonavailability of PICU beds, an intubated patient may remain in the ED for a prolonged period. The pediatric ED physicians should consult with PICU physicians to discuss sedation/analgesia provision in these patients.

Multiple and prolonged procedural sedation commonly occurs outside the operating room in the young and potentially vulnerable population as shown by a study by Kamat et al. [7]. Sedation physicians need to be advocates for infants and children who may not require prolonged (and often repeated for follow-up) magnetic resonance imaging for autism spectrum disorders or febrile seizures. Although certain imaging cannot be avoided, other cases may have the potential to be delayed beyond 3 years of age.

Strategies to Decrease Potential Neurotoxicity from Anesthesia/Sedation Exposure

1. Communication with referring physicians and other stakeholders, including families, to discuss the possibility of delaying nonurgent procedures requiring anesthesia or sedation can be beyond 3 years of life. Often tests are ordered by physicians who are not aware of newer diagnostic modalities or the complexities/difficulties with sedation/anesthesia of infants with syndromes etc. (Cravero reference from fast CT paper).
2. The radiologist must be involved in discussions about alternative or shorter imaging modalities (e.g., ultrasound vs. magnetic resonance imaging). Newer dual-source computed tomography scanners have concise scanning times with radiation exposures below 1 millisievert or less [58]. In addition, decreasing the acquisition of imaging sequences during MRI can potentially reduce anesthesia/sedation exposure.
3. Using child life specialists and nonsedation techniques (feed and wrap, immobilization with swaddling for neonates, etc.) for short procedures [59].
4. Exposure to anesthesia/sedation, especially in young infants, can be delayed or even eliminated if stakeholders adhere to national guidelines or recent evidence from the literature. Cooper et al. have shown a low prevalence of definite pathology in children with ASD undergoing brain MRI. Routine MRIs in such children can be avoided unless there is an abnormal neurologic examination, seizures, or

headaches. Similarly, routine neuroimaging may not be required in infants or children with simple febrile seizures, minor head injuries, abdominal pain, or for evaluation of brain development of premature infants before discharge from the neonatal intensive care unit (NICU) [60].

5. Choice of sedative/anesthetic: Dexmedetomidine has shown neuroprotective properties and is not on the list of drugs with the FDA warning for potential neurotoxicity from anesthetics/sedatives should be considered for radiologic imaging [61].
6. Support for more research in the area of neurotoxicity from anesthetics/sedation should be encouraged by collaboration between various subspecialties, creation of databases, and sharing of data. In addition, educating resident learners from various pediatric subspecialties about potential neurotoxicity is vital [62].

In summary, concerns for potential for neurotoxicity from exposure to anesthesia/sedation are undisputed, especially in animal studies, and its clinical significance in humans remains largely unknown. Single short exposure (<1 hour) to anesthetic/sedation in infants/children is less likely to alter neurodevelopment, which is consistent with findings from preclinical animal studies. While research in humans is ongoing, pediatric providers of anesthesia/sedation in the operating rooms, intensive care units, or outpatient sedation units caring for infants and children should advocate to decrease exposure to medications listed in Table 17.1, use nonsedation methods when possible, delay elective procedures, and decrease exposure length whenever feasible.

References

1. Rappaport B, Mellon RD, Simone A, Woodcock J. Defining safe use of anesthesia in children. N Engl J Med. 2011;364(15):1387–90.
2. Card EB, Wells NL. An introduction to the smart tots consensus statement on the use of anesthetic and sedative drugs in infants and toddlers. J Perianesth Nurs. 2016;31(1):3–10.
3. FDA Drug Safety Communication: FDA review results in new warnings about using general anesthetics and sedation drugs in young children and pregnant women. 2016; https://www.fda.gov/Drugs/DrugSafety/ucm532356.htm.
4. Wilder RT, Flick RP, Sprung J, et al. Early exposure to anesthesia and learning disabilities in a population-based birth cohort. Anesthesiology. 2009;110(4):796–804.
5. FDA Drug Safety Communication: FDA review results in new warnings about using general anesthetics and sedation drugs in young children and pregnant women. 2017; https://www.fda.gov/Drugs/DrugSafety/ucm532356.htm.
6. Kamat PP, Kudchadkar SR, Simon HK. Sedative and anesthetic neurotoxicity in infants and young children: not just an operating room concern. J Pediatr. 2018;204:285–90.
7. Kamat PP, Sulton C, Kudchadkar SR, et al. Procedural sedation outside the operating room and potential neurotoxicity: analysis of an at-risk pediatric population. Acad Pediatr. 2019;19(8):978–84.
8. Curley MAQ, Gedeit RG, Dodson BL, et al. Methods in the design and implementation of the Randomized Evaluation of Sedation Titration for Respiratory Failure (RESTORE) clinical trial. Trials. 2018;19(1):687.

9. Flick RP, Katusic SK, Colligan RC, et al. Cognitive and behavioral outcomes after early exposure to anesthesia and surgery. Pediatrics. 2011;128(5):e1053–61.
10. Ikonomidou C, Bittigau P, Ishimaru MJ, et al. Ethanol-induced apoptotic neurodegeneration and fetal alcohol syndrome. Science. 2000;287(5455):1056–60.
11. Ikonomidou C, Stefovska V, Turski L. Neuronal death enhanced by N-methyl-D-aspartate antagonists. Proc Natl Acad Sci U S A. 2000;97(23):12885–90.
12. Lovinger DM, White G, Weight FF. Ethanol inhibits NMDA-activated ion current in hippocampal neurons. Science. 1989;243(4899):1721–4.
13. Wirkner K, Poelchen W, Koles L, et al. Ethanol-induced inhibition of NMDA receptor channels. Neurochem Int. 1999;35(2):153–62.
14. Olney JW, Wozniak DF, Farber NB, Jevtovic-Todorovic V, Bittigau P, Ikonomidou C. The enigma of fetal alcohol neurotoxicity. Ann Med. 2002;34(2):109–19.
15. Ikonomidou C, Bosch F, Miksa M, et al. Blockade of NMDA receptors and apoptotic neurodegeneration in the developing brain. Science. 1999;283(5398):70–4.
16. Brambrink AM, Evers AS, Avidan MS, et al. Isoflurane-induced neuroapoptosis in the neonatal rhesus macaque brain. Anesthesiology. 2010;112(4):834–41.
17. Andropoulos DB. Effect of anesthesia on the developing brain: infant and fetus. Fetal Diagn Ther. 2018;43(1):1–11.
18. Slikker W Jr, Zou X, Hotchkiss CE, et al. Ketamine-induced neuronal cell death in the perinatal rhesus monkey. Toxicol Sci. 2007;98(1):145–58.
19. Paule MG, Li M, Allen RR, et al. Ketamine anesthesia during the first week of life can cause long-lasting cognitive deficits in rhesus monkeys. Neurotoxicol Teratol. 2011;33(2):220–30.
20. Brambrink AM, Evers AS, Avidan MS, et al. Ketamine-induced neuroapoptosis in the fetal and neonatal rhesus macaque brain. Anesthesiology. 2012;116(2):372–84.
21. Creeley CE. From drug-induced developmental neuroapoptosis to pediatric anesthetic neurotoxicity-where are we now? Brain Sci. 2016;6(32):1–12. https://doi.org/10.3390/brainsci6030032
22. Jevtovic-Todorovic V, Hartman RE, Izumi Y, et al. Early exposure to common anesthetic agents causes widespread neurodegeneration in the developing rat brain and persistent learning deficits. J Neurosci. 2003;23(3):876–82.
23. Loepke AW. Developmental neurotoxicity of sedatives and anesthetics: a concern for neonatal and pediatric critical care medicine? Pediatr Critical Care Med. 2010;11(2):217–26.
24. Zhang L, Zhang J, Yang L, Dong Y, Zhang Y, Xie Z. Isoflurane and sevoflurane increase interleukin-6 levels through the nuclear factor-kappa B pathway in neuroglioma cells. Br J Anaesth. 2013;110(Suppl 1):i82–91.
25. Shen X, Dong Y, Xu Z, et al. Selective anesthesia-induced neuroinflammation in developing mouse brain and cognitive impairment. Anesthesiology. 2013;118(3):502–15.
26. Boscolo A, Ori C, Bennett J, Wiltgen B, Jevtovic-Todorovic V. Mitochondrial protectant pramipexole prevents sex-specific long-term cognitive impairment from early anaesthesia exposure in rats. Br J Anaesth. 2013;110(Suppl 1):i47–52.
27. Hayley S, Poulter MO, Merali Z, Anisman H. The pathogenesis of clinical depression: stressor- and cytokine-induced alterations of neuroplasticity. Neuroscience. 2005;135(3):659–78.
28. Joksovic PM, Lunardi N, Jevtovic-Todorovic V, Todorovic SM. Early exposure to general anesthesia with isoflurane downregulates inhibitory synaptic neurotransmission in the rat thalamus. Mol Neurobiol. 2015;52(2):952–8.
29. Burkhardt U, Sack U, Wild L, Olthoff D. Serum cytokines and cytokine receptors in children after small or larger surgical interventions with halothane anesthesia. Anaesthesiol Reanim. 1997;22(2):50–4.
30. Patanella AK, Zinno M, Quaranta D, et al. Correlations between peripheral blood mononuclear cell production of BDNF, TNF-alpha, IL-6, IL-10 and cognitive performances in multiple sclerosis patients. J Neurosci Res. 2010;88(5):1106–12.

31. Salim S, Chugh G, Asghar M. Inflammation in anxiety. Adv Protein Chem Struct Biol. 2012;88:1–25.
32. Tan H, Cao J, Zhang J, Zuo Z. Critical role of inflammatory cytokines in impairing biochemical processes for learning and memory after surgery in rats. J Neuroinflammation. 2014;11:93.
33. Ing C, DiMaggio C, Whitehouse A, et al. Long-term differences in language and cognitive function after childhood exposure to anesthesia. Pediatrics. 2012;130(3):e476–85.
34. DiMaggio C, Sun LS, Ing C, Li G. Pediatric anesthesia and neurodevelopmental impairments: a Bayesian meta-analysis. J Neurosurg Anesthesiol. 2012;24(4):376–81.
35. Walters JL, Paule MG. Review of preclinical studies on pediatric general anesthesia-induced developmental neurotoxicity. Neurotoxicol Teratol. 2017;60:2–23.
36. Talpos JC, Chelonis JJ, Li M, Hanig JP, Paule MG. Early life exposure to extended general anesthesia with isoflurane and nitrous oxide reduces responsivity on a cognitive test battery in the nonhuman primate. Neurotoxicology. 2019;70:80–90.
37. Walters JL, Zhang X, Talpos JC, et al. Sevoflurane exposure has minimal effect on cognitive function and does not alter microglial activation in adult monkeys. Neurotoxicology. 2019;71:159–67.
38. Hu D, Flick RP, Zaccariello MJ, et al. Association between exposure of Young children to procedures requiring general anesthesia and learning and behavioral outcomes in a population-based birth cohort. Anesthesiology. 2017;127(2):227–40.
39. Warner DO, Zaccariello MJ, Katusic SK, et al. Neuropsychological and behavioral outcomes after exposure of Young children to procedures requiring general anesthesia: the Mayo anesthesia safety in kids (MASK) study. Anesthesiology. 2018;129(1):89–105.
40. Faulk DJ, Twite MD, Zuk J, Pan Z, Wallen B, Friesen RH. Hypnotic depth and the incidence of emergence agitation and negative postoperative behavioral changes. Paediatr Anaesth. 2010;20(1):72–81.
41. Stipic SS, Carev M, Kardum G, Roje Z, Litre DM, Elezovic N. Are postoperative behavioural changes after adenotonsillectomy in children influenced by the type of anaesthesia?: a randomised clinical study. Eur J Anaesthesiol. 2015;32(5):311–9.
42. Alvarado MC, Murphy KL, Baxter MG. Visual recognition memory is impaired in rhesus monkeys repeatedly exposed to sevoflurane in infancy. Br J Anaesth. 2017;119(3):517–23.
43. Coleman K, Robertson ND, Dissen GA, et al. Isoflurane anesthesia has long-term consequences on motor and behavioral development in infant rhesus macaques. Anesthesiology. 2017;126(1):74–84.
44. Stargatt R, Davidson AJ, Huang GH, et al. A cohort study of the incidence and risk factors for negative behavior changes in children after general anesthesia. Paediatr Anaesth. 2006;16(8):846–59.
45. Watson KK, Platt ML. Of mice and monkeys: using non-human primate models to bridge mouse- and human-based investigations of autism spectrum disorders. J Neurodev Disord. 2012;4(1):21.
46. Raper J, Alvarado MC, Murphy KL, Baxter MG. Multiple anesthetic exposure in infant monkeys alters emotional reactivity to an acute stressor. Anesthesiology. 2015;123(5):1084–92.
47. Raper J, De Biasio JC, Murphy KL, Alvarado MC, Baxter MG. Persistent alteration in behavioural reactivity to a mild social stressor in rhesus monkeys repeatedly exposed to sevoflurane in infancy. Br J Anaesth. 2018;120(4):761–7.
48. Sun LS, Li G, Miller TL, et al. Association between a single general anesthesia exposure before age 36 months and neurocognitive outcomes in later childhood. JAMA. 2016;315(21):2312–20.
49. Orser BA, Suresh S, Evers AS. SmartTots update regarding anesthetic neurotoxicity in the developing brain. Anesth Analg. 2018;126(4):1393–6.
50. Davidson AJ, Disma N, de Graaff JC, et al. Neurodevelopmental outcome at 2 years of age after general anaesthesia and awake-regional anaesthesia in infancy (GAS): an international multicentre, randomised controlled trial. Lancet. 2016;387(10015):239–50.
51. Graham MR, Brownell M, Chateau DG, Dragan RD, Burchill C, Fransoo RR. Neurodevelopmental assessment in kindergarten in children exposed to general anes-

thesia before the age of 4 years: a retrospective matched cohort study. Anesthesiology. 2016;125(4):667–77.
52. Glatz P, Sandin RH, Pedersen NL, Bonamy AK, Eriksson LI, Granath F. Association of anesthesia and surgery during childhood with Long-term academic performance. JAMA Pediatr. 2017;171(1):e163470.
53. McCann ME, de Graaff JC, Dorris L, et al. Neurodevelopmental outcome at 5 years of age after general anaesthesia or awake-regional anaesthesia in infancy (GAS): an international, multicentre, randomised, controlled equivalence trial. Lancet. 2019;393(10172):664–77.
54. Backeljauw B, Holland SK, Altaye M, Loepke AW. Cognition and brain structure following early childhood surgery with anesthesia. Pediatrics. 2015;136(1):e1–12.
55. Bartels DD, McCann ME, Davidson AJ, Polaner DM, Whitlock EL, Bateman BT. Estimating pediatric general anesthesia exposure: quantifying duration and risk. Paediatr Anaesth. 2018;28(6):520–7.
56. Best KM, Asaro LA, Curley MAQ. Randomized evaluation of sedation titration for respiratory failure study I. Sedation management for critically ill children with pre-existing cognitive impairment. J Pediatr. 2019;206:204–211 e201.
57. Ikeda KM, Connors R, Lee DH, Khandji AG, Claassen J, Young GB. Isoflurane use in the treatment of super-refractory status epilepticus is associated with hippocampal changes on MRI. Neurocrit Care. 2017;26(3):420–7.
58. Cravero JP, Callahan MJ. The radiological home: pediatric anesthesiologist's role in risk assessment for imaging procedures. Paediatr Anaesth. 2017;27(9):878–9.
59. Bjur KA, Payne ET, Nemergut ME, Hu D, Flick RP. Anesthetic-related neurotoxicity and neuroimaging in children: a call for conversation. J Child Neurol. 2017;32(6):594–602.
60. Cooper AS, Friedlaender E, Levy SE, et al. The implications of brain MRI in autism spectrum disorder. J Child Neurol. 2016;31(14):1611–6.
61. Perez-Zoghbi JF, Zhu W, Grafe MR, Brambrink AM. Dexmedetomidine-mediated neuroprotection against sevoflurane-induced neurotoxicity extends to several brain regions in neonatal rats. Br J Anaesth. 2017;119(3):506–16.
62. Jackson WM, Chen J, Dworkin RH. Engaging stakeholders to promote safe anesthesia and sedation care in young children. J Neurosurg Anesthesiol. 2019;31(1):125–8.

Chapter 18
Sedation and Analgesia for Endotracheal Intubation

Elizabeth Laverriere and Akira Nishisaki

Indication for Tracheal Intubation in Pediatric ICU

General Principles

Tracheal intubation (TI) in pediatric intensive care units (ICUs) is a frequently performed procedure, yet is often associated with high risk. This is fundamentally different from the majority of TIs in operating suites, where the risk is generally much lower due to lower patient acuity. While the incidence of adverse respiratory events during TI for children in the operating suites is reported as 15% [1], and 37% of anesthesia-related cardiac arrests occur at the time of anesthesia induction and airway management [2], the adverse event rates of TI in the pediatric ICU are closer to 20%, in both general and cardiac ICUs [3–6]. Severe adverse events, including cardiac arrests and hypotension, occur in as many as 5% of PICU TIs. Consequently, it is crucial that providers carefully consider what the risks and benefits are for each critically ill child before making the decision to perform TI.

Typical Indications

Indication for TI in pediatric ICUs plays an important role since it determines the risk of TI and reflects local ICU practice. The data from National Emergency Airway Registry for Children (NEAR4KIDS) show that the most common indications are oxygenation and/or ventilation failure, followed by procedural indications. In cardiac patients specifically, hemodynamic instability is second only to oxygenation

E. Laverriere (✉) · A. Nishisaki
Anesthesiology and Critical Care Medicine, Children's Hospital of Philadelphia, Philadelphia, PA, USA
e-mail: laverrieree@email.chop.edu; nishisaki@email.chop.edu

P. P. Kamat, J. W. Berkenbosch (eds.), *Sedation and Analgesia for the Pediatric Intensivist*, https://doi.org/10.1007/978-3-030-52555-2_18

and/or ventilation failure as the indications for TI. The procedural indications account for approximately one in five TIs, and are associated with a lower risk of adverse events or oxygen desaturation [7].

Factors Associated with Safety of Tracheal Intubation in Pediatric ICU

Overall Description: Overall Safety Data and Association with Long-Term Outcomes

Adverse events observed in TIs are classified as severe and nonsevere TI-Associated Events (TIAEs). While not included in this category, another commonly occurring event is oxygen desaturation. These events remain relatively common despite the local and multi-institutional quality improvement efforts. During 2010–2011, any adverse TIAE occurred in 20% and severe adverse TIAEs occurred in 6% of all TIs [7]. Oxygen desaturation to an $SpO_2 < 80\%$ was reported in 13% of all TIs, although a more recent study reported moderate and severe oxygen desaturation rates of 19% and 13%, respectively, suggesting that the rate may be higher than earlier thought [8]. It is important to note that specific patient, provider, and practice factors are closely associated with the occurrence of adverse TIAEs and oxygen desaturation. Not surprisingly, the occurrence of adverse TIAEs and oxygen desaturations are closely associated with each other. In 33% of TIs in which there is an adverse TIAE, oxygen desaturation to <80% also occurs (unpublished data). Similarly, during TIs in which oxygen desaturation to <80% occurs, hemodynamic TIAEs (i.e., cardiac arrest, hypo-/hypertension, dysrhythmia) are more likely to also be experienced (9.8% vs. 4.4% of TIs without oxygen desaturation) [8]. This association remained significant after adjusting for patient conditions and provider levels: The odds ratio for hemodynamic TIAEs were 1.83 (95% CI: 1.34–2.51) in TIs with moderate desaturation ($SpO_2 < 80\%$), and 2.16 (95% CI: 1.54–3.04) in TIs with severe desaturation ($SpO_2 < 70\%$). Occurrence of adverse TIAEs or oxygen desaturation was independently associated with a longer duration of mechanical ventilation +12% (95% CI: 4–21%), and the occurrence of severe TIAEs was independently associated with increased pediatric ICU mortality (odds ratio = 1.80, 95% CI: 1.24–2.60) [9]. While a causal relationship is not established, it makes sense to make every effort to prevent adverse TIAEs, severe TIAEs, and oxygen desaturation during TI of critically ill children.

Tracheal Intubation Procedural Outcomes

The overwhelming majority (98%) of the initial course for TI (the first method of approach, e.g., standard sequence intubation with direct laryngoscopy) is successful [7]. The first attempt was successful in 62%, and the initial provider is ultimately successful in 79% of all TIs. Fourteen percent of TIs require three or more attempts [7].

Specific Factors Associated with Adverse Events and Oxygen Desaturation Events

It is crucial to evaluate the risk of TI using patient, provider, and practice as a conceptual framework. These factors likely interact with each other. The underlying microsystem (ICU safety system and culture) likely modifies the effect of each factor.

Patient Factors

Table 18.1 shows the patient factors associated with the adverse TI-associated events and oxygen desaturations. It is important to note that infants less than 12 months of age are at higher risk for oxygen desaturation [8]. Respiratory failure and hemodynamic instability have an additive effect in putting patients at risk for tracheal intubation-associated cardiac arrest. Both a history of difficult airway and difficult airway features, especially signs of upper airway obstruction, are associated with adverse TIAEs and oxygen desaturation. Of note, 12–16% of children who receive TIs in pediatric ICUs have a history of difficult airway (either difficult mask ventilation or difficult intubation) previously [7]. Procedural indication for TI is associated with fewer adverse TIAEs and oxygen desaturation.

Provider Factors

A series of observational studies documents the difference in TI first-attempt success, overall success, and the occurrence of TIAEs and severe TIAEs across the spectrum of provider experience [7, 10]. An early study demonstrated the pediatric resident first-attempt success rate was approximately half that of critical care fellows (residents 37%, fellows 70%, and attendings 72%) [10]. TIs by residents had 30% of TIAEs while TIs by fellows had 16% and TIs by attendings had 22%.

Table 18.1 Patient factors associated with TIAEs and oxygen desaturation

Patient factors	Association with adverse TIAEs and oxygen desaturation
Patient age	Younger age is associated with oxygen desaturation
History of difficult airway	Presence of history of a difficult airway is associated with adverse TIAE and oxygen desaturation
Difficult airway features	Presence of difficult airway features is associated with adverse TIAE and oxygen desaturation
Patient diagnosis	Respiratory diagnosis is associated with adverse TIAE and oxygen desaturation. Sepsis/shock diagnosis at the time of TI is associated with adverse TIAE
Indication for tracheal intubation	Oxygenation/ventilation failure and upper airway obstruction are associated with adverse TIAEs and oxygen desaturation. Shock is associated with adverse TIAE Neurologic indication is associated with lower occurrence of TIAE and oxygen desaturation Procedural indication is associated with lower occurrence of TIAE and oxygen desaturation

Interestingly severe TIAE rates were the highest in TIs performed by attending providers (9%) as compared to TIs by residents (6%) and fellows (6%), suggesting the provider selection based on anticipated patient risk for severe adverse events.

Practice Factors

From a large observational study, the use of video laryngoscopy was associated with a lower occurrence of TIAEs in pediatric ICU intubations [11]. This is similar to results from a single academic neonatal ICU study [12]. While cricoid pressure is commonly used during pediatric ICU TI (23% of all TIs) after induction with sedatives to prevent gastric regurgitation, its use is not associated with a lower incidence of regurgitation (adjusted odds ratio 1.57, 95% CI: 0.99–2.47, $p = 0.054$) [13]. The incidence of regurgitation during TI is 0.7% in the pediatric ICU, which is seven times higher than that in the operating room. However, cricoid pressure is often used differently in the pediatric ICU, with only 26% of rapid sequence inductions using cricoid pressure and 22% of standard sequence inductions using cricoid pressure. In addition, there are concerns that medical providers do not consistently or correctly apply the cricoid pressure maneuver. Even when applied correctly, cricoid pressure may actually loosen lower esophageal sphincter tone in the patient [14]. Consequently, routine cricoid pressure use is not recommended in pediatric ICU TIs. Sometimes confused with cricoid pressure, external laryngeal manipulation may also be attempted to improve glottic exposure during TI. External laryngeal manipulation is actually associated with a slightly lower initial TI attempt success (adjusted odd ratio = 0.93, 95% CI: 0.9–0.95, $p < 0.001$) [15] and routine use during TI in the pediatric ICU is also not recommended. While there are some concerns among providers to allow family members at bedside during TI, family member presence during TI is not significantly associated with the occurrence of adverse events or an increase in the number of attempts required for successful intubation in both the pediatric ICU [16] and neonatal ICU (unpublished data) settings. We recommend to have one dedicated staff assigned to support family members during TI in the pediatric ICU.

Role of Induction Medications for Tracheal Intubations

There is substantial practice variation in the types of medications administered for TI in the pediatric ICU. Clinicians frequently tailor their choice of medications as well as the dose to optimize the intubation conditions while avoiding hypotension and other potential adverse effects. Few contraindications exist in the choice of medications (and are discussed elsewhere in this textbook). These include avoiding etomidate in children with septic shock due to risk of adrenal suppression, avoiding succinylcholine in children with known risk for malignant hyperthermia, known skeletal myopathy, immediately following burn injury, or with known or at high risk for rhabdomyolysis due to the risk of lethal hyperkalemia-induced ventricular dysrhythmias and avoid medications to which there is a documented allergy or adverse reaction.

There are three categories of induction medications: vagolytics, sedatives/narcotics/hypnotics, and neuromuscular blockers. These medications are used most often in combination.

It is important to know that traditional anesthesia literature uses the term "rapid sequence" induction; however, this term implies different things in different medical disciplines. For emergency medicine providers, it most commonly refers to the administration of both sedative(s) and neuromuscular blockade to a patient in an expeditious fashion during induction, regardless of whether mask ventilation is performed. Neonatologists frequently use this definition as well. For pediatric intensivists as well as anesthesiologists, the classic rapid sequence induction refers to a simultaneous administration of sedative and neuromuscular blockade without mask ventilation to minimize the risk of regurgitation. In PICU patients, a "modified" rapid sequence induction, in which bag-mask ventilation with or without cricoid pressure is provided during the time between administration of sedative/neuromuscular blockade and successful tracheal intubation, is most typically performed. Regardless of medication choice, it is critical to explicitly discuss the induction plan during a "time out" prior to airway management in order to delineate anticipated risks and the plan to mitigate and address them. This "time out" discussion should include the types of medications and dosages, primary and backup devices for TI, as well as first-attempt and backup laryngoscopists and the anticipated timing of the transition (if needed).

Roles and Types of Anticholinergic and Other Adjunctive Medications

The role of anticholinergic medications during pediatric airway management is controversial. Atropine and glycopyrrolate are the two major medications frequently used as a part of induction. Anticholinergic medications have been demonstrated to increase the heart rate during induction. However, their clinical benefit in preventing hemodynamically significant bradycardia and adverse events is questionable. Large observational studies have consistently shown that the addition of an anticholinergic during pediatric TI is associated with a higher risk of hemodynamic adverse events although a significant contribution of patient selection bias (i.e., sicker patients tend to receive anticholinergics more frequently) to this finding may exist [7]. Routine use of anticholinergics to reduce hemodynamic adverse events during tracheal intubation is not supported by evidence. For patients with increased intracranial pressure (ICP), atropine may obscure the clinical examination by causing bilateral mydriasis. Glycopyrrolate is less likely to cause mydriasis since it does not readily cross the blood-ocular barrier.

Intravascular lidocaine has also been used to blunt the ICP spike from laryngoscopy-induced noxious stimulation. However, controversy exists about the duration of this effect (debated to be from 30 seconds to 3 minutes after lidocaine administration), and other studies show that fentanyl can also effectively blunt this intracranial pressure spike. There remains a paucity of data regarding optimal induction medication choice in children at risk of or with documented intracranial hypertension.

Role and Type of Sedatives and Analgesics

Sedative/narcotic/hypnotics are used to provide optimal depth of sedation to immobilize a patient during laryngoscopy, stabilize patient hemodynamics, and provide amnesia. A single medication or a combination of medications can be used to achieve these goals.

Ketamine is a medication that has seen an increase in usage in pediatric ICUs in recent years, especially in children with shock physiology because of its preferable hemodynamic profile (less hypotension due to stimulation of the release of endogenous catecholamines) [17]. Ketamine has both sedative and analgesic effects through its action as an *N*-methyl-D-aspartate (NMDA) receptor antagonist. It is considered a dissociative anesthetic. Ketamine itself does not likely increase ICP based on an observational study in the ICU [18]. Ketamine itself is a direct myocardial depressant, but this effect tends to be clinically insignificant due to ketamine's sympathomimetic effects. In addition, ketamine causes less respiratory depression and maintains protective airway reflexes, making it an attractive option for intubation in patients in whom neuromuscular blockade may be undesired. It is also an effective bronchodilator, making it attractive for use during intubation of patients with significant lower respiratory obstructive processes such as asthma or bronchiolitis.

Propofol is often used for TIs in patients with a lower risk for hemodynamic instability. Propofol is also often used for children with concern for seizure or increased ICP. It has potent anticonvulsive effects, and lowers ICP by decreasing the cerebral metabolic rate for oxygen. Another benefit is a rapid onset of action (often less than 30 seconds). However, propofol also has potent respiratory suppressive effects and, at doses required to create adequate intubation conditions, commonly causes central apnea. Airway providers should be ready to provide mask ventilation immediately after propofol administration. Because propofol is a myocardial depressant and also reduces systemic vascular resistance, propofol should be used with caution (or possibly avoided) in patients requiring intubation with shock physiology or with myocardial dysfunction. The sedating effects of propofol also are short-lived and would be expected to have dissipated before the effects of associated neuromuscular blocker use during TI, so additional sedation should be provided following airway securement in order to avoid awareness underneath residual chemical paralysis.

Midazolam and fentanyl are commonly used medications, and are often used in combination. Their onset of action is relatively slow compared to the ketamine or propofol. The effect of these agents is variable among children, especially those who have experienced prolonged exposure to sedative medications and subsequent tolerance development prior to their administration for TI, in which case higher than usual doses may be required. Whereas midazolam has only sedative effects and fentanyl has predominantly an analgesic effect with very limited sedative effects at a commonly administered dose, combining the two is pharmacodynamically logical. Midazolam has venodilatory effects that may induce hypotension after induction. Rapid injection of fentanyl may be associated with the development of rigid chest syndrome, for which the treatment is neuromuscular blockade administration so this effect may be of less concern during TI scenarios in which neuromuscular blockade is planned.

Etomidate is rarely used in pediatric ICUs (<1%) [7], but it is still commonly used in trauma settings in the emergency department. Etomidate preserves hemodynamics well, but has a relatively short duration of action (10–20 minutes). Similar to with propofol use, undersedation can occur if a child is intubated with etomidate and most of the available neuromuscular blockers since the duration of action of these agents is longer than that of etomidate. This may cause unrecognized agitation in children, and may have a detrimental effect in children with high risk of increased ICP (e.g., traumatic brain injury, stroke). Its use in the pediatric ICUs is limited mostly secondary to concerns due to inhibition of the enzymatic biosynthesis of steroid hormones and studies demonstrating an association of its use with increased mortality in the ICU [19].

Roles and Types of Neuromuscular Blockade

Neuromuscular blockade is used in the overwhelming majority of TIs in pediatric ICUs (90%) [7]. The use of neuromuscular blockade is not associated with lower occurrence of adverse TIAEs and multiple attempts in the pediatric ICU TIs, although the overwhelming majority of TIs utilized neuromuscular blockade (92%). Among critically ill neonates, the use of neuromuscular blockade is less common (only 47%), but its addition is significantly associated with a lower occurrence of adverse TIAEs (adjusted odds ratio = 0.48, 95% CI: 0.34–0.65, compared to TIs without neuromuscular blockade) [20]. In the absence of a contraindication to usage such as an anticipated difficult airway or medication allergy to neuromuscular blockade, the use of neuromuscular blockade is recommended for routine use in TIs in the PICU.

There are two types of neuromuscular blockade medications available: depolarizing and nondepolarizing neuromuscular blockers. The only depolarizing neuromuscular blockade medication available in the United States is succinylcholine. Succinylcholine has rapid onset of action (providing intubating conditions in approximately 30 seconds), and short duration of action (<10 minutes), making it ideal for patients who need neurologic assessments shortly after TI. While short, however, this duration of action is still too long before return of spontaneous ventilation in the event that a patient is unable to be mask ventilated. In addition, the aforementioned contraindications to succinylcholine use must be considered when choosing a neuromuscular blocker.

The three commonly used non-depolarizing neuromuscular blockers available in the United States are rocuronium, vecuronium, and cisatracurium. Rocuronium, at a double dose (1.2 mg/kg), provides an equivalent intubating conditions to succinylcholine within 90–120 seconds, making it the most commonly used neuromuscular blocker for rapid sequence induction. Vecuronium and cisatracurium have a longer onset of action and are used in situations where a rapid sequence induction is not required. Cisatracurium is also particularly attractive for use in situations where renal and hepatic failure are present as its elimination from the body is due to Hoffman elimination without relying on hepatic enzyme function.

The traditional reversal agent for neuromuscular blockade (neostigmine) does not effectively reverse the effects of nondepolarizing neuromuscular blockade unless train-of-four twitch testing is greater than or equal to 1 out of 4. However, sugammadex reliably reverses aminosteroid nondepolarizing neuromuscular blockade (rocuronium and vecuronium) in the absence of a twitch on train-of-four testing. There is a role for sugammadex in the pediatric ICU as an emergency rescue medication in situations under which, following neuromuscular blockade administration, the patient cannot be ventilated or intubated. Use of sugammadex is contraindicated in patients with renal failure, and there are limited data on its use in pediatric populations. Because of in vitro data that indicate that sugammadex may bind to progestogen, the use of sugammadex while using hormonal contraceptives is considered equivalent to missing doses and a back-up method of contraception must be used for 7 days following the sugammadex administration.

Special Considerations for High-Risk Tracheal Intubations in Pediatric ICU

Patients with Hemodynamic Instability

Approximately 10% of TIs in pediatric ICUs occur in patients with hemodynamic instability [8]. This population has a higher risk of hypotension, cardiovascular collapse, and cardiac arrest during intubation. Tracheal intubation planning with (1) optimization of patient hemodynamic condition by fluid resuscitation, correction of metabolic acidosis, and initiation of catecholamine infusions or small boluses, (2) minimizing oxygen desaturation risk by using apneic oxygenation and minimizing apneic time, and (3) intubation by the most skilled laryngoscopist to optimize likelihood of rapid first attempt success are all essential. A thorough "Time Out" should be performed to review patient risk factors, TI approach with specific discussions about providers, medications and devices, and roles should significant hemodynamic collapse occur [21].

Ketamine is often the drug of choice in this population, supported by the data that greater than 50% of children with sepsis or shock as ICU admission diagnosis received ketamine as an induction medication. Its use is associated with lower occurrence of hemodynamic TIAEs (odds ratio = 0.74, 95% CI: 0.58–0.95) [17] in the large observational data from NEAR4KIDS database, although this effect did not reach a level of significance in children with shock (odds ratio = 0.81, 95% CI: 0.58–1.12) [17]. Ketamine dosage (as is similar for all induction agents) needs to be titrated to effect especially in children in shock, since ketamine itself is a direct myocardial depressant and can cause hypotension in a catecholamine depleted shock state.

Patients with a Difficult Airway

Patients with either a history of difficult airway or clinical features suggesting an increased likelihood of a difficult airway (such as signs of upper airway obstruction, limited neck extension, limited mouth opening, small jaw, or midface hypoplasia) require specific attention and planning for safe airway management. Obtaining previous airway management information, if available, is crucial. It is especially important to know if the difficult airway history was due to difficult mask ventilation, difficult tracheal intubation, or both. Based on this airway history and the clinical assessment, the team should make a careful plan for proceeding with the intubation. Patient factors become important when a team is dealing with a child with history of difficult airway with acute respiratory failure. The level of support with noninvasive ventilation and the threshold to transition to invasive ventilation may need to be different. Given the risk of acute deterioration and failure to rescue by tracheal intubation, a lower threshold for the transition may be necessary. Also it may be prudent to avoid a natural airway sedation for procedures in some high-risk patients. Skilled airway providers, such as anesthesiologists or otolaryngologists, may need to be present before airway management begins. Airway management may need to take place in the operating room, which can provide better lighting, space, specialized equipment and personnel, particularly if a fiberoptic or surgical airway is emergently required. If an approach has previously been identified as successful for the patient, this is often the ideal initial approach. If patients can be ventilated via a supraglottic airway (such as a laryngeal mask airway), it should be available as part of a rescue plan. For some difficult intubations, ventilation with laryngeal mask airway between laryngoscopy attempts may reduce the patient's risk for oxygen desaturation and further hemodynamic derangement. The laryngeal mask airway can also provide a conduit for intubation with flexible fiberoptic bronchoscope. From a system perspective, these patients should be flagged as "difficult airway" in the electronic medical record, and detailed information about the airway management should be updated every time these patients undergo sedation and/or TI. A letter with a detailed difficult airway description can be generated and handed to patients and caregivers from the airway management team.

Patient with Increased Intracranial Pressure

Patients with known or at high risk for elevated intracranial pressure (ICP) require specific attention. The airway management plan should avoid any precipitating factors known to increase ICP. These include hypercarbia, hypoxemia, and painful stimulation, among others. The cerebral blood flow has a linear positive correlation with partial pressure of carbon dioxide ($PaCO_2$). Therefore, any $PaCO_2$ increase may directly increase ICP. A prolonged apneic time from a classic rapid sequence induction and long laryngoscopy time will place the patient at risk for an increase in $PaCO_2$ and ICP. To avoid this, continued ventilation immediately before laryngoscopy as well as shortening laryngoscopy time in skilled provider's hands are essential. Minimizing laryngoscopy time and consideration for apneic oxygenation use may also assist in decreasing the risk of hypoxemia. Patients with traumatic brain injury with transient hypoxemia tend to have worse neurologic outcomes compared to patients without hypoxemia during initial resuscitation (including airway management) [22]. To minimize ICP elevations during laryngoscopy, the use of fentanyl or lidocaine as an adjunctive medication should be considered. Atropine may obscure the clinical examination by causing bilateral mydriasis as described earlier. Ketamine use is no longer considered contraindicated in this population and provides a favorable hemodynamic profile for induction but should still be used with caution. An appropriately deep level of sedation is essential to prevent an ICP surge.

Other Special Considerations

Patients with external tracheal compression should be considered a special case of difficult airway. While direct visualization of the larynx itself (depending on the anatomic location of the airway compression), tracheal intubation of the upper trachea may not relieve distal airway compression and may be associated with inability to maintain a patent airway. Neuromuscular blockade will likely worsen the airway compression due to loss of airway tone. Avoidance of neuromuscular blockade, maintenance of spontaneous ventilation, use of noninvasive ventilation, and turning the patient to their side or prone position may be necessary [23]. If tracheal intubation is performed, a deep mainstem intubation bypassing the compressed segment may be required.

It is important to note that anterior mediastinal mass compression of the airway may also compress the pulmonary arteries or superior vena cava that can induce obstructive shock physiology. Concomitant pericardial effusion and development of cardiac tamponade may occur if the mediastinal mass is from an oncologic origin. In a large case series, these children with anterior mediastinal masses were managed safely by anesthesiologists for their diagnostic workup with preserved spontaneous ventilation. Patients who cannot lie flat on the bed likely have substantial airway compression or hemodynamic compromise, and should be considered high risk for acute deterioration and cardiorespiratory collapse. These patients may need extracorporeal membranous oxygenation (ECMO) circuit standby when requiring sedation or airway management. Consideration should be given to providing empirical treatment with steroids to reduce the tumor burden if the mass is likely a lymphoma on the imaging study.

Summary

It is crucial to evaluate the risk of TIs using a patient, provider, and practice-based conceptual framework. A careful plan should be made to address each of these categories. The initial risk assessment with planning, timeout immediately before the procedure, and debriefing are key for the continuous safe airway management for critically ill children.

References

1. von Ungern-Sternberg BS, Boda K, Chambers NA, et al. Risk assessment for respiratory complications in paediatric anaesthesia: a prospective cohort study. Lancet. 2010;376(9743):773–83. https://doi.org/10.1016/S0140-6736(10)61193-2.
2. Zgleszewski SE, Graham DA, Hickey PR, et al. Anesthesiologist- and system-related risk factors for risk-adjusted pediatric anesthesia-related cardiac arrest. Anesth Analg. 2016;122(2):482–9. https://doi.org/10.1213/ANE.0000000000001059.
3. Lee JH, Nuthall G, Ikeyama T, et al. Tracheal Intubation Practice and Safety Across International PICUs: A Report From National Emergency Airway Registry for Children. Pediatr Crit Care Med. 2019;20(1):1–8.
4. Rehder KJ, Giuliano JS Jr, Napolitano N, et al. Increased occurrence of tracheal intubation-associated events during nights and weekends in the PICU. Crit Care Med. 2015;43(12):2668–74.
5. Gradidge EA, Bakar A, Tellez D, et al. Effect of location on tracheal intubation safety in cardiac disease-are cardiac ICUs safer? Pediatr Crit Care Med. 2018;19(3):218–27. https://doi.org/10.1097/PCC.0000000000001422.
6. Gradidge EA, Bakar A, Tellez D, et al. Safety of tracheal intubation in the presence of cardiac disease in paediatric ICUs. Cardiol Young. 2018;28(7):928–37. https://doi.org/10.1017/S1047951118000495.
7. Nishisaki A, Turner DA, Brown CA 3rd, et al. A national emergency airway registry for children: landscape of tracheal intubation in 15 PICUs. Crit Care Med. 2013;41(3):874–85.
8. Li S, Hsieh T, Rehder KJ, et al. Frequency of desaturation and association with hemodynamic adverse events during tracheal intubations in PICUs. Pediatr Crit Care Med. 2018;19(1):e4–e50.
9. Parker MM, Nuthall G, Brown C 3rd, et al. Relationship Between Adverse Tracheal Intubation Associated Events and PICU Outcomes. Pediatr Crit Care Med. 2017;18(4):310–18.
10. Sanders RC Jr, Giuliano JS Jr, Sullivan JE, et al. Level of trainee and tracheal intubation outcomes. Pediatrics. 2013;131(3):821.
11. Grunwell JR, Kamat PP, Miksa M, et al. Trend and outcomes of video laryngoscope use across PICUs. Pediatr Crit Care Med. 2017;18(8):741–9.

12. Pouppirt NR, Nassar R, Napolitano N, et al. Association between video laryngoscopy and adverse tracheal intubation-associated events in the neonatal intensive care unit. J Pediatr. 2018;201:28–284.e1.
13. Kojima T, Harwayne-Gidansky I, Shenoi AN, et al. Cricoid pressure during induction for tracheal intubation in critically ill children: a report from national emergency airway registry for children. Pediatr Crit Care Med. 2018;19(6):528–37. https://doi.org/10.1097/PCC.0000000000001531.
14. Tournadre JP, Chassard D, Berrada KR, Bouletreau P. Cricoid cartilage pressure decreases lower esophageal sphincter tone. Anesthesiology. 1997;86(1):7–9. https://doi.org/10.1097/00000542-199701000-00003.
15. Kojima T, Laverriere EK, Owen EB, et al. Clinical impact of external laryngeal manipulation during laryngoscopy on tracheal intubation success in critically ill children. Pediatr Crit Care Med. 2018;19(2):106–14. https://doi.org/10.1097/PCC.0000000000001373.
16. Sanders RC, Nett ST, Davis KF, et al. Family presence during pediatric tracheal intubations. JAMA Pediatr. 2016;170(3):e154627. https://doi.org/10.1001/jamapediatrics.2015.4627.
17. Conway JA, Kharayat P, Sanders RC Jr, et al;. Ketamine Use for Tracheal Intubation in Critically Ill Children Is Associated With a Lower Occurrence of Adverse Hemodynamic Events. Crit Care Med. 2020;48(6):e489-e497. https://doi.org/10.1097/CCM.0000000000004314
18. Cohen L, Athaide V, Wickham ME, Doyle-Waters MM, Rose NG, Hohl CM. The effect of ketamine on intracranial and cerebral perfusion pressure and health outcomes: a systematic review. Ann Emerg Med. 2015;65(1):4–51.e2. https://doi.org/10.1016/j.annemergmed.2014.06.018.
19. den Brinker M, Joosten KF, Liem O, et al. Adrenal insufficiency in meningococcal sepsis: bioavailable cortisol levels and impact of interleukin-6 levels and intubation with etomidate on adrenal function and mortality. J Clin Endocrinol Metab. 2005;90(9):5110–7. doi: jc.2005-1107 [pii]
20. Ozawa Y, Ades A, Foglia EE, et al. Premedication with neuromuscular blockade and sedation during neonatal intubation is associated with fewer adverse events. J Perinatol. 2019;39(6):848–56. https://doi.org/10.1038/s41372-019-0367-0.
21. Li S, Rehder KJ, Giuliano JS, et al. Development of a quality improvement bundle to reduce tracheal intubation–associated events in pediatric ICUs. Am J Med Qual. 2016;31(1):47–55.
22. Rosario BL, Horvat CM, Wisniewski SR, et al. Presenting characteristics associated with outcome in children with severe traumatic brain injury: a secondary analysis from a randomized, controlled trial of therapeutic hypothermia. Pediatr Crit Care Med. 2018;19(10):957–64. https://doi.org/10.1097/PCC.0000000000001676.
23. Stricker PA, Gurnaney HG, Litman RS. Anesthetic management of children with an anterior mediastinal mass. J Clin Anesth. 2010;22(3):159–63. https://doi.org/10.1016/j.jclinane.2009.10.004.

Part V
PICU Environment and Sedation/Analgesia

Chapter 19
Sleep in the Pediatric Intensive Care Unit

Jessica A. Berger and Sapna R. Kudchadkar

Introduction

It is widely accepted that an adequate quantity of high-quality sleep is integral to the comprehensive health of children and adolescents. In the otherwise healthy developing child, sleep derangements can have far-reaching and life-altering effects on the extent to which children meet typical neurocognitive milestones, the way they follow standards of behavior, and how they perform academically [1, 2]. Poor sleep quality has been linked to the development of metabolic dysregulation—such as insulin resistance—in children and adolescents [3], and a growing body of literature describes the complex interactions between poor sleep and chronic pain in youth with sickle cell disease, juvenile idiopathic arthritis, and other conditions that predispose individuals to pain and insomnia [4–9].

Given how vital sleep is to the functioning of a healthy body, it stands to reason that it would play a particularly significant role during periods of extreme physical and psychological vulnerability, such as when children and adolescents are hospitalized for acute illness, particularly in an intensive care unit (ICU). In this chapter, we aim to summarize the current literature describing sleep in the pediatric critical care setting. Specifically, we will focus on how sleep promotes recovery, the ways in which poor sleep can be detrimental to critically ill children, and the validated tools we have at our disposal to measure sleep quantity and categorize sleep quality in these patients. We will review the medical and environmental factors that put

J. A. Berger
Anesthesiology and Critical Care Medicine, Pediatrics, Johns Hopkins Hospital, Baltimore, MD, USA
e-mail: jberge34@jhmi.edu

S. R. Kudchadkar (✉)
Pediatric Anesthesiology and Critical Care Medicine, Pediatrics, Physical Medicine and Rehabilitation, Johns Hopkins Hospital, Baltimore, MD, USA
e-mail: sapna@jhmi.edu

P. P. Kamat, J. W. Berkenbosch (eds.), *Sedation and Analgesia for the Pediatric Intensivist*, https://doi.org/10.1007/978-3-030-52555-2_19

critically ill patients at risk for sleep disturbance in the pediatric ICU (PICU), as well as some of the initiatives that PICUs are undertaking to ameliorate these risks.

The Importance of Sleep in Critically Ill Pediatric Patients

Sleep disturbances can be categorized into sleep deprivation, or decreased total sleep time, and sleep fragmentation, whereby frequent awakenings or interruptions occur, often with preserved total sleep time. Both can contribute to the physiologic and metabolic derangements described in this chapter. Sleep is an essential component of the recovery from critical illness, and disruptions in sleep can severely disturb the cardiovascular, endocrine, and immune systems [10–13].

Inadequate sleep quantity and/or quality contributes to catecholamine surges and increased cortisol levels, elevated blood glucose, and increased insulin sensitization [10, 11]. Some evidence suggests that the metabolic rate increases when sleep is poor, which is compounded by the fact that the body is unable to adequately perform restorative functions in the absence of normal sleep architecture [10, 11, 13, 14]. In particular, children in the PICU have been shown to lack the ultradian variability of slow wave activity seen in healthy children that is believed to promote healing, neurocognitive development, and synaptic maturity [14]. Additionally, a pro-inflammatory milieu prevails in the sleep-deprived patient, with elevated serum C-reactive protein and interleukins 1, 2, and 6 despite a relatively immunosuppressed state, leading to poor wound healing [10, 11].

Promotion of high-quality sleep during a patient's ICU stay is critically important beyond the initial phase of recovery. Many patients recovering from the acute phase of illness are subject to persistent sleep disturbances in the months after ICU hospitalization. A systematic review of adult patients by Altman et al. [15] identified 22 studies of post-ICU sleep quality that used a combination of subjective and objective measures to describe overall sleep disturbance rates of 50–66.7% in the first month after discharge and 22–57% between months 3 and 6 after discharge. These findings have also been reported in discharged PICU patients. When compared with healthy, age-matched controls, a sample of 88 children hospitalized in a United Kingdom PICU had a significantly higher risk of post-discharge sleep impairment (72% vs 49%, $p = 0.009$), with the most notable effects being found on bedtime resistance and nighttime awakenings. Multivariable analysis did not yield any additional independent predictors for these phenomena, suggesting that critical illness and hospitalization in and of themselves may have the strongest impact [16]. One study by Colville et al. [17] further illustrates this point. In a 3-month follow-up study of PICU survivors, those with the highest pediatric index of mortality at admission score, a measure of illness severity, actually reported significantly less fatigue on the Pediatric Quality of Life Inventory Multidimensional Fatigue Scale than the rest of the cohort [17]. Though much evidence point toward the PICU stay as a negative predictor for post-hospitalization sleep quality, these data are reminders that recovering a child from a severe, sleep-altering, and potentially life-threatening illness may, in fact, normalize the child's quality of life.

The importance of preventing sleep disturbances and promoting healthy sleep in the ICU is now recognized on a national organizational level, with the inclusion of sleep as a pillar of high-quality critical care. In 2018, improving sleep and reducing immobility were added to the 2013 Pain, Agitation, and Delirium (PAD) guidelines of the Society of Critical Care Medicine to form the adult-oriented Pain, Agitation, Delirium, Immobility, and Sleep (PADIS) clinical practice guidelines [18].

The Study of Sleep

Before delving deeper into the hospital- and PICU-specific risk factors for sleep impairment, it is important to understand the metrics and tools we use to evaluate sleep in children and adolescents. The instruments used in sleep research are heterogeneous but can generally be divided into two groups: quantitative and qualitative. Quantitative measures of sleep, namely polysomnography (PSG, including sleep electroencephalography, or EEG) and actigraphy, aim to use objective data and defined criteria to determine when a patient is asleep or awake, the length of time in each state, and whether sleep meets a particular standard for quality and quantity. Qualitative measures of sleep, which include patient- or parent-completed diaries, as well as a multitude of validated questionnaires and tools, tend to focus on retrospective assessments of sleep patterns, behaviors, and subjective impressions of disturbances [19].

Quantitative Measures of Sleep

PSG and Sleep EEG

PSG, colloquially referred to as a "sleep study," integrates EEG, electrooculography, and electromyography to categorize a patient's state as awake, rapid eye movement (REM) sleep, non-REM sleep, or slow wave sleep. A significant advantage of PSG, widely considered the gold standard of sleep evaluation for both clinical practice and research, is its ability to identify stages of sleep. However, PSG has several limitations, both in practicality of use and in data interpretation for critically ill patients. The placement of electrodes for accurate data measurement requires time and skilled staff. Data recording and interpretation also necessitate trained staff and can be very time-consuming. Additionally, because the equipment can cause relative discomfort, sleep at the start of a study period may be especially disrupted. However, as it is technically challenging to maintain the electrodes for an extended length of time, PSG studies are often short and may be terminated before a patient adjusts to the electrodes on the body. Therefore, it can be difficult and potentially inaccurate to generalize PSG data to a patient's entire day, let alone an entire hospitalization [20].

Traditionally, a trained physician or sleep technician classifies the sleep stages with PSG by visual inspection of the EEG waveform. Application of these techniques may be limited by use of sedative medications, neuromuscular blockade, and/or critical illness encephalopathy, all of which may cause EEG abnormalities that affect interpretation. Kudchadkar and colleagues characterized the sleep EEG in eight PICU patients, using power spectral analysis of bilateral central and occipital EEG electrodes to measure the average power at five frequencies during a 24-hour period. All the patients had a diagnosis of acute respiratory distress syndrome without an underlying neurologic disorder or known sleep-disordered breathing. The EEGs of these PICU patients were compared to those of healthy age-matched controls and showed a loss of normal ultradian variability and increased power in select frequencies in the daytime. Using a quantitative analysis of the sleep EEG that accompanies PSG, this group was also able to adjust for the potential impact of benzodiazepine and opiate use [14]. Additionally, a study by Ducharme and colleagues evaluated the presence of sleep spindles on EEG in pediatric patients within 24 hours after the return of spontaneous circulation after cardiac arrest. They found an association with better neurocognitive outcomes at 6 months as compared to those without sleep spindles [21].

Actigraphy

Though PSG remains the gold standard for sleep research, the limitations in its practical use have more recently increased the use of actigraphy, or wearable accelerometry, to assign sleep or awake states based on a computerized algorithm's assessment of body movement in one or more axes [20, 22, 23]. Actigraphy has several advantages over PSG. The actigraphs are small, can be worn continuously for days to weeks with little interference in daily life, and are relatively inexpensive [12].

Although the primary outcome of actigraphy is a binary "asleep" or "awake" assignment, the data can be extrapolated to provide further detail and to estimate variables, such as sleep latency, total sleep time, wake after sleep onset, and sleep efficiency—a ratio of total sleep time to total time in bed [22, 23]. In contrast to PSG, actigraphy cannot be used to determine what stage of sleep (e.g., REM or non-REM) a patient is in [20, 22, 23]. Actigraphy may be prone to spurious data, as when a child is in a stroller or moving vehicle but asleep or when a child is awake but laying still [24], though corroboration with a sleep diary can adjust for this phenomenon when it occurs [24, 25]. Most of the time, actigraphy data agree with data from sleep diaries, and the differences are often so slight as to be insignificant [24].

As actigraphy began to increase in prevalence in the pediatric literature, many sleep researchers sought to advance its use in studies in a wide range of pediatric populations. Such efforts included studies to validate actigraphy against the gold standard of PSG. One critique of many of these early studies was that they were validated against adult PSG data and lacked available norms across the spectrum of pediatric ages and developmental stages [25]. One study by Gottschlisch and colleagues showed that actigraphy data closely approximated PSG data in a population of pediatric burn patients [11], but confirmed limitations, particularly in overestimating sleep and not accurately detecting periods of wakefulness [11, 20, 25]. Additionally, there is evidence that variability in the particular device and algorithm used may invite significant inconsistencies in study outcomes [26].

More recent studies have sought to establish normal values for actigraphic sleep data in healthy children and adolescents across a wide range of ages and settings [27], including normal values for movement in the nighttime hours [28]. It is important to recognize, however, that healthy children and adolescents behave differently from those who are critically ill, and the normal variability seen on weeknights and weekends in adolescents [27] may not be present in the ICU, where differences between weekdays and weekend days are blurred. Clinical practice guidelines produced by the American Academy of Sleep Medicine in 2018 also note that patients with periodic limb movement disorders may not be accurately assessed by actigraphy [22, 23].

To adjust for the fact that critically ill PICU patients spend a larger proportion of both day and night in bed compared to healthy norms, Kudchadkar et al. [12] introduced the daytime activity ratio estimate (DARE), a measure of daytime movement (08:00–20:00) divided by movement over 24 hours. The DARE serves to facilitate comparisons between subjects and controls as well as between subjects and themselves across multiple days of a study. The DARE has utility in patients with underlying weakness [12], which has been a recognized limitation of actigraphy in the past [20]. The use of the DARE as a measure of sleep fragmentation in critically ill children first emerged in the literature in 2019; its application will be discussed further in a subsequent section of this chapter [12].

Qualitative Measures of Sleep

Many studies utilize qualitative, or subjective, measures of sleep either alone or in conjunction with quantitative measures. Dozens of tools exist, ranging from a simple diary noting bedtime and wake time to complex, multidimensional tools that are considered well established and use evidence-based criteria from the American Psychological Association [19]. Limitations to patient- and nurse-reported measures of sleep include recall bias, poor judgment of sleep, especially if circadian rhythms are altered, and cognitive impairment, such as delirium [20].

Data regarding how well these subjective measures align with objective measures are conflicting. Whereas some studies suggest a high degree of correlation between sleep diaries and actigraphy [24] and generally recommend using the two measures in tandem [24, 25]; other studies in both pediatric [29] and adult patients [20] describe significant discordance between observational assessments of sleep and PSG data. In fact, patients and their nurses often have different perceptions of when and how well the patients are sleeping [20]. Some of the limitations caused by poor judgment or delirium, which can impact how an adult patient completes a questionnaire, may be minimized in the pediatric patient if his or her parent is the survey responder, though parents may not be able to assess a child's sleep or symptomatology accurately 100% of the time. We make mention here of a few tools used frequently in the pediatric population. An important limitation of all of these tools is that they all seek primarily to identify the presence or absence of sleep and are less sensitive at differentiating between sleep depths/stages.

Brief Infant Sleep Questionnaire (BISQ)

The Brief Infant Sleep Questionnaire (BISQ), developed in 2003, remains the best and most well-established qualitative measure of sleep for infants and toddlers up to the age of 29 months. The BISQ was developed to evaluate this unique population of children, using developmentally appropriate questions, as infants do not have a consolidative sleep pattern as older children do. Outcomes include sleep time and nighttime awakenings. BISQ data have been validated against actigraphy data in a comparable population [19, 30].

Anderson Behavioral State Scale

The Anderson Behavioral State Scale is frequently used in neonatal intensive care populations, with particular focus on the preterm infant. This scale, based on observations by nurses or other trained staff, assigns neonates to behavioral states based on clearly defined descriptions, including deep sleep, light sleep, drowsiness, quiet alert, active alert, and crying. Though the assignments are made based on subjective assessments, interrater reliability is high. The amount of time infants spend in each state, and the number of state transitions, can be measured and used as a quantitative outcome in response to a research intervention [31].

Other Multidimensional Measures

Some of the other frequently used qualitative measures of sleep include the Children's Sleep Habits Questionnaire (CSHQ), the Pediatric Sleep Questionnaire (PSQ), and the Sleep Disturbance Scale for Children (SDSC). All of these tools were validated primarily in children over the age of 2 years and are especially useful for diagnosing sleep disorders, including medical sleep disorders, such as sleep-disordered breathing, restless legs, and parasomnias. Of these tools, the CSHQ has been used in a population of children with comorbidities, including obesity, attention-deficit hyperactivity disorder, autism spectrum disorders, and intellectual disability [19].

Risk Factors for Poor Sleep

As described above, pediatric patients in the hospital, especially those in the PICU, are at high risk for sleep disturbances. The causes of derangements in the normal sleep–wake pattern in these patients are multifactorial and products of the underlying illness, medical interventions to treat the illness, and the hospital or ICU environment (Fig. 19.1). Physiologic derangements in many critical illnesses, including hypoxia, sepsis and inflammation, and traumatic brain injury, can alter sleep–wake cycles [32]. Additional risk factors for sleep disturbance include need for mechanical ventilation, need for sedation, prolonged immobility, and other invasive interventions, such as urinary catheters [32–34].

The hospital environment is often not conducive to high-quality sleep, as patients are frequently interrupted during nighttime hours for checks of vital signs, medication administration, and other reasons. Children hospitalized on even low-acuity medical wards experience an average of 7.3 room entries by staff between the nighttime hours of 23:00 and 07:00 [35]. Noise pollution caused by equipment, alarms, and voices is omnipresent and challenging to overcome [13, 36]. Many of these environmental factors are reported by adult ICU patients in qualitative assessments of their perceived barriers to sleep. Interruptions and loud noises during the night can cause intense disorientation, which may intersect with fear. For some patients, alarms at night might trigger worry that a life-sustaining machine is malfunctioning or that another patient is dying nearby. Some fear not waking up from sleep, which leads to sleep hesitancy. Weakness, being connected to many cables or tubes, and having equipment in the mouth were also cited by patients as obstacles to

Medical Conditions	Environmental Factors
Sepsis	Light
Hypoxia	Noise pollution
Burns	*Alarms*
Recent surgery	*Voices*
Pain	Nighttime awakenings
Delirium	Vital signs and daily weights
	Bathing
	Lab draws
	Imaging studies
	Early morning rounds
Medical Therapies	**Psychological/Emotional Factors**
Invasive lines and tubes	Fear
Endotracheal tubes	Anxiety
Urinary catheters	Abandonment
Monitoring cables	Disorientation to time
Sedative medications	
Benzodiazepines	
Anticholinergics	

Fig. 19.1 Risk factors for sleep disturbances [12, 13, 15–18, 32, 35, 37, 47]

movement, comfort, or asking for help, and in turn, negatively impacted sleep [37]. Patients in the PICU are also at high risk for delirium, which is both a contributor to and a consequence of sleep fragmentation during periods of critical illness [12, 13, 33, 36, 38]. Delirium will be covered in greater detail later in this chapter and elsewhere in this text.

The Impact of Medications on Sleep

The medications administered to PICU patients can have a significant impact on sleep and should be selected and dosed with care. Medications that are commonly used for patient comfort and sedation include opiates, benzodiazepines, alpha-2 agonists, ketamine, barbiturates, and antipsychotics. Deciding which class of medication to administer and how to titrate to effect can be challenging, particularly when patient feedback is limited. For example, patients who are chemically paralyzed during use of neuromuscular blockade are at high risk for oversedation [13, 39]. One study of pediatric cardiac intensive care nurses suggested that the triggers for increasing analgesic or sedative medications were heterogeneous and based on a wide range of clinical changes, from behaviors to vital signs. While the goals of treatment are always the same, i.e., patient comfort and hemodynamic stability, lack of standardization among providers can lead to inconsistent interventions and results [40]. Lack of standardization can also contribute to significant polypharmacy and prolonged weaning from multiple classes of medications, thus, further exacerbating sleep deficits [13].

Benzodiazepines have long been a mainstay of PICU sedation protocols, and a survey of pediatric intensivists in 2014 suggested that they are still used frequently, particularly as continuous infusions with additional as-needed intermittent boluses available in mechanically ventilated patients [39]. Substantial evidence from the adult critical care literature, however, suggests that benzodiazepines negatively affect sleep architecture, place patients at high risk for delirium [13, 39, 41], and increase patient-ventilator dyssynchrony [42]. The Safety and Efficacy of Dexmedetomidine Compared with Midazolam (SEDCOM) study group revealed that mechanically ventilated adults receiving dexmedetomidine infusions for sedation developed delirium at lower rates than those receiving continuous infusions of midazolam and had shorter courses of mechanical ventilation and fewer episodes of hypertension and tachycardia. There were no differences in time spent at a targeted level of sedation [43]. The Maximizing Efficiency of Targeted Sedation and Reducing Neurologic Dysfunction (MENDS) trial also revealed that dexmedetomidine reduced rates of delirium when compared to a different benzodiazepine, such as lorazepam. Patients in this trial who received dexmedetomidine spent more time at goal sedation levels than did patients in the lorazepam group [44].

A growing body of literature supports the use of dexmedetomidine for sedation and as an analgesic adjunct in the PICU. Dexmedetomidine is believed to facilitate a more natural sleep state, with fewer disruptions to sleep architecture [42]. However, only 1% of providers cited it as their preferred sedative in a 2014 survey by Kudchadkar and colleagues [39]. Since then, many studies have further demonstrated the safety and efficacy of dexmedetomidine in noninvasively ventilated [45] and intubated pediatric patients [46]. It is important to note that children may show signs of withdrawal after discontinuation of dexmedetomidine, with increased pain, agitation, and impaired sleep [46], necessitating a slow wean and/or supplementation with adjunctive medications, such as enteral clonidine.

Untreated pain has a negative impact on sleep in hospitalized and critically ill children and adults [12, 37, 47]. Paradoxically, both the sensation of poorly treated pain and the administration of many analgesics to avoid pain undertreatment can affect sleep quality and quantity. In adult patients, opiates have been shown to disrupt normal sleep architecture, leading to decreased slow wave and REM sleep [13]. Ketamine, an N-methyl-D-aspartate receptor antagonist with both sedative and analgesic properties was also shown to decrease REM sleep in pediatric burn patients compared to those burn patients who did not receive ketamine for a debridement procedure that same day. Of note, both the subjects and controls already had impaired REM sleep prior to the study [48].

Other medications, including antipsychotics, such as haloperidol; dedicated sleep aids, such as zolpidem; and antihistamines, such as diphenhydramine, have been studied in pediatric burn patients, who are particularly vulnerable to sleep disturbances while in the ICU. In light of the severity of the sleep derangements in the majority of burn patients treated with haloperidol or zolpidem, even small statistically significant improvements leave the patients meaningfully impaired [10]. Similarly, diphenhydramine improved total sleep time in the burn patients studied but did not improve sleep quality [49]. In the present day, the overwhelming conclusion of both the adult and pediatric critical care literature is that benzodiazepines and anticholinergic medications should be avoided, if at all possible, given their deleterious effects on healthy sleep architecture.

Special Populations at Risk

Mechanically Ventilated Patients

It can be particularly challenging to ensure that mechanically ventilated patients get an adequate amount of quality sleep while in the ICU. Part of the challenge relates to the difficulty of accurately measuring sleep in a subset of children requiring continuous sedation and, at times, neuromuscular blockade. A small pilot study in intubated children treated with neuromuscular blockers showed that PSG is feasible, but electrooculography and electromyography are affected by chemical paralysis, particularly impairing the identification of REM sleep. The patients in the study showed EEG evidence of sleep, but the ability to interpret the data was limited [50].

Providing safe and compassionate care to mechanically ventilated patients is one of the most significant challenges of clinical care for physician and nurse providers. Although immobility is sometimes necessary for safety, many frontline providers fear that the provision of neuromuscular blockade increases the risk of awareness. This concern raises the downstream probability of oversedation and delirium [13, 32, 39], prolonging the need for mechanical ventilation [42]. Owing to high clinical acuity, the ICU environments of mechanically ventilated patients are often more noisy and chaotic. PICU patients typically require more hands-on care and are subject to more invasive and potentially disruptive monitoring [13]. Once delirium emerges as a consequence of medical and environmental factors, it can be difficult to distinguish ventilator-associated agitation from an altered sensorium, potentially prolonging the detrimental cycle [13, 39, 42].

Postsurgical Patients

Much of what has been outlined above applies to the pediatric critical care patient in general, whether admitted for medical care, postsurgical care, or some combination. Several recent studies have aimed to understand the way that sleep is affected in the postsurgical state. Kudchadkar et al. [12] collected over 2000 days of actigraphy data in children and adolescents who underwent cardiac, urologic, or orthopedic surgery and were admitted to the PICU postoperatively. The postoperative population as a whole had a lower mean DARE than did healthy matched subjects, consistent with sleep fragmentation. In particular, the patients undergoing urologic and orthopedic surgeries fared worse than those undergoing cardiac surgery. As a group, the patients in the PICU had a lower mean DARE than those on the inpatient floor later in the hospitalization, but sleep improved only slightly on the day of transfer [12]. This study did not adjust for pain and analgesic medication as covariates, but the authors commented on the likely impact of postsurgical pain on sleep in these patients. Other studies suggest that sleep impairments that originate in the acute postoperative period and persist after discharge can contribute to the development of subacute and chronic pain that endures for weeks [47].

Delirium

Any summary of sleep disturbances in the PICU would be incomplete without a more in-depth discussion of delirium. The revised fifth edition of the Diagnostic and Statistical Manual of Mental Disorders (DSM-V) defines delirium as an acute change in attention and awareness, accompanied by cognitive impairment, that waxes and wanes over time. These impairments are directly attributable to an active medical condition, medication, or intoxication and cannot be explained by a preexisting neurocognitive disorder [32, 51]. Patients may present with hyperactive (agitation, restlessness, and hallucinations), hypoactive (fatigue and lethargy), or mixed manifestations [32].

In pediatrics, several tools exist to complement the clinical diagnosis of delirium. The Pediatric Confusion Assessment Method for the ICU (pCAM-ICU) has been validated in intubated and non-intubated children over the age of 5 years and can assist with diagnosis when combined with an appropriate index of suspicion on the part of the provider. Additional tools are available for use in younger children to account for age-appropriate behavioral changes. The Cornell Assessment of Pediatric Delirium can be used for patients of all ages through 21 years and is more sensitive than the pCAM-ICU, but less specific, particularly in children with underlying developmental delay [32, 34]. Routine screening and a keen clinical eye are essential to identifying delirium early. Evidence suggests that many frontline providers are underinformed or misinformed about the risk factors for delirium, and this unfamiliarity can increase the likelihood of delayed or missed diagnoses [33].

Many of the risk factors for delirium in PICU patients are identical to those for sleep disturbances, a fact that highlights the synergistic relationship between sleep disturbances and delirium in the PICU. Patients with acute delirium may experience striking loss of normal circadian rhythms, agitation, and restlessness during nighttime hours. Symptoms of delirium, which wax and wane, may emerge at night without adequate localizing clues [32–34].

Mainstays of treatment for delirium focus on eliminating triggers and attempting to return patients to their baseline mental status. The pillars of treatment are both environmental and pharmacologic. The unfamiliarity of the PICU environment is a clear trigger for delirium, and, as such, surrounding a child with familiar people and objects can help the child localize to place and reduce anxiety. Restoration of circadian rhythms can be facilitated by turning lights on and opening window shades in the daytime and turning lights off in the evening. Reducing immobility in patients whose condition does not require it can also help when it is deemed safe. Minimizing unnecessary nighttime interruptions to allow for uninterrupted periods of sleep is critical to recovery [32, 34]. Medications can assist in returning children with delirium to baseline. These include supplemental melatonin and atypical antipsychotics. Quetiapine may have advantages over haloperidol, because it has a more favorable side effect profile. Safely weaning sedative medications that predispose patients to delirium is also important. Medications should be titrated to a sedation level appropriate for the individual child's condition. Analgesics, though potentially sedating, should not be withheld, as untreated pain can trigger delirium [32, 34]. For a more complete discussion on delirium in critically ill children, the reader is referred to Chapter_____.

Sleep Promotion in the PICU

Many of the strategies for treating delirium can be used empirically to prevent it and help promote healthy sleep in critically ill children. In the past several years, many PICUs have developed "delirium bundles," early mobilization strategies, and other measures to reduce the incidence of delirium and return children to normal functioning (Fig. 19.2). Though evidence-based clinical practice

Medical	**Environmental**
Target sedation Avoid benzodiazepines and anticholinergics Consider dexmedetomidine for sedation Provide adequate analgesia Reevaluate the need for invasive therapies and monitors daily Use empiric delirium screening	Reduce noise pollution *"Quiet time" at night* Provide appropriate lighting for time of day Limit nighttime awakenings *Daytime bathing and daily weights* *Timed lab drawsand imaging* Limit sensory deprivation *Provide glasses and hearing aids* Limit screen time appropriate with age Initiate early mobility when safe Provide familiar people and objects Frequently reorient patient to time and place

Fig. 19.2 Strategies for promoting healthy sleep [13, 18, 32, 34, 36, 39, 41, 42, 53]

guidelines for sleep have not yet been produced for the pediatric population, most of the current PICU initiatives to promote sleep and reduce delirium reflect the recommendations of the PADIS guidelines, including fostering an environment conducive to sleep [18]. Because children tend to sleep better at home than in the hospital, optimizing the hospital environment to simulate home is an integral step in optimizing sleep hygiene. These steps include reducing sensory deprivation by providing children with their eyeglasses and hearing aids, setting daytime and nighttime hours with appropriate lighting, completing cares, such as bathing and daily weights during the daytime, encouraging upright positioning and ambulation during the day, and limiting television commensurate with American Academy of Pediatrics Guidelines [36, 52, 53]. Frequently reorienting patients to their environment, including the alarms and equipment that surround them, can provide reassurance and decrease fear, which may help reduce psychological barriers to sleep [37]. The PADIS guidelines also suggest paying attention to the mode of mechanical ventilation to avoid patient discomfort and ventilator dyssynchrony at night [18].

Rational use of medications plays a role in promoting healthy sleep and circadian rhythms in the PICU. Using validated scales for sedation, such as the State Behavioral Scale (SBS) or Richmond Agitation and Sedation Scale (RASS), to titrate sedatives can help avoid oversedation and create a shared mental model among physicians, nurses, and other providers as to the patient's goals of care [13, 36]. Benzodiazepines and anticholinergic medications, such as diphenhydramine, should be avoided in favor of less deliriogenic medications [13, 32, 34, 36, 42]. Opiates do not need to be restricted and can be used carefully to provide analgesia and minimize sedation. Saliski and Kudchadkar [41] advocate for a patient-controlled analgesia pump with a low-dose morphine infusion, for example, which reduces pain and noxious stimuli from the endotracheal tube but facilitates participation in early mobility.

Conclusion

Promotion of healthy sleep in the PICU is a challenging but critically important endeavor. Critical illness and the ICU environment are both disruptive to normal sleep architecture, and sleep disruption can, in turn, impair recovery and return to function. The field of pediatric sleep research has numerous tools for evaluating sleep disturbances, though critically ill children pose additional challenges to the performance of sleep research and the interpretation of sleep data. Many risk factors for impaired sleep have already been identified, with especially high rates of sleep fragmentation in children who are mechanically ventilated. The need for frequent interventions and sedation puts these children at an additional risk for delirium, which is directly associated with dysregulated sleep. Many PICUs are now focusing on quality measures to reduce the incidence of sleep impairment and delirium in their patients. Close attention to sleep hygiene promotion for critically ill children could have a significant impact on both short- and long-term outcomes.

References

1. Bathory E, Tomopoulos S. Sleep regulation, physiology and development, sleep duration and patterns, and sleep hygiene in infants, toddlers, and preschool-age children. Curr Probl Pediatr Adolesc Health Care. 2017;47:29–42.
2. El-Sheikh M, Philbrook LE, Kelly RJ, Hinnant JB, Buckhalt JA. What does a good night's sleep mean? Nonlinear relations between sleep and children's cognitive functioning and mental health. Sleep. 2019;42(6):zsz078;
3. De Bernardi Rodrigues AM, da Silva Cde C, Vasques AC, et al. Association of Sleep Deprivation with Reduction in insulin sensitivity as assessed by the hyperglycemic clamp technique in adolescents. JAMA Pediatr. 2016;170:487–94.
4. Holley AL, Wilson AC, Palermo TM. Predictors of the transition from acute to persistent musculoskeletal pain in children and adolescents: a prospective study. Pain. 2017;158:794–801.
5. Law EF, Dufton L, Palermo TM. Daytime and nighttime sleep patterns in adolescents with and without chronic pain. Health Psychol. 2012;31:830–3.
6. Lewandowski AS, Palermo TM, De la Motte S, Fu R. Temporal daily associations between pain and sleep in adolescents with chronic pain versus healthy adolescents. Pain. 2010;151:220–5.
7. Lewandowski AS, Ward TM, Palermo TM. Sleep problems in children and adolescents with common medical conditions. Pediatr Clin N Am. 2011;58:699–713.
8. Palermo TM, Law E, Churchill SS, Walker A. Longitudinal course and impact of insomnia symptoms in adolescents with and without chronic pain. J Pain. 2012;13:1099–106.
9. Valrie CR, Bromberg MH, Palermo T, Schanberg LE. A systematic review of sleep in pediatric pain populations. J Develop Behavior Pediatr. 2013;34:120–8.
10. Armour A, Gottschlich MM, Khoury J, Warden GD, Kagan RJ. A randomized, controlled prospective trial of zolpidem and haloperidol for use as sleeping agents in pediatric burn patients. J Burn Care Res. 2008;29:238–47.
11. Gottschlich MM, Mayes T, Khoury J, Simakajornboon N, Kagan RJ. Comparison of sleep parameters obtained from actigraphy and polysomnography during the rehabilitative phase after burn. J Burn Care Res. 2013;34:183–90.

12. Kudchadkar SR, Aljohani O, Johns J, et al. Day-night activity in hospitalized children after major surgery: an analysis of 2271 hospital days. J Pediatr. 2019;209:190–197.e1.
13. Kudchadkar SR, Aljohani OA, Punjabi NM. Sleep of critically ill children in the pediatric intensive care unit: a systematic review. Sleep Med Rev. 2014;18:103–10.
14. Kudchadkar SR, Yaster M, Punjabi AN, et al. Temporal characteristics of the sleep EEG power spectrum in critically ill children. J Clin Sleep Med. 2015;11:1449–54.
15. Altman MT, Knauert MP, Pisani MA. Sleep disturbance after hospitalization and critical illness: a systematic review. Ann Am Thorac Soc. 2017;14:1457–68.
16. Als LC, Picouto MD, Hau SM, et al. Mental and physical well-being following admission to pediatric intensive care. Pediatr Critical Care Med. 2015;16:e141–9.
17. Colville GA, Pierce CM, Peters MJ. Self-reported fatigue in children following intensive care treatment. Pediatr Critical Care Med. 2019;20:e98–e101.
18. Devlin JW, Skrobik Y, Gelinas C, et al. Clinical practice guidelines for the prevention and management of pain, agitation/sedation, delirium, immobility, and sleep disruption in adult patients in the ICU. Crit Care Med. 2018;46:e825–e73.
19. Lewandowski AS, Toliver-Sokol M, Palermo TM. Evidence-based review of subjective pediatric sleep measures. J Pediatr Psychol. 2011;36:780–93.
20. Bourne RS, Minelli C, Mills GH, Kandler R. Clinical review: sleep measurement in critical care patients: research and clinical implications. Crit Care. 2007;11:226.
21. Ducharme-Crevier L, Press CA, Kurz JE, Mills MG, Goldstein JL, Wainwright MS. Early presence of sleep spindles on electroencephalography is associated with good outcome after pediatric cardiac arrest. Pediatr Critical Care Med. 2017;18:452–60.
22. Smith MT, McCrae CS, Cheung J, et al. Use of Actigraphy for the evaluation of sleep disorders and circadian rhythm sleep-wake disorders: an American Academy of sleep medicine systematic review, meta-analysis, and GRADE assessment. J Clin Sleep Med. 2018;14:1209–30.
23. Smith MT, McCrae CS, Cheung J, et al. Use of Actigraphy for the evaluation of sleep disorders and circadian rhythm sleep-wake disorders: an American Academy of Sleep Medicine Clinical Practice Guideline. J Clin Sleep Med. 2018;14:1231–7.
24. Tetreault E, Belanger ME, Bernier A, Carrier J. Actigraphy data in pediatric research: the role of sleep diaries. Sleep Med. 2018;47:86–92.
25. Meltzer LJ, Montgomery-Downs HE, Insana SP, Walsh CM. Use of actigraphy for assessment in pediatric sleep research. Sleep Med Rev. 2012;16:463–75.
26. Quante M, Kaplan ER, Cailler M, et al. Actigraphy-based sleep estimation in adolescents and adults: a comparison with polysomnography using two scoring algorithms. Nat Sci Sleep. 2018;10:13–20.
27. Galland BC, Short MA, Terrill P, et al. Establishing normal values for pediatric nighttime sleep measured by actigraphy: a systematic review and meta-analysis. Sleep. 2018;41(4).
28. Meltzer LJ, Short M, Booster GD, et al. Pediatric motor activity during sleep as measured by actigraphy. Sleep. 2019;42(1):zsy196.
29. Armour AD, Khoury JC, Kagan RJ, Gottschlich MM. Clinical assessment of sleep among pediatric burn patients does not correlate with polysomnography. J Burn Care Res. 2011;32:529–34.
30. Sadeh A. A brief screening questionnaire for infant sleep problems: validation and findings for an Internet sample. Pediatrics. 2004;113:e570–7.
31. McGrath J, Vittner D. Behavioral assessment. In: Tappero EP, Honeyfield ME, editors. Physical assessment of the newborn: a comprehensive approach to the art of physical examination. Petaluma, CA: NICU INK Book Publishers; 2015. p. 193–219.
32. Calandriello A, Tylka JC, Patwari PP. Sleep and delirium in pediatric critical illness: what is the relationship? Med Sci (Basel). 2018;6(4):90.
33. Flaigle MC, Ascenzi J, Kudchadkar SR. Identifying barriers to delirium screening and prevention in the pediatric ICU: evaluation of PICU staff knowledge. J Pediatr Nurs. 2016;31:81–4.
34. Smith HA, Brink E, Fuchs DC, Ely EW, Pandharipande PP. Pediatric delirium: monitoring and management in the pediatric intensive care unit. Pediatr Clin N Am. 2013;60:741–60.

35. Erondu AI, Orlov NM, Peirce LB, et al. Characterizing pediatric inpatient sleep duration and disruptions. Sleep Med. 2019;57:87–91.
36. Kawai Y, Weatherhead JR, Traube C, et al. Quality improvement initiative to reduce pediatric intensive care unit noise pollution with the use of a pediatric delirium bundle. J Intensive Care Med. 2019;34:383–90.
37. Mattiussi E, Danielis M, Venuti L, Vidoni M, Palese A. Sleep deprivation determinants as perceived by intensive care unit patients: findings from a systematic review, meta-summary and meta-synthesis. Intensive Crit Care Nurs. 2019;53:43–53.
38. Brahmbhatt K, Whitgob E. Diagnosis and Management of Delirium in critically ill infants: case report and review. Pediatrics. 2016;137:e20151940.
39. Kudchadkar SR, Yaster M, Punjabi NM. Sedation, sleep promotion, and delirium screening practices in the care of mechanically ventilated children: a wake-up call for the pediatric critical care community*. Crit Care Med. 2014;42:1592–600.
40. Staveski SL, Lincoln PA, Fineman LD, Asaro LA, Wypij D, Curley MA. Nurse decision making regarding the use of analgesics and sedatives in the pediatric cardiac ICU. Pediatr Critical Care Med. 2014;15:691–7.
41. Saliski M, Kudchadkar SR. Optimizing sedation management to promote early mobilization for critically ill children. J Pediatr Intensive Care. 2015;4:188–93.
42. Barnes SS, Kudchadkar SR. Sedative choice and ventilator-associated patient outcomes: don't sleep on delirium. Ann Translation Med. 2016;4:34.
43. Riker RR, Shehabi Y, Bokesch PM, et al. Dexmedetomidine vs midazolam for sedation of critically ill patients: a randomized trial. JAMA. 2009;301:489–99.
44. Pandharipande PP, Pun BT, Herr DL, et al. Effect of sedation with dexmedetomidine vs lorazepam on acute brain dysfunction in mechanically ventilated patients: the MENDS randomized controlled trial. JAMA. 2007;298:2644–53.
45. Venkatraman R, Hungerford JL, Hall MW, Moore-Clingenpeel M, Tobias JD. Dexmedetomidine for sedation during noninvasive ventilation in pediatric patients. Pediatr Critical Care Med. 2017;18:831–7.
46. Whalen LD, Di Gennaro JL, Irby GA, Yanay O, Zimmerman JJ. Long-term dexmedetomidine use and safety profile among critically ill children and neonates. Pediatr Critical Care Med. 2014;15:706–14.
47. Rabbitts JA, Zhou C, Narayanan A, Palermo TM. Longitudinal and temporal associations between daily pain and sleep patterns after major pediatric surgery. J Pain. 2017;18:656–63.
48. Gottschlich MM, Mayes T, Khoury J, McCall J, Simakajornboon N, Kagan RJ. The effect of ketamine administration on nocturnal sleep architecture. J Burn Care Res. 2011;32:535–40.
49. Yangzom N, Gottschlich MM, Ossege J, Wangmo T, Kagan RJ. The effect of diphenhydramine on sleep in pediatric burn patients: a secondary analysis. J Burn Care Res. 2015;36:266–71.
50. Carno MA, Hoffman LA, Henker R, Carcillo J, Sanders MH. Sleep monitoring in children during neuromuscular blockade in the pediatric intensive care unit: a pilot study. Pediatr Critical Care Med. 2004;5:224–9.
51. APA. Diagnostic and statistical manual of mental disorders, fifth edition. Arlington: American Psychiatric Association; 2013.
52. Media and young minds. Pediatrics. 2016;138(5):e20162591.
53. Wieczorek B, Ascenzi J, Kim Y, et al. PICU up!: impact of a quality improvement intervention to promote early mobilization in critically ill children. Pediatr Critical Care Med. 2016;17:e559–e66.

Chapter 20
Delirium

Veronica Ramirez-Ramon and Chani Traube

What Is Delirium?

Delirium is a behavioral syndrome that manifests as acute, global cerebral dysfunction. Delirium occurs frequently in the pediatric intensive care unit (PICU) and is strongly associated with poor outcomes, such as increased mortality, prolonged time on mechanical ventilation, additional PICU days, and increased costs [1–5]. It is defined in the *Diagnostic and Statistical Manual of Mental Disorders, Fifth Edition (DSM-V)* as a disturbance in attention or awareness accompanied by a change in baseline cognition that develops acutely and tends to fluctuate in severity throughout the day. Delirium develops as the direct physiological consequence of an underlying medical condition or in response to exposure to certain drugs or toxins [6–9]. Although delirium itself is generally reversible, research studies have highlighted its strong association with increased morbidity and mortality. For this reason, the Society of Critical Care Medicine (SCCM) published guidelines in 2013 advocating for routine screening for delirium in adult ICU patients as standard of care [10]. Numerous recent studies suggest that these guidelines should be extended to the pediatric critical care population as well [1, 11].

Clinical Presentation

There are three distinct subtypes of delirium: hyperactive, hypoactive, and mixed. Hyperactive delirium is characterized by agitation, mood lability, and poor cooperation. These patients may be incorrectly labeled as the "difficult to sedate" children. In

V. Ramirez-Ramon (✉) · C. Traube
Department of Pediatrics, Division of Pediatric Critical Care Medicine, Weill Cornell Medical College, New York, NY, USA
e-mail: ver9022@med.cornell.edu; chr9008@med.cornell.edu

P. P. Kamat, J. W. Berkenbosch (eds.), *Sedation and Analgesia for the Pediatric Intensivist*, https://doi.org/10.1007/978-3-030-52555-2_20

contrast, hypoactive delirium is notable for sluggishness and lethargy which can be easily misdiagnosed as oversedation or clinical depression. In mixed delirium, patients have fluctuating levels of psychomotor activity, often vacillating between hyperactive and hypoactive delirium in the same day. More recently, two "variants" of delirium have also been described: the "catatonic variant," which represents an extreme form of hypoactive delirium, and the "excited variant," which represents an extreme form of hyperactive delirium [12]. While hyperactive delirium is the most recognizable subtype, mixed and hypoactive delirium are much more common and associated with the poorest prognosis [1, 13, 14]. In a longitudinal study that followed 1547 pediatric patients over more than 7500 patient days, hypoactive and mixed delirium comprised >90% of the cases (46% and 45% respectively). In contrast, hyperactive delirium was only found in 8% of patients [1]. Delirium usually has an acute course, lasting hours to days. However, persistent or chronic delirium has also been described, which can last from weeks to months, and is also associated with worse outcomes [14].

Disturbances in the sleep–wake cycle are extremely common in delirium. They may manifest as difficulty in falling asleep, intermittent or frequent episodes of wakefulness throughout the night, often accompanied by agitation, daytime sleepiness, and in some cases, a complete reversal of the sleep–wake cycle. Studies in the adult population suggest that sleep disorganization is both a key risk factor in the development of delirium, and a core symptom [15]. In the pediatric population, this relationship has not been definitively established and may, instead, reflect the cyclical relationship between delirium and sleep in that sleep deprivation can trigger delirium which then further disrupts subsequent sleep [16].

Etiology

The pathophysiologic mechanisms behind the development of delirium are complex and multifactorial. It is helpful to think of delirium as the result of both precipitating factors (medical illness, secondary treatment effects, sedative exposure, and ICU environment) and patient-related predisposing factors (age, underlying disease, and genetics). There are multiple pathways that are thought to play important roles in the evolution of pediatric delirium.

One of the first pathways examined suggests that acute, systemic inflammation (from trauma, surgery, or infection) induces activation of pro-inflammatory substances in the brain and alteration in blood-brain barrier permeability [17]. This is known as the *neuroinflammatory hypothesis*. It describes activation of cytokines, with generation of reactive oxygen species (ROS), nitric oxide (NO), and other inflammatory mediators that cause neurotoxic effects on microglia, astrocytes, and neurons [18]. Many studies have found elevated levels of pro-inflammatory cytokines in delirious patients when compared to non-delirious patients, despite controlling for multiple confounders [19–21]. Evidence of dysregulated proteins and acute phase response elements have also been identified in the cerebrospinal fluid (CSF) of delirious patients [22].

In the *oxidative stress hypothesis*, delirium is considered the clinical expression of a cerebral metabolic defect [17, 23]. Inadequate oxidative metabolism, due to either tissue hypoxia or hypoperfusion, generates reactive oxygen species that induce cerebral damage leading to the neurobehavioral changes seen in delirium. Specifically, an inability to maintain ionic gradients causes widespread cortical cellular depolarization, abnormalities in neurotransmitter synthesis and metabolism, and free radical production with accumulation of neurotoxic by-products [24–27]. Multiple studies have demonstrated a correlation between hypoxia and delirium in both adults and children [2, 28, 29].

The *neurotransmitter hypothesis* was proposed after delirium was observed with the use of drugs that alter neurotransmitter function and availability [17]. In particular, use of anticholinergic medications has been strongly linked to delirium in the geriatric population because of age-related decrease in acetylcholine synthesis [30, 31]. The cholinergic system is known to modulate activities that depend on selective attention and conscious awareness (two key factors affected in the diagnosis of delirium). Multiple studies have revealed impairment in cholinergic neurotransmission as well as excess dopaminergic activity in several models of encephalopathy and delirium [32–34]. In addition to acetylcholine and dopamine, other neurotransmitter changes that have been implicated in development of delirium include reduced melatonin, excess norepinephrine and glutamate, and alterations in serotonin, histamine, and/or gamma-aminobutyric acid levels [12].

Several other hypotheses have also been proposed related to neuronal aging (i.e., vulnerability to oxidative stress), the neuroendocrine axis (specifically, the role of glucocorticoids) as well as dysregulation of the circadian rhythm [17]. In 2017, Maldonado published an updated literature review with the objective of consolidating the various proposed pathophysiologic theories and how they interact with each other to produce the different phenotypes of delirium. In this novel interpretation, known as the *systems integration failure hypothesis*, he describes the various contributions from each pathway into a complex web with multiple areas of intersection and overlap [12]. The neurobehavioral changes characterized as delirium are the end result of the interactions between a susceptible patient and multiple precipitating factors.

Epidemiology

In adults, delirium has been recognized as a major public health concern that affects more than 30% of all critically ill patients and up to 80% of those that are mechanically ventilated, with costs ranging between 4 and 16 billion dollars annually in the United States alone [35–37]. Research in pediatrics has trailed behind due to decreased awareness and lack of validated screening tools. However, in the past decade, a plethora of studies have demonstrated that critically ill children often become delirious during their stay in the PICU [38, 39]. Frequency of delirium varies between institutions, and specific patient populations may be affected differently [39]. In the largest point-prevalence study to date, 994 subjects from 25 separate pediatric intensive care units across the world were screened for delirium during two different time points using a validated tool. Twenty-five percent of patients were found to be delirious. This rate increased to 38% in children who had been in the PICU for more than 5 days [39]. Higher delirium rates have also been reported in cardiac (49–57%) and postsurgical (65%) pediatric critical care units [40–42].

Outcomes

Similar to findings in the adult population, pediatric delirium has been independently associated with substantial short-term morbidity. Delirious children can be more difficult to wean from invasive mechanical ventilation (median 4 vs 1 day; $p < 0.001$) [1]. They also have longer stays in the intensive care unit and in the hospital. In one study, after controlling for severity of illness on admission and need for mechanical ventilation, the adjusted relative length of stay (LOS) was more than doubled [odds ratio (OR) 2.3, CI 2.1–2.5] in delirious patients [1]. In a cardiac ICU cohort, delirium was an independent predictor of prolonged ICU LOS, with patients who were ever delirious having a 60% increase in ICU days compared to patients who were never delirious ($p < 0.01$) [40]. Pediatric delirium also has a significant impact on costs of care and resource utilization. Hospital charges associated with pediatric delirium in the United States can exceed 500 million dollars per year. A delirious day in the PICU costs 23% more than a delirium-free day [5].

A more significant and alarming finding may be that despite controlling for underlying severity of illness, delirium in critically ill children has been strongly and independently associated with in-hospital mortality with an adjusted OR of 4.4 ($p < 0.001$) [1]. Interestingly, in this particular cohort, delirium was a stronger predictor of mortality than the well-validated Pediatric Index of Mortality 3 (PIM-3) score (OR 3.2 for patients in the highest tertile). While this is merely an association and not indicative of causality, it is consistent with adult studies where delirium is now part of prognostic scores [43]. Increased awareness is needed as pediatric delirium may be an important means of identifying patients who are at risk for worse in-hospital outcomes.

Further research is needed to investigate the long-term effects of delirium on cognitive outcomes in children after discharge as well as possible impact on psychological and emotional health. In a pilot study of 47 patients who developed delirium postsurgically, no significant long-term impact on global cognition, executive functions, or behavior was seen at 2 years after discharge from the PICU [44]. This is the first study published of this nature with several important limitations. Further prospective investigations that take into account baseline cognition and which better limit biases are needed.

Risk Factors

Multiple risk factors have been associated with delirium in critically ill adults, such as elderly age, dementia, hypertension, high severity-of-illness score on admission, alcoholism, and cigarette use. Depth of sedation, exposure to benzodiazepines, and use of physical restraints are also known hospital-acquired risk factors [12]. In delirious children, similar susceptibilities have been described. It is helpful to divide the risk factors for pediatric delirium into two distinct categories: predisposing (non-modifiable) factors and precipitating (modifiable) factors (Fig. 20.1). This distinction is important to understand since avoidance of precipitating factors, particularly in high-risk subgroups, may help us decrease the incidence of delirium in children.

Predisposing Factors

Most studies demonstrate that preschool-aged children (<5 years old) are at higher risk for developing delirium, as are children with underlying neurodevelopmental disabilities [1, 2, 39, 40]. Developing and abnormal brains, respectively, may be more vulnerable to delirium in a way analogous to adults with dementia, a well-known, high-risk group in adult critical care.

Delirium rates are also higher in children who require invasive mechanical ventilation [1, 2, 39]. This could be related to the need for sedatives in this subpopulation, a potential modifiable risk factor as clinicians can choose which drugs to use and how deeply sedated they want their patient to be [2]. Finally, children with a

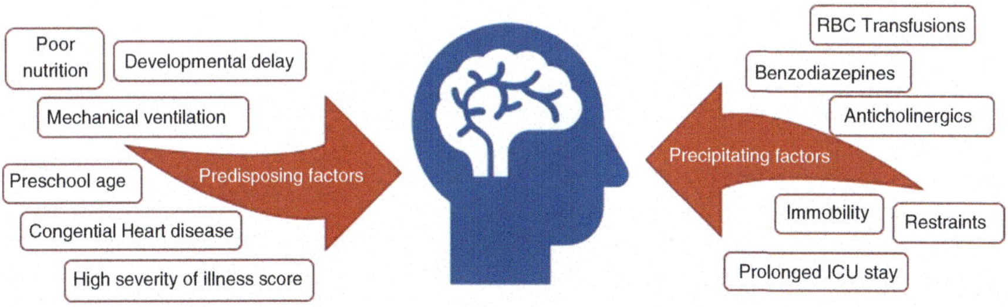

Fig. 20.1 Delirium in critically ill children is often multifactorial, with a complex interplay of predisposing and precipitating factors

higher severity-of-illness score on admission are also more likely to develop delirium, even after controlling for multiple variables [1, 40, 42, 45].

The congenital heart disease subpopulation has also been found to represent a particularly high-risk group. Chiefly, the exposure to cardiopulmonary bypass, which is itself characterized by the initiation of a significant inflammatory response, is a strong risk factor for development of delirium. Longer bypass time and increasingly complex surgical repairs are independently associated with delirium incidence. Children with cyanotic congenital lesions as well as those with poor nutritional status preoperatively may also be at increased risk for developing delirium; this is consistent with the previously discussed oxidative stress and metabolic etiologic pathways [40, 41].

Precipitating Factors

With the recent boom in pediatric delirium research, several potentially modifiable risk factors for delirium have been identified. Most significantly, the use of benzodiazepine-based sedation has been strongly linked to delirium in critically ill children [1, 39–41, 45–48]. In a prospective, observational study using multivariable analysis that included 1547 children, patients exposed to benzodiazepines had a five-fold increased risk of delirium (CI 3.7–7.5) [1]. Because the relationship between use of opiates, use of sedatives such as benzodiazepines, mechanical ventilation, and delirium poses an intricate web of potential confounders, a systematic, longitudinal assessment was needed to establish a causal effect. This was achieved in a subsequent

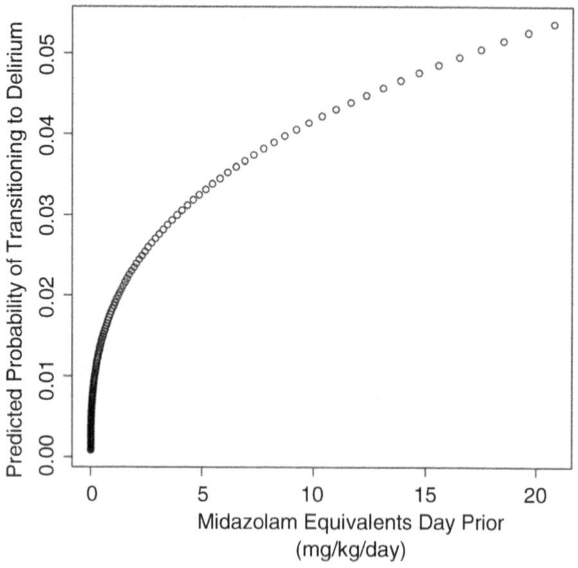

Fig. 20.2 Children with normal cognitive status who received benzodiazepines had an adjusted odds ratio of 3.3 for developing delirium, with a clear dose–response relationship demonstrating a biological gradient. (Reproduced with permission from: Mody et al. [46])

study using marginal structural modeling to control for time-dependent variables. In that study, benzodiazepines were strongly associated with transition from normal cognitive status to delirium, with an odds ratio of 3.3 (CI 1.4–7.8), after controlling for cognitive status, mechanical ventilation, and opiates. In addition, a dose-response effect was described with 43% increase in risk for subsequent delirium with every one-log increase in benzodiazepine exposure ($p < 0.001$) (Fig. 20.2) [46].

Immobilization and use of physical restraints represent another potentially modifiable risk factor for pediatric delirium. An international point-prevalence study showed that the odds of delirium were four times higher for patients who were physically restrained. This is consistent with data in adults; however, it is possible that children were restrained after developing delirium, as temporality could not be assessed in this study due to its design [39].

Another interesting, recent finding was an association between red blood cell (RBC) transfusions and development of delirium. In a nested cohort study, children who were transfused RBCs were more than twice as likely to be delirious during their admission compared with children who were never transfused, after controlling for other known predictors of delirium development (adjusted OR 2.16; 95% CI 1.38–3.37; $p = 0.001$) [49].

Diagnosis

Conventionally, pediatric intensivists had to depend on psychiatrists to perform a comprehensive interview and exam before establishing the diagnosis of delirium. This likely led to a significant under-recognition of delirium as psychiatrists were only consulted in the most extreme or disruptive cases [50]. The increasing awareness of delirium as a significant health problem in critical care has highlighted the need for well-validated bedside screening tools in the pediatric population [51].

Two types of validated pediatric delirium screening tools are currently available and they both require that the patient be arousable to verbal stimuli for their administration. The pediatric and preschool versions of the Confusion Assessment Method for the ICU (pCAM-ICU and psCAM-ICU, respectively) are point-in-time, interactive tools designed to assess for delirium in the moment the test is being administered. The pCAM-ICU is designed for patients older than 5 years, and the psCAM-ICU is designed for children aged 6 months to 5 years [52, 53]. They are both scored as "delirium present" or "delirium absent." The Cornell Assessment for Pediatric Delirium (CAPD) is a strictly observational tool that provides a longitudinal picture of a pediatric patient over the course of a nursing shift (Fig. 20.3). It can be used in children of all ages, developmental stages and cognitive abilities. A score of 9 or higher is consistent with a delirium diagnosis. By trending the CAPD score over time, a child's delirium trajectory can be established as can their response to interventions [54]. Studies from various institutions have demonstrated that use of the CAPD is both feasible and reliable in units across different nations with varying cultures and practices [39, 55–57]. Furthermore, the European Society of Pediatric

Please answer the following questions based on your interactions with the patient over the course of your shift:						
	Never 4	Rarely 3	Sometimes 2	Often 1	Always 0	Score
1. Does the child make eye contact with the caregiver?						
2. Are the child's actions purposeful?						
3. Is the child aware of his/her surroundings?						
4. Does the child communicate needs and wants?						
	Never 0	Rarely 1	Sometimes 2	Often 3	Always 4	
5. Is the child restless?						
6. Is the child inconsolable?						
7. Is the child underactive—very little movement while awake?						
8. Does it take the child a long time to respond to interactions?						
					TOTAL	

Fig. 20.3 Cornell Assessment of Pediatric Delirium, a valid and reliable observational screening tool designed for use in critically ill children. A score of 9 or higher is consistent with a diagnosis of delirium. (Reproduced with permission from: Traube et al. [54])

and Neonatal Intensive Care has released clinical practice guidelines calling for use of the CAPD as standard of care to screen all critically ill children for delirium (Grade A level recommendation) [11]. Both tools, however, have been shown to have a high sensitivity and specificity from delirium identification in critically ill children.

Treatment

It is important to remember that delirium in itself is not a psychiatric condition, but rather acute cerebral dysfunction in response to certain triggers. Clinically, delirium can be thought of as a product of the interplay between the underlying disease, iatrogenic effects of treatment, and the ICU environment. Management should be focused, in a stepwise fashion, on addressing these three factors.

Underlying Disease

A positive delirium screen should prompt the ICU team to assess the patient with a comprehensive physical exam, and perform laboratory studies and imaging as clinically indicated. Specific questions the clinician should ask include the following. Is the patient hypoxic? Is there concern for a new infectious process (delirium may precede fever in these scenarios)? Is there evolving new organ dysfunction leading to metabolic disturbances? Additionally, alteration in mental status should not be attributed to delirium automatically, but should prompt a careful neurological examination to rule out a new primary central nervous system (CNS) disease [58].

Iatrogenic Factors

After assessing for a new or worsening underlying disease process, focus should shift toward identification and management of the multiple modifiable factors associated with delirium. Inadequate pain control, which includes both under- and over-treatment, should be remedied. Sedation should be minimized as much as clinically appropriate, particularly limiting the exposure to benzodiazepines [10, 46]. The patient's medication list should be reviewed sensibly for other potential deliriogenic drugs such as anticholinergics and steroids, which should also be discontinued when feasible [2, 10, 58]. Opioid and benzodiazepine withdrawal can also precipitate delirium. Clinicians should aim to prevent withdrawal using appropriate weaning strategies. However, prompt identification and management is required if it still develops. Many of the physiologic signs of abstinence overlap with symptoms of hyperactive delirium [59, 60]. Opiates should be replaced judiciously, but not excessively, as inappropriately escalating the opioid dose may just prolong the delirium [2]. Environmental modifications and even pharmacological management may be required for a hyperactive delirium that was triggered by withdrawal.

Environment

Optimization of the patients' environment in the ICU is integral to both treatment and prevention of delirium [61]. Simple interventions such as use of the patient's eyeglasses or hearing aids, repeated reorientation to the surroundings and personnel, noise reduction, bringing favorite items from home, and keeping a daily schedule are feasible and should be encouraged. Cares should be clustered and preferably done during the daytime as much as possible [2, 39, 58]. Close attention should be paid to minimizing disruption of sleep and promotion of normal circadian rhythms. Lights should be off at nighttime (preferably at a time close to the child's established bedtime) and bedside interruptions should be minimized [62].

During the daytime, the patient's room should remain well-lit and a routine that includes both cognitive and physical activity ought to be followed as much as the clinical situation allows. In adult ICUs, early mobilization has been shown to improve functional outcome and reduce delirium [63]. A recently published quality-improvement intervention demonstrated that implementation of a structured early mobilization program in the PICU was achievable without adverse events even in neonates and children who were mechanically ventilated [64]. Another single-center PICU study demonstrated a decrease in delirium rates with implementation of an early mobilization program [56]. Further large-scale research is needed to replicate this finding and investigate the effectiveness of early mobilization on decreasing pediatric delirium rates.

Pharmacological Intervention

The vast majority of cases of pediatric delirium improve with the above stated interventions. However, in severe or persistent cases of delirium, pharmacological therapy may be indicated. There are currently no medications approved by the United States Food and Drug Administration (FDA) to treat delirium in either adults or children; therefore, all therapies are off-label [10]. In children, case series describe the use of atypical antipsychotics for treatment of pediatric delirium. This drug class has a favorable side effect profile and may be related to an overall improvement in cognition [10, 65, 66]. When starting antipsychotics, one should monitor for extrapyramidal symptoms, QT prolongation and dysrhythmias [66]. A single-site retrospective review of the short-term use of quetiapine to treat delirium in 50 critically ill children showed that it was safe with no serious, adverse events reported [67]. Limited data exist regarding use of either haloperidol or other atypical antipsychotics including risperidone in critically ill children [4] although due to side effects, use of haloperidol is increasingly discouraged. Further prospective, randomized, placebo-controlled trials are necessary to better understand efficacy and superiority of available options.

Prevention

Traditionally, an admission to the critical care unit, particularly if mechanical-ventilation was required, was accompanied by sedation, immobility, and an environment surrounded by the noisy beeping of machinery and lights throughout day and night. For children, parental time at the bedside might have been limited to specific visiting hours. Fortunately, it is now well understood that this approach to patient care is suboptimal and may, in fact, be harmful. Consequently, and appropriately, there has been a shift in culture toward environments that are less disruptive [38, 56, 68]. The first step toward culture change is recognizing that delirium prevention is

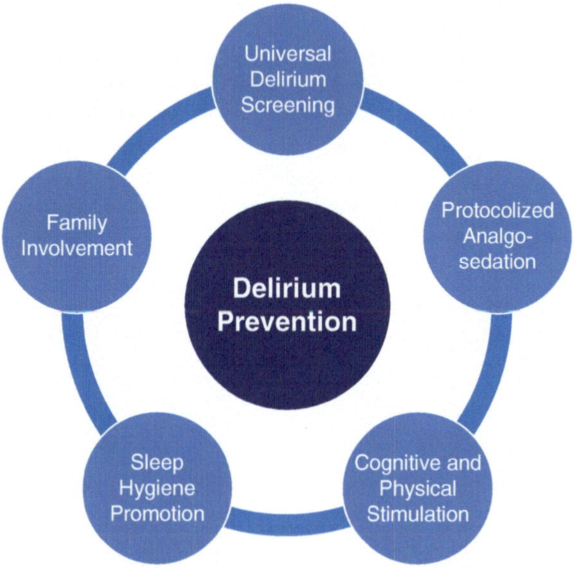

Fig. 20.4 A multidisciplinary approach can decrease delirium rates in the pediatric intensive care unit

a multidisciplinary endeavor that involves unit-wide education of nurses, physicians, pharmacists, house staff, physical and occupational therapists, respiratory therapists, and child-life specialists [10]. Universal delirium screening, protocols aimed at minimizing sedation, sleep hygiene, and early mobilization programs are being adopted as routine care (Fig. 20.4) [68].

The SCCM has endorsed an "analgo-sedation" approach in adult ICUs that is also gaining traction in the pediatric community [10]. Many mechanically ventilated patients do not need sedation as first-line therapy and would benefit from an analgesic-driven approach. More alert patients can communicate their pain better which leads to better pain control. Being less sedated also facilitates participation in early mobilization. Decreased exposure to sedatives, particularly benzodiazepines, reduces the risk of iatrogenic delirium. When sedation is required, consideration should be given to using alternatives to benzodiazepines. A randomized controlled trial by Pandharipande and colleagues found that in mechanically ventilated adult ICU patients, the use of a dexmedetomidine infusion (rather than a benzodiazepine infusion) resulted in more days alive without delirium or coma and more time at the targeted level of sedation [69]. This is biologically plausible, as benzodiazepines have high affinity for $GABA_A$ receptors, and activation of these receptors can alter levels of numerous neurotransmitters believed to be deliriogenic. Benzodiazepines also suppress slow-wave sleep thus affecting the quality of sleep [70–72]. Dexmedetomidine, however, acts at the level of the locus ceruleus, with a different neurotransmitter profile and preserves slow-wave (deep nonrapid eye movement) sleep in its neuronal pathway [73, 74].

Prevention of delirium in at-risk children is achievable if we follow a step-wise approach geared toward: (1) enhanced awareness and screening for pediatric delirium, (2) implementation of a protocolized analgo-sedation approach, (3) incorporation of early mobilization, (4) promotion of sleep hygiene, and (5) involvement of family members in daily care. For example, a single-center prospective PICU study demonstrated a reduction in monthly delirium prevalence after systematic introduction of three bundles of care (routine delirium screening, protocolized analgo-sedation, and early mobilization) over a 22-month period. Before implementation of this quality-improvement initiative, this unit did not screen for delirium, yet they were able to document feasibility, sustainability (compliance >95% with screening after 22 months), and effectiveness of their interventions, reporting a 39% decrease in their delirium rates throughout the course of the project [56]. In addition, a recently published case series has described the feasibility and utility of operationalizing family members as part of a PICU's delirium prevention program [75].

Conclusions

Delirium is a frequent complication of pediatric critical illness that is associated with significant short-term morbidity and mortality. Universal screening for delirium has proven to be feasible and necessary, as early recognition leads to identification of potential triggers and prompt interventions that may decrease the burden of delirium. Benzodiazepines have been strongly associated with development of delirium in children, with a dose–response effect. Adopting an analgo-sedation approach may help decrease exposure to sedatives, and consequently reduce risk of delirium. Further studies are needed to assess the long-term effects of pediatric delirium and establish best practices for treatment and prevention of delirium in critically ill children.

References

1. Traube C, Silver G, Gerber LM, Kaur S, Mauer EA, Kerson A, et al. Delirium and mortality in critically ill children: epidemiology and outcomes of pediatric delirium. Crit Care Med. 2017;45(5):891–8.
2. Silver G, Traube C, Gerber LM, Sun X, Kearney J, Patel A, et al. Pediatric delirium and associated risk factors: a single-center prospective observational study*. Pediatr Crit Care Med. 2015;16(4):303–9.
3. Turkel SB, Tavare CJ. Delirium in children and adolescents. J Neuropsychiatry Clin Neurosci. 2003;15(4):431–5.
4. Schieveld JNM, Leroy PLJM, Os J, Nicolai J, Vos GD, Leentjens AFG. Pediatric delirium in critical illness: phenomenology, clinical correlates and treatment response in 40 cases in the pediatric intensive care unit. Intensive Care Med. 2007;33(6):1033–40.
5. Traube C, Mauer EA, Gerber LM, Kaur S, Joyce C, Kerson A, et al. Cost associated with pediatric delirium in the ICU. Crit Care Med. 2016;44(12):e1175–9.
6. American Psychiatric Association: Diagnostic and Statistical Manual of Mental Disorders: Diagnostic and Statistical Manual of Mental Disorders, Fifth Edition. Arlington, VA: American Psychiatric Association, 2013.

7. Patel AK, Bell MJ, Traube C. Delirium in pediatric critical care. Pediatr Clin N Am. 2017;64(5):1117–32.
8. Zaal IJ, Devlin JW, Peelen LM, Slooter AJ. A systematic review of risk factors for delirium in the ICU. Crit Care Med. 2015;43:40–7.
9. Silver G, Traube C, Kearney J, Kelly D, Yoon MJ, Nash Moyal W, et al. Detecting pediatric delirium: development of a rapid observational assessment tool. Intensive Care Med. 2012;38(6):1025–31.
10. Barr J, Fraser GL, Puntillo K, Ely EW, Gélinas C, Dasta JF, et al. Clinical practice guidelines for the management of pain, agitation, and delirium in adult patients in the intensive care unit. Crit Care Med. 2013;41(1):278–80.
11. Harris J, Ramelet A-S, van Dijk M, et al. Clinical recommendations for pain, sedation, withdrawal and delirium assessment in critically ill infants and children: an ESPNIC position statement for healthcare professionals. Intensive Care Med. 2016;42:972–86.
12. Maldonado JR. Acute brain failure: pathophysiology, diagnosis, management, and sequelae of delirium. Crit Care Clin. 2017;33(3):461–519.
13. Smith HAB, Fuchs DC, Pandharipande PP, Barr FE, Ely EW. Delirium: an emerging frontier in the management of critically ill Children. Anesthesiol Clin. 2011;29(4):729–50.
14. Peterson JF, Pun BT, Dittus RS, Thomason JWW, Jackson JC, Shintani AK, et al. Delirium and its motoric subtypes: a study of 614 critically ill patients: delirium subtypes in the critically ill. J Am Geriatr Soc. 2006;54(3):479–84.
15. Jabbar F, Leonard M, Meehan K, et al. Neuropsychiatric and cognitive profile of patients with DSM-IV delirium referred to an old age psychiatry consultation-liaison service. Int Psychogeriatr. 2011;23(7):1167–74.
16. Calandriello A, Tylka J, Patwari P. Sleep and delirium in pediatric critical illness: what is the relationship? Med Sci. 2018;6(4):90.
17. Maldonado JR. Neuropathogenesis of delirium: review of current etiologic theories and common pathways. Am J Geriatr Psychiatry. 2013;21:1190–222.
18. Cerejeira J, Firmino H, Vaz-Serra A, et al. The neuroinflammatory hypothesis of delirium. Acta Neuropathol. 2010;119:737–54.
19. Van Munster BC, Korevaar JC, Korse CM, Bonfrer JM, Zwinderman AH, de Rooij SE. Serum S100B in elderly patients with and without delirium. Int J Geriatr Psychiatry. 2010;25(3):234–9.
20. De Rooij SE, van Munster BC, Korevaar JC, Levi M. Cytokines and acute phase response in delirium. J Psychosom Res. 2007;62(5):521–5.
21. McGrane S, Girard TD, Thompson JL, Shintani AK, Woodworth A, Ely EW, et al. Procalcitonin and C-reactive protein levels at admission as predictors of duration of acute brain dysfunction in critically ill patients. Crit Care. 2011;15(2):R78.
22. Poljak A, Hill M, Hall RJ, et al. Quantitative proteomics of delirium cerebrospinal fluid. Transl Psychiatry. 2014;4(11):e477.
23. Engel GL, Romano J. Delirium, a syndrome of cerebral insufficiency. J Chronic Dis. 1959;9(3):260–77. 531–2
24. Somjen GG, Aitken PG, Balestrino M, Herreras O, Kawasaki K. Spreading depression-like depolarization and selective vulnerability of neurons. A brief review. Stroke. 1990;21(11 Suppl):III179–83.
25. Globus MY, Busto R, Dietrich WD, Martinez E, Valdes I, Ginsberg MD. Effect of ischemia on the in vivo release of striatal dopamine, glutamate, and gamma-aminobutyric acid studied by intracerebral microdialysis. J Neurochem. 1988;51(5):1455–64.
26. Busto R, Globus MY, Dietrich WD, Martinez E, Valdes I, Ginsberg MD. Effect of mild hypothermia on ischemia-induced release of neurotransmitters and free fatty acids in rat brain. Stroke. 1989;20(7):904–10.
27. Globus MY, Alonso O, Dietrich WD, Busto R, Ginsberg MD. Glutamate release and free radical production following brain injury: effects of posttraumatic hypothermia. J Neurochem. 1995;65(4):1704–11.
28. Seaman J, Carroll D, Brown T. Impaired oxidative metabolism precipitates delirium: a study of 101 ICU patients. Psychosomatics. 2006;47(1):56–61.

29. Schoen J, Meyerrose J, Paarmann H, Heringlake M, Hueppe M, Berger K-U. Preoperative regional cerebral oxygen saturation is a predictor of postoperative delirium in on-pump cardiac surgery patients: a prospective observational trial. Crit Care. 2011;15(5):R218.
30. Flacker JM, Cummings V, Mzach JR, Bettin K, Kiely DK, Wei J. The association of serum anticholinergic activity with delirium in elderly medical patients. Am J Geriatr Psychiatry. 1999;6(1):31–41.
31. Tune LE. Serum anticholinergic activity levels and delirium in the elderly. Semin Clin Neuropsychiatry. 2000;5(2):149–53.
32. Trzepacz PT, Leavitt M, Ciongoli K. An animal model for delirium. Psychosomatics. 1992;33:404e415.
33. Trzepacz PT. Is there a final common neural pathway in delirium? Focus on acetylcholine and dopamine. Semin Clin Neuropsychiatry. 2000;5:132–48.
34. Hshieh TT, Fong TG, Marcantonio ER, et al. Cholinergic deficiency hypothesis in delirium: a synthesis of current evidence. J Gerontol A Biol Sci Med Sci. 2008;63:764–72.
35. Milbrandt EB, Deppen S, Harrison PL, et al. Costs associated with delirium in mechanically ventilated patients. Crit Care Med. 2004;32:955–62.
36. McNicoll L, Pisani MA, Zhang Y, et al. Delirium in the intensive care unit: occurrence and clinical course in older patients. J Am Geriatr Soc. 2003;51:591–8.
37. Ouimet S, Kavanagh BP, Gottfried SB, et al. Incidence, risk factors and consequences of ICU delirium. Intensive Care Med. 2006;33(1):66–73.
38. Schieveld JN, Janssen NJ. Delirium in the pediatric patient: on the growing awareness of its clinical interdisciplinary importance. JAMA Pediatr. 2014;168:595–6.
39. Traube C, Silver G, Reeder RW, et al. Delirium in critically ill children: an international point prevalence study. Crit Care Med. 2017;45:584–90.
40. Patel AK, Biagas KV, Clarke EC, Gerber LM, Mauer E, Silver G, et al. Delirium in children after cardiac bypass surgery. Pediatr Crit Care Med. 2017;18(2):165–71.
41. Alvarez RV, Palmer C, Czaja AS, Peyton C, Silver G, Traube C, et al. Delirium is a common and early finding in patients in the pediatric cardiac intensive care unit. J Pediatr. 2018;195:206–12.
42. Meyburg J, Dill M-L, Traube C, Silver G, Von Haken R. Patterns of postoperative delirium in children. Pediatr Crit Care Med. 2017;18(2):128–33.
43. Scarpi E, Maltoni M, Miceli R, et al. Survival prediction for terminally ill cancer patients: revision of the palliative prognostic score with incorporation of delirium. Oncologist. 2011;16(12):1793–9.
44. Meyburg J, Ries M, Zielonka M, Koch K, Sander A, von Haken R, Reuner G. Cognitive and behavioral consequences of pediatric delirium. Pediatr Crit Care Med. 2018;19:e531–7.
45. Schieveld JNM, Lousberg R, Berghmans E, Smeets I, Leroy PLJM, Vos GD, et al. Pediatric illness severity measures predict delirium in a pediatric intensive care unit. Crit Care Med. 2008;36(6):1933–6.
46. Modi K, Kaur S, Mauer E, Gerber L, Greenwald B, Silver G, et al. Benzodiazepines and development of delirium in critically ill children: estimating the causal effect. Crit Care Med. 2018;46:1486–91.
47. Traube C, Ariagno S, Thau F, Rosenberg L, Mauer EA, Gerber LM, et al. Delirium in hospitalized children with Cancer: incidence and associated risk factors. J Pediatr. 2017;191:212–7.
48. Smith HAB, Gangopadhyay M, Goben CM, Jacobowski NL, Chestnut MH, Thompson JL, et al. Delirium and benzodiazepines associated with prolonged ICU stay in critically ill infants and young children. Crit Care Med. 2017;45(9):1427–35.
49. Nellis ME, Goel R, Feinstein S, Shahbaz S, Kaur S, Traube C. Association between transfusion of RBCs and subsequent development of delirium in critically ill children. Pediatr Crit Care Med. 2018;19(10):925–9.
50. Ely EW, Siegel MD, Inouye SK. Delirium in the intensive care unit: an underrecognized syndrome of organ dysfunction. Semin Respir Crit Care Med. 2002;22(02):115–26.

51. Silver G, Kearney J, Traube C, et al. Delirium screening anchored in child development: the Cornell assessment for pediatric delirium. Palliat Support Care. 2015;13(4):1005–11.
52. Smith HAB, Gangopadhyay M, Goben CM, Jacobowski NL, Chestnut MH, Savage S, et al. The preschool confusion assessment method for the ICU: valid and reliable delirium monitoring for critically ill infants and children. Crit Care Med. 2015;1
53. Smith HAB, Boyd J, Fuchs DC, Melvin K, Berry P, Shintani A, et al. Diagnosing delirium in critically ill children: validity and reliability of the pediatric confusion assessment method for the intensive care unit. Crit Care Med. 2011;39(1):150–7.
54. Traube C, Silver G, Kearney J, Patel A, Atkinson TM, Yoon MJ, et al. Cornell assessment of pediatric delirium: a valid, rapid, observational tool for screening delirium in the PICU. Crit Care Med. 2014;42(3):656–63.
55. Meyburg J, Dill M-L, von Haken R, Picardi S, Westhoff JH, Silver G, et al. Risk factors for the development of postoperative delirium in pediatric intensive care patients. Pediatr Crit Care Med. 2018;19(10):e514–21.
56. Simone S, Edwards S, Lardieri A, Walker LK, Graciano AL, Kishk OA, et al. Implementation of an ICU bundle: an interprofessional quality improvement project to enhance delirium management and monitor delirium prevalence in a single PICU. Pediatr Crit Care Med. 2017;18(6):531–40.
57. Valdivia HR, Carlin KE. Determining interrater reliability of the Cornell assessment of pediatric delirium screening tool among PICU nurses. Pediatr Crit Care Med. 2019;5, e216-e220. https://doi.org/10.1097/PCC.0000000000001896.
58. Smith HAB, Brink E, Fuchs DC, Ely EW, Pandharipande PP. Pediatric delirium: monitoring and management in the pediatric intensive care unit. Crit Care Pediatr Patient. 2013;60(3): 741–60.
59. Franck LS, Harris SK, Soetenga DJ, Amling JK, Curley MA. The Withdrawal Assessment Tool-1 (WAT-1): an assessment instrument for monitoring opioid and benzodiazepine withdrawal symptoms in pediatric patients. Pediatr Crit Care Med. 2008;9(6):573–80.
60. Traube C, Greenwald B. Iatrogenic withdrawal syndrome, or undiagnosed delirium? Crit Care Med. 2017;45(6):e622–3.
61. Hshieh TT, Yue J, Oh E, et al. Effectiveness of multicomponent nonpharmacological delirium interventions: a meta-analysis. JAMA Intern Med. 2015;175(4):512.
62. Kudchadkar SR, Yaster M, Punjabi NM. Sedation, sleep promotion, and delirium screening practices in the care of mechanically ventilated children: a wake-up call for the pediatric critical care community. Crit Care Med. 2014;42(7):1592–600.
63. Schweickert WD, Pohlman MC, Pohlman AS, et al. Early physical and occupational therapy in mechanically ventilated, critically ill patients: a randomised controlled trial. Lancet. 2009;373(9678):1874–82.
64. Wieczorek B, Ascenzi J, Kim Y, et al. PICU up!: impact of a quality improvement intervention to promote early mobilization in critically ill children. Pediatr Crit Care Med. 2016;17(12):e559–66.
65. Silver GH, Kearney JA, Kutko MC, Bartell AS. Infant delirium in pediatric critical care settings. Am J Psychiatry. 2010;167(10):1172–7.
66. Turkel SB, Jacobson J, Munzig E, et al. Atypical antipsychotic medications to control symptoms of delirium in children and adolescents. J Child Adolesc Psychopharmacol. 2012;22(2):126–30.
67. Joyce C, Witcher R, Herrup E, et al. Evaluation of the safety of quetiapine in treating delirium in critically ill children: a retrospective review. J Child Adolesc Psychopharmacol. 2015;25(9):666–70.
68. Traube C, Greenwald BM. "The times they are A-Changin": universal delirium screening in pediatric critical care. Pediatr Crit Care Med. 2017;18(6):594–5.
69. Pandharipande PP, Pun BT, Herr DL, et al. Effect of sedation with dexmedetomidine vs lorazepam on acute brain dysfunction in mechanically ventilated patients: the MENDS randomized controlled trial. JAMA. 2007;298:2644–53.

70. Mihic SJ, Harris RA. GABA and the GABAA receptor. Alcohol Health Res World. 1997;21(2):127–31.
71. van der Mast RC. Delirium: the underlying pathophysiological mechanisms and the need for clinical research. J Psychosom Res. 1996;41(2):109–13.
72. van der Mast RC. Pathophysiology of delirium. J Geriatr Psychiatry Neurol. 1998;11(3):138–45.
73. Pandharipande P, Ely EW. Sedative and analgesic medications: risk factors for delirium and sleep disturbances in the critically ill. Crit Care Clin. 2006;22(2):313.
74. Nelson LE, Lu J, Guo T, Saper CB, Franks NP, Maze M. The α_2-adrenoceptor agonist dexmedetomidine converges on an endogenous sleep-promoting pathway to exert its sedative effects. Anesthesiology. 2003;98(2):428–36.
75. Silver G, Traube C. A systematic approach to family engagement: feasibility pilot of a pediatric delirium management and prevention toolkit. Palliat Support Care. 2019;17(1):42–5.

Chapter 21
Mobility in the PICU

Kristina A. Betters and Sapna R. Kudchadkar

The Consequences of Critical Illness

With the advancements in medicine, science, and technology, the landscape of pediatric intensive care is rapidly changing. Over the past several decades, mortality in the pediatric intensive care unit (PICU) has continued to decline [1, 2]. A large cohort study of over 4000 PICU patients that compared mortality in the years 1982, 1995, and 2005–2006 showed that, despite the similar acuity of illness and length of stay, mortality decreased from 11% in 1982 to approximately 5% in 2005–2006 [1]. In a more recent study of five US teaching hospital PICUs, the 2010 mortality rates were even lower, at an average of 2.4% [2]. With such a decline in the mortality rates, PICU clinicians must and are shifting focus from survival to morbidity and quality of life after critical illness.

An unfortunate potential consequence of improved survival from critical illness is the development of new or worsening comorbidities. In the last decade, research has further characterized the impairments experienced by adult ICU survivors as post-intensive care syndrome (PICS). PICS refers to the combination of physical, cognitive, and psychiatric deficits experienced by many ICU survivors [3–5]. Studies of adult patients have shown that more than 25% of ICU survivors experience physical disability [6], 25–75% experience cognitive deficits, and up to 62% experience psychiatric illness [6].

K. A. Betters
Department of Pediatrics; Division of Critical Care Medicine,
Vanderbilt Univerisity, Nashville, TN, USA
e-mail: kristina.betters@vanderbilt.edu

S. R. Kudchadkar (✉)
Departments of Anesthesiology and Critical Care Medicine; Pediatrics; Physical Medicine and Rehabilitation, Johns Hopkins University School of Medicine, Baltimore, MD, USA
e-mail: sapna@jhmi.edu

P. P. Kamat, J. W. Berkenbosch (eds.), *Sedation and Analgesia for the Pediatric Intensivist*, https://doi.org/10.1007/978-3-030-52555-2_21

Although the diagnosis of PICS has not been studied in children as it has been in adults, emerging data suggest that children who survive the ICU are at a similar risk of experiencing PICS [1, 7–17]. In a systematic review of outcomes of PICU survivors, Herrup and colleagues analyzed 19 different pediatric studies and found that children who survive critical illness also suffer from physical, neurocognitive, and psychological morbidities [7]. A lack of standardized assessments and tools for pediatric patients makes it difficult to ascertain the true incidence of such deficits post-PICU stay. However, large multicenter studies have established the deleterious effects of an ICU stay on pediatric patients by using validated scales, such as the Functional Status Scale (FSS), Pediatric Overall Performance Category (POPC) scale, Pediatric Cerebral Performance Category (PCPC) scale, Pediatric Evaluation of Disabilities Inventory Computer Adaptive Test (PEDI-CAT), and others [9, 11–14, 16]. Even more concerning is that many of these studies have shown that children with underlying disabilities have significant exacerbations after a PICU admission [9, 13, 16], and regardless of the baseline status, many patients have long-standing deficits months after their PICU discharge [11, 16].

Even before PICS was acknowledged as an important diagnostic consideration, physical deficits after an ICU stay were long described in adult patients [18–20]. More recently, pediatric data have shown similar findings of ICU-acquired weakness in children [21–25] and raised concerns that such sequelae are under-recognized and under-diagnosed in the pediatric population [26]. Serial bedside ultrasound and electrical impedance myography in 34 PICU patients receiving mechanical ventilation showed that diaphragm and quadriceps thickness decreased by an average of 2% and 1% per day, respectively [23]. About 83% of study patients had documented atrophy (defined as ≥10% decrease in thickness) in at least one muscle group, and 47% in at least two or more muscle groups [23]. Retrospective cohort studies have shown much lower frequencies of ICU-acquired weakness in children, although these results are likely influenced by under-recognition and underreporting [22, 26, 27]. In a large retrospective database study of over 200,000 PICU admissions from 2009 to 2013, a documented diagnosis of critical illness myopathy was rare (0.02%) and, after controlling for severity of illness, was associated with respiratory illness and infection, mechanical ventilation requirement, renal replacement therapy, extracorporeal life support, and tracheostomy [27]. Regardless of the low incidence of reporting, a diagnosis of critical illness myopathy was associated with worse outcomes, including longer PICU length of stay, higher number of ICU admissions requiring mechanical ventilation, tracheostomy placement, and discharge to an intermediate, chronic care, or rehabilitation care unit [27].

Other pediatric studies that used validated clinical scales have shown that motor and mobility deficits are the leading causes of disability in PICU survivors [11, 13, 16]. Choong and colleagues found that mobility domain deficits were the leading baseline functional deficit upon PICU admission, with 39% of patients being below 2 standard deviations for age [16]. On PICU discharge and at 3 months post-discharge, mobility continued to be a leading disability, illustrating that a PICU stay can exacerbate baseline mobility issues and lead to new motor morbidities [16]. Similar trends were observed in a large cohort study that used the FSS to characterize new morbidities of PICU patients [10]. In patients with new morbidities and FSS domain increases of 2 or more, motor domain deficits were the second highest new morbidity [10].

In an effort to ameliorate the harmful patient effects and prolonged consequences of an ICU stay, the Society of Critical Care Medicine created the ICU Liberation initiative [28]. Using critical care evidence, mostly derived from adult studies, the ABCDEF bundle was created to empower multidisciplinary providers to facilitate improvement in patient outcomes [29, 30]. The ABCDEF bundle specifically refers to the following six components: *A*ssess, prevent, and manage pain; *B*oth spontaneous awakening and spontaneous breathing trials; *C*hoice of analgesia and sedation; *D*elirium assessment, prevention, and management; *E*arly mobility and exercise; and *F*amily engagement and empowerment [29, 30]. In a landmark study of over 15,000 adults in 68 different ICUs, increased bundle compliance was associated with improvements in survival, mechanical ventilation use, coma, delirium, ICU readmissions, and

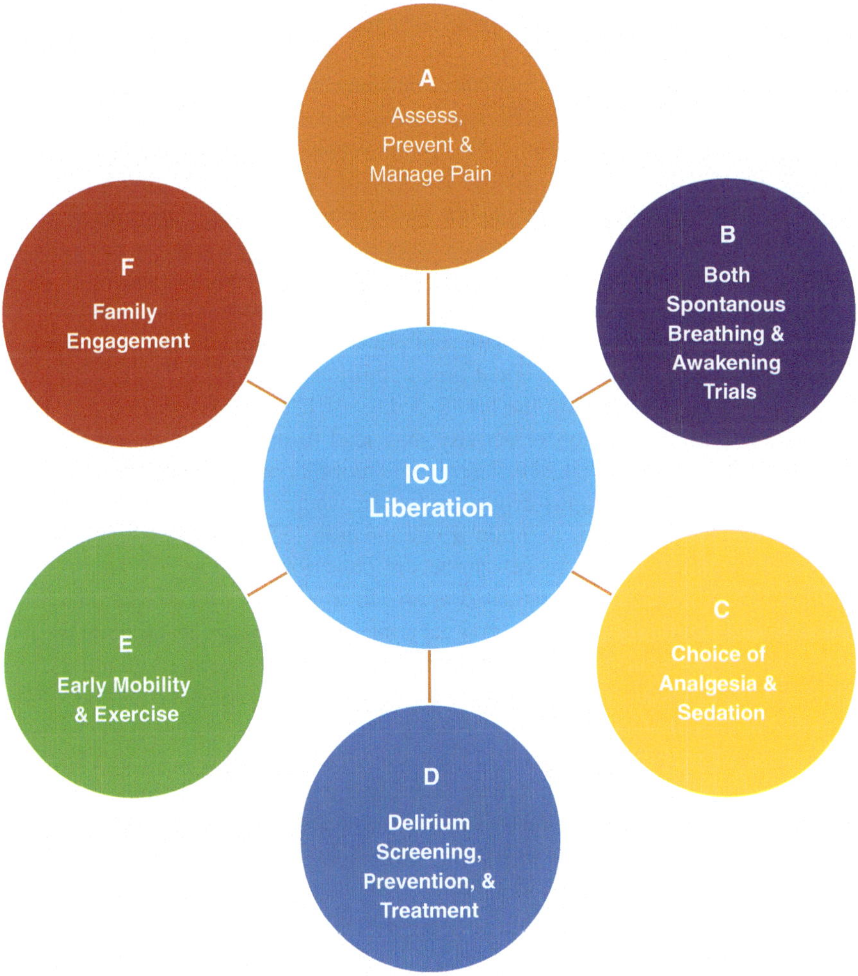

Fig. 21.1 Components of the ICU Liberation Bundle

post-ICU discharge disposition [31]. Early mobility is an integral element of the ICU Liberation initiative. Figure 21.1 shows the components of the ICU Liberation Bundle.

The Benefits of Early Mobility Versus Bedrest: Unpacking the Evidence

A compelling body of literature has illuminated the negative effects of immobility and bedrest in adults. Not only does immobility predispose patients to ICU-acquired weakness [18, 19, 32–35]; it is also associated with increased inflammatory marker concentrations [36, 37], glucose intolerance and insulin resistance [37–39], joint contractures [37, 40–42], skin ulcers [37], microvascular disease [37, 39], venous thromboembolism [42], atelectasis [43], delirium [44], and cognitive decline [45]. Although literature from the past two decades has detailed the detriments of immobility, such concepts are not new. In 1899, Dr. Emil Reis made the following comment regarding early activity of patients after intra-abdominal surgery: "what they do need is the use of their muscles, and if we do not prevent them from using their muscles we have no atrophy [46]." These sentiments were shared by many physicians in the 1900s [47–49], and the concept of "early rising" after surgery is described in medical literature during the World War II era [50]. Unfortunately with the advent of ICU medicine, bedrest became a common practice for critically ill patients, and not until the late 20th century did the ICU community begin to question the consequences of such practice [51].

Early mobility refers to the initiation of physical movement early on in critical illness. Although no widely accepted time definition exists, most sources consider early mobility to mean within the first 2–5 days of ICU admission [52, 53]. Data suggest that earlier initiation of activity may lead to higher patient benefit [54]. Numerous ICUs have published different early mobility protocols. Many are physical and occupational therapist-driven protocols, whereas others may be nursing-driven, physician-managed, or often a combination [55]. Some protocols group patients by clinical factors to determine the prescribed activity levels [56, 57], whereas others use a single graduated approach to activities for all patients [58]. Pediatric early mobility protocols may take into consideration developmental and age-based activity goals [59]. Protocols may include passive range of motion activities, but some consider early mobility to be only active range of motion [51].

With the advent of early mobility protocols, researchers have sought to elucidate the benefits of mobilizing critically ill patients. Protocols tend to be unit-specific and driven by a hospital's resources or needs; therefore, great variation exists from center to center. This heterogeneity has led to most research studies being single center in nature. Regardless, several adult studies have illustrated numerous benefits of early mobility, including increased muscle fiber cross-sectional area [32], earlier achievement of activities of daily living [56, 60], fewer ventilator days [60], decreased ICU length of stay [56, 58, 61], decreased hospital length of stay [58, 61, 62], and less delirium [60, 61, 63].

In one of the earlier studies to examine the effects of early mobility, Needham and colleagues instituted a quality improvement project in the medical ICU that focused on increasing physical and occupational therapy staffing, establishing rehabilitation consultation guidelines, and decreasing sedative use [61]. Post-protocol patients had a greater median number of rehabilitation treatments (1 vs. 7 treatments), achieved higher functional mobility in their sessions (56% vs. 78% sitting or greater), had significantly decreased sedative use and exposure, had shorter lengths of ICU and hospital stay (decreased by 2 and 3 days, respectively), and had more delirium-free days [61].

Another single-center study examined the effects of early mobility in a prospective cohort of adult ICU patients [58]. An early mobility team, consisting of a critical care nurse, nursing assistant, and physical therapist, rotated through seven different ICUs for a period of time and assigned patients to standard care or an intervention arm via block allocation. [58] Protocol patients had therapy initiated in the ICU more often (91% vs. 13%), were out of bed earlier (day 5 vs. day 11), and had a shorter length of ICU (6 vs. 7 days) and hospital stay (11 vs. 15 days), even after adjustment for severity of illness and body mass index [58]. Although absolute hospital costs per patient were lower for the protocol group, including mobility team costs, it was not a statistically significant difference [58].

In a 2009 study conducted at two university hospitals, 104 mechanically ventilated adults with known baseline functional independence were randomized to early mobilization during a daily sedation interruption or daily sedation interruption with therapy as ordered by clinician discretion [60]. The intervention group had passive range of motion activities performed daily, as well as active sessions, as tolerated with physical and occupational therapy [60]. About 60% of patients in the intervention group returned to independent functional status at hospital discharge (defined as the ability to perform six activities of daily living and walk independently) vs. 35% in the control group [60]. The intervention patients were also noted to have significantly shorter duration of delirium (2 vs. 4 days) and more ventilator-free days (24 vs. 21 days) [60]. Despite these positive outcomes, no significant difference was noted between groups in ICU length of stay, hospital length of stay, or mortality [60].

Schaller and colleagues completed a randomized international multicenter trial at five different surgical ICUs [56]. A cohort of 200 adult patients was randomized to standard care or early goal-directed mobilization. Study patients were functionally independent at baseline and had received mechanical ventilation for less than 48 hours at study enrollment [56]. The intervention group had a defined mobility goal set in morning rounds, and a multidisciplinary team with an assigned facilitator performed the daily goal [56]. When compared with the control group, the intervention group reached a significantly higher mobility level, as defined by the surgical ICU optimal mobility scale [56]. ICU length of stay was decreased in the intervention group (7 vs. 10 days), and intervention patients had higher functional mobility at hospital discharge, as defined by the mini-modified functional independence measure score [56].

In a smaller trial, 19 adult patients with septic shock were randomized within 72 hours of admission to a control group, which received 30 minutes of manual passive or active mobilization daily, or an intervention group, which received two mobility sessions daily (manual mobilization and chair or bed cycling) [32]. Participants had skeletal muscle biopsies at days 1 and 7 [32]. Muscle fiber cross-sectional area showed better preservation of fibers in the intervention group than in the control group [32].

Although the emerging pediatric data on early mobility has focused primarily on its safety and feasibility, as discussed in the next section, two studies have investigated the effect of mobility on outcomes in children. A Japanese study of pediatric patients who underwent liver transplant examined the benefits of early mobility in children [62]. In a 70-month retrospective study, patients ages 2–18 years who walked prior to transplant were analyzed before and after the implementation of an early mobility protocol [62]. A total of 35 patients were treated before the early mobility protocol, and 40 were treated after the introduction of the protocol [62]. As expected, protocol patients were more likely to receive physical therapy in the PICU and spent more time on therapy activities [62]. Patients in the post-protocol period were able to walk 50 yards without a rolling walker earlier (28 vs. 23 days, $p = 0.015$) and had a shorter hospital length stay (55 vs. 40 days, $p = 0.012$) [62]. In another pediatric study conducted in a 19-bed PICU, early mobility was implemented as part of a quality improvement program that included delirium screening and a sedation protocol [63]. Over the course of the study period, the mean delirium rate decreased from 19% to 12% [63]. Outside of these few studies, there is a paucity of pediatric outcome data. Future efforts should focus on defining the true impact of early mobility in the PICU population.

Barriers to Early Mobility in the PICU

Despite our knowledge of the benefits of early mobility, mostly derived from adult studies, challenges in initiating and sustaining PICU early mobility programs persist. The PARK-PICU study (Prevalence of Acute Rehabilitation for Kids in the PICU), a point prevalence study of early mobility practices in over 80 United States PICUs, showed a point prevalence of physical or occupational therapy provided mobility of only 35%. Older age and male gender increased likelihood to receive mobility, whereas children with higher baseline function less often had rehabilitation consultation within the first 72 hours of ICU stay [71]. In a large retrospective cohort study of 600 children in six different Canadian PICUs, only 26% received mobility therapy, and less than 10% received early mobility (defined as occurring within the first 48 h of admission) [64]. The most common documented reason for deferring mobility was lack of a physician's order [64]. Several other pediatric studies have described barriers to pediatric early mobility, including lack of equipment [57, 65], safety concerns [59, 65, 66], staff availability [59, 65], patient mental status [59], and unit culture [65]. Although barriers in adult studies have been well documented [67], safety concerns may be more pronounced in pediatrics given the higher rates of unplanned extubation correlated to younger age [68, 69] and smaller size [69] and more frequent line dislodgement [70] compared with that in adult patients.

Safety and Feasibility of Early Mobility in the PICU

Even with such documented barriers, several PICUs have successfully implemented early mobility programs, enriching the evidence base for safety and feasibility in the pediatric population. Using a quality improvement framework and a tiered activity plan, Wieczorek and colleagues increased physical and occupational therapy consults and mobility interventions in 100 PICU patients [57]. Patients in the post-quality improvement group were more likely than those in the control group to have engaged in mobilization activities by day 3 of admission, including active bed positioning ($p < 0.001$) and ambulation ($p = 0.04$). Moreover, the median number of mobilizations per patient increased from 3 to 6 ($p < 0.001$) during the first 3 days of PICU admission [57]. No adverse events were reported, and no mobilization events were aborted early as a result of patient intolerance [57].

With a multidisciplinary team and staff education, another academic PICU documented 130 mobility sessions with intubated PICU patients [59]. Mobilized patients were receiving a median positive end-expiratory pressure of 6 cm H_2O (25th–75th IQR: 5–8) and median fraction of inspired oxygen of 30% (25th–75th IQR: 30–40%) and were mobilized for an average of 35 minutes per session. No serious adverse events, defined as unplanned extubation, hemodynamic instability during mobility session, loss of central venous line, loss of arterial line, or cardiopulmonary arrest, occurred during mobilization of over 70 intubated PICU patients [59]. Two patients had a desaturation episode mitigated with ventilator changes, and in one patient, a nasogastric tube was inadvertently dislodged [59].

A multicenter randomized controlled trial increased ICU mobility sessions across three PICUs with a formalized protocol [72]. Fifty-eight children with a new brain insult were randomized to an early intervention protocol versus usual care. The intervention protocol consisted of consultation to physical therapy, occupational therapy, and speech language therapy within 72 h of PICU admission [72]. Protocol patients were more likely to receive evaluation by occupational therapy (26 of 26 protocol patients vs. 23 of 32 usual care patients, $p = 0.003$) and speech therapy (26 of 26 vs. 17 of 32, $p = 0.011$) [72]. Patients in the intervention group were evaluated by all three rehabilitation services earlier (physical therapy: 2 vs. 8 days, $p = 0.001$; occupational therapy: 2 vs. 7 days, $p = 0.001$; speech therapy: 2 vs. 13 days, $p = 0.026$) and had significantly more PICU sessions with each of these disciplines compared with the usual care group ($p < 0.001$) [72]. Of the hundreds of documented early mobility sessions, only seven were discontinued early due to patient instability (five for change in systolic blood pressure and two for increased intracranial pressure), and instability events did not impact the overall patient outcome [72].

Colwell and colleagues conducted a quality improvement project in which they instituted a PICU-wide early mobility protocol with mobility goals based on patient age and severity of illness [66]. They analyzed more than 500 patient encounters over a 9-month timespan and found that 52% of encounters reached goal mobilization. Those who met goal mobilization were younger ($p = 0.04$), had higher severity of illness ($p < 0.001$), and were less likely to have barriers ($p < 0.001$) [66]. The study reported a complication rate of less than 3%, with no difference in complications between patients who met goal mobilization and those who did not [66]. No serious adverse events (unplanned extubation or hemodynamic instability) occurred, and the most common complication was transient oxygen desaturation [66].

In a 30-patient pilot study, the use of an in-bed cycler increased the days mobilized and time mobilized in PICU patients [73]. No adverse events were reported in either arm in the study [73]. Another small pilot study used virtual reality gaming to increase upper body limb activity in PICU patients [74]. Four of the eight study patients were mechanically ventilated during the activity, and no adverse events occurred [74].

Cuello-Garcia and colleagues conducted a systematic review in which they analyzed 11 pediatric early mobility studies, including two pilot studies and nine observational studies [75]. In these studies, the timing of "early" mobility was defined as a range (48–72 h) after admission to the ICU or when clinical safety criteria were met [75]. Unfortunately a lack of outcomes data precluded an efficacy analysis, but available data suggested that early mobility is safe and feasible in the pediatric population [75]. In the pooled data of approximately 1100 patients, adverse events occurred in only 13, for an incidence of about 1% [75].

Facilitating Early Mobility in the PICU

Although proven to be feasible in published studies, creating a sustainable PICU early mobility protocol can be challenging. Current PICU culture hinders early mobility through a variety of mechanisms [8, 76–78]. Various factors have shaped this culture. An emphasis on patient safety and avoidance of hospital-acquired conditions has led to a more sedated and immobile PICU population [8]. Education surrounding the benefits and safety of early mobility is integral to culture change. Beyond safety concerns, the heterogeneous nature of PICU patients, with their varied developmental and cognitive levels, complicates early mobility protocols [8, 77]. In addition, pediatric-specific resources to support early mobility culture may be insufficient. Adult data suggest a significant cost-savings to support early mobility programs [79], but pediatrics is lacking comparable data to support increased staffing and equipment.

When creating a PICU early mobility protocol, each center should take into consideration unit- and hospital-specific resources and needs. A one-size-fits-all approach may not fit every unit, but utilizing basic implementation strategies may aid in the success. First and foremost, securing support from administration and hospital leadership is essential. Subsequently, a multidisciplinary committee with key stakeholders from each clinical field can be formed to help with protocol creation, education, and implementation. Representation from multiple fields ensures

Table 21.1 Multidisciplinary components of the pediatric early mobility team

Discipline	Role
Physical therapy	Improve mobility through exercises and activities focused on body biomechanics, including strength, balance, flexibility, and positioning
Occupational therapy	Focus on helping patients complete activities of daily living, including physical activities, environmental modifications, and cognitive/social interactions
Bedside nurse	Ensure patient tolerance and safety during early mobility activities and may be the primary provider of many early mobility activities
Respiratory therapy	Help secure respiratory support devices and monitor patient tolerance during early mobility sessions
Speech language pathology	Improve communication and cognitive communication deficits in patients
ICU providers (physician/nurse practitioner/physician assistant)	Evaluate patient safety and readiness for early mobility, advocate for patient early mobility
Child life specialists	Encourage early mobility participation by helping children and families cope with hospitalization and critical illness and facilitating play
Family members	Support and motivate child to participate in early mobility
Ancillary staff (chaplaincy, music therapy, art therapy, pet therapy)	Provide motivation and support for children to participate in early mobility

that all aspects of the protocol are taken into consideration; it also allows for stakeholders to take ownership of educating their peers. When instituting the early mobility protocol, patience is key. Culture change in the PICU may take years, and as such small successes should be celebrated. One pediatric study illustrated a positive provider perception change over the course of 2 years, with more than a 30% increase in the number of staff who believed it was safe to mobilize an intubated patient [59]. As with any new protocol or practice change, care should be taken to assess issues or concerns, routinely reassess and identify areas for improvement, and proactively attempt to identify unintended undesired consequences. Revisions based on resources or staffing may be necessary to ensure success. Table 21.1 shows the multidisciplinary components of the pediatric early mobility team. Figure 21.2 shows the steps for starting an early mobility program.

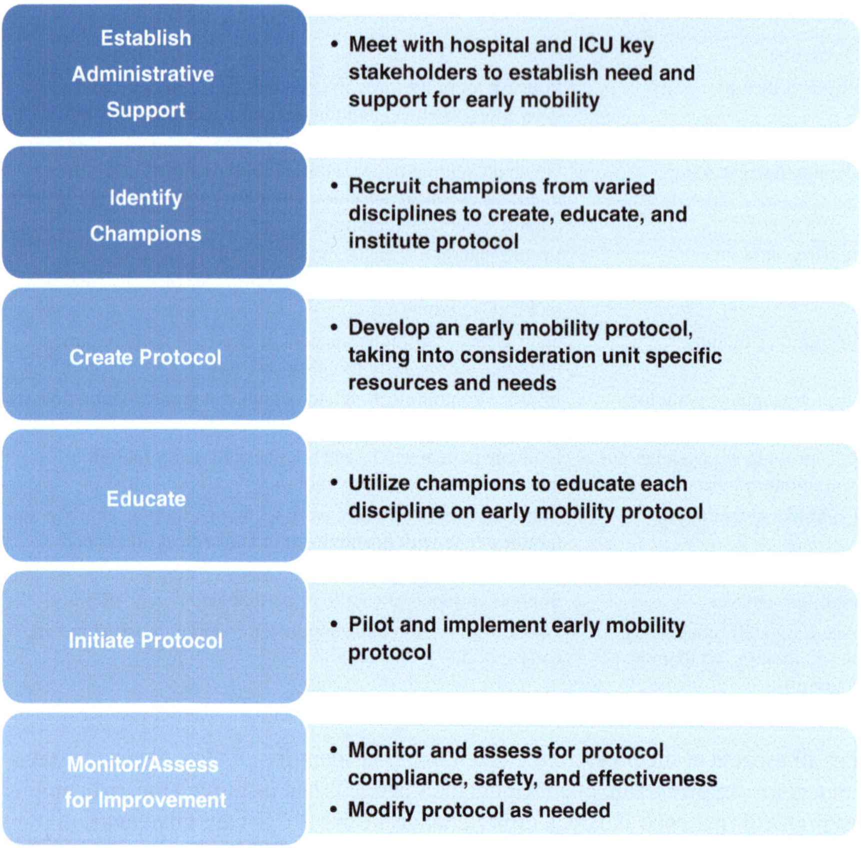

Fig. 21.2 Starting an early mobility program

Conclusions

As mortality in the PICU declines, our efforts should shift toward optimizing quality of life and minimizing morbidities in PICU survivors. After a PICU stay, a substantial portion of children will experience new or worsening functional deficits. Research suggests that motor decline may be one of the most pronounced effects of an ICU stay, and early mobility may help mitigate these effects. While early mobility in the pediatric population appears to be safe and feasible, more robust research on the effects of early mobility in children is required, as is support for resources while more pediatric programs work toward instituting their own programs.

References

1. Namachivayam P, Shann F, Shekerdemian L, Taylor A, Van Sloten I, Delzoppo C, et al. Three decades of pediatric intensive care: who was admitted, what happened in intensive care, and what happened afterward. Pediatr Crit Care Med. 2010;11(5):549–55.
2. Burns JP, Sellers DE, Meyer EC, Lewis-Newby M, Truog RD. Epidemiology of death in the PICU at Five U.S. teaching hospitals. Crit Care Med. 2014;42(9):2101–8.
3. Brummel N, Sidiqi S, Pandharipande P, Thompson J, Vasilevskis E, Girard T, et al. Overlap of cognitive, physical and mental health impairments in the post-intensive care syndrome. Crit Care Med. 2014;42(12):A358.
4. Marra A, Pandharipande PP, Girard TD, Patel MB, Hughes CG, Jackson JC, et al. Co-occurrence of post-intensive care syndrome problems among 406 survivors of critical illness. Crit Care Med. 2018;46(9):1393–401.
5. Elliott D, Davidson JE, Harvey MA, Bemis-Dougherty A, Hopkins RO, Iwashyna TJ, et al. Exploring the scope of post–intensive care syndrome therapy and care. Crit Care Med. 2014;42(12):2518–26.
6. Rawal G, Yadav S, Kumar R. Post-intensive care syndrome: an overview. J Transl Intern Med. 2017;5(2):90–2.
7. Herrup EA, Wieczorek B, Kudchadkar SR. Characteristics of postintensive care syndrome in survivors of pediatric critical illness: a systematic review. World J Crit Care Med. 2017;6(2):124–34.
8. Hopkins R, Choong K, Zebuhr C, Kudchadkar S. Transforming PICU culture to facilitate early rehabilitation. J Pediatr Intensive Care. 2015;4(4):204–11.
9. Bone MF, Feinglass JM, Goodman DM. Risk factors for acquiring functional and cognitive disabilities during admission to a PICU. Pediatr Crit Care Med. 2014;15(7):640–8.
10. Pinto NP, Rhinesmith EW, Kim TY, Ladner PH, Pollack MM. Long-term function after pediatric critical illness: results from the survivor outcomes study. Pediatr Crit Care Med. 2017;18(3):e122–30.
11. Jones S, Rantell K, Stevens K, Colwell B, Ratcliffe JR, Holland P, et al. Outcome at 6 months after admission for pediatric intensive care: a report of a National Study of Pediatric Intensive Care Units in the United Kingdom. Pediatrics. 2006;18(3):e122–30.
12. Fiser DH, Tilford JM, Roberson PK. Relationship of illness severity and length of stay to functional outcomes in the pediatric intensive care unit: a multi-institutional study. Crit Care Med. 2000;28(4):1173–9.
13. Pollack MM, Holubkov R, Funai T, Clark A, Berger JT, Meert K, et al. Pediatric intensive care outcomes: development of new morbidities during pediatric critical care. Pediatr Crit Care Med. 2014;15(9):821–7.
14. Alievi PT, Carvalho PRA, Trotta EA, Filho RM. The impact of admission to a pediatric intensive care unit assessed by means of global and cognitive performance scales. Jornal de Pediatria. 2007;83(6):505–11.
15. Ong C, Lee JH, Leow MKS, Puthucheary ZA. Functional outcomes and physical impairments in pediatric critical care survivors: a scoping review. Pediatr Crit Care Med. 2016;17(5):e247–59.
16. Choong K, Fraser D, Al-Harbi S, Borham A, Cameron J, Cameron S, et al. Functional recovery in critically ill children, the "WeeCover" multicenter study. Pediatr Crit Care Med. 2018;19(2):145–54.
17. Nelson LP, Lachman SE, Li SW, Gold JI. The effects of family functioning on the development of posttraumatic stress in children and their parents following admission to the PICU*. Pediatr Crit Care Med. 2019;20(4):e208–15.
18. Kramer CL. Intensive care unit–acquired weakness. Neurol Clin. 2017;35(4):723–36.
19. Jolley SE, Bunnell AE, Hough CL. ICU-acquired weakness. Chest [Internet]. 2016;150(5):1129–40. Available from: https://doi.org/10.1016/j.chest.2016.03.045

20. Kress JP, Hall JB. ICU-acquired weakness and recovery from critical illness. N Engl J Med [Internet]. 2014;370(17):1626–35. Available from: http://www.nejm.org/doi/10.1056/NEJMra1209390
21. Banwell BL, Mildner RJ, Hassall AC, Becker LE, Vajsar J, Shemie SD. Muscle weakness in critically ill children. Neurology. 2003;61(12):1779–82.
22. Kukreti V, Shamim M, Khilnani P. Intensive care unit acquired weakness in children: critical illness polyneuropathy and myopathy. Indian J Crit Care Med. 2014;18(2):95–101.
23. Johnson RW, Ng KWP, Dietz AR, Hartman ME, Baty JD, Hasan N, et al. Muscle atrophy in mechanically-ventilated critically ill children. PLoS One. 2018;13(12):e0207720.
24. Valla FV, Young DK, Rabilloud M, Periasami U, John M, Baudin F, et al. Thigh ultrasound monitoring identifies decreases in quadriceps femoris thickness as a frequent observation in critically ill children. Pediatr Crit Care Med. 2017;18(8):e339–47.
25. Glau CL, Conlon TW, Himebauch AS, Yehya N, Weiss SL, Berg RA, et al. Progressive diaphragm atrophy in pediatric acute respiratory failure. Pediatr Crit Care Med. 2018;19(5):406–11.
26. Colleti J, De Carvalho WB. PICU-acquired weakness: underestimated and underreported. Pediatr Crit Care Med. 2016;17(4):381.
27. Field-Ridley A, Dharmar M, Steinhorn D, McDonald C, Marcin JP. ICU-acquired weakness is associated with differences in clinical outcomes in critically ill children. Pediatr Crit Care Med. 2016;17(1):53–7.
28. Society of Critical Care Medicine. ICU Liberation [Internet]. Available from: https://www.sccm.org/ICULiberation/Home
29. Ely EW. The ABCDEF bundle: science and philosophy of how ICU liberation serves patients and families. Crit Care Med. 2017;45(2):321–30.
30. Marra A, Ely EW, Pandharipande PP, Patel MB. The ABCDEF bundle in critical care. Crit Care Clin. 2017;33:225–43.
31. Pun BT, Balas MC, Barnes-Daly MA, Thompson JL, Aldrich JM, Barr J, et al. Caring for critically ill patients with the ABCDEF bundle. Crit Care Med. 2019;47(1):3–14.
32. Hickmann CE, Castanares-Zapatero D, Deldicque L, Van den Bergh P, Caty G, Robert A, et al. Impact of very early physical therapy during septic shock on skeletal muscle. Crit Care Med [Internet]. 2018;46(9):1. Available from: http://insights.ovid.com/crossref?an=00003246-900000000-96229
33. Thabet Mahmoud A, Tawfik MAM, Abd El Naby SA, Abo El Fotoh WMM, Saleh NY, Abd El Hady NMS. Neurophysiological study of critical illness polyneuropathy and myopathy in mechanically ventilated children; additional aspects in paediatric critical illness comorbidities. Eur J Neurol. 2018;25(7):991–8.
34. Finn PJ, Plank LD, Clark MA, Connolly AB, Hill GL. Progressive cellular dehydration and proteolysis in critically ill patients. Lancet. 1996;347(9002):654–6.
35. Ferrando AA, Lane HW, Stuart CA, Davis-Street J, Wolfe RR. Prolonged bed rest decreases skeletal muscle and whole body protein synthesis. Am J Physiol Endocrinol Metab. 1996;270(4 Pt 1):E627–33.
36. Truong AD, Fan E, Brower RG, Needham DM. Bench-to-bedside review: mobilizing patients in the intensive care unit – from pathophysiology to clinical trials. Crit Care. 2009;13(4):216.
37. Brower RG. Consequences of bed rest. Critical Care Medicine. 2009;37(10 Suppl):S422–8.
38. Patel BK, Pohlman AS, Hall JB, Kress JP. Impact of early mobilization on glycemic control and ICU-acquired weakness in critically ill patients who are mechanically ventilated. Chest. 2014;146(3):583–9.
39. Hamburg NM, McMackin CJ, Huang AL, Shenouda SM, Widlansky ME, Schulz E, et al. Physical inactivity rapidly induces insulin resistance and microvascular dysfunction in healthy volunteers. Arterioscler Thromb Vasc Biol. 2007;146(3):583–9.
40. Clavet H, Hébert PC, Fergusson D, Doucette S, Trudel G. Joint contracture following prolonged stay in the intensive care unit. CMAJ. 2008;178(6):691–7.
41. G J, M K, G R, H R, K K, E P, et al. Pediatric contractures in burn injury: a burn model system national database study. J Burn Care Res. 2017;38(1):e192–9.

42. Dittmer DK, Teasell R. Complications of immobilization and bed rest. Part 1: musculoskeletal and cardiovascular complications. Can Fam Physician. 1993;39:1428–32.
43. Teasell R, Dittmer DK. Complications of immobilization and bed rest. Part 2: other complications. Can Fam Physician. 1993;39:1440–2.
44. NICE Guidelines. Delirium: pre prevention, diagnosis and management. Natl Collaborating Cent Acute Chronic Cond. 2010. https://www.nice.org.uk/guidance/cg103, Published date: 28 July 2010 Last updated: 14 March 2019, page 13/21 of guideline.
45. Lipnicki DM, Gunga HC. Physical inactivity and cognitive functioning: results from bed rest studies. Eur J Appl Physiol. 2009;105(1):27–35.
46. Ries E. Some radical changes in the after-treatment of celiotomy cases. J Am Med Assoc. 1899;XXXIII(8):454–6.
47. Ghormley RK. The abuse of rest in bed in orthopedic surgery. J Am Med Assoc. 1944;54:330–3.
48. Dock W. The evil sequelae of complete bed rest. J Am Med Assoc. 1944;125(16):1083–5.
49. Powers JH. The abuse of rest as a therapeutic measure in surgery: early postoperative activity and rehabilitation. J Am Med Assoc. 1945;6:544–6.
50. Ashkins J. Early rising after surgical operations. N Engl J Med. 1945;233:33–7.
51. Hashem MD, Nelliot A, Needham DM. Early mobilization and rehabilitation in the ICU: moving back to the future. Respir Care. 2016;61(7):971–9.
52. Cameron S, Ball I, Cepinskas G, Choong K, Doherty TJ, Ellis CG, et al. Early mobilization in the critical care unit: a review of adult and pediatric literature. J Crit Care. 2015;30(4):664–72.
53. Hodgson CL, Berney S, Harrold M, Saxena M, Bellomo R. Clinical review: early patient mobilization in the ICU. Crit Care. 2012;17(1):207.
54. Johnson AM, Henning AN, Morris PE, Tezanos AGV, Dupont-Versteegden EE. Timing and amount of physical therapy treatment are associated with length of stay in the cardiothoracic icu. Sci Rep. 2017;7(1):17591.
55. Bakhru RN, Wiebe DJ, McWilliams DJ, Spuhler VJ, Schweickert WD. An environmental scan for early mobilization practices in U.S. ICUs. Crit Care Med. 2015;43(11):2360–9.
56. Schaller SJ, Anstey M, Blobner M, Edrich T, Grabitz SD, Gradwohl-Matis I, et al. Early, goal-directed mobilisation in the surgical intensive care unit: a randomised controlled trial. Lancet. 2016;388(10052):1377–88.
57. Wieczorek B, Ascenzi J, Kim Y, Lenker H, Potter C, Shata NJ, et al. PICU Up! Pediatr Crit Care Med [Internet]. 2016;17(12):e559–66. Available from: http://insights.ovid.com/crossref?an=00130478-201612000-00021
58. Morris PE, Goad A, Thompson C, Taylor K, Harry B, Passmore L, et al. Early intensive care unit mobility therapy in the treatment of acute respiratory failure. Crit Care Med. 2008;36(8):2238–43.
59. Betters KA, Hebbar KB, Farthing D, Griego B, Easley T, Turman H, et al. Development and implementation of an early mobility program for mechanically ventilated pediatric patients. J Crit Care. 2017;41
60. Schweickert WD, Pohlman MC, Pohlman AS, Nigos C, Pawlik AJ, Esbrook CL, et al. Early physical and occupational therapy in mechanically ventilated, critically ill patients: a randomised controlled trial. Lancet [Internet]. 2009;373(9678):1874–82. Available from: https://doi.org/10.1016/S0140-6736(09)60658-9
61. Needham DM, Korupolu R, Zanni JM, Pradhan P, Colantuoni E, Palmer JB, et al. Early physical medicine and rehabilitation for patients with acute respiratory failure: a quality improvement project. Arch Phys Med Rehabil. 2010;91(4):536–42.
62. Tsuboi N, Hiratsuka M, Kaneko S, Nishimura N, Nakagawa S, Kasahara M, et al. Benefits of early mobilization after pediatric liver transplantation. Pediatr Crit Care Med. 2019;20(2):e91–7.
63. Simone S, Edwards S, Lardieri A, Walker LK, Graciano AL, Kishk OA, et al. Implementation of an ICU bundle: an Interprofessional quality improvement project to enhance delirium management and monitor delirium prevalence in a single PICU. Pediatr Crit Care Med. 2017;18(6):531–40.

64. Choong K, Koo KKY, Clark H, Chu R, Thabane L, Burns KEA, et al. Early mobilization in critically ill children: a survey of Canadian practice. Crit Care Med. 2013;41(7):1745–53.
65. Joyce CL, Taipe C, Sobin B, Spadaro M, Gutwirth B, Elgin L, et al. Provider beliefs regarding early mobilization in the pediatric intensive care unit. J Pediatr Nurs [Internet]. 2018;38:15–9. Available from: https://doi.org/10.1016/j.pedn.2017.10.003
66. Colwell BRL, Williams CN, Kelly SP, Ibsen LM. Mobilization therapy in the pediatric intensive care unit: a multidisciplinary quality improvement initiative. Am J Crit Care. 2018;27(3):194–203.
67. Dubb R, Nydahl P, Hermes C, Schwabbauer N, Toonstra A, Parker AM, et al. Barriers and strategies for early mobilization of patients in intensive care units. Ann Am Thorac Soc. 2016;13(5):724–30.
68. Razavi SS, Nejad RA, Mohajerani SA, Talebian M. Risk factors of unplanned extubation in pediatric intensive care unit. Tanaffos. 2013;12(3):11–6.
69. Vats A, Hopkins C, Hatfield KM, Yan J, Palmer R, Keskinocak P. An airway risk assessment score for unplanned extubation in intensive care pediatric patients. Pediatr Crit Care Med. 2017;18(7):661–6.
70. Ullman AJ, Marsh N, Mihala G, Rickard CM, Cooke M. Complications of central venous access devices: a systematic review. Pediatrics. 2015;136(5):e1331–44.
71. Kudchadkar SR, Nelliot A, Awojoodu R, Vaidya D, Traube C, Walker T, et al. Physical Rehabilitation in Critically Ill Children: A Multicenter Point Prevalence Study in the United States. Crit Care Med. 2020;48(5):634–44.
72. Fink EL, Beers SR, Houtrow AJ, Richichi R, Burns C, Doughty L, et al. Early protocolized versus usual care rehabilitation for pediatric neurocritical care patients: a randomized controlled trial. Pediatr Crit Care Med. 2019;20(6):540–50.
73. Choong K, Awladthani S, Khawaji A, Clark H, Borhan A, Cheng J, et al. Early exercise in critically ill youth and children, a preliminary evaluation: the wEECYCLE pilot trial. Pediatr Crit Care Med. 2017;18(11):e546–54.
74. Abdulsatar F, Walker RG, Timmons BW, Choong K. "Wii-Hab" in critically ill children: a pilot trial. J Pediatr Rehabil Med. 2013;6(4):193–204.
75. Cuello-Garcia CA, Mai SHC, Simpson R, Al-Harbi S, Choong K. Early mobilization in critically ill children: a systematic review. J Pediatr [Internet]. 2018.; Available from: https://doi.org/10.1016/j.jpeds.2018.07.037
76. Walker T, Kudchadkar SR. Early mobility in the pediatric intensive care unit: can we move on? J Pediatr. 2018;203:10–2.
77. Walker TC, Kudchadkar SR. Early mobilization in the pediatric intensive care unit. Transl Pediatr. 2018;7(4):308–13.
78. Saliski M, Kudchadkar S. Optimizing sedation management to promote early mobilization for critically ill children. J Pediatr Intensive Care. 2015;4(4):188–93.
79. Lord RK, Mayhew CR, Korupolu R, Mantheiy EC, Friedman MA, Palmer JB, et al. ICU early physical rehabilitation programs: financial modeling of cost savings. Crit Care Med. 2013;41(3):717–24.

Chapter 22
Palliative Sedation

Eileen Rhee, Efrat Lelkes, and Wynne Morrison

Introduction

The term "palliative sedation" has been used to refer to a wide range of therapies. The concept is often disconcerting for clinicians, due to ethical, legal, or procedural worries about the process. Generally, there are three types of palliative sedation that have been described in the literature: ordinary sedation, proportionate palliative sedation, and palliative sedation to unconsciousness [3]. However, these three ideas have been interchanged and conflated, which has added to the confusion [4–6]. In this chapter, we will use the term palliative sedation, and it will conceptually most align with proportionate palliative sedation (Table 22.1), with the understanding that sedation to unconsciousness may be an unintended effect of this practice [3, 7, 8].

The American Academy of Hospice and Palliative Medicine, American Medical Association, National Hospice and Palliative Care Organization, and the European Association for Palliative Care have endorsed principles and guidelines to help inform the practice of palliative sedation [9–12].

E. Rhee (✉)
Department of Pediatrics, Division of Pediatric Critical Care Medicine, Division of Bioethics and Palliative Care, Seattle Children's Hospital and University of Washington School of Medicine, Seattle, WA, USA
e-mail: eileen.rhee@seattlechildrens.org

E. Lelkes
Department of Pediatrics, Division of Critical Care Medicine, Integrated Pediatric Pain and Palliative Care, University of California San Francisco, San Francisco, CA, USA

W. Morrison
Department of Anesthesiology and Critical Care Medicine, Pediatric Advanced Care Team, The Children's Hospital of Philadelphia and Perelman School of Medicine at the University of Pennsylvania, Philadelphia, PA, USA

P. P. Kamat, J. W. Berkenbosch (eds.), *Sedation and Analgesia for the Pediatric Intensivist*, https://doi.org/10.1007/978-3-030-52555-2_22

Table 22.1 Definitions

Palliation	Treatment of pain and suffering with no intent to hasten death [13].
Euthanasia	Administration of medication with the specific intent to hasten death [13].
Physician aid-in-dying	The practice of prescribing a lethal dose of medication to a patient to self-administer if he or she chooses to do so near the end-of-life in order to hasten death [14, 15].
Doctrine of double effect	An ethical argument to support acts that have both intended and unintended consequences [23–27].
Proportionate palliative sedation	Treatment of end-of-life symptoms with medications that are proportionately increased to effect, resulting in increasing levels of sedation during both waking and sleeping hours to help relieve symptoms [3].

Ethical Considerations

The use of sedation, especially to the point of unconsciousness, at the end-of-life often raises ethical questions about how to distinguish the palliative management of symptoms from the process of euthanasia [13]. Palliation, euthanasia, and physician aid-in-dying (PAD) describe three different and distinct modes of providing sedation at the end-of-life. Palliation differs from the latter two acts in that the goal is not to hasten death, yet there is clear intent to avoid prolonging the dying process unnecessarily. Table 22.1 provides definitions of these terms. Several US states have legal procedures for the provision of PAD in adult patients, but none have included children as an eligible population for PAD [1, 2]. There are several terms used for PAD, including "physician-assisted suicide" and "physician-assisted dying," and our preference is for "physician aid-in-dying" as it captures the descriptive nature of this complex end-of-life procedure most wholly [14, 15]. Euthanasia differs from PAD in that the medications are administered by the physician; euthanasia is not legal in the US (although some European countries allow it) [16].

There is a long-standing legal and moral precedent that pain and suffering at the end-of-life can and should be treated. In a Supreme Court opinion, Justice Sandra Day O'Connor stated that "a patient who is suffering from a terminal illness and who is experiencing great pain has no legal barriers to obtaining medication, from qualified physicians, to alleviate that suffering, even to the point of causing unconsciousness and hastening death" [17]. Fears of legal repercussions should not prevent physicians from treating pain or other symptoms at the end-of-life. Distinguishing euthanasia from palliative sedation is therefore important because of these legal and ethical considerations. One of the key distinguishing features between the two practices is that palliative sedation is titrated to effect – medications are escalated until symptoms are controlled and then not escalated further once the patient is comfortable. Clinicians begin with the safest medications and proceed to the use of "riskier" medications only if symptoms cannot be controlled with first-tier agents [14]. In practice, most studies have shown that the quantity of opioids and benzodiazepines administered for end-of-life symptoms do not appear to be associated with time of death [18–22].

The doctrine of double effect is often invoked to support acts that have both intended and unintended consequences [23]. In the case of end-of-life care, double effect is an ethical principle used to argue for providing medications to treat pain and suffering, when there is a risk that these same medications will hasten death [24–27]. The components that make the unintended consequence acceptable include:

1. The act itself (treating suffering) must be inherently good.
2. The agent intends the good effect (treating suffering) rather than the bad effect (hastening death).
3. The good effect must outweigh the bad effect (e.g., hastening death by many years for mild pain would be unacceptable).

Many ethicists add that the bad effect must not be a means to the good effect – i.e., death is not used as the means to end suffering. If death occurs, however, as an unfortunate side effect of actions that are necessary to relieve suffering, it is acceptable. Practically, these arguments elucidate what medications may be appropriate to use at the end-of-life. Medications that treat pain or other symptoms should be used in reasonable doses based on the patient's prior exposure and expected tolerance. The medications may be escalated (rapidly if needed) for untreated symptoms. If the only way to control suffering is to escalate sedation to the point of unconsciousness, doing so may be appropriate or even morally necessary. Unacceptable medications are those that would merely hasten the dying process without treating suffering (e.g., neuromuscular blockade and potassium chloride) [28].

These concepts can make sense to patients and families as well – when a patient is suffering at the end-of-life, the team can commit to trying to titrate medications to keep the patient both comfortable and interactive. If that becomes impossible, however, it might be necessary to accept "comfortable and sleepy" or "comfortable and unconscious" when there is no other choice.

Symptom Management

In palliative sedation, some clinicians may only feel comfortable escalating sedation in slowly progressive increments. However, we would advocate that the rate of titration is specific to the patient and clinical situation. In some cases, severe, uncontrolled symptoms at the end-of-life may require rapid escalation of medications in order to treat symptoms that are distressing to the patient. As medications are titrated, whether gradually or rapidly, a responsible clinician must be readily available in order to direct/administer bolus dosing of sedatives at short, regular intervals. Deliberate palliative sedation to unconsciousness for extreme, uncontrolled pain, should be an even more rare practice, as most pain can usually be managed by close attention to symptom management.

In the pediatric critical care or inpatient setting, palliative sedation is ideally administered through a continuous infusion, augmented by intermittent, frequently available bolus dosing (equivalent to the dose administered over 1 hour via the infusion) – generally every 5–10 minutes when initiating treatment for severe symptoms. We recommend starting with a single agent, although a combination of medications or a combination of continuous and intermittent dosing may become necessary. Once symptom control is achieved, the sum total of continuous and bolus dosing over 1–3 hours of management may be used to estimate a new, higher continuous hourly rate. The ultimate goal is to reach a point where, if possible, the patient only requires additional bolus dosing every few hours.

Medications typically used for palliative sedation are discussed in detail elsewhere in this book. First-tier medications are typically benzodiazepines, such as midazolam or lorazepam. Both medications have quick onset of action and good bioavailability, and they are easily titratable and work well as an infusion at the end-of-life [22, 29]. Infusions of opioids may also be used, but they may not achieve a similar degree of sedation. Opioids may, however, be a part of the palliative sedation regimen as extreme or intractable pain is often the indication for palliative sedation [7]. Second-tier agents include propofol, ketamine, and dexmedetomidine. These agents may be considered when first-tier agents are insufficient. Ketamine and dexmedetomidine may allow for a preserved respiratory drive and hemodynamic stability, as can propofol in low doses [29–32]. Less commonly, barbiturates, including pentobarbital and phenobarbital, may also be used as infusions or as intermittent bolus dosing for palliative sedation [29, 33].

When death is imminent, typically described as days to weeks, and severe symptoms are likely, palliative sedation to unconsciousness may be required [12, 34, 35]. Transparency with the patient and/or family about this potential situation is essential. Severe symptoms could be caused by acute airway obstruction, severe agitated delirium, massive hemoptysis, hematemesis, or rapid exsanguination due to erosion by a tumor into a large blood vessel. Often, in these situations, the use of second-tier agents, such as propofol or ketamine, will be indicated [30].

Delirium is a complex neurocognitive disorder that may be difficult to control at the end-of-life [36]. It can manifest as hallucinations or agitation, often with a waxing and waning level of alertness, and it is often very distressing to caregivers. It can be a side effect of chronic sedative and analgesic medications, secondary to the disease process itself, the result of electrolyte or metabolic disturbances, or a terminal symptom at the end-of-life [36]. Once all of the treatable physiologic causes have been assessed and addressed, typical and atypical antipsychotics, such as haloperidol, olanzapine, or quetiapine, may be required [36–39]. Generally, standard dosing of these medications will provide a benefit within 30–60 minutes. If no clear improvement is seen, an additional dose may be given after 30 minutes. At that point, if relief of symptoms has not been achieved, then we would endorse focusing on palliation with first- or second-tier agents. While the management of delirium for a recoverable illness often involves minimizing benzodiazepine use, in the last hours to days of life they may be necessary [40]. Escalating sedation to the point of unconsciousness may be indicated if the delirium leads to the potential for self-harm or severe distress.

Guidelines and Protocols

In the US, palliative sedation is rarely used in adult patients, and its use is even more rare in pediatrics [33]. Challenges in developing standardized protocols in pediatrics include the variability in diagnoses, symptoms, and illness trajectory, and institutions may not be likely to have protocols for this rare need. Guidelines can, however, be helpful in identifying shared goals between the medical team and family/patient, selecting medications, titrating therapy to effect, and assessing efficacy in order to improve care for patients at the end-of-life [32, 41–45] (Table 22.2).

Table 22.2 Best practices for palliative sedation

Assessment
Assess whether the patient's condition is terminal, and death is imminent (days to weeks)
Establish consensus between clinicians and patient/family that intractable suffering is present
Assess whether standard palliative therapies (pain control, anxiolysis, and psychosocial support) have failed to adequately manage the symptoms
Assess if delirium is contributing to symptoms and if delirium treatment is warranted
Determine if assistance from palliative care or ethics consultants would be helpful
Review relevant institutional policies regarding palliative sedation or end-of-life care
Document assessment and indications for palliative sedation in the medical record
Preparation
Educate patient, family, and medical team regarding goals of sedation (symptom control rather than hastening death)
Ensure adequate supervision by clinicians experienced with the process of palliative sedation
Prepare patient and family regarding signs/symptoms of dying and uncertainty of time course
Ensure adequate supply of medications for symptom management, including sufficient amounts for escalation of doses or agents
Consider discontinuation of any medications that are not symptom-focused
Consider whether artificial nutrition and hydration is likely to prevent or worsen symptoms, and discontinue if it is not beneficial
Prepare as calm and quiet a setting as feasible for the patient and family
Establish roles of team members and ensure adequate staffing for close attention to symptom management
Place orders for limitations on resuscitation/invasive interventions as appropriate
Administration
Choose the "safest" regimen first (proceed to second-tier therapies only if first-tier therapies are inadequate)
Escalate doses or add agents as needed, based on frequent patient assessments
Once symptoms are controlled, maintain doses
Escalate medications to levels that decrease level of consciousness only when necessary to control symptoms
Avoid actions that would merely hasten death without a symptom benefit
Identify teams/team members to provide emotional and logistical support to family
Identify and address staff concerns, particularly if the dying process continues through multiple staff handoffs

The first step is to establish that a patient is at the end-of-life. Both the family and medical team must be in agreement that the symptoms (such as pain, anxiety, dyspnea, nausea, or delirium) cannot be controlled with any other modality. Prior to initiating palliative sedation, we recommend consulting a multidisciplinary team, including palliative care, pain or anesthesiology specialists, child life specialists, chaplaincy, social work, and clinical pharmacy, to work with the family (and child if appropriate) and clearly communicate the goals of palliative sedation and establish informed consent. A clinical ethics team may be helpful to determine if palliative sedation is appropriate. It is necessary to discuss code status and clarify goals as comfort-directed measures only.

Critical elements of a practice guideline include documentation for all reasons leading to the decision for palliative sedation, including the nature of the symptoms and the alternative or primary palliative treatments that were attempted, consultations obtained, and a palliative care team consultation, as well as documentation of the informed consent and code status. Ideally, in the process leading to the provision of palliative sedation, the patient would be transferred to a private room, and a formalized care plan will be discussed with the bedside care team prior to the initiation of palliative sedation [32, 41, 44]. The care plan would provide recommendations for objectively assessing appropriate level of sedation, reference guidelines for titration of medications, and guidance on key communication points for the caregivers, patient, and family.

Moral Distress

Moral distress is "the pain or anguish affecting the mind, body or relationships in response to a situation in which the person is aware of a moral problem, acknowledges moral responsibility, and makes a moral judgment about the correct action; yet, as a result of real or perceived constraints, participates, either by act or omission, in a manner he or she perceives to be morally wrong" [46]. Members of the health care team, including bedside nurses, respiratory therapists, trainees, and ancillary staff, are at risk for developing moral distress if they are asked to administer or participate in palliative sedation for a patient, and they find the practice to be morally wrong.

This distress may be secondary to a belief that palliative sedation itself is wrong or may be a result of deeply held convictions about what a "good death" should look like, such as ensuring a patient's capacity for awareness and interaction with loved ones until the time of death [44–49]. Distress may occur if providers or staff view that medications are being used to hasten death or if they perceive that they are being coerced, either from the family or other members of the medical team, to increase sedation beyond the level of symptom control [50–51]. In pediatrics, an additional layer of distress is associated with the inherent surrogate decision-making required of parents/guardians for their child who may have never been able to assert or ascertain his or her own values. Thus, there may be a concern that palliative sedation would not have been desired by the child.

Distress may also occur when a patient or family member is asking for palliative sedation for psychological or existential distress. In Europe, some countries allow the practice of palliative sedation for this indication, but from our standpoint, doing so would be inconsistent with US practice and guidelines. The underlying reasons that may be contributing to the existential distress need to be addressed and treated thoroughly (e.g., inadequately managed pain or depression), as providing palliative sedation for this indication would be non-proportionate. Consultation with the bioethics and palliative care teams may be considered for these complex situations [32, 41, 44, 52, 53].

Further, in palliative sedation, it is appropriate to discontinue life-prolonging therapies, including artificial nutrition and hydration, renal replacement therapy, and antibiotics [26]. The goal of selectively removing these interventions is not to hasten death but rather to discontinue therapies that are ineffective in achieving comfort and the relief of suffering [7, 30, 54]. The discontinuation of these therapies may be ethically justified but may also add to the level of distress of those caring for the patient. In this situation, certain therapies may need to be removed more gradually or not at all.

As described in the previous section, a formal guideline or policy may help to address moral distress, as the inclusion of a multidisciplinary team and careful documentation will provide guidance and ensure excellent communication for all members of the medical team as well as for the patient and family. Continuous transparent communication about the palliative sedation plan must be maintained throughout the duration of the patient's end-of-life management, and presumably through his or her death [55, 56].

Though palliative sedation for a patient may be ethical and appropriately indicated, it is important to support all members of the team, especially those that feel distressed by the procedure. We urge centers to allow for conscientious objection and allow those who disagree with palliative sedation to be removed from the care of the patient if feasible and be allowed to meet with members of the palliative care and ethics teams to voice their concerns. Allowing for avenues of open and honest communication, and an ability to opt out of care that feels discordant with one's belief system, may ease the moral anguish that may result in burnout of healthcare providers while still allowing for continued appropriate care of patients. The opt-out avenue also ensures that the family and patient will not be exposed to the distress of others while they are actively proceeding through their own grief and bereavement process.

Final Considerations

Palliative sedation can be confusing and distressing based on misconceptions from an ethical or moral perspective. Guidelines that direct goals of care, decision-making, medication administration and titration, documentation, and communication may help address many of the issues that impede appropriate and effective palliative sedation.

Embedded in the care of a patient requiring palliative sedation at the end-of-life is the fundamental need to ensure trust between the patient, family, and medical team, as well as between the different members of the multidisciplinary teams [57–59]. Depending on the patient's and family's experience, they may have developed misconceptions about specific medications or clinical care or endured biases in their personal lives that may contribute to misinterpretation or mistrust of the team's recommendations. Similarly, any assumptions that clinicians make about a patient or family that are not clarified in transparent and non-agenda-based communication will lead to judgment, non-compassion, and ineffectively guided decision-making, which will only create discordance between the medical team and patient/family, as well as limit the care and comfort that is needed by the patient and family in such a high-stake situation. A multidisciplinary care team may help guide and direct management of a patient's end-of-life care and will help to ensure that all members of the bedside team and family are fully informed about the underlying decision-making process and goals of palliative sedation.

References

1. Oregon Death With Dignity Act, OR. REV. STAT. §127.800–127.995 (2015).
2. Hedberg K, New C. Oregon's death with dignity act: 20 years of experience to inform the debate. Ann Intern Med. 2017;167:579–83. https://doi.org/10.7326/M17-2300.
3. Quill TE, Lo B, Brock DW, et al. Last-resort options for palliative sedation. Ann Intern Med. 2009;151(6):421–4. https://doi.org/10.7326/0003-4819-151-6-200909150-00007.
4. Henderson CM, FitzGerald M, Hoehn KS, Weidner N. Pediatrician ambiguity in understanding palliative sedation at the end of life. Am J Hosp Palliat Care. 2017;34(1):5–19. https://doi.org/10.1177/1049909115609294journals.sagepub.com/home/ajh.
5. Putman MS, Yoon JD, Rasinski KA, Curlin FA. Intentional sedation to unconsciousness at the end of life: findings from a National Physician Survey. J Pain Symptom Manag. 2013;46(3):326–34. https://doi.org/10.1016/j.jpainsymman.2012.09.007.
6. Maiser S, Estrada-Stephen K, Sahr N, Gully J, Marks S. A survey of hospice and palliative care clinicians' experiences and attitudes regarding the use of palliative sedation. J Palliat Med. 2017;20(9):915–21. https://doi.org/10.1089/jpm.2016.0464.
7. Quill TE, Byock IR. Responding to intractable terminal suffering: the role of terminal sedation and voluntary refusal of food and fluids. ACP-ASIM end-of-life care consensus panel. American College of Physicians-American Society of Internal Medicine. Ann Intern Med. 2000;132(5):408–14. Review. Erratum in: Ann Intern Med. 2000 Jun 20; 132(12):1011. https://doi.org/10.7326/0003-4819-132-5-200003070-00012.
8. Jansen LA, Sulmasy DP. Sedation, alimentation, hydration, and equivocation: careful conversation about care at the end of life. Ann Intern Med. 2002;136(11):845–9. https://doi.org/10.7326/0003-4819-136-11-200206040-00014.
9. American Academy of Hospice and Palliative Medicine: Position Statements: Statement on Palliative Sedation. December 5, 2014. Chicago, IL. http://aahpm.org/positions/palliative-sedation. Acessed 2 Apr 2019.
10. American Medical Association. AMA code of medical ethics' opinions on sedation at the end of life. Virtual Mentor. 2013;15(5):428–9. https://doi.org/10.1001/virtualmentor.2013.15.5.coet1-1305.
11. Kirk TW, Mahon MM. National Hospice and Palliative Care Organization (NHPCO) position statement and commentary on the use of palliative sedation in imminently dying ter-

minally ill patients. J Pain Symptom Manag. 2010;39(5):914–23. https://doi.org/10.1016/j.jpainsymman.2010.01.009.
12. Cherny NI, Radbruch L, The Board of the European Association for Palliative Care. European Association for Palliative Care (EAPC) recommended framework for the use of sedation in palliative care. Palliat Med. 2009;23(7):581–93. https://doi.org/10.1177/0269216309107024.
13. Morrison W, Kang T. Judging the quality of mercy: drawing a line between palliation and euthanasia. Pediatrics. 2014;133:S31–6. https://doi.org/10.1542/peds.2013-3608F.
14. Quill TE, Lee BC, Nunn S. Palliative treatments of last resort: choosing the least harmful alternative. Ann Intern Med. 2000;132(6):488–93. https://doi.org/10.7326/0003-4819-132-6-200003210-00011.
15. Campbell CS, Black AM. Dignity, death, and dilemmas: a study of Washington hospices and physician-assisted death. J Pain Symptom Manag. 2014;47:137e153. https://doi.org/10.1016/j.jpainsymman.2013.02.024.
16. Goligher EC, Ely EW, Sulmasy DP, et al. Physician-assisted suicide and euthanasia in the ICU: a dialogue on core ethical issues. Crit Care Med. 2017;45:149–55. https://doi.org/10.1097/CCM.0000000000001818.
17. Menikoff J. Law and bioethics: an introduction. Washington DC: Georgetown University Press; 2001.
18. Vitetta L, Kenner D, Sali A. Sedation and analgesia-prescribing patterns in terminally ill patients at the end of life. Am J Hosp Palliat Care. 2005;22(6):465–73. https://doi.org/10.1177/104990910502200601.
19. Maltoni M, Scarpi E, Rosati M, Derni S, Fabbri L, Martini F, Amadori D, Nanni O. Palliative sedation in end-of-life care and survival: a systematic review. J Clin Oncol. 2012;30(12):1378–83. https://doi.org/10.1200/JCO.2011.37.3795. Epub 2012 Mar 12.
20. Wilson WC, Smedira NG, Fink C, et al. Ordering and administration of sedatives and analgesics during the withholding and withdrawal of life support from critically ill patients. JAMA. 1992;267(7):949–53. https://doi.org/10.1001/jama.1992.03480070065032.
21. Mazer MA, Alligood CM, Wu Q. The infusion of opioids during terminal withdrawal of mechanical ventilation in the medical intensive care unit. J Pain Symptom Manag. 2011;42(1):44–5. https://doi.org/10.1016/j.jpainsymman.2010.10.256.
22. Chan JD, Treece PD, Engleberg RA, et al. Narcotic and benzodiazepine use after withdrawal of life support: association with time to death? Chest. 2004;126:286–93. https://doi.org/10.1378/chest.126.1.286.
23. Beauchamp TL, Childress JF. Principles of biomedical ethics. 7th ed: Oxford University Press; 2012.
24. Gamblin V, Chevalier L, Pierrat M, et al. Sedation or limits of palliative care - ethical questions. Ethic Med Public Heath. 2017;3:343–8. https://doi.org/10.1016/j.jemep.2017.05.007.
25. ten Have H, Welie JVM. Palliative sedation Verus euthanasia: an ethical assessment. J Pain Sympom Manag. 2014;47(1):123–36. https://doi.org/10.1016/j.jpainsymman.2013.03.008.
26. Hahn MP. Review of palliative sedation and its distinction from euthanasia and lethal injection. J Pain Pall Pharm. 2012;26(1):30–9. https://doi.org/10.3109/15360288.2011.650353.
27. Rady MY, Verheijde JL, McGregor JL. Palliation or euthanasia and end-of-life care: is it in the eye of the beholder? Am J Respir Crit Care Med. 2008;178:775–6. https://doi.org/10.1164/ajrccm.178.7.775a.
28. Truog RD, Campbell ML, Curtis JR, Haas CE, Luce JM, Rubenfeld GD, Rushton CH, Kaufman DC. Recommendations for end-of-life care in the intensive care unit: a consensus statement by the American College of Critical Care Medicine. Crit Care Med. 2008;36:953–63. https://doi.org/10.1097/CCM.0B013E3181659096.
29. Schildmann EK, Schildmann J, Kiesewetter I. Medication and monitoring in palliative sedation therapy: a systematic review and quality assessment of published guidelines. J Pain Symtpom Manag. 2015;49:734–46. https://doi.org/10.1016/j.jpainsymman.2014.08.013.
30. Johnson LM, Frader J, Wolfe J, et al. Palliative sedation with propofol for an adolescent with a DNR order. Pediatrics. 2017;140(2):e20170487. https://doi.org/10.1542/peds.2017-0487.

31. Anghelescu DL, Knapp E, Johnson LM, et al. The role of the pediatric anesthesiologist in relieving suffering at the end of life: when is palliative sedation appropriate in pediatrics? Paediatr Anaesth. 2017;27(4):443–4. https://doi.org/10.1111/pan.13103.
32. Reid TT, Demme RA, Quill TE. When there are no good choices: illuminating the borderland between proportionate palliative sedation and palliative sedation to unconsciousness. Pain Manag. 2011;1(1):31–40. https://doi.org/10.2217/pmt.10.1.
33. Lux MR, Protus BM, Kimbrel J, Grauer P. A survey of hospice and palliative care physicians regarding palliative sedation practices. Am J Hosp Palliat Care. 2017;34(3):217–22. https://doi.org/10.1177/1049909115615128. Epub 2016 Jul 11.
34. Lynch M. Palliative sedation. Clin J Oncol Nurs. 2003;7(6):653–7. https://doi.org/10.1188/03.CJON.653-657.
35. Braun TC, Hagen NA, Clark T. Development of a clinical practice guideline for palliative sedation. J Palliat Med. 2003;(3):345–50. https://doi.org/10.1089/109662103322144655.
36. Wu Y, Tseng P, Tu Y, et al. Association of Delirium Response and Safety of Pharmacological Interventions for the Management and Prevention of Delirium: a network meta-analysis. JAMA Psychiatry. Published online February 27, 2019. https://doi.org/10.1001/jamapsychiatry.2018.4365.
37. Agar MR, Lawlor PG, Quinn S, et al. Efficacy of oral risperidone, haloperidol, or placebo for symptoms of delirium among patients in palliative care: a randomized controlled trial. JAMA Intern Med. 2012;117(1):34–42.
38. Grassi L, Caraceni A, Mitchell AJ, et al. Management of Delirium in palliative care: a review. Curr Psychiatry Rep. 2015;17:13. https://doi-org.offcampus.lib.washington.edu/10.1007/s11920-015-0550-8
39. Bodnar J. A review of agents for palliative deep sedation: pharmacology and practical applications. J Pain Palliat Care Pharmacother. 2017;31(1):16–37. https://doi.org/10.1080/15360288.2017.1279502.
40. Hui D, Frisbee-Hume S, Wilson A, et al. Effect of lorazepam with haloperidol vs haloperidol alone on agitated delirium in patients with advanced cancer receiving palliative care: a randomized clinical trial. JAMA. 2017;318(11):1047–56. https://doi.org/10.1001/jama.2017.11468.
41. Abarshi E, Rietjens J, Robijn L, Caraceni A, Payne S, Deliens L, Van den Block L, EURO IMPACT. International variations in clinical practice guidelines for palliative sedation: a systematic review. BMJ Support Palliat Care. 2017;7(3):223–9. https://doi.org/10.1136/bmjspcare-2016-001159. Epub 2017 Apr 20. Review. Erratum in: BMJ Support Palliat Care. 2018 Jun; 8(2):239.
42. Gurschick L, Mayer DK, Hanson LC. Palliative sedation: an analysis of international guidelines and position statements. Am J Hosp Pall Med. 2015;32(6):660–71. https://doi.org/10.1177/1049909114533002.
43. Cellarius V. A pragmatic approach to palliative sedation. J Palliat Care. 2014;30(3):173–8. PMID:25265741.
44. De Graeff A, Dean M. Palliative sedation therapy in the last weeks of life: a literature review and recommendations for standards. J Palliat Med. 2007;10(1):67–85. https://doi.org/10.1089/jpm.2006.0139.
45. Forde R, Materstvedt LJ, Markestad T, et al. Palliative sedation at the end of life – revised guidelines. Tidsskr Nor Legeforen. 2015;3:135. https://doi.org/10.4045/tidsskr.14.1116.
46. Nathaniel A. Moral reckoning in nursing. West J Nurs Res. 2006;28(4):419–38. https://doi.org/10.1177/0193945905284727.
47. Maeda S, Morita T, Ikenaga M, Abo H, Kizawa Y, Tsuneto S. Changes in opinions on palliative sedation of palliative care specialists over 16 years and their effects on clinical practice. Support Care Cancer. 2018; https://doi.org/10.1007/s00520-018-4497-2. [Epub ahead of print].
48. Davis MS. Palliative sedation: four questions. Prog Palliat Care. 2009;17:203–4. https://doi.org/10.1179/096992609X12455871936946.

49. Henry B. A systematic literature review on the ethics of palliative sedation: an update (2016). Curr Opin Support Palliat Care. 2018;10:201–7. https://doi.org/10.1097/SPC.0000000000000224.
50. Tycross R. Reflections on palliative sedation. Palliat Care. 2019;12:1–16. https://doi.org/10.1177/1178224218823511.
51. Lokker ME, Swart SJ, Rietjensa JAC, et al. Palliative sedation and moral distress: a qualitative study of nurses. App Nurs Res. 2018;40:157–61. https://doi.org/10.1016/j.apnr.2018.02.002.
52. Quill TE. Doctor, I want to die. Will you help me? JAMA. 1993;270(7):870–3. https://doi.org/10.1001/jama.1993.03510070092043.
53. Quill TE. The ambiguity of clinical intentions. N Engl J Med. 1993;329(14):1039–40. https://doi.org/10.1056/NEJM199309303291414.
54. van Deijck RHPD, Hasselaar JGJ, Verhagen SCA, et al. Level of discomfort decreases after the administration of continuous palliative sedation: a prospective multicenter study in hospices and palliative care units. J Pain Symptom Manag. 2016;52(3):361–9. https://doi.org/10.1016/j.jpainsymman.2016.05.008.
55. Zuleta-Benjumea A, Munoz SM, Velez MC, Krikorian A. Level of knowledge, emotional impact and perception about the role of nursing professionals concering palliative sedation. J Clin Nurs. 2018;27:3968–78. https://doi.org/10.1111/jocn.14582.
56. Tursunov O, Cherny NI, Ganz FD. Experiences of family members of dying patients receiving palliative sedation. Oncol Nurs Forum. 2016;43(6):E226–32. https://doi.org/10.1188/16.ONF.E226-E232.
57. Clement de Ciety S, Friedel M, Verhagen E, et al. Please do whatever it takes to end our daughter's suffering! Pediatrics. 2016;137(1):e20153812. https://doi.org/10.1542/peds.2015-3812.
58. Bruinsma S, Rietjens J, van der Heide A. Palliative sedation: a focus group study on the experiences of relatives. J Palliat Med. 2013;16(4):349–55. https://doi.org/10.1089/jpm.2012.0410.
59. Bruinsma SM, Rietjens JAC, Seymour JE, et al. The experiences of relatives with the practice of palliative sedation: a systematic review. J Pain Symptom Manage. 2012; 44:e431–e445. https://doi.org/10.1016/j.jpainsymman.2011.09.006.

Chapter 23
Child Life in the Pediatric ICU

Jessie E. Gordon and Elizabeth Sanders Martin

Child Life Profession Defined

Every day children within the United States, and around the world, find themselves in a hospitalized environment. Visits and admissions can run the gamut from simple blood draws and X-rays to major surgeries, life-changing diagnoses, and, in some cases, PICU admissions. As a whole, the medical field has advanced itself particularly well in recognizing that children are not just "miniature adults" but rather a special subset of patients who need and deserve their own specialists. With the advancement of pediatric specific trained medical specialists from the clinical perspective, the field has also taken a turn to begin recognizing the importance of treating the child's issues from an overall perspective—meaning physically, psychologically, emotionally, socially, developmentally, and spiritually. This framework for treating children has brought about the fundamental idea that while the medical interventions are focused on the child, the overall care is centered on the family. Family-centered care indeed infuses individuals into the interdisciplinary team to address the needs in all of these highly important and recognized areas. One group of individuals working within the interdisciplinary team to address many of these areas of need is child life specialists. In 2014, the American Academy of Pediatrics Committee on Hospital Care released a statement recognizing the overall importance of including these specialists, and child life programs in general, as a standard of care in all US pediatric hospitals [3].

Child life specialists are trained professionals with strong backgrounds in child development and family systems. These individuals also have extensive

J. E. Gordon (✉)
"Just For Kids" Critical Care Center, Norton Children's Hospital, Louisville, KY, USA
e-mail: Jessie.Gordon@Nortonhealthcare.org

E. S. Martin
Norton Children's Hospital, Louisville, KY, USA
e-mail: Elizabeth.SandersMartin@nortonhealthcare.org

P. P. Kamat, J. W. Berkenbosch (eds.), *Sedation and Analgesia for the Pediatric Intensivist*, https://doi.org/10.1007/978-3-030-52555-2_23

clinical experiences within the hospital setting and greatly understand the associated impacts of hospitalization on children and families. Child life specialists' goals surround encouraging positive coping techniques and outcomes for infants, children, adolescents, and young adults [3]. These are accomplished through developmentally appropriate interventions, often including play, to address hospital related fears. Interventions can be centered around, but are not limited to, preparing children for procedures, providing diagnosis specific education, normalizing the hospital environment, providing medical play, encouraging family involvement, providing family or sibling support, and assisting with pain management. Interventions are selected based on a specialist's assessment of the child and situation, which takes into consideration a number of factors. Interventions will vary from child to child and professional to professional based on style and need, but key variables of child development are always kept foundational.

Role of Child Development

In order to meet the needs of a hospitalized child appropriately, we must first have a thorough understanding of how a child's mind thinks and develops. We must not treat a child as a miniature version of an adult but as an individual whose brain and body are still in a constant state of development. It is through two key models of thought that child life specialists utilize expertise in the field of child development. Erik Erikson and Jean Piaget are both thought to be renowned thinkers and foundational within their field of study. Jean Piaget's theory of cognitive development is a stage theory that promotes children as active participants in the learning process and deduces that the formation of intelligence can be separated into four main stages [34]. Erik Erikson's theory of psychosocial development maintains that individuals in infancy through adult develop their personality as they make their way through eight distinct stages, or crises [34]. It is through the lenses of both these theories that child life specialists hone in on what should be considered a normal developmental behavior for a child, and hand in hand with other stress and coping theories, are able to determine and understand the role hospitalization can have on development.

In order to optimize PICU care by all providers, opportunities for staff education on child development are warranted at all levels. For clinical and nonclinical professionals working in the inpatient PICU setting, it is of the utmost importance to have a basic working knowledge of the common reactions we see based on a patient's age or developmental level. At any and all levels, understanding these commonly seen reactions will allow providers to better function as a cooperative member of the interdisciplinary healthcare team and, ultimately, meet the growing and multifaceted needs of the child [15]. Each unit's child life specialist can provide both general and detailed information surrounding development and how it relates specifically to a patient's behavior and reaction within the PICU.

General Principles of Child Life

Procedure-Specific (Refer to "Child Life for Procedural Sedation", Chap. 33)

Diagnosis Education and Preparation

From the age of 5, if not sooner, we send US children to schools to begin formal education in an effort to prepare to send them out into the world to begin their future, a future which they will have prepared for by gaining knowledge and mastery over certain skills to optimize their chances for success. This same practice is implemented by child life professionals within hospital settings as well. When children are given an opportunity to be educated on procedures and diagnoses, they receive the tools they need to set them up for successful coping. By providing hands on, developmentally appropriate education, as well as preparation, we can help dispel misconceptions, provide concrete and realistic information, and even help rehearse and role-play how a scenario might play out [30].

Providing preparation or education for a procedure specifically can involve various modalities, including opportunities for medical play. Medical play involves putting appropriate medical equipment into children's hands to allow them to have control over how it is to be used [21]. In some instances, depending on age and experience, medical play can be reflective of a child's own experiences or perhaps even showcase misconceptions a child might currently have. Having a child demonstrate by "teaching back" and showing on a stuffed animal or doll is an excellent way to assess what the child has been able to retain from the education.

In a critical care setting, while time is often of the essence, when it is in fact available, providing education and/or preparation from the onset is idyllic. The sooner we are able to begin providing support or preparation to a patient, the better. In some instances, children are able to be prepared prior to a planned intubation or other invasive procedure. However, while preparation is often the priority and the standard, education has the opportunity to be beneficial no matter the timing. What is paramount is that the child is provided truthful and consistent information, all while coming from a reliable and trusting source.

Role and Value of Play

Play is without a doubt a powerful tool when working with children. Many often state that play is the work of children and that it is how they learn about the world around them [13]. Child life specialists take this notion to be exceptionally true. Knowing that play is fundamentally a part of who a child is, it therefore becomes fundamental to ensure play is infused into a children's hospital environment, even in critical care. Play has the ability to take on many roles. It can be engaging, silly, educational or informative, dramatic, medically based, and even therapeutic. No matter which of these forms play may take on within a hospital setting, it is always one thing: normalizing. Child life specialists aim to bring normalization into an environment that is far from normal. Therefore, we infuse play, in all its many forms, into all areas of the hospital. Play can help a child act out what they are incapable of verbally expressing, thereby giving providers an understanding into their emotional and coping states. By giving children the freedom to play, child life specialists are again infusing an opportunity to build positive coping skills while facing challenging circumstances.

Stress-Induced PICU Outcomes

Critical illness is often associated with long-lasting negative outcomes after hospital discharge, some that can be lifelong. As members of the interdisciplinary team, child life specialists can play an active role in helping to lessen these outcomes for the patient and family, through non-pharmacological interventions over periods of time while patients are admitted in the PICU. These outcomes and interventions are outlined further in sections below.

Environmental Stressors for Patients

For patients, many of the stressors are related to the environment such as the noise level and bright lights, causing sensory overload. For children of all ages, these can interrupt sleep patterns, influence heart rate and blood pressure, and create a lack of awareness of day- and nighttime cycles. Noise control studies have been conducted in the PICU to increase awareness of staff to the frequency of noise increases for the patients and families. Ear plugs, earphones, and soothing music can help reduce the impact on the patient if appropriate per diagnosis and treatment.

The layout of the rooms can add stress due to the open visibility for medical personnel to monitor. This reduces privacy for adolescents and family members who want to maintain some modesty and confidentiality. Child life specialists can advocate for personal privacy for adolescent patients by using curtains, advocating for closing doors when appropriate, and generally increasing awareness of medical staff about patient's modesty and privacy needs. The size of the room can inhibit parents from feeling welcome and comfortable to remain at the bedside, causing increased anxiety of both parent and patient due to separation. It is encouraging that many hospitals and PICUs are increasingly facilitating family presence at the bedside by expanding visitation hours and changing room designs to incorporate a sleep space, showers, and sitting areas for parents and caregivers to encourage them to stay with their child. Child life specialists can provide activities that encourage the parent or caregiver to engage with the patient in an effort to allow the parent to fulfill their caregiving role. This is especially helpful as caregivers of children in the PICU may 1) feel anxiety about engaging with their child due to the presence of devices or fear regarding their overall medical status and 2) feel somewhat helpless as they perceive that they are failing to fulfill their role as the child's normal caregiver.

Separation from siblings and parents can also add anxiety for the patient, as well as for the healthy sibling(s). Child life specialists can support healthy siblings as they visit their brother/sister in the PICU, as seeing their sibling as patient who is critically ill may be anxiety-invoking. Preparation is key to helping siblings in the PICU environment. Encouraging siblings to speak to and gently touch their brother or sister can not only provide them with a role in the patient's healing, but may also aid in reducing sibling anxiety by providing some "normalization" to their interactions. Education about the hospital and treatment gives the sibling more comfort to be present with their ill and possibly sedated brother or sister. Child life specialists offer play opportunities for siblings and patients to engage with medical equipment to gain mastery and understanding of the medical environment.

Manning et al. [18] wrote that self-esteem and perceived amount of control are stunted up to 6 months following discharge from the PICU. This may impact their behaviors, memory, attention span, and self-confidence. Child life specialists work with the patient using play to give the patient more control and success to build their self-esteem. Talking openly about their hospital admission gives the patient the permission to express their perceptions of their experience. Play allows this to happen in a safe, therapeutic milieu. Giving the patient opportunities to participate in their care, such as putting on their own blood pressure cuff, holding their own thermometer, and administering their own oral medications, also gives them a sense of control over their treatment and their body, helping them to reconnect.

Developmental Stressors for Patients

As children develop, they gain cognitive skills that can influence their ability to encode, recall, and adapt to traumatic events [5]. Their lack of knowledge and experience may negatively impact their understanding of the present world. The result can result in omissions and misconceptions in their perceptions of their environment and interactions. Dow et al. [5] noted that younger children encode with less detail and may be more forgetful than older children. As language, emotional regulation, cognitive inhibition, memory, and reasoning develop, children have a better means of encoding, factual recall, and adaptive coping. Child life specialists and integrative therapies work directly with the developmental level of the child to encourage emotional regulation, factual recall, and positive coping techniques to minimize the possible negative outcomes of pediatric critical care.

The medical equipment required can limit the amount of positive interpersonal touch that parents and family members can provide to enhance developmental growth. These patients also often experience painful or uncomfortable touch from the squeeze of the blood pressure cuff to the daily blood draws, incisions required for surgical procedures or device insertions (chest tubes, intravenous catheters) and non-surgical devices such as urinary or nasogastric catheters. Staveski et al. [28] conducted a study on the use of massage and reading after cardiac surgeries to reduce anxiety and the use of opioids and benzodiazepines in their patients. Intervention patients required less opioids and benzodiazepines, which could have the benefit of decreasing PICU delirium development as well as other adverse outcomes, such as abnormal hippocampal growth, cognitive dysfunction, or abnormal brain development. Those patients receiving massage therapy also scored lower at discharge on Spielberger's State-Trait Anxiety Inventory Child measurement. Peterson [22] noted that infant massage and maternal touch have been shown to lessen the physiological and behavioral responses of stress and pain, reduce levels of cortisol, strengthen the maternal-infant interaction, and increase developmental scores. A study by Guan et al. [10] found that repeated sessions of hand and foot massages increased the amount of parasympathetic activity for critically ill children, slowing the heart rate to allow rest. Significantly, massage therapy can be treatments provided by educated parents or other caregivers, which can allow them to provide both beneficial therapy to their child and aid in the child's recovery.

Minimizing the amount of invasive procedures and bundling nursing care helps the child and the parents reduce their amount of anxiety and delirium [26]. For infants, nursing staff practice of clustering care, meaning they perform multiple tasks together and then allow the child to rest and physically recover, results in improvements in vital signs (lower blood pressure, lower respiratory rate, and lower heart rate). This also allows the parents to plan on when to be present to assist and when to step away to meet their physical needs such as eating and personal care. Child life specialists can work with the nurses and medical team to post times for treatment and medications on the daily schedule.

Hearing a familiar voice can sooth the sedated patient. Child life specialists can record a parent singing or reading a book to their child if they are not able to be present. Books at the bedside allow the siblings and visitors to engage with the patient. Listening to familiar music can aid the older patient in feeling like they have some control over their environment and the younger patient by soothing/comforting.

Patients also bring with them their past experiences and coping styles learned within their family system and other aspects of their home environment. If they have experienced past traumas, the reactions they experienced will tend to develop during their admission, so the hospitalization may be looked upon as akin to an additional trauma. In addition, sedation delays the cognitive and emotional processing that occurs naturally within our brain and body, leaving gaps in the child's linear memory. Consequently, these patients may struggle to understand what is happening to them as well as their emotions that arise during the admission. Sedation reduces the amount of cognitive and emotional processing that can occur in the PICU and creates a disconnection from the body and mind as awareness decreases [36]. Child life specialists can collaborate with integrative therapies to incorporate various narrative interventions such as a PICU diary, journaling, and scrapbooking. Documenting the patient's story helps the patient gain a better understanding of what actually happened to them and why. Another technique that can be helpful is for parents and staff to maintain a PICU diary for the patient as a reflection of their experience [11]. The diary is designed to remain at the bedside and is used to document important moments or events in the patient's care. Dryden-Palmer [6] noted the diaries must remain nontechnical and true to the caregiver's interaction. Nursing staff are encouraged to write down facts about the treatment of the day and any responses the patient may have displayed. The parents are also encouraged to share their thoughts and experiences during their stay in the PICU. An extension of this is the use of scrapbooking as a way to photo document the patient's admission and for the parents to journal their emotions and thoughts for the patient [24]. Outpatient counseling following discharge can also help those 25–40% of patients and families who develop post-traumatic stress disorder and other negative psychosocial outcomes associated with post-intensive care syndrome [7].

Early Mobility

Early mobility or "EM" is a term used to describe physical activity and rehabilitation early on in critical illness [2]. While EM has yet to become the standard in care across all PICU settings, much research is being performed within the field to show clinical significance for this population. Some hospitals have gone as far as to develop multidisciplinary Early Mobility Committee(s) in an effort to assist with protocols related to EM within the PICU [2]. Child life specialists can play an active role in instituting opportunities for patients to engage in EM, even while ventilated, on ECMO, or a VAD device. Foremost, allowing the child life specialist time to establish rapport with the child will help them build a sense of trust with the individual. When obstacles or new opportunities that often bring about fear for a child are involved, having a trusted individual involved can be of the utmost importance and help achieve patient buy-in with the new intervention. Child life specialists can assist members of the healthcare team with providing opportunities for positive encouragement, appropriate play based on current abilities, caregiver involvement, and affirmation. Utilizing knowledge of behavior will allow the child life specialist to help guide the team in what to possibly expect from the child and assist with the incorporation of appropriate expectations for EM sessions. Further, if the child is viewed as becoming under too much duress, the child life specialist may also advocate for the shortening of length of time, or perhaps a different activity, etc.

PICU Delirium

The word delirium is used in many ways and settings, but when referenced in the context of the PICU, it is described as having an acute onset of symptoms, including change or fluctuation in baseline mental status, inattention, and either disorganized thinking or an altered level of consciousness [1]. While statistics vary, some data show that up to 66% of patients in the PICU are estimated to be diagnosed with delirium [1, 16, 19, 27, 32]. While pharmacological means are often a priority for preventing or managing delirium, there are also a number of nonpharmacological methods of environment modification that can contribute to delirium care as well.

All clinical and nonclinical staff have an opportunity to assist with PICU delirium care, but parents and caregivers also play a very important role. Child life specialists have the ability to provide education about delirium in an effort to make caregivers better understand the condition and, therefore, be able to assist with environmental modifications. Delirium teaching sheets and handouts can be very helpful in spelling out what the condition is, why it is caused, and what specifically can be done. Clinical bedside staff can also benefit from education, specifically about developmental milestones, as they assess the patient for delirium. While several delirium screening tools exist, including the Cornell Assessment for Pediatric Delirium (CAPD) [31] and the pediatric Confusion Assessment Method for the ICU (pCAM-ICU) [27], due to its ease of use, the CAPD has become the more widely used tool across the field and has become the standard screening method in numerous PICUs [25]. Since part of the standard assessment tools for delirium look at behavior, knowledge of age and developmentally appropriate behavior for children assist with giving nurses an appropriate baseline.

Along with education, overall environmental modifications are one of the best ways child life specialists can help parents and caregivers engage in strategies for delirium prevention and management. Helping to provide a calm and reassuring environment within the room with things like pictures that are familiar can be beneficial. It is also encouraged to allow the child to have favorite toys, blankets, music, and other personal items. Reminders of where the child is, what they are doing there, and the date can also be helpful to assist when appropriate.

"Mixing up days and nights" is another significant factor associated with PICU delirium. Child life specialists can work with families and caregivers on creating daily schedules to help assist with re-coordinating sleep cycles. Of additional help can be reminders to keep lights on during daytime hours and set specific times for lights out to facilitate sleep. Having all healthcare team members on board with day-night routines is of the utmost importance as we strive to return a patient to a normal day-night cycle.

Pain Management

It is of no surprise that pain is often a major negative experience for pediatric patients in the critical care setting. It is of vital importance that the clinical team consistently assesses as well as effectively treats a child's pain. However, children's understanding and perceptions of pain as well as their ability to describe and accurately report it can make pain evaluation and, therefore, appropriate treatment challenging. Many times, children confuse the specific differences between pain, agitation or discomfort, and anxiety [28]. Once again, while pharmacological means are often the priority in addressing a child's pain, child life specialist's interventions can also make a powerful impact.

As mentioned in previous sections, play is the most natural form of communication for a child. Even in the midst of pain, we can often find a child engaged in play. What we know to be true is that when compared to other children, a child who is relatively calm, with pain that is being managed, is less likely to be anxious or fearful of the PICU environment and may respond better to comforting and distraction by familiar staff and family members [1]. All in all, distraction through play has the ability to help breakthrough bouts of certain levels of pain.

Another opportunity to engage patients in pain control is through deep and controlled breathing exercises. Our brain and our body are without a doubt interconnected. It is important to recognize that how we feel impacts our breathing and, conversely, how we are breathing impacts how we feel [14]. Our natural inclination when pain is present is to hold our breath, when in fact deep breathing may actually be less restricting and more beneficial in helping with relaxation [14]. Child life specialists use child-friendly techniques such as "blowing out the candle" or even blowing bubbles to teach children to take long deep breaths. With slightly older school-age and adolescent children, belly breathing and square breathing, techniques that both utilize counting, can be beneficial. All of these interventions cause children to focus internally on their breath, in a way that is developmentally appropriate, and can lead to better pain control in some contexts.

Finally, guided imagery can also be offered as an intervention technique to help assist with pain management. Imagery is defined as either the spontaneous or deliberate mental reconstructions of things, such as sights, sounds, smells, tastes, and even feelings, in a manner as if they were actually occurring [14]. Guided imagery is when an individual helps facilitate or *guide* someone through this process. The goal of guided imagery with children and adolescents is to help promote feelings of relaxation, which in turn will help with pain receptors, breathing, and the management of pain in general. There are several guided imagery books and scripts available over the Internet or in print form that are appropriate to be utilized with children. While guided imagery intervention attempts are not successful with all individuals, it can be a very beneficial pain management technique for some populations.

Positive Touch, Swaddling, and Infant Massage

It is without hesitation that we admit most of the physical touch that happens within the confines of a PICU has a negative association. And furthermore, this touch is often associated with pain. Positive touch is associated with healthy development for a child along with being an important aspect of nonverbal communication (*The Handbook of Child Life*). Therefore, it is imperative that we infuse elements of positive touch whenever possible into a child's daily routine.

Encouraging parents and caregivers to engage in positive touch can often be blocked by the physical barrier of medical devices that are on or near children in a critical care environment. Many times, a child is intertwined with so many devices that it can be overwhelming to a caregiver to know where they can touch their child or if it is even allowed. It is important that we advocate to bedside clinical staff that they show family caregivers places they can provide light, gentle soothing touch on a patient that is in a critical state. Gentle strokes, hand-holding, and brushing hair can all be examples of positive touch. Further, medical caregivers can also engage in positive touch by using verbal communication to narrate what they are going to do. Sometimes, the anticipation of something negative about to happen is more overwhelming than the procedure or event that will actually take place. If bedside clinical staff can use positive, calming words to explain their actions, there is an opportunity to lessen the fear of possible oncoming negative touch occurring.

For infants that are admitted to the intensive care unit, positive touch from caregivers may also come in the form of both swaddling and infant massage. It is well known that close body contact along with being carried reduces infant distress and crying (Kuttner, et al., 2010). However, these two forms of soothing are often not options while an infant is in a critical care environment. However, newer studies are showing that swaddling (wrapping snugly in a blanket or cloth) also makes an infant feel more secure and has the possibility to reduce the pulse rate in response to procedural pain [8]. Therefore, even when holding or skin-to-skin contact is not an option for an intubated patient, swaddling or facilitated tucking can still be done in an effort to reduce possible pain. Infant massage, when approved by an attending physician, also has the opportunity to serve as an intervention to possibly reduce infant pain. Individuals who are trained as infant massage instructors can help teach parents or caregivers simple techniques to provide infant massage to age appropriate children. These techniques have the ability to also offer positive touch, provide soothing, and in some cases reduce levels of pain. Furthermore, they provide parents and caregivers the opportunity for an involved participatory role in the care of their child while admitted to the hospital, which can both alleviate parental anxiety and provide them the acknowledgement that they can, indeed, play a real role in their child's healing and recovery.

Communication

Communication can also become a major difficulty for patients while in the PICU. Due to many patients being intubated, verbal communication becomes impeded and other forms of communication must be found. In conjunction with speech language pathologists, child life specialists are able to work in developmentally appropriate ways to find interventions that will assist patients in communicating with caregivers and members of their family. For some, standard written communication boards are used. While for others, personalized boards are made, or even high-tech iPad applications can be utilized. The goal is always similar in that we want to ensure the patient has a way to communicate their needs and feelings as simply as possible.

Family Stressors

Parents and Caregivers

Parents have their own set of stressors when their child is admitted to the PICU. Studies have shown that parents of children admitted to the PICU have greater anxiety than those whose children are admitted to the general pediatric wards. Rzucidlo and Campbell [23] stated "parental traumatic stress has been found to contribute to child traumatic stress symptoms" (p. 132). Davidson et al. [4] added that 25–50% of family members of critically ill children experience psychological symptoms during and after the PICU admission. They call these symptoms (acute stress, generalized anxiety, depression, and post-traumatic stress) "Post-Intensive Care Syndrome –Family" (104).

Often the parents have to make difficult decisions. Stremler et al. [29] found that parents who lived near the hospital had greater decisional conflict than those who lived further away (31–60 km). The same study showed that parents who lived nearby demonstrated less anxiety than those who live a greater distance from the hospital. Stremler et al. [29] added that more than half of the parents displayed signs of major depression within the first few days of admission.

Hill et al. [12] and Stremler et al. [29] mention the PICU environment as a stressor for parents, factors including the limited space in the patient room, the lack of privacy in the waiting rooms, and limited bathroom access for parents. Studies have shown that proximity to the patient is extremely important to the parent and helps to decrease some anxiety. Many of these rooms are open or separated only by a curtain, which allows both care personnel and other families to hear private conversations. Conversely, this openness exposes families to noise or distressing sounds from other patients and/or their family members. It can be particularly distressing for parents to witness another patient acutely deteriorating or even coding, and the multiple staff required to stabilize or resuscitate the child is often chaotic, loud, and intense and concerns for parents that the events could be occurring in their child are almost certainly present, even if subconsciously. Hill et al. [12] noted that the waiting room may be filled with anxious and upset family members, who may display distressing or threatening behaviors, and often no one is present or available to help maintain emotional regulation and control. Parents also find entering the PICU from the waiting room to be time-consuming per Hill et al. [12].

Seeing their child for the first time after surgery from injury or intubation from respiratory distress may greatly increase anxiety and depression for the parents. When initially admitted to the PICU, many children are (or become) swollen and may be attached to multiple life-assisting machines or devices. This can be overwhelming to parents. Concern about the prognosis for their child can also cause anxiety and inability of the healthcare team to be able to provide assurances in many cases may worsen this anxiety. After several days, the realization that their child may not regain their prior abilities may lead to additional depression and despair in the parents. Studies have noted the benefit of linking families within the PICU as a way to express their emotions and reduce the isolation parents felt within the PICU environment [4, 29]. Having a trained staff member to facilitate may also allow the parents to relate with a mental health professional that can offer more one-on-one assistance if needed. Providing refreshments in a quiet area near the PICU may increase more participation as the parents can remain close to their child while meeting some personal needs. Encouraging peer-to peer support can help parents relate to each other and share what they may not be able to express or ask the medical team or their own family members.

Lack of sleep has psychological impact on parents, and studies consistently report disruption in sleep patterns, quality, and amount of sleep, leading to sleep deprivation in parents of PICU patients. This can lead to hypersensitivity to pain and cognitive dysfunction in parents who are often asked to make life-altering decisions. Child life specialists can encourage parents to use the daily schedule set for their child as a way to schedule rest for themselves, helping with day and night awareness. Finding avenues for parents to get outside and possibly exercise may help with sleep patterns also. Offering soothing music with headphones can encourage rest.

Communication has been a well-described factor contributing to stress for parents in the PICU, as many of them have never been in a hospital or have familiarity/understanding of medical terminology. Limited and sporadic information poses a barrier for parents to gain meaning of their child's illness or injury and, therefore, feel like they can make adequately informed decisions regarding the care of the patient. Including the parents in daily rounds shows respect towards the parents in making decisions about their child's future. One study focused on the value of parental intuition as well as relying on the medical staff to make these important decisions [17]. This study also noted the value of spirituality in making decisions about their child's care. When parents do not speak English or have differing cultural beliefs, they may receive very little information even with an interpreter [35]. Some parents have noted the amount, frequency, style, and content of the communication from medical staff are beneficial in reducing anxiety. Studies have shown that clear goals and treatment plans are essential for patients and families. These goals and plans can be implemented in writing on dry erase boards in the patient room to help remind parents and motivate the patient. Using "layman's language" helps the patient and parent to better understand what is expected. These boards can also include comfort measures such as pacifier or favorite blanket or stuffed animal to help inform about ways to soothe patient. Studies have shown that frequent medical updates, understandable language, and education about the patient help reduce the anxiety experienced by the patient. Davidson et al. [4] recommend the use of routine interdisciplinary family conferences in the PICU to improve family satisfaction, to build trust with the medical team, and to meet family needs as they arise. Child life and integrative therapies can participate in these meetings to advocate for the family and provide services as needed.

Often families are torn between the hospital and home, especially if they have multiple children. Finding someone they trust to care for their other children can cause more stress, especially if they are a single parent or have recently moved. Some families experience injuries while traveling, which forces them to stay in an unfamiliar location. Parents who work full time may exhibit more decisional conflict than parents on parental leave [29]. Parents often have to juggle many roles and responsibilities, such as child care, employment, and care of the house and pets. Advocating for parents to take a break from the hospital and take care of some of these responsibilities can reassure them and reduce anxiety. Referring parents to the chaplain, psychologist, or social worker may give the parents some reprieve from the guilt of not being able to meet all needs at the present and to help prioritize.

Very few studies have shown that medical personnel directly ask the parents and family members about any past traumas that either the parents or the patient have experienced. These past traumas may influence how well the parents are able to comprehend any medical information about the patient and cope within the intensive care environment. The previous traumas may also cause distrust by the parents toward the medical team. Learning this trauma history may be helpful in understanding the parents and how they relate with the staff, their sedated child, and the medical treatment [37]. Many parents may experience vicarious traumatization as they view their children as a part of themselves. Many studies have shown that parental stress, whether acute or chronic, will impact their child negatively if not addressed [20, 23, 37]. Parents can benefit from many of the narrative and expressive therapies provided by child life and integrative therapies, to cope not only with the current crisis in the PICU but also their previous traumas that are impacting this admission.

Scrapbooking provides parents with an outlet to meet other parents, share their stories verbally, photo document their stories, and journal their thoughts and emotions [24]. The final product can become a treasured memoir about their experience in the hospital. From leaving the room to receive a new heart to the first skin-to-skin contact with their newborn, the parents can not only show the photograph but also then add their reactions to the milestone their child experienced. Many parents choose to incorporate the medical staff that became part of their PICU "family" during their extended admission. One family used their scrapbook to show the patient what he missed while he was unconscious for 2 weeks, which can be a significant aid in helping the child cope with their PICU experience once discharged and the resources of the hospital are no longer as present.

Siblings

For siblings, the stressors include lack of knowledge about the patient's health condition and treatment required, leaving them to create their own ideas that are often misconceptions and based on egocentric development. Many times, the parents are fearful of clearly informing the siblings about the patient's condition. In addition, the parents may be fearful of bringing the siblings to the PICU to visit the patient. The siblings are influenced by the parents' anxiety so they become fearful as well. Child life specialists are trained to educate and prepare siblings to visit the patient within the hospital. They can also speak with the parents about how to tell the sibling of the patient's injuries or illness, using language that is developmentally appropriate. This can relieve the burden from already stressed parents of explaining to their other children situations and conditions that they themselves might not fully understand, and, for siblings, demystification of their siblings condition can be anxiety reducing and better aid their ability to remain at home and cope until the PICU process is completed.

The admission in the PICU causes disruptions in the family routine. The parents feel torn about being at the hospital, while so many of the siblings are forced to take on family activities that the parents performed prior. With prolonged admissions, the siblings may begin to feel emotionally neglected by the parents. Some children will act out to show their frustrations and struggle, especially when their vocabulary is still developing. With parents torn between home and hospital, the siblings may have changes in their routine, beginning with who is caring for them if both parents are present with the patient during the initial admission to PICU. An important factor to remember is the siblings may have a trauma history, which can be triggered with the admission of the patient. These children may also behave with similar trauma reactions they have learned from their parents. Some hospitals provide sibling groups or meet individually with a sibling to explore their understanding and provide emotional outlets to express concerns. Child life specialists may host family meals on the unit to encourage time together with the siblings and should, additionally, be encouraged by the PICU team to engage with siblings throughout the hospital admission to identify coping issues and directly provide support or direct caregivers to get them the support they additionally need before maladaptive behaviors become ingrained.

End-of-Life Care

While the ultimate outcome for a critical care patient is always curative and based on returning to a life of normalcy and quality at home, that is unfortunately not the case for all patients [33]. When we do have patients that transition to end-of-life care, child life specialists can play a very important role in supporting the patient, family, and in many cases even the staff.

Death and Dying

Child life specialists have received extensive training in understanding developmental concepts of death and dying in an effort to best meet the needs of children. Whether it be the patient themselves, or a sibling, friend, cousin, etc., recognizing how a child understands and views death is of the utmost importance. This brings us back to models of coping and child development theories in an effort to understand how a child's brain is processing. Assisting a child during this time requires extensive assessment and minute attention to detail in order to meet the needs most appropriately. There is not simply a "one-size-fits-all" approach but rather sets of parameters that must be considered before working with a child. Variables to consider include, but are not limited to, age and developmental level, prior experiences with death, spiritual beliefs of family, presence or involvement in trauma, the context of the current death, the patient's current and preexisting health condition, and the wishes of the family. All of these variables combined will determine what interventions from the child life specialist will look like.

Memory Making and Legacy Building

One dynamic opportunity that is commonly presented to end-of-life families no matter the variables or circumstances surrounding the death is memory making. Memory making constitutes interventions whose goals are to provide tangible items to families and caregivers to help them remember their loved one. Specific memory-making interventions vary from facility to facility but typically capture things such as a patient's handprint, footprint, fingerprints, or even their voice or heartbeat. Memory making can be completed pre- or postmortem depending on the physician, family, and facility's choice in the matter. Memory making as a whole has limited quantitative data to support its clinical significance. However, from a qualitative feedback perspective, the results are most commonly positive. Memory making should always be offered to families as an option, not as an obligation they must agree to, as some families choose to decline this offering based on their own personal preferences about remembering their child or spiritual beliefs.

Legacy building provides another dynamic opportunity to create tangible items for families to remember their loves one by, but it does require involvement of the patient themselves. According to [9], when there are children and adolescents who are living with a terminal illness, efforts to build memories and confirm they are loved and will indeed be remembered are important. Again, while there is little quantitative data to support its use, legacy building provides a planned opportunity for a patient to utilize their creativity in leaving a "legacy" for their loved ones. This can be through the writing of letters, creating a piece of meaningful artwork, using photography, leaving their wishes, etc., all in an effort to leave an imprint of their legacy behind. While in hospital, child life specialists can work with patients able to participate with them in building some of these legacy pieces.

Post-intensive Care Syndrome

Recently, research has focused on post-intensive care syndrome and its impact on patients and families. Post-intensive care syndrome is described as the new development or increased presence of physical, cognitive, or psychological impairments shortly after a critical illness or injury and lasting for a period of time after discharge

[7]. Studies have shown that upwards of one third of PICU survivors develop this syndrome [11]. This may impact not only the patient but also the caregivers and the family members. Symptoms include sleep deprivation, anxiety, depression, complex grief, and PTSD. As many patients may be admitted to the PICU due to an injury or critical illness, the parents may experience vicarious traumatization as they often consider their child as a piece or extension of themselves. Some patients may sustain life-changing injuries or treatment that will alter their care afterward. This may be considered by some as traumatic, such as receiving a tracheostomy or gastric tube. Post-traumatic stress disorder can impact cognitive functioning and development as well as deregulate emotions. As a result, physical abilities can be impacted negatively. These symptoms can persist for months or years.

Bessel van der Kolk [36] adds that many traumas within our history can be retriggered. Many parents have experienced some sort of trauma within their childhood. So, when their child is hurt or seriously ill, these parents may display behavior that is either uncharacteristic or even irrational, leaving the staff to define them as difficult or unruly. Rzucidlo and Campbell [23] point out that most families have some preexisting coping styles that can utilized with medical staff, extended family, and members of their community. Child life specialists learn about these coping mechanisms (strengths) and use them to help the family and patient through their admission.

Utilizing various integrative therapies within the hospital setting can help reduce the impact of the PICU syndrome for patients and families. Expressive therapies can offer narrative therapy, which helps to reduce PTSD by telling their stories and giving the patient and/or parent a sense of understanding. Using the diaries or journal technique can help fill in memory gaps that trauma can cause. For patients, positive touch can be very effective for bonding of the parent and patient. The use of body movement through yoga, art, music, and dance has been found helpful in reducing PTSD in adults and children. Expression of emotions through art and music interventions are known to reduce anxiety and depression. Research has shown that social connection has been helpful during the PICU admission. A trained professional can facilitate a parent group to allow parents to connect and share about their experiences.

Areas for Future Growth

When comparing the child life profession to others within the field of medicine, the field itself is still in its infancy. Like anything in this stage, we have made exceptional gains and also have room for exceptional growth. With the backing and support of the American Academy of Pediatrics, the expectation is now clear that child life specialists should be found in every pediatric hospital facility within the United States. Further, the AAP and the Association of Child Life Professionals are laying out unit and population-specific expectations and even patient to specialist ratios for hospital administrations to use as best practices. But what is lacking in all of these recommendations is the current quantitative and qualitative data to support the actual changes. What difference are child life specialists actually making? The field itself is built on principals of child developmental theorists that will withhold the test of time. But to remain current and applicable, research and data are desperately needed.

With incorporation of quality, scholarly research, there is a hope to have a better illustration of the stressors that exist within the critical care environment—for patients and family members and caregivers. When we have this fully illustrated picture of stressors, we then must also recognize that child life specialists are not the only answer. The answer draws out more broadly to an overarching multidisciplinary team approach. There is an opportunity to integrate multiple therapeutic modalities into pediatric critical care environments, and we must simply showcase the need. Art therapy, music therapy, psychology, etc. all have a significant role they can play in supporting the needs of hospitalized families as they cope with the various stressors, and each in their own unique way.

References

1. Bettencourt A, Mullen JE. Delirium in children: identification, prevention, and management. Crit Care Nurse. 2017;37(3):e9–e18. https://doi.org/10.4037/ccn2017692.
2. Betters KA, Hebbar KB, Farthing D, et al. Development and implementation of an early mobility program for mechanically ventilated pediatric patients. J Crit Care. 2017;41:303–8. https://doi.org/10.1016/j.jcrc.2017.08.004.
3. Committee on Hospital Care and Child Life Council, Pediatrics. 2014;133(5):e1471–e1478. https://doi.org/10.1542/peds.2014-0556.
4. Davidson JE, Aslakson RA, Long AC, et al. Guidelines for family-centered care in the neonatal, pediatric, and adult PICU. Crit Care Med. 2017;45(1):103–28. http://search.ebscohost.com/login.aspx?direct=true&db=mdc&AN=27984278&site=ehost-live. Accessed March 29, 2019
5. Dow BL, Kenardy JA, Long DA, Le Brocque RM. Cognitive/affective factors are associated with children's acute posttraumatic stress following pediatric intensive care. Psychol Trauma Theory Res Pract Policy. 2019;11(1):55–63. https://doi.org/10.1037/tra0000349.
6. Dryden-Palmer. Karen Dell PICU Diaries: A simple and promising family-centered intervention. Pediatric Crit Care Med. 2019;20(2):p. 208–09. https://doi.org/10.1097/PCC.0000000000001838.
7. Esses S, Small S, Rodemann A, Hartman M. Post-intensive care syndrome: educational interventions for parents of hospitalized children. Am J Crit Care. 2019;28(1):19–27.
8. Fearon I, Kisilevsky BS, Mains SM, Muir DW, Tranmer J. Swaddling after heel lance. J Dev Behav Pediatr. 1997;18(4) https://doi.org/10.1097/00004703-199708000-00002.
9. Foster TL, Dietrich MS, Friedman DL, Gordon JE, Gilmer MJ. Legacy-making activities survey. PsycTESTS Dataset. 2012; https://doi.org/10.1037/t36811-000.
10. Guan L, Collet JP, Yuskiv N, Skippen P, Brant R, Kissoon N. The effect of massage therapy on autonomic activity in critically ill children. Evid Based Complement Alternat Med. 2014;2014:656750.
11. Herrup EA, Wieczorek B, Kudchadkar SR. Feasibility and perceptions of PICU diaries. Pediatr Critical Care Med. 2019;20(2):e83–90. https://doi.org/10.1097/PCC.0000000000001814.
12. Hill C, Knafl KA, Santacroce SJ. Family-centered care from the perspective of parents of children cared for in a pediatric intensive care unit: an integrative review. J Pediatr Nurs. 2017; https://doi.org/10.1016/j.pedn.2017.11.007.
13. Jessee P, Gaynard L. Paradigms of play. In: Thompson R, editor. The Handbook of child life: a guide for pediatric psychosocial care. Springfield: Charles C Thomas Publisher Ltd.; 2009. p. 220–37.
14. Kuttner L. A child in pain: what health professionals can do to help. Wales: Crown House; 2010.
15. Lisanti AJ, Cribben J, Connock EM, Lessen R, Medoff-Cooper B. Developmental care rounds: an interdisciplinary approach to support developmentally appropriate care of infants born with complex congenital heart disease. Clin Perinatol. 2016;43(1):147–56. https://doi.org/10.1016/j.clp.2015.11.010.
16. Luetz A, Gensel D, Muller J, et al. Validity of different delirium assessment tools for critically ill children: covariates matter. Crit Care Med. 2016;44(11):2060–9.

17. Madrigal V, Carroll K, Faerber J, Walter J, Morrison W, Feudtner C. Parental sources of support and guidance when making difficult decisions in the pediatric intensive care unit. J Pediatr. 2019;169:221–226.e4.
18. Manning J, Redsell S, Latour J. Should out of sight mean out of mind? Challenging the role of paediatric intensive care in understanding and supporting children and families following childhood critical illness. Br Assoc Critical Care Nurses. 2016;21(5):262–4.
19. Meyburg J, Dill ML, Traube C, Silver G, von Haken R. Patterns of postoperative delirium in children. Pediatr Crit Care Med. 2017;18(2):128–33.
20. Nugent N, Ostrowski S, Christopher N, Delahanty D. Parental posttraumatic stress symptoms as a moderator of child's acute biological response and subsequent posttraumatic stress symptoms in pediatric injury. J Pediatr Psychol. 2007;32(3):309–18.
21. Pearson L. Child life interventions in critical care and at the end of life. In: Thompson R, editor. The Handbook of child life: a guide for pediatric psychosocial care. Springfield: Charles C Thomas Publisher Ltd.; 2009. p. 220–37.
22. Peterson JK. Supporting optimal neurodevelopmental outcomes in infants and children with congenital heart disease. Crit Care Nurse. 2018;38(3):68–74. https://doi.org/10.4037/ccn2018514.
23. Rzucidlo S, Campbell M. Beyond the physical injuries: child and parent coping with medical traumatic stress after pediatric trauma. J Trauma Nurs. 2009;16(3):130–5.
24. Schwarz B, Fatzinger C, Meier P. RUSH special Kare keepsakes: families celebrating the NPICU journey. Am J Matern Child Nurs. 2004;29(6):354–61.
25. Silver G, Kearney J, Traube C, Hertzig M. Delirium screening anchored in child development: the Cornell assessment for pediatric delirium. Palliat Support Care. 2015;13(4):1005–11. https://doi.org/10.1017/S1478951514000947.
26. Simone S, Edwards S, Lardieri A, et al. Implementation of an PICU bundle: an interprofessional quality improvement project to enhance delirium management and monitor delirium prevalence in a single PICU. Pediatr Critical Care Med. 2017;18(6):531–40. https://doi.org/10.1097/PCC.0000000000001127.
27. Smith HA, Boyd J, Fuchs DC, et al. Diagnosing delirium in critically ill children: validity and reliability of the pediatric confusion assessment method for the intensive care unit. Crit Care Med. 2011;39(1):150–7.
28. Staveski SL, Boulanger K, Erman L, et al. The impact of massage and reading on children's pain and anxiety after cardiovascular surgery: a pilot study. Pediatr Critical Care Med. 2018;19(8):725–32. https://doi.org/10.1097/PCC.0000000000001615.
29. Stremler R, Haddad S, Pullenayegum E, Parshuram C. Psychological outcomes in parents of critically ill hospitalized children. J Pediatr Nurs. 2017;34:36–43.
30. Squires V, Allen K. The emergency department and ambulatory care. In: Thompson R, editor. The Handbook of child life: a guide for pediatric psychosocial care. Springfield: Charles C Thomas Publisher Ltd.; 2009. p. 220–37.
31. Traube C, Silver G, Kearney J, et al. Cornell assessment of pediatric delirium: a valid, rapid, observational tool for screening delirium in the PICU*. Crit Care Med. 2014;42(3):656–63.
32. Traube C, Silver G, Reeder RW, et al. Delirium in critically ill children: an international point prevalence study. Crit Care Med. 2017;45(4):584–90.
33. Truog RD, Meyer EC, Burns JP. Toward interventions to improve end-of-life care in the pediatric intensive care unit. Crit Care Med. 2006;34(Suppl) https://doi.org/10.1097/01.ccm.0000237043.70264.87.
34. Turner J. Theoretical foundations of child life practice. In: Thompson R, editor. The Handbook of child life: a guide for pediatric psychosocial care. Springfield: Charles C Thomas Publisher Ltd.; 2009. p. 220–37.
35. Van Cleave A, Roosen-Runge M, Miller A, Milner L, Karkazis K, Magnus D. Quality of communication in interpreted versus noninterpreted PICU family meetings. Crit Care Med. 2014;42:1507–17.
36. Van der Kolk B. The body keeps the score. New York: Viking Penguin; 2014.
37. Watson RS, Choong K, Colville G, Crow S, Dervan L, Hopkins R, Knoester H, Pollack M, Rennick J, Curley MQ. Life after critical illness in children-toward an understanding of pediatric post-intensive care syndrome. J Pediatr. 2018;198:16–24.

Part VI
Procedural Sedation

Chapter 24
Introduction to Procedural Sedation Within and Outside the ICU

Kristin A. Tiedt, Juan P. Boriosi, and Gregory A. Hollman

Pediatric procedural sedation conducted outside of the operating room setting has increased steadily in the past couple of decades and is ubiquitous in any hospital that cares for children. While no one pediatric subspecialty inherently owns sedation, sedation is a prominent part of Pediatric Critical Care Medicine (PCCM) practice both within and outside the PICU. Within the PICU, performing invasive and stressful procedures on children at bedside is a routine part of day-to-day care [1]. Outside the PICU, PCCM physicians are frequently at the center of providing procedural sedation within an institution. Indeed, most sedation programs belonging to the Pediatric Sedation Research Consortium (PSRC), a group of over 30 sedation centers that prospectively record sedation encounters, are based out of critical care medicine programs [2–4].

On the surface, PCCM physicians, by virtue of their training, experience, and expertise, are well suited to perform procedural sedation on children. Yet, like many skills and competencies required in critical care, procedural sedation poses a number of special requirements and challenges to the PCCM practitioner. This chapter will provide an overview of pediatric procedural sedation and discuss the monitoring and management guidelines developed by the American Academy of Pediatrics (AAP). The subsequent sections will discuss the necessary components that are the basis of high-quality procedural sedation.

K. A. Tiedt · J. P. Boriosi · G. A. Hollman (✉)
Department of Pediatrics, University of Wisconsin School of Medicine and Public Health, Madison, WI, USA
e-mail: ghollman@pediatrics.wisc.edu

P. P. Kamat, J. W. Berkenbosch (eds.), *Sedation and Analgesia for the Pediatric Intensivist*, https://doi.org/10.1007/978-3-030-52555-2_24

Overview of Pediatric Procedural Sedation

With the rising number of procedures performed on pediatric patients outside of the operating room, there has been an increased need for awareness and guidance of procedural sedations by non-anesthesiologists. These settings include inpatient units, outpatient clinics, imaging centers, and dental offices, with sedations conducted by individuals from various medical backgrounds, including the PCCM physician. The 2016 American Academy of Pediatrics (AAP) guidelines outline the necessary components required in the selection, monitoring, and management of pediatric patients in order to promote safe and effective procedural sedation [5]. Adherence to these guidelines, which are based on the intended level of sedation depth for a pediatric patient, highlights the importance of vigilant monitoring to promote rapid recognition of changes in respiratory and cardiovascular status [5, 6]. The guidelines further emphasize that the depth of sedation for a given patient exists on a continuum and that the provider conducting the sedation must possess the skills to rescue a patient from a level of sedation deeper than originally intended [5, 7].

The Sedation Continuum

In 1985, the AAP released consensus guidelines for the use of elective sedation and general anesthesia in the pediatric patient [8]. These guidelines defined three distinct levels of sedation – conscious, deep, and general anesthesia – based upon a patient's level of consciousness and response to external stimuli while receiving sedation medications. Since the release of this document, the terms used to describe a patient's level of sedation have evolved into the currently used terminology of minimal, moderate, and deep sedation and general anesthesia [5, 6]. Despite clear distinctions made between levels of sedation, it is largely recognized that a degree of fluidity and overlap exists between the levels, with the risk of airway compromise and respiratory depression increasing with greater sedation depth and illness severity (Fig. 24.1).

Patients may have variable responses to sedative drugs, and what may lead to minimal sedation in one patient could result in moderate sedation in another. Additionally, patients may fluctuate between different levels of sedation during any given procedure due to a number of factors, including dosing and timing of drug administration and the degree of stimulation. The ability for a patient to drift into a level of sedation deeper than intended requires timely recognition of these shifts on the part of the provider and competency of that provider to adjust monitoring and management accordingly in order to detect and respond to changes in cardiorespiratory status [7]. Failure to recognize changes in sedation depth could result in a delayed response to a critical respiratory event, leading to serious consequences, such as hypoxemic brain injury, cardiovascular decompensation, and even death [5].

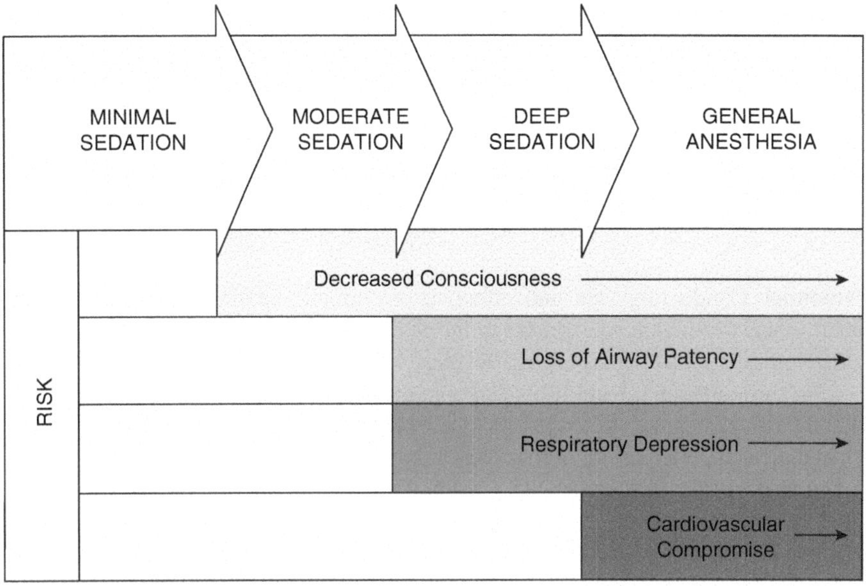

Fig. 24.1 Levels of sedation and categories of risk for ASA Class I and II. Greater risk in each of the categories increases with increasing depth of sedation. Note: Patients ASA Class III or greater are at greater risk at lower levels of sedation

Minimal Sedation Minimal sedation is a drug-induced state (e.g. anxiolysis) during which patients otherwise remain awake. Cardiovascular and respiratory functions remain generally unaffected, though patients may display impairment in their cognition and coordination. Minimal sedation is considered a low risk clinical activity though patients require observation and assessment of sedation level, as they can transition into a state of moderate sedation. Patients meeting criteria for moderate sedation should be managed according to moderate sedation guidelines [5, 6, 9].

Moderate Sedation Moderate sedation is a drug-induced depression in consciousness during which patients maintain a purposeful response to verbal and light tactile stimuli. Despite this depression in consciousness, patients remain able to maintain a patent airway and adequate ventilation. Cardiovascular function is typically not affected [5, 6, 9].

Deep Sedation Deep sedation is a drug-induced depression of consciousness during which patients are unable to respond purposefully to verbal or light tactile stimuli. Though difficult to arouse, patients maintain a present but blunted response to repeated tactile and painful stimuli. Airway patency, protective airway reflexes, and spontaneous ventilation may be impaired, requiring additional assistance from the sedation provider for maintenance of adequate respiratory function. Cardiovascular function is typically preserved [5, 6, 9].

General Anesthesia General anesthesia is a drug-induced loss of consciousness during which patients are unarousable to verbal, tactile, or painful stimuli. Patients often lose the ability to maintain a patent airway and require additional support to maintain adequate ventilation. Cardiovascular function may be depressed [5, 6].

Standardized Monitoring

Personnel Conducting safe and effective procedural sedation requires a skilled practitioner, who is knowledgeable in the selection and delivery of sedation drugs, competent in monitoring a patient's level of sedation, and capable of managing the cardiorespiratory complications of sedation, including rescuing a patient from a level of sedation deeper than intended [5, 6]. Proficiency in advanced pediatric airway management is required, including the skills required to detect and manage apnea, laryngospasm, airway obstruction, hypoventilation, and airway secretions. The provider must be capable of administering pediatric advanced life support in the event of cardiorespiratory decompensation. For moderate and deep sedation, a second individual must be present to monitor patient status and assist the primary provider should resuscitative measures be required. The AAP recommends that this individual be capable of providing advanced airway skills and have a working knowledge of the location and use of emergency equipment. During moderate sedation, it is acceptable for this individual to assist with short interruptible tasks related to the sedated procedure. However, during deep sedation, one provider must be solely responsible for consistent monitoring of patient vital signs, airway patency, and ventilation and direct the titration and delivery of sedation medications. It is recommended that one provider present during the sedation also be competent in establishing vascular access should an IV be lost or the need arises for a second site of access [5, 6].

Monitoring and Equipment The use of objective monitoring techniques to evaluate patient oxygenation, ventilation, and hemodynamic status is critical in conducting safe procedural sedation. Monitoring these variables through the use of pulse oximetry, capnography, direct auscultation, and blood pressure allows the practitioner to rapidly recognize changes in patient status, perform earlier interventions, and decrease the incidence of sedation-related adverse events [5]. Multiple professional specialty organizations have published guidelines to direct the use of physiologic monitoring during procedural sedation, including the American Society of Anesthesiologists (ASA), American College of Emergency Physicians (ACEP), and the AAP [5, 6, 9]. These guidelines serve as a fundamental resource for both programs and individual providers to use in order to promote delivery of safe sedation practices.

Respiratory Monitoring The AAP guidelines recommend continuous pulse oximetry monitoring for all patients undergoing moderate and deep sedation. Pulse oximetry should be equipped with variable-pitched tonal notification of changes in oxygenation to alert the provider. While the use of pulse oximetry has been associated with improved detection of respiratory events, there can be a lag time of up to

30 seconds between arterial oxygen desaturation and detection by pulse oximetry, particularly if supplemental oxygen is administered [10–12]. Additionally, pulse oximetry is unable to provide direct information on CO_2 exchange or ventilation [11, 12]. Therefore, the AAP recommends the use of either capnography or direct auscultation with a pretracheal or precordial stethoscope to provide information on patient ventilatory status. For moderately sedated patients, the APP recommends providers be able to maintain bidirectional communication in addition to one of these modalities. For instances where this may not be possible, the AAP requires the use of one of these objective measures. Capnography is required during all deep sedations [5]. The use of capnography, which provides practitioners both a continuous waveform and numeric reading of expired CO2 to monitor ventilation, has been shown to allow for the earlier detection of respiratory depression and airway obstruction when compared to continuous observation in patients undergoing procedural sedation. This earlier detection may lead to decreased episodes of hypoxia in patients under moderate and deep sedation, particularly in patients receiving supplemental oxygen [13–15]. Furthermore, the addition of the pretracheal stethoscope to pulse oximetry and capnography has been shown to aid in the earlier detection of respiratory events, particularly in the setting of upper airway obstruction [16].

Hemodynamic Monitoring Many of the sedative and analgesic agents used in procedural sedation have the potential to cause hemodynamic changes through altered vascular tone, negative inotropic effects, and blunted or enhanced responses of the autonomic nervous system. These effects, in addition to the autonomic stress responses that may result in an inadequately sedated patient, carry the risk of a cardiovascular complication if not detected and intervened upon in a timely fashion. Therefore, close monitoring of heart rate and blood pressure is recommended in all patients undergoing moderate and deep sedation [5]. Additionally, electrocardiographic monitoring should be used in moderately sedated patients with a history of cardiovascular disease and in patients undergoing procedures with an increased risk for dysrhythmias (e.g., PICC placement). All patients undergoing deep sedation require electrocardiographic monitoring [5, 6].

Documentation Documentation of vital signs is recommended during all moderate and deep sedations in order to improve awareness of the provider to changes in patient status that could indicate the need for an intervention. Pertinent vital signs, including heart rate, blood pressure, respiratory rate, oxygen saturation, and end-tidal carbon dioxide, should be recorded prior to the administration of sedative medications, at regularly scheduled intervals during the procedure, during recovery, and prior to discharge. These vital signs, in addition to the level of consciousness, should be captured every 10 minutes during moderate sedation and every 5 minutes during deep sedation [5]. There are several published scales to assist in monitoring a patient's level of consciousness during procedural sedation. Though no one scale is recommended for its use, the AAP and ASA agree that patients undergoing moderate and deep sedation should be monitored for response to verbal commands and stimuli as a means to classify a patient's level of sedation and adjust monitoring and pharmacologic intervention accordingly [5, 6].

Components of Quality Sedation Practice

The elements of quality procedural sedation practice require a concentric, integrated system that begins with the practitioner's skills and competencies, followed by the structural elements and function of the work system and process (Fig. 24.2).

The Practitioner Skills and Competencies

Pediatric procedural sedation is a multifaceted high-risk clinical activity that requires a set of diverse yet interconnected skills and competencies. To perform pediatric procedural sedation proficiently through all three phases of the sedation encounter requires the integration of specific skills and competencies well beyond simply administering a sedative drug during the procedure.

Education and training in procedural sedation is an expected component of the educational curriculum during PCCM fellowship [18]. As part of the fellowship, PCCM fellows also receive education, training, and experience germane to procedural sedation practice, including cardiorespiratory monitoring, advanced airway management skills, and cardiopulmonary resuscitation. By virtue of their training, experience, and expertise, PCCM physicians are frequently considered to have the requisite skills and competencies to safely and effectively perform pediatric procedural sedation. Yet, specific sedation training objectives and determination of sedation proficiency are lacking in many, if not most, PCCM training programs [18]. In a survey of PCCM fellowship programs, Hooper et al. found only 38% of respondents reported receiving formal training in pediatric procedural sedation during

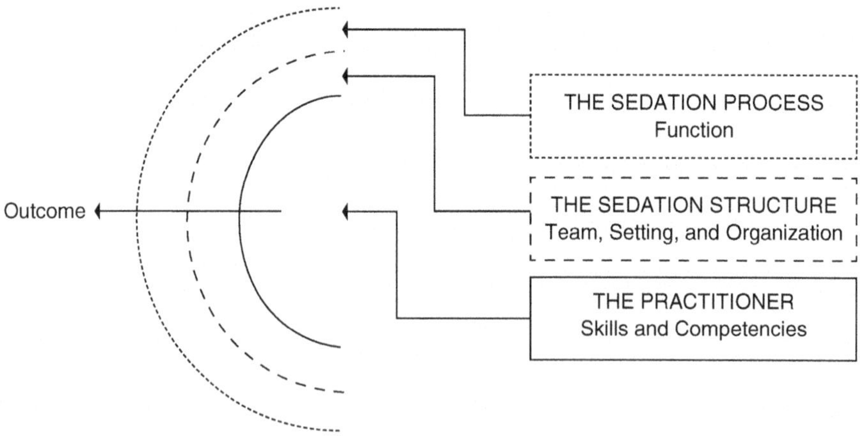

Fig. 24.2 Components of quality procedural sedation practice encompass the practitioner's skills and competencies, the tangible components of the sedation structure, and the work system process of delivering sedation. Adapted from Donabedian [17]

PCCM fellowship. Of those who received training, 25% required further training and mentoring to conduct sedation independently [18]. These findings illustrate the variability in procedural sedation training in PCCM fellowship programs and bring to light the complex nature of establishing the skills and competencies for PCCM practitioner to be proficient in conducting pediatric procedural sedation.

Procedural Sedation Skills Skills are hierarchically ordered and comprise the building blocks of higher-order skills and competencies [19, 20]. A practitioner's cognitive, psychomotor, and affective skills are the primary ingredients of medical competency in procedural sedation (Fig. 24.3).

Basic to all three of these domains is the ability and willingness to receive information.

Cognitive Skills Cognitive skills comprise a practitioner's intellectual abilities and begin with a knowledge base providing the ability to recognize and recall previously learned information. The ability to comprehend data, apply information, and solve complex problems is progressively higher orders of intellectual skills [20]. The large-scale report from the PSRC of sedation encounters performed by PCCM physicians with propofol finds that 5.0% of procedural sedations were associated with

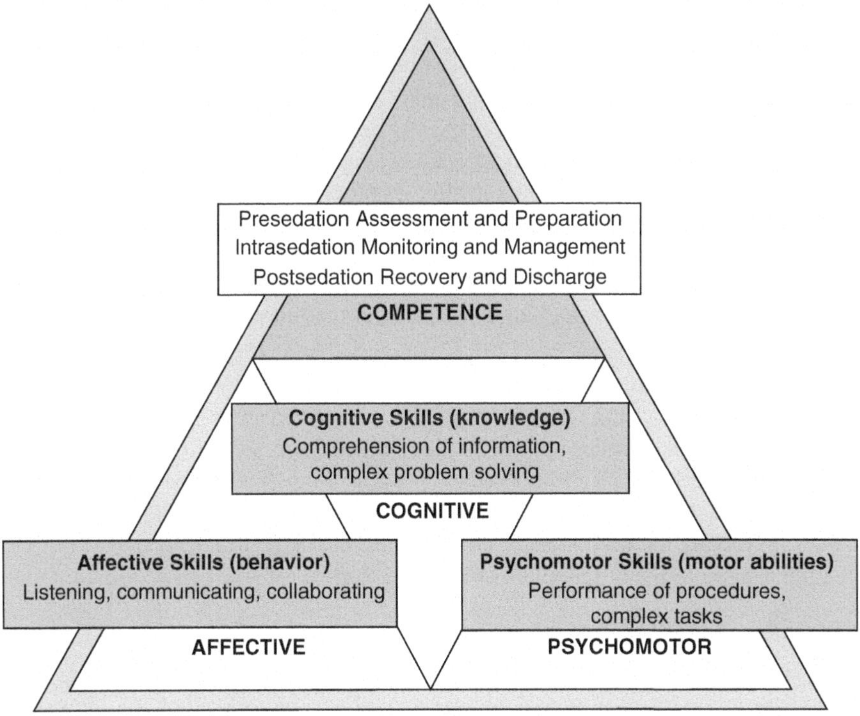

Fig. 24.3 Practitioner skills and competencies required to perform pediatric procedural sedation. The cognitive, psychomotor, and affective skills comprise the building blocks of higher-order sedation competencies

an adverse event [4]. Respiratory depression was the contributing factor to the vast majority of sedation-related complications, including oxygen desaturation, upper airway obstruction, apnea, coughing, airway secretions, and laryngospasm [1–3]. Consequently, the PCCM practitioner must have knowledge about a sedative drug's respiratory depressant effects and be ready to recognize and respond to changes in a patient's cardiorespiratory status [21–23]. Cognitive abilities are the basis of procedural sedation education and provide the foundation for developing a practitioner's psychomotor and affective (behavioral) abilities.

Psychomotor Skills Psychomotor abilities encompass the motor-skill aspects of sedation practice and, like intellectual abilities, proceed from simpler to more complex levels of performance. Psychomotor skills begin with *perceiving* a cue that sets *the stage* for performing a particular action. At higher levels of motor activity, practitioners demonstrate ability to perform and adapt to complex tasks under diverse situations. Results from the PSRC clarify many of the necessary motor skills to proficiently perform procedural sedation and include oxygen administration; airway repositioning; bag-mask ventilation; airway suctioning; oral, nasopharyngeal, or laryngeal mask airway placement; and endotracheal tube intubation [2–4].

Affective Skills The affective aspect of sedation practice pertains to a practitioner's behavior and attitude. Affective skills begin with the ability to *receive* information (e.g., listening attentively) and progresses to the higher levels of active participation (*responding)* and a commitment to high quality (*valuing*). The ability to effectively listen, communicate, and collaborate with medical staff, patients, and families during the procedural sedation encounter is an example of affective skills. The importance of affective skills like communication cannot be overstated as the majority of serious medical errors reported to the Joint Commission can be attributed to breakdowns in communication between team members [24].

Procedural Sedation Competency Competency is both outcome and context dependent [25–27]. To say a practitioner is competent to perform procedural sedation indicates they are able to apply the necessary cognitive, psychomotor, and behavioral skills to a desired outcome within the context of their clinical practice. Published sedation monitoring and management recommendations from various national societies [5, 6, 28, 29] outline the general competencies required by practitioners to safely and effectively conduct procedural sedation. In general, recommendations specify that practitioners be competent to perform all aspects of care during the three phases of the sedation encounter to include:

1. *Pre-sedation risk assessment, planning, and preparation*, including obtaining informed consent and performance of a "time-out."
2. *Intra-sedation monitoring and management* of a patient's level of consciousness and cardiorespiratory status, including rescuing patients from a deeper-than-planned level of sedation.
3. *Post-sedation recovery and discharge* planning and education, including knowledge of discharge criteria.

The Sedation Structure

While establishment of practitioner competency and subsequent institutional privileging in pediatric procedural sedation is essential for promoting safe and effective care, the quality of procedural sedation rests on a system with (1) a sedation team knowledgeable and experienced in providing sedation, (2) an environment with the space and resources conducive to conducting procedural sedation, and (3) a set of policies and procedures that govern the sedation practice. The sedation team (human resources), setting (material resources), and organization (administrative resources) comprise the tangible elements of providing high-quality sedation [17, 30] (Fig. 24.4).

The Sedation Team (Human Resources) Considerable variation in procedural sedation practice and sedation team composition exists in children's hospitals across the country. At a minimum, the sedation team should consist of a sedation provider and a support person, often a sedation nurse. The function and goals of the sedation team must provide a safe and effective procedural sedation environment regardless of the specific makeup and setting [5, 6, 29]. The team must be composed of indi-

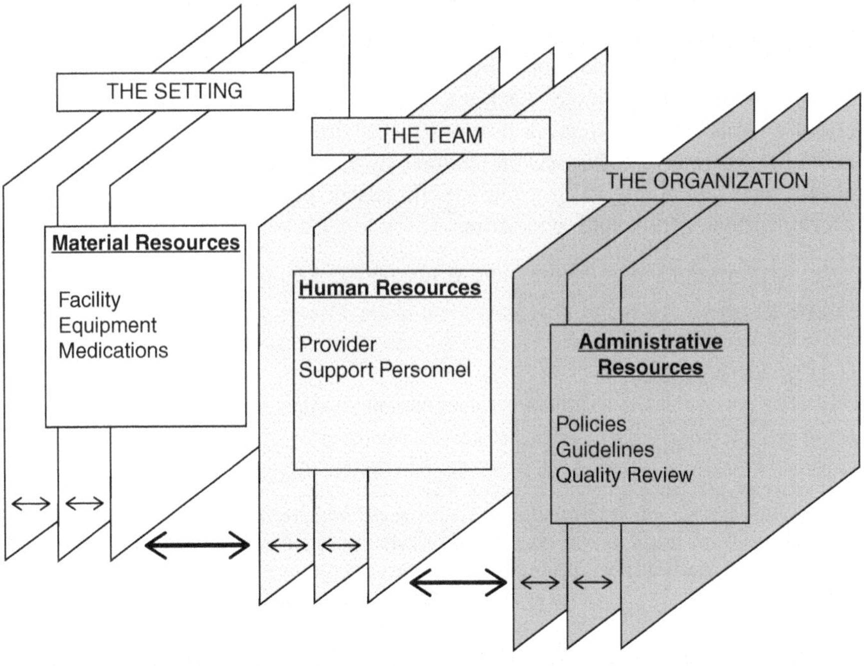

Fig. 24.4 The sedation structure comprises the tangible components of sedation practice and includes the sedation team, setting, and organization. Examples of resources in each of these areas are outlined in the boxes. Key functions and processes within and between components important to coordination of care are represented by arrows. (Adapted from Donabedian's quality of care categories [17])

viduals who possess the knowledge, skills, and experience to care for patients during all phases of the sedation process. Sufficient number of staff members must also be present to perform a pre-sedation assessment, administer and monitor sedation, and recover and discharge the patient. The practitioner conducting sedation is ultimately responsible for and must be competent to conduct all aspects of the sedation encounter as described above, including sedative drug administration and monitoring and management of the patient. In addition, this individual should be dedicated solely to patient monitoring and not be the individual person who performs the procedure [5, 28, 29]. Specific roles of additional personnel must be clear and may include patient monitoring and documentation, assistance in treatment measures, and sedative drug administration under the supervision of the sedation provider. Despite the importance of individual roles, the sedation team must function as a cohesive, collaborative team. Communication between team members must be fluid and timely, particularly in regard to drug titration, monitor interpretation, and adverse event response.

The Sedation Setting (Material Resources) The pediatric procedural sedation setting comprises the physical environment and the necessary monitoring and resuscitative equipment to safely perform sedation. Ideally the setting is child safe and friendly and family centered. Regardless of setting context (e.g., radiology suite vs intensive care unit), the environment must be conducive to providing safe and effective procedural sedation and managing emergency situations. Settings outside the PICU must have an adequate "back up" system in the event of serious sedation-related complications. Unique aspects of the environment (e.g., MRI), including specific tasks greatly influence the context in which sedation is delivered [31]. Indeed, type and acuity of procedure, skill sets of personnel, and patient illness severity will vary from setting to setting.

At a minimum, monitoring and resuscitative equipment must include the following:

Monitoring equipment (BEEPS)	Resuscitative equipment (SOAP)
Blood pressure (noninvasive) **E**lectrocardiogram **E**nd-tidal carbon dioxide (capnography) **P**ulse oximeter **S**tethoscope (pretracheal, precordial)	**S**uction source and equipment **O**xygen supply and delivery equipment including self-inflating reservoir bag-valve-mask system **A**irway equipment: towel roll, oral and nasopharyngeal airways, laryngeal mask airways, and endotracheal tubes **P**harmacologic agents: emergency medications, reversal agents, and additional sedation medications

The Sedation Organization (Administrative Resources) The organization defines the "rules" for the sedation practice and includes the program's policies and procedures and quality assurance processes. The provision of high-quality procedural sedation is guided by institution-specific policies and procedures and includes defining who is qualified to administer sedation, monitoring requirements, fasting protocols, recovery and discharge criteria, and the frequency and nature of documentation. Documentation during the pre-sedation phase should include that informed consent was obtained according to local, state, and institutional requirements and patient/caregiver information was provided that stated the objectives, options, and risks of sedation. Records should indicate that a health evaluation was performed that included the patient's age, weight, vital signs, ASA classification, and dietary status. In addition, documentation should indicate that a "time-out" was completed and that the patient was assessed just prior to the procedural sedation. While professional medical organizations have published guidelines for the monitoring and management of pediatric patients during and after sedation [5, 6, 32], each institution must have its own policies and procedures that take into consideration the unique environment where sedation is provided. Finally, a multidisciplinary sedation committee must exist in the institution that oversees quality metrics (e.g., adverse sedation events), training, and privileging for procedural sedation within the institution.

The Sedation Process and Work System

The staff, including practitioner competency, setting, and organization comprise the tangible elements of procedural sedation. However, they do not specifically address the process of care, that is, *how* care is delivered. Fully developing a safe procedural sedation environment requires integrating the structural elements to the processes of the system.

Threats to Safety Delivering high-quality sedation is complicated and despite an institution's best efforts to put barriers to patient harm in place, threats to patient safety still exist. Clinical practices, like procedural sedation, that are high risk, complex, and dynamic are particularly vulnerable to weaknesses in a system. Unlike the delivery of anesthesia, where highly trained subspecialists (i.e., anesthesiologists) consistently provide care in a structured, well-controlled environment, provision of pediatric sedation is delivered in an array of settings, by a wide range of provider types and teams with varying levels of cohesiveness, training, and experience [33, 34]. Differences exist not so much in what is done, per se, but *how* it is done, who does it, and the environment in which it is conducted. Consequently, there is every reason to believe that procedural sedation outside the operating room is less controlled and more vulnerable to poor team function, substandard ergonomics, and extraneous disruptions. Closed claims reports of sedation/anesthesia performed outside the operating room provide information about inadequacies in care that lead to poor outcomes [21–23]. Cote et al. found that poor outcomes, including severe neurological injury and death, during procedural sedation were connected to poor overall care and included inadequate performance of a pre-sedation risk assessment, insufficient knowledge of sedative drug pharmacology, incomplete understanding and use of monitoring tools, lack of appropriate response to monitoring information, and insufficient recovery and discharge procedures [22]. Similar findings have been observed from closed claims reports of anesthesia conducted outside the operating room setting [21, 23]. Common, to each of these reports, was that most injuries were judged as being preventable by better monitoring, including greater vigilance in recognizing and responding to an adverse event by the sedation team and practitioner.

Understanding threats to safety requires an understanding of the safety measures built into the system and the vulnerabilities that still exist. The "Swiss Cheese" model of medical error, originally described by Reason, modified by Carayon, and recently applied to sedation safety outside the operating room by Webster, et al., takes into account the weaknesses within the system that jeopardize patient safety [30, 33, 35, 36]. In the context of procedural sedation, components of sedation practice (team, setting and structure) have been described earlier and can be visualized as barriers between "threats" (e.g., disruptions) in the system and patient injury (Fig. 24.5).

While these safeguards usually prevent patient harm, there are often inherent weaknesses within a system (holes) that are exposed when deviations in care occur. These hazards to patient safety frequently occur as a result of ergonomic (human factors) shortfalls that include environment deficiencies, team dysfunction, and extraneous disruptions [33, 34, 37, 38].

Ergonomic (Human Factors) Considerations Human factors is the field concerned with understanding the interactions between humans and the elements of a system (workplace) in which they function, in an effort to optimize overall system

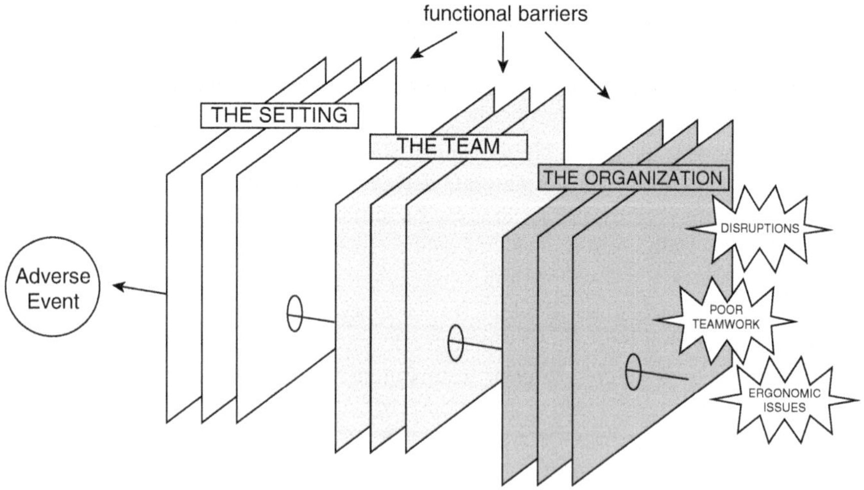

Fig. 24.5 Weaknesses (holes) within and between components allow threats (e.g., poor teamwork) to cause sedation-related adverse events and potential patient harm. Adapted from Reason's "Swiss Cheese" model of medical error [35] and Webster [33]

performance [39]. Ergonomics incorporates virtually all aspects of a system's design and function and its impact on human welfare and performance by evaluating physical issues (e.g., room layout), cognitive issues (e.g., mental workload, attentiveness), and organizational issues (e.g., team communication). Even within the controlled environment of the operating room, however, ergonomic shortcomings in the form of team function, physical layout, and distractions are a leading cause of disturbance to workflow and patient care. Inadequacies in human factors are likely to be a greater issue in sedation conducted outside the operating room setting.

Teamwork (Organizational Aspects) Most serious medical errors reported to the Joint Commission can be attributed to breakdowns in communication and coordination between team members. Recent studies demonstrate the important link between teamwork communication and coordination, quality of care, and patient safety [31, 37, 40]. Analysis of factors contributing to critical adverse events in sedation and anesthesia in patients demonstrates a causal role of poor team functioning and communication [37]. Observational studies in the operating room reveal that when teamwork and communication is poor, patient complications and even death increase significantly [31, 41, 42]. Wiegmann et al. found that medical errors in the operating room increased significantly with greater numbers of disruptions and were particularly vulnerable to problems in teamwork communication and coordination [43].

The pediatric sedation team must function as a dynamic, *tightly coupled* unit, particularly during the actual procedural sedation. The desire and ability to function as a cohesive, collaborative team are critical to providing safe and effective sedation. A shared mental model of teamwork among team members is important in effective team function [37]. Similarly, some evidence exists that teams that perceive a positive teamwork environment have better patient outcomes [37]. While few studies have yet to directly link effective teamwork to patient safety and outcome, the general consensus is that team communication and collaboration (e.g., role clarification, procedure expectations, structured handovers, checklists) are critical to promoting an effective and safe work system [44, 45].

Design Layout – Setup (Physical Aspects) The workplace layout; arrangement of monitors, equipment, and furniture; lighting; and noise level distinguish the procedural sedation environment outside the operating room and PICU as much as any ergonomic quality the PCCM physician will be exposed to. Following analysis of 1080 disruptions, Palmer et al. developed a standardized human factors methodology for classifying flow disruptions in the operating room that were potential threats to safety [46]. The majority of disruptions were related to layout issues that included positioning of equipment and furniture, space constraints, and visibility problems. For safety and efficiency purposes, a great deal of attention has been given to the physical components of the operating room work environment [38]. It is important to give similar attention to the procedural sedation setting in designing a user-friendly environment that reduces time to perceive a problem, decide on a plan, and act with an intervention while at the same time optimizing efficiencies in physical movement [39].

Distractions (Cognitive Aspects) Distractions are intrusions of unexpected secondary events that occur during the performance of a primary task [47]. Distracting events are both pervasive and insidious in the healthcare environment. As such, healthcare workers are frequently unaware of their presence and the impact they have on their workflow. Factors that influence the impact of a distracting event include the "internal" psychological and cognitive state of the individual, the context of the activity, and the complexity of the task [48]. Distracting events that occur during high working-memory load (e.g., complex tasks, time constraints, multitasking), critical periods of task execution, and conditions in which staff feel less control over their working environment are more likely to have a negative impact on patient care [49–51]. Comprehensive management of factors like distractions that lead to medical error is best dealt with from a systems standpoint aimed at strategies that impact the entire picture, the individual and team, the primary tasks, the workplace setting, and the institution as a whole [30, 52, 53]. Areas in which the simultaneous integration of cognitive, psychomotor, and affective skills (team work) are required to deliver high-quality patient care are particularly vulnerable to the negative impact of distracting events and the occurrence of a medical error. Focusing specifically on the anesthesia team, Campbell et al. found that distracting events to the team led to negative consequences (e.g., adverse physiologic events) 22% of the time [54]. Savoldelli et al. observed 209 distracting events during anesthetic induction, of which 173 (82.8%) resulted in the anesthesia team either being distracted, multitasking, or switching tasks. Of note, 22% of distractions resulted in a negative patient impact [55]. Recently developed standardized human factors methodology for classifying flow disruptions in the operating room has been utilized to define workflow disruptions as any event that disturbed the performance of the anesthesiologist's or nurse's primary tasks [46, 56]. In 878 events, 25% of time was devoted to resolving disruptions to care, in which 49% were accounted for by extraneous distractions.

To date, no studies have evaluated distractions during pediatric procedural sedation and the impact they have on the sedation team workflow and individual performance. Yet, there is every reason to believe that distracting events are more frequent and have a more negative impact in procedural sedation outside the operating room. For one, as described above, there is much greater variance in practice and subsequently less organization, consistency, and order to the process. Implementation of targeted strategies, mindful practice, checklists, and "rules" to the game have been shown to improve team communication and coordination, reducing the frequency of extraneous distractions and the negative impact of distractions and multitasking in healthcare settings [49, 50, 57–61].

Delivering High-Quality Procedural Sedation

Organized sedation services are preferred because they provide consistent, safe, and effective care. Studies show that highly motivated and organized sedation services have the capability to deliver safe and effective sedation, with very low adverse event rates [2, 3]. Whether procedural sedation is conducted in the PICU, by a *mobile sedation service* or a *stand-alone sedation unit*, the principles of delivering quality care should be the same. However, the sedation team must understand the significant differences that may exist from one location to another. The team composition, skills and competencies, physical layout and setup, and procedural personnel characteristics, and tasks will vary considerably whether sedation is conducted in a burn unit, radiology suite, or inpatient pediatric ward. Below are the basic requirements in any environment/institution conducting procedural sedation:

- The Sedation Team Personnel and Function:
  - Personnel qualifications: Practitioners must have the necessary skills, competencies, and experience and according to institutional policy be privileged to conduct procedural sedation. Support personnel must have the necessary skills, competencies, and experience to conduct sedation under the supervision of a practitioner based on the context of the setting.
  - Personnel number: Sufficient number of personnel must be present to safely and effectively conduct the sedation and procedure.
  - Sedation team: The sedation team must have experience working together and be able to function as a cohesive, collaborative team where communication is open and coordination of care is clear. The sedation team must be attentive and mindful to limiting the negative impact of extraneous distractions.
- The Sedation Setting and Layout:
  - The sedation setting must be child friendly and safe and family centered.
  - Room layout must be designed with safety and efficiency in mind. Equipment, monitors, and furniture must be positioned, and lighting and noise adjusted to optimize detection and reaction times. Room layout must be designed for efficiency in physical movement for the sedation, the procedure, and resuscitative measures.
  - Room setup must be designed to optimize sedation team communication and coordination between members and with procedure personnel.
  - The sedation setting must be conducive to limiting the number and impact of irrelevant external events.
  - Facilities and backup emergency services: the environment must have a design adequate for the provision of sedation (i.e., oxygen source, suction, monitors, etc.). In addition, if needed, backup anesthesia and PICU should be readily available.
- The Sedation Organization and Oversight:
  - The organization must include institution-approved protocols and policies that promote, support, and guide safe and effective procedural sedation.
  - Adequate institutional oversight of procedural sedation practice, outcomes, and standards must exist in the hospital and consist of a committee composed of pediatric subspecialists in anesthesiology, critical care, emergency medicine, hospital medicine, nursing, and administration.

- Ideally, the sedation service consists of schedulers, medical assistants, coders, child life specialists, and other ancillary staff with sedation experience.
- Quality improvement initiatives must be in place to optimize outcomes for all patients undergoing procedural sedation.

Conclusion

PCCM practitioners have assumed a greater role in providing pediatric procedural sedation outside the traditional operating room setting. While PCCM practitioners have many of the skills and competencies well suited for performing procedural sedation, significant deficiencies in educational curriculums and training, specific for procedural sedation, exist. Providing high-quality procedural sedation within and outside the PICU requires knowing the necessary components of the sedation team, setting, and organization and appreciating the importance of human factors in delivering high-quality care.

References

1. Baarslag MA, Jhingoer S, Ista E, Allegaert K, Tibboel D, van Dijk M. How often do we perform painful and stressful procedures in the paediatric intensive care unit? A prospective observational study. Aust Crit Care. 2019;32(1):4–10.
2. Cravero JP, Beach ML, Blike GT, Gallagher SM, Hertzog JH, Pediatric Sedation Research C. The incidence and nature of adverse events during pediatric sedation/anesthesia with propofol for procedures outside the operating room: a report from the Pediatric Sedation Research Consortium. Anesth Analg. 2009;108(3):795–804.
3. Cravero JP, Blike GT, Beach M, Gallagher SM, Hertzog JH, Havidich JE, et al. Incidence and nature of adverse events during pediatric sedation/anesthesia for procedures outside the operating room: report from the Pediatric Sedation Research Consortium. Pediatrics. 2006;118(3):1087–96.
4. Kamat PP, McCracken CE, Gillespie SE, Fortenberry JD, Stockwell JA, Cravero JP, et al. Pediatric critical care physician-administered procedural sedation using propofol: a report from the Pediatric Sedation Research Consortium Database. Pediatr Crit Care Med. 2015;16(1):11–20.
5. Cote CJ, Wilson S, American Academy of P, American Academy of Pediatric D. Guidelines for monitoring and management of pediatric patients before, during, and after sedation for diagnostic and therapeutic procedures: update 2016. Pediatrics. 2016;138:1.
6. American Society of Anesthesiologists Task Force on S, Analgesia by N-A. Practice guidelines for sedation and analgesia by non-anesthesiologists. Anesthesiology. 2002;96(4):1004–17.
7. Department of Health and Human Services CfMaMS. Revised hospital anesthesia services interpretive guidelines 2011. Available from: www.cms.gov/SurveyCertificationgeninfo/downloads/SCLetter11_10.pdf.
8. Guidelines for the elective use of conscious sedation, deep sedation, and general anesthesia in pediatric patients. Committee on Drugs Section on anesthesiology. Pediatrics. 1985;76(2):317–21.

9. Godwin SA, Caro DA, Wolf SJ, Jagoda AS, Charles R, Marett BE, et al. Clinical policy: procedural sedation and analgesia in the emergency department. Ann Emerg Med. 2005;45(2):177–96.
10. Becker DE, Casabianca AB. Respiratory monitoring: physiological and technical considerations. Anesth Prog. 2009;56(1):14–20; quiz 1-2.
11. Fu ES, Downs JB, Schweiger JW, Miguel RV, Smith RA. Supplemental oxygen impairs detection of hypoventilation by pulse oximetry. Chest. 2004;126(5):1552–8.
12. Sammartino M, Volpe B, Sbaraglia F, Garra R, D'Addessi A. Capnography and the bispectral index-their role in pediatric sedation: a brief review. Int J Pediatr. 2010;2010:828347.
13. Deitch K, Miner J, Chudnofsky CR, Dominici P, Latta D. Does end tidal CO2 monitoring during emergency department procedural sedation and analgesia with propofol decrease the incidence of hypoxic events? A randomized, controlled trial. Ann Emerg Med. 2010;55(3):258–64.
14. Langhan ML, Shabanova V, Li FY, Bernstein SL, Shapiro ED. A randomized controlled trial of capnography during sedation in a pediatric emergency setting. Am J Emerg Med. 2015;33(1):25–30.
15. Lightdale JR, Goldmann DA, Feldman HA, Newburg AR, DiNardo JA, Fox VL. Microstream capnography improves patient monitoring during moderate sedation: a randomized, controlled trial. Pediatrics. 2006;117(6):e1170–8.
16. Boriosi JP, Zhao Q, Preston A, Hollman GA. The utility of the pretracheal stethoscope in detecting ventilatory abnormalities during propofol sedation in children. Paediatr Anaesth. 2019;29(6):604–10.
17. Donabedian A. The quality of care. How can it be assessed? JAMA. 1988;260(12):1743–8.
18. Hooper MC, Kamat PP, Couloures KG. Evaluating the need for pediatric procedural sedation training in pediatric critical care medicine fellowship. Pediatr Crit Care Med. 2019;20(3):259–61.
19. Leung WC. Competency based medical training: review. BMJ. 2002;325(7366):693–6.
20. Swing SR, International CC. Perspectives on competency-based medical education from the learning sciences. Med Teach. 2010;32(8):663–8.
21. Bhananker SM, Posner KL, Cheney FW, Caplan RA, Lee LA, Domino KB. Injury and liability associated with monitored anesthesia care: a closed claims analysis. Anesthesiology. 2006;104(2):228–34.
22. Cote CJ, Notterman DA, Karl HW, Weinberg JA, McCloskey C. Adverse sedation events in pediatrics: a critical incident analysis of contributing factors. Pediatrics. 2000;105(4 Pt 1):805–14.
23. Metzner J, Posner KL, Domino KB. The risk and safety of anesthesia at remote locations: the US closed claims analysis. Curr Opin Anaesthesiol. 2009;22(4):502–8.
24. Hunt EA, Shilkofski NA, Stavroudis TA, Nelson KL. Simulation: translation to improved team performance. Anesthesiol Clin. 2007;25(2):301–19.
25. Epstein RM. Assessment in medical education. N Engl J Med. 2007;356(4):387–96.
26. Klass D. Reevaluation of clinical competency. M J Phys Med Rehabil. 2000;79:481–6.
27. Okuyama A, Martowirono K, Bijnen B. Assessing the patient safety competencies of healthcare professionals: a systematic review. BMJ Qual Saf. 2011;20(11):991–1000.
28. Sury M, Bullock I, Rabar S, Demott K, Guideline Development G. Sedation for diagnostic and therapeutic procedures in children and young people: summary of NICE guidance. BMJ. 2010;341:c6819.
29. Zielinska M, Bartkowska-Sniatkowska A, Becke K, Hohne C, Najafi N, Schaffrath E, et al. Safe pediatric procedural sedation and analgesia by anesthesiologists for elective procedures: a clinical practice statement from the European Society for Paediatric Anaesthesiology. Paediatr Anaesth. 2019;29(6):583–90.
30. Carayon P, Schoofs Hundt A, Karsh BT, Gurses AP, Alvarado CJ, Smith M, et al. Work system design for patient safety: the SEIPS model. Qual Saf Health Care. 2006;15(Suppl 1):i50–8.

31. Rosen MA, DiazGranados D, Dietz AS, Benishek LE, Thompson D, Pronovost PJ, et al. Teamwork in healthcare: key discoveries enabling safer, high-quality care. Am Psychol. 2018;73(4):433–50.
32. Godwin SA, Burton JH, Gerardo CJ, Hatten BW, Mace SE, Silvers SM, et al. Clinical policy: procedural sedation and analgesia in the emergency department. Ann Emerg Med. 2014;63(2):247–58 e18.
33. Webster CS, Mason KP, Shafer SL. Threats to safety during sedation outside of the operating room and the death of Michael Jackson. Curr Opin Anaesthesiol. 2016;29(Suppl 1):S36–47.
34. Youn AM, Ko YK, Kim YH. Anesthesia and sedation outside of the operating room. Korean J Anesthesiol. 2015;68(4):323–31.
35. Reason J. Human error: models and management. BMJ. 2000;320(7237):768–70.
36. Reason J. Safety in the operating theatre – Part 2: human error and organisational failure. Qual Saf Health Care. 2005;14(1):56–60.
37. Manser T. Teamwork and patient safety in dynamic domains of healthcare: a review of the literature. Acta Anaesthesiol Scand. 2009;53(2):143–51.
38. Raghavendra Rao RS. Ergonomical aspects of anaesthetic practice. Indian J Anaesth. 2016;60(5):306–11.
39. Carayon P, Xie A, Kianfar S. Human Factors and Ergonomics. Making health care safer II: an updated critical analysis of the evidence for patient safety practices 2013. p. 325–50.
40. Schmutz J, Manser T. Do team processes really have an effect on clinical performance? A systematic literature review. Br J Anaesth. 2013;110(4):529–44.
41. Mazzocco K, Petitti DB, Fong KT, Bonacum D, Brookey J, Graham S, et al. Surgical team behaviors and patient outcomes. Am J Surg. 2009;197(5):678–85.
42. Wilson RM, Runciman WB, Gibberd RW, Harrison BT, Newby L, Hamilton JD. The quality in Australian health care study. Med J Aust. 1995;163(9):458–71.
43. Wiegmann DA, ElBardissi AW, Dearani JA, Daly RC, Sundt TM 3rd. Disruptions in surgical flow and their relationship to surgical errors: an exploratory investigation. Surgery. 2007;142(5):658–65.
44. Funk E, Taicher B, Thompson J, Iannello K, Morgan B, Hawks S. Structured handover in the Pediatric Postanesthesia Care Unit. J Perianesth Nurs. 2016;31(1):63–72.
45. Hagerman NS, Varughese AM, Kurth CD. Quality and safety in pediatric anesthesia: how can guidelines, checklists, and initiatives improve the outcome? Curr Opin Anaesthesiol. 2014;27(3):323–9.
46. Palmer G 2nd, Abernathy JH 3rd, Swinton G, Allison D, Greenstein J, Shappell S, et al. Realizing improved patient care through human-centered operating room design: a human factors methodology for observing flow disruptions in the cardiothoracic operating room. Anesthesiology. 2013;119(5):1066–77.
47. Ahmed A, Ahmad M, Stewart CM, Francis HW, Bhatti NI. Effect of distractions on operative performance and ability to multitask–a case for deliberate practice. Laryngoscope. 2015;125(4):837–41.
48. Reason J. Beyond the organisational accident: the need for "error wisdom" on the frontline. Qual Saf Health Care. 2004;13(Suppl 2):ii28–33.
49. Grundgeiger T, Sanderson P. Interruptions in healthcare: theoretical views. Int J Med Inform. 2009;78(5):293–307.
50. Li SY, Magrabi F, Coiera E. A systematic review of the psychological literature on interruption and its patient safety implications. J Am Med Inform Assoc. 2012;19(1):6–12.
51. Westbrook JI, Raban MZ, Walter SR, Douglas H. Task errors by emergency physicians are associated with interruptions, multitasking, fatigue and working memory capacity: a prospective, direct observation study. BMJ Qual Saf. 2018;27(8):655–63.
52. Healey AN, Primus CP, Koutantji M. Quantifying distraction and interruption in urological surgery. Qual Saf Health Care. 2007;16(2):135–9.
53. Makary MA, Daniel M. Medical error-the third leading cause of death in the US. BMJ. 2016;353:i2139.

54. Campbell G, Arfanis K, Smith AF. Distraction and interruption in anaesthetic practice. Br J Anaesth. 2012;109(5):707–15.
55. Savoldelli GL, Thieblemont J, Clergue F, Waeber JL, Forster A, Garnerin P. Incidence and impact of distracting events during induction of general anaesthesia for urgent surgical cases. Eur J Anaesthesiol. 2010;27(8):683–9.
56. Cohen TN, Cabrera JS, Sisk OD, Welsh KL, Abernathy JH, Reeves ST, et al. Identifying workflow disruptions in the cardiovascular operating room. Anaesthesia. 2016;71(8):948–54.
57. Kuo CY, Yeh YY. Reset a task set after five minutes of mindfulness practice. Conscious Cogn. 2015;35:98–109.
58. Lindsay EK, Creswell JD. Mechanisms of mindfulness training: monitor and acceptance theory (MAT). Clin Psychol Rev. 2017;51:48–59.
59. Mrazek MD, Franklin MS, Phillips DT, Baird B, Schooler JW. Mindfulness training improves working memory capacity and GRE performance while reducing mind wandering. Psychol Sci. 2013;24(5):776–81.
60. D'Esmond LK. Distracted practice and patient safety: the healthcare team experience. Nurs Forum. 2017;52(3):149–64.
61. Henrickson SE, Wadhera RK, Elbardissi AW, Wiegmann DA, Sundt TM 3rd. Development and pilot evaluation of a preoperative briefing protocol for cardiovascular surgery. J Am Coll Surg. 2009;208(6):1115–23.

Chapter 25
Screening of Children for Procedural Sedation Outside the Operating Room

Jocelyn R. Grunwell

Introduction

Children often require analgesia, anxiolysis, and sedation prior to undergoing procedures outside of the operating room. These procedures are varied and include radiologic studies, such as magnetic resonance imaging (MRI), computed tomography (CT), and positron emission tomography (PET scans). Sedation is also required for repeated lumbar puncture and bone marrow aspiration procedures for children with oncologic diagnoses. Other children require sedation for painful procedures such as fracture reduction, incision and drainage of an abscess, or suturing of a laceration. Children with special needs, such as those with autism, developmental delay, and behavioral issues, may need non-pharmacological coping strategies in addition to sedation to complete relatively minor or routine procedures such as phlebotomy, physical examination, or echocardiography, in addition to the procedures described. Sedation outside the operating room is common and often performed by advanced practice nurse practitioners, pediatric hospitalists, pediatric emergency medicine physicians, and pediatric intensivists.

Physician-nurse sedation teams must assess each child's risk profile and decide which child is appropriate for procedural sedation versus which child should be referred to anesthesiology. Inaccurate screening of children for sedation results in same-day cancellations that delay care, decrease parental satisfaction, and lost school and workdays. Hospital resources are used inefficiently and wasted. To improve pediatric sedation efficiency, clinicians need an accurate and practical means to assess sedation risk. The goal of pre-sedation risk assessment is to prevent children from experiencing adverse events, not being able to complete sedation due to adverse events, and to reduce the frequency of same-day cancellations. This

J. R. Grunwell (✉)
Pediatrics, Emory University School of Medicine/Children's Healthcare of Atlanta at Egleston, Atlanta, GA, USA
e-mail: jgrunwe@emory.edu

P. P. Kamat, J. W. Berkenbosch (eds.), *Sedation and Analgesia for the Pediatric Intensivist*, https://doi.org/10.1007/978-3-030-52555-2_25

chapter describes the risk factors associated with incomplete sedations due to increased sedation-related adverse events and same-day cancellations. Based on these factors to guide sedation risk, we describe a questionnaire and point system to discriminate which children should be referred to anesthesia to complete their procedure. Where available, the literature supporting these risk factors is discussed.

Risk Factors Associated with Sedation-Related Adverse Events

Retrospective studies from single centers and multiple centers associated with the Pediatric Sedation Research Consortium (PSRC) have identified several risk factors associated with sedation-related adverse events, resulting in the inability to complete the radiologic study or procedure [1–5]. These factors are discussed below and include the following: (1) current upper respiratory tract infection (URI), (2) congenital heart disease, (3) sleep-disordered breathing (SDB)/obstructed sleep apnea (OSA), (4) obesity, (5) premature birth, and (6) an American Society of Anesthesiologists physical status (ASA-PS) of 3 or more [3]. In addition, the textbook edited by Keira Mason on Procedural Sedation Outside the Operating Room and the references therein contain excellent detailed discussions of patient characteristics to assess to help prevent sedation-related complications [6].

Based on the literature and experience in a high-volume outpatient sedation center, a pediatric sedation assessment questionnaire was developed and tested at the Children's Healthcare of Atlanta at Egleston campus. The conceptual framework for the questionnaire is shown in Fig. 25.1 [7]. Using this framework as a guide, a questionnaire consisting of nine questions with points awarded to each question is detailed in Table 25.1 [8]. This questionnaire may be used as an interview guide for a prescreening call to parents in the week prior to sedation, and, if the child has been seen before by the sedation service or hospitalized, the information may be abstracted from the child's electronic health record.

To evaluate the performance of this screening questionnaire, we performed a case-control study of children who were successfully sedated ($n = 104$) by a primarily propofol-based seditionist service, who were not able to complete their procedure due to a sedation-related adverse event – defined as a "failed" sedation ($n = 72$), and who were referred to anesthesiology ($n = 101$) to anesthesia (GA) [8]. Composite scores were calculated (score range: 9 [no risk factors] to 42 [many risk factors]) and compared using the Kruskal-Wallis analysis of variance test for multiple comparisons using Bonferroni corrections [8]. Test characteristics were calculated based on different threshold scores for referral to anesthesiology. The median (25th–75th interquartile range) score for children who were successfully sedated was 11 (9–13), failed sedation was 18 (16–19), and referred to anesthesiology was 18 (17–21) (Fig. 25.2a) [8]. For children with a screening score of 15 or more, the PSAT had a sensitivity of 94.4%, a specificity of 83.7%, a positive likelihood ratio of 5.81, and a negative likelihood ratio of 0.06 of children needing a referral to anesthesiology [8].

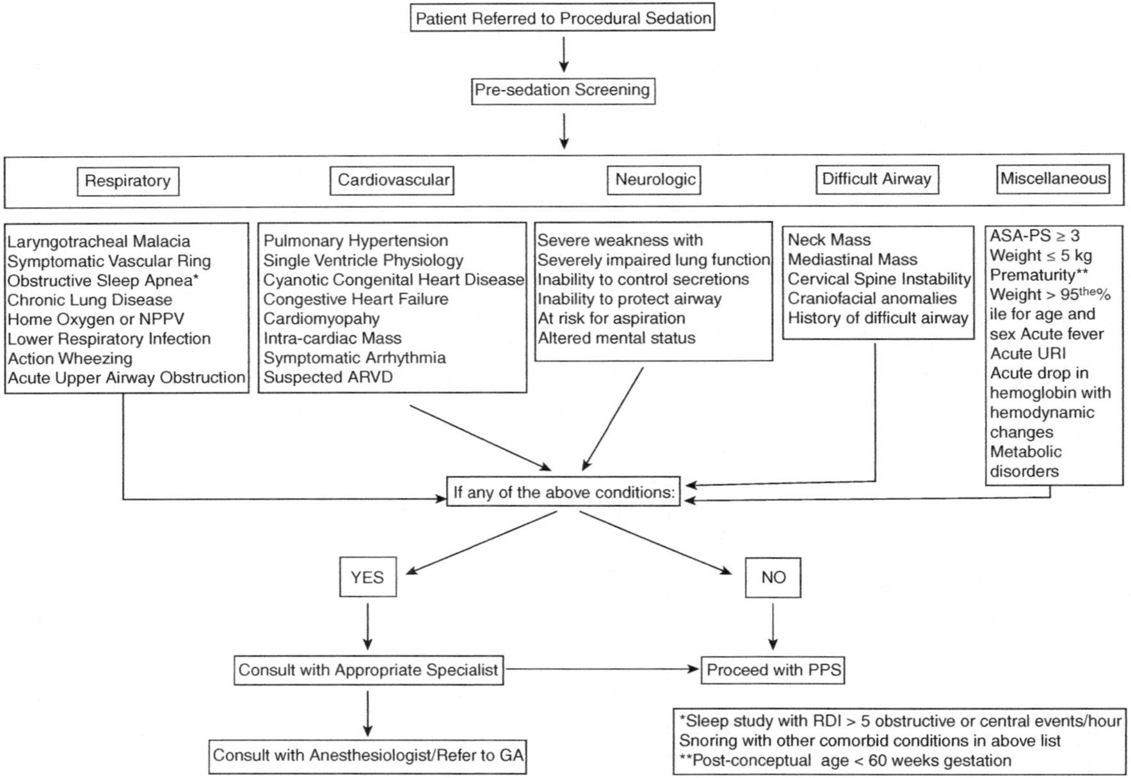

Fig. 25.1 Flow diagram of pre-sedation screening guide for pediatric procedural sedation (PPS). Once children are referred to PPS, they undergo a screening interview with a trained sedation nurse by phone prior to PPS. Children at risk for having the potential for sedation-related complications are categorized by respiratory, cardiovascular, neurologic, difficult airway, and other characteristics or conditions listed. Consultation with specialists and an anesthesiologist are recommended prior to PPS. This list is a suggested list of conditions and is not exhaustive. Abbreviations include ARVD arrhythmogenic right ventricular dysplasia, ASA-PS American Society of Anesthesiologists physical status, GA general anesthesia, PPS pediatric procedural sedation, RDI respiratory disturbance index, URI upper respiratory tract infection (Permission to use this figure was obtained from the publisher of Ref. [7])

Table 25.1 Pediatric sedation assessment tool (PSAT) questionnaire and scoring rubric

Question	Score
1. *Which of the following apply?*	
Prior successful sedation	1
No prior sedation or general anesthesia	3
Prior general anesthesia for the same procedure	5
2. *Is there a history of the following breathing problems?*	
None	1
Recent lower respiratory tract infection[a]	4
Airway malacia[b, c]	5
Recent croup, wheezing, cough, purulent rhinitis, acute sinusitis[b]	5
Home oxygen use	5
3. *Is there a history of heart problems?*	
None or repaired acyanotic congenital heart disease and is not shunt dependent	1
Recent history of arrhythmias or on therapy for an unstable arrhythmia	4
Congestive heart failure	5
Myocarditis/cardiomyopathy	5
History of or taking medications to treat pulmonary hypertension	5
History of a vascular ring	5
History of unrepaired cyanotic congenital heart disease, including staged repair with shunt dependence[d]	5
4. *Is there a history of neurologic problems?*	
None	1
Inability to control secretions or feed by mouth due to aspiration risk	4
Generalized neuromuscular weakness or cerebral palsy	4
Abnormal computed tomography scan with a large intracranial mass, acute hydrocephalus, or midline shift	5
5. *Is there a history of trouble breathing while sleeping?*	
None	1
Recent sleep study positive for obstructive sleep apnea	7
Snoring with respiratory pauses during sleep, wakes up to breathe, or stops breathing	7
Is an infant with loud noisy breathing during sleep	7
6. *Is there a history of any of the following genetic or metabolic disorders?*	
None	1
Down syndrome	4
Any genetic syndrome with a difficult airway: achondroplasia, Apert, Beckwith-Wiedemann, Goldenhar, Pierre Robin, Treacher Collins, Duchenne muscular dystrophy, mitochondrial disorder, mucopolysaccharidosis, or Williams syndrome	5
7. *Was the child born prematurely?*	
No, born at full term (≥37 weeks' gestational age)	1
Yes, born at <37 weeks' gestational age	4
8. *Is the child's weight ≥95th percentile for age and height[e]?*	
No	1
Yes, BMI ≥95th percentile with a z score >2.5	5

(continued)

Table 25.1 (continued)

Question	Score
9. *Has there been a recent illness where medical treatment was sought?*	
No	1
Ill and admitted to the hospital less than a week ago	4
Visited an emergency department in the past 48 hours for cough, vomiting, or diarrhea	4

[a]Airway malacia includes laryngomalacia, tracheomalacia, bronchomalacia
[b]Recent is within the past 7 days
[c]Lower respiratory tract infections include pneumonia and bronchiolitis
[d]Includes Blalock-Taussig shunt and Glenn shunt
[e]Body mass index (BMI) is calculated by obtaining the weight (kg) and height (m) = weight/(height)^2

Implementation of this rapid and simple telephone nurse-led sedation screening tool was assessed in 549 children by retrospective review of prospectively collected data of children undergoing nursing-led screening for procedural sedation at the Children's Healthcare of Atlanta at Egleston and Scottish Rite campuses from January 1, 2018, to March 31, 2018 [8]. Anesthesiologists were surveyed on the appropriateness of the child referred to their service to complete MRI. Of these children, 55 (10.0%) did not require any sedation to complete their procedure and were excluded from analysis [8]. The median (25th–75th interquartile range) score for children who were successfully sedated (n = 343) was 11 (9–12; $p < 0.0001$ vs. cancelled and referred to anesthesia), who were cancelled on the same day (n = 39) was 19 (18–20), and who were referred to anesthesiology (n = 54) was 18 (14.75–20.25 $p = 0.089$ vs. cancelled) (Fig. 25.2b) [8]. The area under the receiver operating curve (AUROC) to predict same-day cancellations based on the scored questionnaire was 0.986 [8]. For children with a screening score of 15 or more, the screening questionnaire had a sensitivity of 82.8%, a specificity of 95.3%, a positive likelihood ratio of 17.6, and a negative likelihood ratio of 0.06 of children needing a referral to anesthesiology [8]. Surveyed anesthesiologists indicated that 85.5% of the referred patients were appropriate for the anesthesiologists due to the risks of airway obstruction (28/54), need for positive pressure ventilation (7/54), anticipated difficult airway (5/54), and/or risk of aspiration (5/54) [8]. Seventy-five percent (6/8) of the children who were deemed inappropriate anesthesia referrals were managed with a laryngeal mask airway and volatile anesthesia to complete their MRI [8]. Implementation of this screening tool led to a decrease in same-day cancellation below 10% (Fig. 25.2c) [8].

The following sections highlight the patient characteristics that are important to consider when sedating a child outside the operating room with a noninvasive airway strategy.

Previous Sedation History

Children with prior successful sedation for the same or a similar procedure are sedation candidates. Children who received anesthesia for the same procedures should, in general, be scheduled with anesthesia. The majority of children screened will

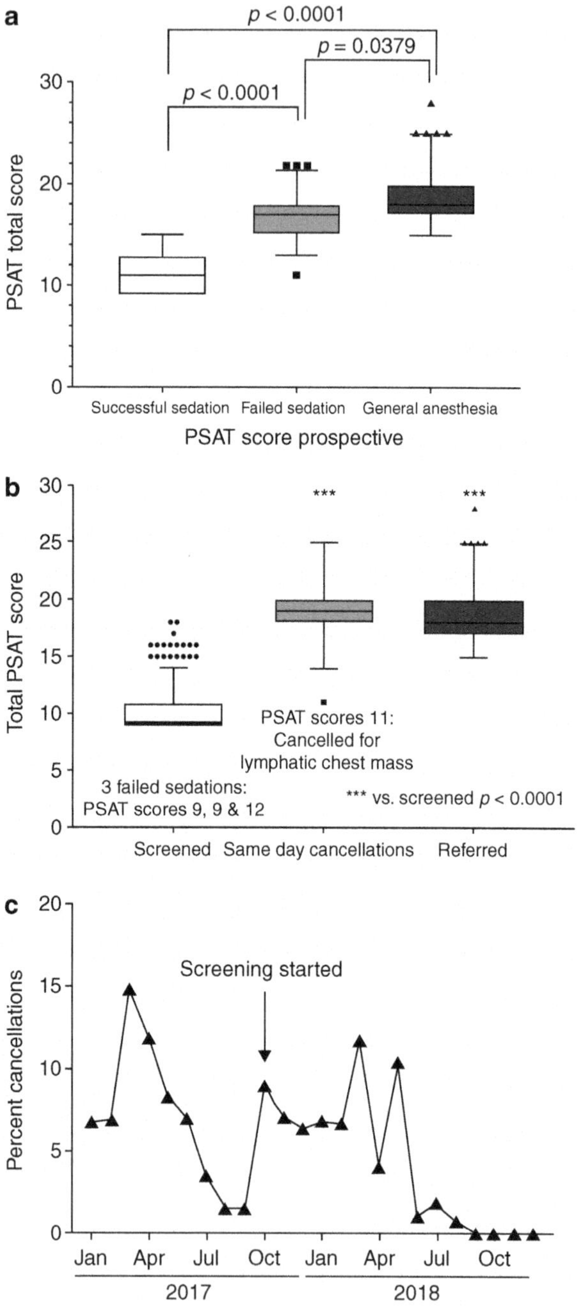

Fig. 25.2 Total pediatric sedation assessment tool (PSAT) scores and outcomes. (**a**) The total PSAT scores of children undergoing successful or failed sedation versus general anesthesia were calculated retrospectively by review of the sedation or anesthesia encounter in the electronic medical record. (**b**) The total PSAT scores of children undergoing successful sedation (screened), those whose procedure was cancelled on the same day (same-day cancellations), and those who went to anesthesia (referred) were retrospectively scored using a prospectively collected nurse-led screening data through telephone interview with the parent or caregiver prior to the sedation appointment. The center line is the median total PSAT score, box edges are the 25th to 75th percentile (interquartile ranges), and whiskers denote fifth to 95th percentile ranges of scores. (**c**) Run chart of quality day showing that implementation of a nurse-led telephone screening process led to a decrease in the frequency of same-day cancellations for procedural sedation

have had no prior sedation or general anesthesia experience, and the subsequent answers to the following screening questions may be used to help determine candidacy for sedation versus anesthesia.

Airway and Breathing History

Children with no prior airway or breathing issues are good sedation candidates. Children with pneumonia or bronchiolitis within the 7 days prior to sedation are at increased risk of adverse events due to secretions, coughing, and parenchyma lung disease, resulting in hypoxia during noninvasive airway sedation. Children with airway malacia, including laryngomalacia, tracheomalacia, and bronchomalacia, are at increased risk of airway obstruction due to dynamic airway collapse from muscle relaxation during sedation. Children with active wheezing, croup within the past 7 days of sedation, purulent rhinitis, active sinusitis, or home oxygen use are also at risk for airway adverse events during sedation, and their procedures may need to be postponed due to intercurrent illness for an elective outpatient procedure.

Recent Illness

Children with recent illness, particularly upper respiratory tract infections (URIs), pose a dilemma to nurse-physician teams of whether to proceed or postpone an elective procedure requiring sedation. Most of the data regarding the risk of perioperative respiratory complications are on children with URIs receiving general anesthesia after presenting to the operating room for surgical procedures [9–18]. Retrospective analysis of approximately 83, 500 children in a large prospectively collected pediatric sedation database showed that a recent or current upper respiratory tract infection (URI) was associated with increased frequency of airway adverse events and interventions after controlling for multiple patient, drug, and procedure characteristics [19]. Despite an increase in adverse airway events and interventions, the frequency of these events was low and could be managed with an experienced and prepared nurse-physician sedation teams [19].

Cardiac History

Children with repaired acyanotic congenital heart disease and those children who are not cardiac shunt dependent are sedation candidates [20–22]. Due to the cardiac depressant nature of propofol, children with congestive heart failure, myocarditis, and cardiomyopathy or those who have either unrepaired cyanotic congenital heart disease or who are shunt dependent, including those children who have had

Blalock-Taussig or Glenn shunt procedures, are better served with an anesthesiologist for their procedure. Retrospective chart reviews of children with palliation for single ventricle physiology prior to a bidirectional Glenn procedure were analyzed and demonstrated that nearly 12% of patients had adverse events including intraoperative arrhythmias, conversion from sedation to general anesthesia, difficult airway, hypotension and desaturation, and cardiac arrest [23]; however, this population of children were inpatients, many of whom arrived to the operative room on vasopressors and are not a comparable population for children undergoing outpatient procedural sedation outside of the operating room [23]. The majority of these children were undergoing central line insertion, percutaneous endoscopic gastrostomy tube or airway surgery, or major intra-abdominal and thoracic operations [23]. By contrast, a retrospective review from a single center of children with repaired congenital heart disease undergoing cardiac MRI using propofol as the sedative-hypnotic agent showed that a procedural sedation service staffed by pediatric intensivists and emergency medicine physicians achieved a similar success rate of completing the imaging study with no difference in adverse events [21]. Similarly, a 10-year single-institution experience of cardiac MRI and contrast angiography for neonates and infants 4 months of age or less showed that adverse events were not related to patient age, complexity of heart disease, type of anesthesia (general anesthesia vs. deep sedation), or dependence on prostaglandin infusion [24]. Nevertheless, children with unrepaired congenital heart disease, vascular ring, myocarditis, cardiomyopathy, and heart failure should have careful consideration to the type and duration of anesthetic and close monitoring by a physician and sedation team that can rescue the child from a sedation-related emergency. Because of these considerations, children with the aforementioned cardiac histories are scored higher than children without these conditions. Children with pulmonary hypertension, regardless of the cause, are at increased risk of perioperative complications and cardiac arrest during and immediately following cardiac catheterization procedures [25]. The more severe the baseline pulmonary arterial hypertension (super-systemic PAH), the higher the risk of major perioperative cardiovascular complications such as cardiac arrest, pulmonary hypertensive crisis, and death [26].

Neurologic History

Information from the PSRC has shown that airway obstruction and adverse respiratory events are more common in children with neurologic conditions [1, 27]. The majority of articles supporting the sedation of children with neurologic disorders discuss caring for children with autism spectrum disorders and other behavior disorders [28, 29]. Aside from an increase in the number of sedation team members for intravenous placement and anesthesia induction, there were no increase adverse events in children with versus without autism spectrum disorders using either propofol or dexmedetomidine as the sedative agent [29, 30]. In a single-center retrospective review of developmentally disabled children compared to normally developing children undergoing brain MRI using pentobarbital and fentanyl, the delayed children were threefold more likely to experience hypoxia [31]; however, prospective study of developmentally delayed versus normally developing children by the same investigators did not show any difference in adverse events between groups [32]. The lack of detection of a difference in adverse events between delayed and normally developing children was due to an increase in adverse events in the control group [32]. In summary, while there is not enough evidence-based data to support specific clinical guidelines with regard to sedative or analgesia choice for the sedation of children with intellectual disabilities and neurologic disorders, physicians providing sedation and analgesia to these children should be vigilant for airway compromise [27].

Sleep-Disordered Breathing

Sleep-disordered breathing (SDB) includes a continuum of upper airway disorders, ranging from primary snoring to obstructive sleep apnea (OSA) [33]. We and others have consistently identified airway obstruction as one of the most frequent complications of sedation, which often requires various airway maneuvers to relieve the obstruction [34–36]. Despite SDB occurring with a frequency of 4–12% in school-aged children [33], it is often underrecognized by parents/caregivers and not adequately assessed in children undergoing anesthesia or sedation [37, 38]. Although perioperative airway complications in children with polysomnogram-quantified SDB have been studied, there has, to our knowledge, been no similar description of polysomnogram-quantified SDB in the pediatric procedural sedation literature.

Many children who require sedation have symptoms consistent with SDB. Some children will have undergone a polysomnogram before presenting for sedation, but most children with SDB will not have been formally evaluated and are more likely to experience sedation-related adverse events [39, 40]. Formal sleep study testing by polysomnogram is the gold standard for diagnosing sleep-disordered breathing, but it is expensive, time-consuming, and impractical for screening large numbers of children needing procedural sedation [39, 41]. Parental questioning of their child's snoring and breathing during sleep is subjective and lacks standardized questionnaires that are consistently implemented by sedation physicians and nurses during the pre-sedation screening process. To address this knowledge gap, we performed a retrospective cohort study of children who had a polysomnogram to identify those with SDB before they underwent a magnetic resonance imaging (MRI) study, a common, long exam requiring sedation or anesthesia to complete in many children [42]. The objective was to determine whether an abnormal sleep study result indicating SDB was associated with higher odds of adverse events and interventions.

We reviewed the sedation encounters of children with a polysomnogram before MRI performed with sedation or anesthesia from 2012 to 2017 at our institution [42]. A total of 305 patients (sedation = 119, anesthesia = 186) were evaluated. The majority of sedated patients (86/119 [72.9%]) were ASA-PS class II [42]. The median AHI for sedated patients was 1.0 (IQR: 0.4–3.1), with 97/119 (84.4%) having an AHI ≤5 [42]. There were 32 sedation-related adverse events, and 110/119 (92.4%) patients needed at least one intervention [42]. On multivariate analysis, only moderate/severe snoring was associated with increased adjusted odds of an adverse event or intervention (Table 25.2) [42].

Table 25.2 Univariate and multivariate logistic regression of characteristics and comorbidities associated with presence of a sedation-related adverse event/intervention, $n = 119$

Characteristic	Odds ratio 95% confidence interval	*p*-value	Adjusted odds ratio 95% confidence interval	*p*-value
Age at time of sedation, years	1.16		1.15	
	1.05–1.29	0.005	1.00–1.32	0.055
ASA-PS (n = 304)				
>II	1.50		1.26	
<II	0.50–4.44 Reference	0.469	0.23–6.83	0.791
Comorbidities				
Asthma	1.64			
	0.69–3.87	0.261		
Autism	1.84			
	0.48–6.99	0.371		
Bronchopulmonary dysplasia[a]	NA	NA		
Congestion	1.79			
	0.29–11.20	0.536		
Developmental delay	0.86			
	0.17–4.49	0.858		
Difficulty swallowing	0.85			
	0.25–2.85	0.793		
Obesity	5.18		3.96	
	1.56–17.28	0.007	0.89–17.58	0.070
Congenital heart disease	0.49			
	0.10–2.37	0.375		
Cough	1.52			
	0.51–4.50	0.454		
Prematurity	0.44			
	0.15–1.26	0.124		
URI	1.32			
	0.23–7.59	0.754		
Wheezing	0.87			
None	0.09–8.62 Reference	0.901		

Table 25.2 (continued)

Characteristic	Odds ratio 95% confidence interval	p-value	Adjusted odds ratio 95% confidence interval	p-value
Apnea-hypopnea index				
>5	0.47		0.79	
≤5	0.13–1.74 Reference	0.26	0.14–4.50	0.791
Snoring quality				
Moderate or severe	3.47		3.69	
Mild	1.21–9.90 Reference	0.020	1.07–12.67	0.038

Sedation-related adverse event: presence of airway obstruction, apnea >15 seconds, coughing, desaturation, stridor, laryngospasm, snoring, or hypoxia
Intervention: bag-valve-mask ventilation, chin-lift/jaw thrust, CPAP/PEEP, ETT, laryngeal mask airway placed, nasopharyngeal tube placed, repositioning/neck roll, or suctioning
NA not applicable
[a]There were very few bronchopulmonary dysplasia cases ($n = 1$) to estimate an odds ratio

Several previous studies have noted airway obstruction as one of the most frequently occurring adverse events during pediatric procedural sedation [1, 4, 5]. Although airway obstruction and other adverse respiratory events can be managed by a well-trained sedation nurse-physician team, some of these events, especially if unrecognized, can be life-threatening. No prior studies, to our knowledge, have assessed whether stratification by polysomnogram-derived AHIs is associated with increased odds of anesthesia referral versus sedation to complete MRI studies. Although some children with severe snoring (AHI >10) who have no additional comorbidities may complete procedural sedation without any adverse events, the combination of SDB, even if mild, with other comorbidities, such as obesity, premature birth history, asthma, bronchopulmonary dysplasia, and congenital heart disease, may be more than additive in increasing the odds of airway-related adverse events during procedural sedation [43–45].

Sleep-disordered breathing is common but often underrecognized in children [38, 40]. We noted that just over one-third of children at our institution had no report of SDB symptoms, but some of those children had polysomnogram results consistent with SDB. Because most children presenting for sedation may have underrecognized symptoms of SDB and because our data suggest that the polysomnogram may be an inefficient screening tool to help anticipate respiratory adverse events during sedation, a standardized, rapid screening tool, as has been described in the anesthesia literature, may provide a rapid, efficient screening tool to reliably diagnose a child's propensity for increased sedation-related airway events [38]. Various questionnaires have been developed to identify children with symptoms consistent with SDB and perioperative respiratory adverse events [46]. The snoring, trouble breathing, and unrefreshed (STBUR) questionnaire consists of five parental/caregiver questions, and if three STBUR questions are answered affirmatively, there is a 3.80 (95% CI: 1.83–8.04) odds of predicting perioperative respiratory adverse events in children with an ASA-PS ≤II [38, 47, 48]. Another pediatric questionnaire that takes very little time to complete is the OSA3/8 (OSA quick test), which focuses on three key symptoms of nighttime breathing patterns and asks parents/caregivers whether their child (1) regularly snores at night, (2) has labored breathing during sleep, or (3) has breathing pauses during sleep [49]. If at least two of these three core questions are answered affirmatively, the child is suspected of having SDB [49]. The STBUR and OSA3/8 questionnaires have not been tested in settings requiring anesthesia or sedation outside the operating room.

Although the risk of serious adverse events, especially life-threatening respiratory events, is rare in sedation, SDB should nevertheless be identified before the sedation or anesthesia encounter in anticipation of children at higher odds of adverse respiratory events and need for interventions during sedation. Children with SDB are also more sensitive to the respiratory-depressant and sedating effects of opioids and benzodiazepines; thus, identification of children with SDB may alter anesthetic management for children presenting for either sedation or anesthesia [50, 51]. For example, dexmedetomidine has been used in procedural sedation to maintain upper airway tone and decrease airway obstruction events in part by enabling smaller doses of coadministered propofol [52, 53]. Many patients undergoing anesthesia may receive both a benzodiazepine and an opioid, and the dosing of these medications may need to be reduced to mitigate peri-anesthetic adverse respiratory events. Because characterization of snoring is not a reliable means to diagnose SDB, a quick, standardized questionnaire-based screening of children for SDB is needed to ensure appropriate referral to anesthesia and sedation management to assess risk and maintain vigilance for respiratory events.

Genetic and Metabolic Conditions

Children with genetic disorders, multiple congenital anomalies, and metabolic disorders, such as mitochondrial disease, presenting for procedural sedation are at risk for complications due to associated characteristics of their syndrome. These risk factors include severe hypotonia, anatomical airway obstruction, vertebral anomalies, and skeletal anomalies that result in altered respiratory mechanics. Sedation nurse-physician teams must be aware of drug sensitivity to opioids, benzodiazepines, and succinylcholine in children with diseases such as muscular dystrophy or those with altered clearance due to liver or kidney dysfunction. Some syndromes, such as muscular dystrophy or glycogen storage disorders, have the potential for associated cardiomyopathies or arrhythmias. Children with mitochondrial disorders have a propensity for hypoglycemia and lactic acidosis (metabolic crisis) that can be associated when exposed to sedative hypnotics, such as propofol, leading to the potential for a higher risk of propofol infusion syndrome. Many syndromes are associated with a difficult airway due to defects in the upper or lower airways including cleft lip/palate, small chin or mouth, macroglossia, choanal stenosis/atresia, tracheomalacia, tracheoesophageal fistula, or craniofacial deformities, and management of an obstructed airway following administration of sedative medications may lead to serious complications and life-threatening emergencies. A selection of specific syndromes is comprehensively discussed in Chapter 4 of the procedural sedation textbook edited by Mason [6]. Because some of these syndromes are rare, most reports are limited to case reports and experience with specific incidences; however, there is an excellent review by Butler et al. on specific genetic diseases at risk for sedation/anesthesia complications [54]. Readers are also referred to the most current edition of *Smith's Recognizable Patterns of Human Malformation* [55], the main textbook used in the clinical practice of genetics, to aid in the identification of syndrome with features that include a high likelihood of airway obstruction or other anomalies associated with characteristics of having a difficult airway.

Premature Birth

Infants born prematurely, defined as being born before the 37th week of gestation, have an increase frequency of postoperative apnea induced by analgosedation medications especially when less than 60 weeks postgestational age [56–59]. Premature birth may also be complicated by other comorbidities such as neurologic disabilities, developmental delays, swallowing dysfunction leading to feeding issues and gastroesophageal reflux disease, chronic lung disease, and frequent episodes of apnea and bradycardia that can compound the risk of sedation-related adverse events. In a prospective observational study of approximately 57, 200 children from birth through 21 years of age receiving sedation/anesthesia procedures outside of the operating room, mainly for MRI studies, children with a history of preterm birth had higher nearly twice the frequency of sedation-related airway and respiratory adverse event rates compared with children born at term [60]. The reasons for apnea associated with prematurity are not understood but are postulated to be related to immaturity of the respiratory and central nervous systems, blunted carotid chemoreceptor responses to hypoxia and hypercarbia, neurotransmitters, a genetic predisposition, and laryngeal chemoreflexes [61–64]. Procedural sedation data also show that preterm children, regardless of age, have higher odds of adverse sedation-related adverse events with two age peaks in children less than 6 months of age and in preadolescent children between 10 and 13 years of age [60]. Children with a history of premature birth, especially those who are less than 6 months of age and less than 60 weeks conceptual age with apnea, with a home apnea monitor, or who are prescribed caffeine to treat apnea of prematurity may be better served by an anesthesiologist and a planned overnight admission for observation in a pediatric intensive care unit.

Obesity

Obesity is an independent risk factor for sedation-related airway adverse events and airway interventions during procedural sedation [65]. These adverse events included prolonged recovery and inability to complete sedations due to sedation-related adverse events [65]. Both retrospective and prospective studies on obese children undergoing general anesthesia had a higher frequency of intraoperative oxygen desaturation, bronchospasm, laryngospasm, and postoperative airway obstruction [34, 66–69]. In a large multicenter cohort of children undergoing procedural sedation, obesity is an independent risk factor associated with sedation-related adverse events and need for any airway intervention [65]; however, a major limitation of that study is the lack of evaluation of the presence of OSA as a colinear variable with obesity [65].

Contraindications for Sedation/Reasons to Refer to Anesthesiology

There are some children with specific diseases or medical issues that are of such high risk of potential airway compromise that they are not sedation candidates and should be referred to anesthesia to complete their procedure. Children with the following conditions and features are not sedation candidates: (1) anterior mediastinal mass, (2) neck mass with airway compromise (hoarse voice, weak cry, difficulty breathing), (3) vascular ring with airway compromise, (4) craniofacial anomalies (e.g., Treacher Collins syndrome, Pierre Robin sequence), (5) cervical neck instability (achondroplasia, some children with Down syndrome), (6) high intracranial pressure (drowsiness, headache, vomiting), (7) respiratory failure (apnea, tachypnea, high oxygen requirement), and (8) high likelihood of aspiration (vomiting, delayed gastric emptying, abdominal distension, large amount of drainage from a nasogastric tube).

Sedation of Hospitalized Patients

Children who are hospitalized for an acute illness frequently require magnetic resonance imaging (MRI) and painful procedures that require procedural sedation. The general pediatricians and pediatric hospitalists must assess each hospitalized patient's risk profile to decide whether sedation is appropriate for that patient or if the patient should be referred to an anesthesiology service for the procedure. Inaccurate screening of children for sedation may result in same-day cancellations that delay care, decreased parental satisfaction, and inefficient use of hospital resources [7, 70, 71]. To improve pediatric sedation efficiency, general pediatricians and pediatric hospitalists need an accurate assessment tool. In teaching hospitals, residents are often the first-line screeners who assess a child's candidacy for sedation or general anesthesia to complete a procedure.

We developed a pediatric sedation assessment history and physical examination template (Table 25.3) and retrospectively scored the 222 children who had undergone sedation screening by a resident physician [8]. Of these 222 children, 148 (66.7%) were deemed sedation candidates, and 38 (17.1%) were referred to anesthesia services [8]. The median (IQR) score for the 148 children who were referred to sedation services was 11 (11–15), whereas the median (IQR) for the 38 children referred to anesthesia services was 18 (14–20) ($P < .0001$) (Fig. 25.3a) [8]. The area under the receiver-operating curve is 0.78 (95% CI, 0.69–0.86) for children being evaluated for sedation versus anesthesia candidacy ($P < .0001$) (Fig. 25.3b) [8]. In children with a screening score of 15 or higher, there is a positive likelihood ratio of 2.60 (95% CI, 1.89–3.57), with a sensitivity of 73.7 (95% CI, 56.9–86.6) and a specificity of 71.6 (95% CI, 63.6–78.7) [8]. Anesthesiologist review of the medical records of children referred to anesthesia was deemed appropriate in all cases; however, in 9/38 (23.7%) of cases, the anesthesiologist believed that while the child was appropriately referred given the current illness level, the child could be a sedation

Table 25.3 Patient history and physical examination sedation evaluation template[a]

Category	Findings	Score if yes[a]
General	Past requirement for general anesthesia	5
	Obesity (z score >2.5)	5
Syndromes	Down (especially with uncorrected heart defect, macroglossia, C-spine instability, obstructive sleep apnea, or pulmonary hypertension)	4
	Beckwith-Wiedemann	5
	Pierre Robin	5
	Goldenhar	5
	Apert	5
	Mucopolysaccharidoses	5
	Treacher Collins	5
	Achondroplasia	5
	Williams	5
	Any syndrome with dysmorphic features that affect mouth or upper airway (may or may not be listed above but, e.g., macroglossia with Down and Beckwith-Wiedemann or micrognathia with Pierre Robin)	5
Head, eyes, ears, nose, and throat	Inability to control secretions	4
	Vocal cord dysfunction, injury, or stridor	5
	Cystic hygroma	5
	Micrognathia	5
	Macroglossia	5
	Unable to open mouth fully	5
Neck	Cervical spine instability (e.g., Down syndrome, injury)	5
	Abscess (e.g., retropharyngeal abscess), any mass, or organ enlargement with potential to obstruct airway	5

(continued)

Table 25.3 (continued)

Category	Findings	Score if yes[a]
Lungs	Any evidence of lower respiratory tract infection (pneumonia, bronchiolitis)	4
	Any respiratory infection in the past 4 weeks (<1 year old)	4
	Any respiratory infection in the past 2 weeks (>1 year old)	4
	Evidence of recent purulent rhinitis or sinusitis	5
	Oxygen requirement	5
	Airway malacia	5
	Bronchopulmonary dysplasia corrected (<6 months old)	5
	Wheezing now	5
	Aspiration history of or failed oropharyngeal motor study	5
	Restrictive lung disease (e.g., muscular dystrophy, spinal muscular atrophy)	5
	Pulmonary hypertension	5
	Obstructive sleep apnea (by history or sleep study)	5
Heart	Any cardiac disease (e.g., congestive heart failure, myocarditis, cyanotic heart disease, coronary disease, arrhythmias, vascular ring)	5
Gastrointestinal	Gastrointestinal reflux disease that requires treatment beyond proton-pump inhibitors or histamine$_2$ blocker (e.g., smart monitor or nasogastric tube feeds)	5
	Any child receiving nasogastric tube feeds	5
Hematology	Hemoglobin <8 g/dL	4

[a]If a category is marked "no" for condition not present, then the score for that category is assigned a score of 1

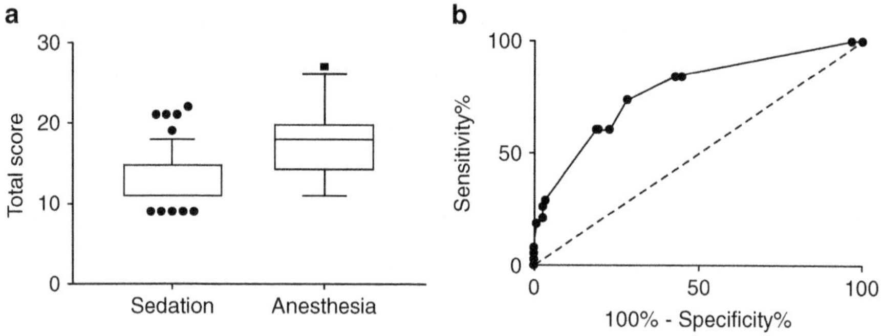

Fig. 25.3 Total sedation assessment scores comparing children undergoing successful or failed sedation and general anesthesia. (**a**) Boxplots of the total scores for children evaluated for sedation versus anesthesia. Center line is median total score, box edges are the 25th to 75th percentile (interquartile ranges), and whiskers denote fifth to 95th percentile ranges of scores ($P < .0001$). (**b**) Area under the receiver operating curve is 0.78 (95% CI, 0.69–0.86) for children being evaluated for sedation versus anesthesia candidacy ($P < .0001$)

candidate for future elective procedures [8]. A survey of 70 pediatric resident physicians and fellows, with a 100% response rate, regarding the use of the sedation assessment history and physical examination template demonstrated that 52 (74.3%) agreed that the tool helped them care for patients, and 49 (70.0%) believed it increased their understanding of risk factors associated with sedation [8]. Implementation of a pediatric resident-led sedation screening tool improves communication among teams to determine which hospitalized children are appropriate for sedation versus anesthesia services.

Conclusions

Sedation physician-nurse teams should be well versed in assessing characteristics that place a child at increased odds for sedation-related adverse events. Running an efficient sedation service line that ensures the safety and well-being of the children who require sedation can be accomplished by screening patients prior to the procedure. Screening tools aid in this process and not only help minimize adverse events during sedation but also reduce the frequency of same-day sedation cancellations by appropriately referring children to anesthesia.

References

1. Cravero JP, Beach ML, Blike GT, Gallagher SM, Hertzog JH, Pediatric Sedation Research Consortium. The incidence and nature of adverse events during pediatric sedation/anesthesia with propofol for procedures outside the operating room: a report from the Pediatric Sedation Research Consortium. Anesth Analg. 2009;108:795–804.
2. Cravero JP, Blike GT, Beach M, Gallagher SM, Hertzog JH, Havidich JE, Gelman B, Pediatric Sedation Research Consortium. Incidence and nature of adverse events during pediatric sedation/anesthesia for procedures outside the operating room: report from the Pediatric Sedation Research Consortium. Pediatrics. 2006;118:1087–96.
3. Grunwell JR, McCracken C, Fortenberry J, Stockwell J, Kamat P. Risk factors leading to failed procedural sedation in children outside the operating room. Pediatr Emerg Care. 2014;30:381–7.
4. Kamat PP, McCracken CE, Gillespie SE, Fortenberry JD, Stockwell JA, Cravero JP, Hebbar KB. Pediatric critical care physician-administered procedural sedation using propofol: a report from the Pediatric Sedation Research Consortium Database. Pediatr Crit Care Med. 2015;16:11–20.
5. Mallory MD, Baxter AL, Yanosky DJ, Cravero JP, Pediatric Sedation Research Consortium. Emergency physician-administered propofol sedation: a report on 25,433 sedations from the Pediatric Sedation Research Consortium. Ann Emerg Med. 2011;57:462–468 e461.
6. Mason KP, editor. Pediatric sedation outside of the operating room. New York: Springer; 2015.
7. Grunwell JR, Marupudi NK, Gupta RV, Travers CD, McCracken CE, Williamson JL, Stockwell JA, Fortenberry JD, Couloures K, Cravero J, Kamat PP. Outcomes following implementation of a pediatric procedural sedation guide for referral to general anesthesia for magnetic resonance imaging studies. Paediatr Anaesth. 2016;26:628–36.

8. Balkam K, Kamat P, Grunwell J, Mallory M, Thompson B. 1394: a nursing screening tool to assess a child's appropriateness for sedation versus need for anesthesia. Crit Care Med. 2019;47:673.
9. Cohen MM, Cameron CB. Should you cancel the operation when a child has an upper respiratory tract infection? Anesth Analg. 1991;72:282-288.
10. Malviya S, Voepel-Lewis T, Siewert M, Pandit UA, Riegger LQ, Tait AR. Risk factors for adverse postoperative outcomes in children presenting for cardiac surgery with upper respiratory tract infections. Anesthesiology. 2003;98:628–32.
11. Parnis SJ, Barker DS, Van Der Walt JH. Clinical predictors of anaesthetic complications in children with respiratory tract infections. Paediatr Anaesth. 2001;11:29–40.
12. Rachel Homer J, Elwood T, Peterson D, Rampersad S. Risk factors for adverse events in children with colds emerging from anesthesia: a logistic regression. Paediatr Anaesth. 2007;17:154–61.
13. Tait AR. Anesthetic management of the child with an upper respiratory tract infection. Curr Opin Anaesthesiol. 2005;18:603–7.
14. Tait AR, Knight PR. The effects of general anesthesia on upper respiratory tract infections in children. Anesthesiology. 1987;67:930–5.
15. Tait AR, Knight PR. Intraoperative respiratory complications in patients with upper respiratory tract infections. Can J Anaesth. 1987;34:300–3.
16. Tait AR, Malviya S. Anesthesia for the child with an upper respiratory tract infection: still a dilemma? Anesth Analg. 2005;100:59–65.
17. Tait AR, Malviya S, Voepel-Lewis T, Munro HM, Seiwert M, Pandit UA. Risk factors for perioperative adverse respiratory events in children with upper respiratory tract infections. Anesthesiology. 2001;95:299–306.
18. Tait AR, Reynolds PI, Gutstein HB. Factors that influence an anesthesiologist's decision to cancel elective surgery for the child with an upper respiratory tract infection. J Clin Anesth. 1995;7:491–9.
19. Mallory MD, Travers C, McCracken CE, Hertzog J, Cravero JP. Upper respiratory infections and airway adverse events in pediatric procedural sedation. Pediatrics. 2017;140:e20170009.
20. Abbas SM, Rashid A, Latif H. Sedation for children undergoing cardiac catheterization: a review of literature. J Pak Med Assoc. 2012;62:159–63.
21. Jain R, Petrillo-Albarano T, Parks WJ, Linzer JF Sr, Stockwell JA. Efficacy and safety of deep sedation by non-anesthesiologists for cardiac MRI in children. Pediatr Radiol. 2013;43:605–11.
22. Lam JE, Lin EP, Alexy R, Aronson LA. Anesthesia and the pediatric cardiac catheterization suite: a review. Paediatr Anaesth. 2015;25:127–34.
23. Brown ML, DiNardo JA, Odegard KC. Patients with single ventricle physiology undergoing noncardiac surgery are at high risk for adverse events. Paediatr Anaesth. 2015;25:846–51.
24. Rangamani S, Varghese J, Li L, Harvey L, Hammel JM, Fletcher SE, Duncan KF, Danford DA, Kutty S. Safety of cardiac magnetic resonance and contrast angiography for neonates and small infants: a 10-year single-institution experience. Pediatr Radiol. 2012;42:1339–46.
25. Bernier ML, Jacob AI, Collaco JM, McGrath-Morrow SA, Romer LH, Unegbu CC. Perioperative events in children with pulmonary hypertension undergoing non-cardiac procedures. Pulm Circ. 2018;8:2045893217738143.
26. Carmosino MJ, Friesen RH, Doran A, Ivy DD. Perioperative complications in children with pulmonary hypertension undergoing noncardiac surgery or cardiac catheterization. Anesth Analg. 2007;104:521–7.
27. Kilbaugh TJ, Friess SH, Raghupathi R, Huh JW. Sedation and analgesia in children with developmental disabilities and neurologic disorders. Int J Pediatr. 2010;2010:189142.
28. Kamat PP, Bryan LN, McCracken CE, Simon HK, Berkenbosch JW, Grunwell JR. Procedural sedation in children with autism spectrum disorders: a survey of current practice patterns of the society for pediatric sedation members. Paediatr Anaesth. 2018;28:552–7.
29. Lubisch N, Roskos R, Berkenbosch JW. Dexmedetomidine for procedural sedation in children with autism and other behavior disorders. Pediatr Neurol. 2009;41:88–94.

30. Kamat PP, Karaga MK, Wisniewski BL, McCracken CE, Simon HK, Sidhu R, Grunwell JR. Outpatient procedural sedation of patients with autism spectrum disorders for magnetic resonance imaging of the brain using propofol. J Child Neurol. 2018;33:313–9.
31. Kannikeswaran N, Mahajan PV, Sethuraman U, Groebe A, Chen X. Sedation medication received and adverse events related to sedation for brain MRI in children with and without developmental disabilities. Paediatr Anaesth. 2009;19:250–6.
32. Kannikeswaran N, Sethuraman U, Sivaswamy L, Chen X, Mahajan PV. Children with and without developmental disabilities: sedation medication requirements and adverse events related to sedation. Pediatr Emerg Care. 2012;28:1036–40.
33. Marcus CL, Brooks LJ, Draper KA, Gozal D, Halbower AC, Jones J, Schechter MS, Sheldon SH, Spruyt K, Ward SD, Lehmann C, Shiffman RN, American Academy of Pediatrics. Diagnosis and management of childhood obstructive sleep apnea syndrome. Pediatrics. 2012;130:576–84.
34. Tait AR, Voepel-Lewis T, Burke C, Kostrzewa A, Lewis I. Incidence and risk factors for perioperative adverse respiratory events in children who are obese. Anesthesiology. 2008;108:375–80.
35. Tait AR, Voepel-Lewis T, O'Brien LM. Postsurgical behaviors in children with and without symptoms of sleep-disordered breathing. Perioper Med (Lond). 2014;3:8.
36. Hillman DR, Chung F. Anaesthetic management of sleep-disordered breathing in adults. Respirology. 2017;22:230–9.
37. Carroll JL, McColley SA, Marcus CL, Curtis S, Loughlin GM. Inability of clinical history to distinguish primary snoring from obstructive sleep apnea syndrome in children. Chest. 1995;108:610–8.
38. Tait AR, Bickham R, O'Brien LM, Quinlan M, Voepel-Lewis T. The STBUR questionnaire for identifying children at risk for sleep-disordered breathing and postoperative opioid-related adverse events. Paediatr Anaesth. 2016;26:759–66.
39. Sinha R, Bose S, Thangaswamy CR. Unrecognized obstructive sleep apnea in children: caught on the wrong foot and lessons learnt!!! Paediatr Anaesth. 2008;18:984–6.
40. Tait AR, Voepel-Lewis T. Sleep-disordered breathing--not just for grownups anymore. J Perianesth Nurs. 2015;30:566–70.
41. Brown KA. Outcome, risk, and error and the child with obstructive sleep apnea. Paediatr Anaesth. 2011;21:771–80.
42. Miniet A, Karaga K, Grunwell J, McCracken C, Simon H, Guglani L, Kamat P. 1210: sedation versus general anesthesia for procedures in pediatric patients with sleep-related concerns. Crit Care Med. 2019;47:581.
43. Schwengel DA, Sterni LM, Tunkel DE, Heitmiller ES. Perioperative management of children with obstructive sleep apnea. Anesth Analg. 2009;109:60–75.
44. Cote CJ. Anesthesiological considerations for children with obstructive sleep apnea. Curr Opin Anaesthesiol. 2015;28:327–32.
45. Wolfe RM, Pomerantz J, Miller DE, Weiss-Coleman R, Solomonides T. Obstructive sleep apnea: preoperative screening and postoperative care. J Am Board Fam Med. 2016;29:263–75.
46. Bauer EE, Lee R, Campbell YN. Preoperative screening for sleep-disordered breathing in children: a systematic literature review. AORN J. 2016;104:541–53.
47. Tait AR, Voepel-Lewis T, Christensen R, O'Brien LM. The STBUR questionnaire for predicting perioperative respiratory adverse events in children at risk for sleep-disordered breathing. Paediatr Anaesth. 2013;23:510–6.
48. Terry KL, Disabato J, Krajicek M. Snoring, Trouble Breathing, Un-Refreshed (STBUR) screening questionnaire to reduce perioperative respiratory adverse events in Pediatric surgical patients: a quality improvement project. AANA J. 2015;83:256–62.
49. Schnoor J, Busch T, Turemuratov N, Merkenschlager A. Pre-anesthetic assessment with three core questions for the detection of obstructive sleep apnea in childhood: an observational study. BMC Anesthesiol. 2018;18:25.
50. Brown KA, Laferriere A, Moss IR. Recurrent hypoxemia in young children with obstructive sleep apnea is associated with reduced opioid requirement for analgesia. Anesthesiology. 2004;100:806–10; discussion 805A.

51. Ehsan Z, Mahmoud M, Shott SR, Amin RS, Ishman SL. The effects of anesthesia and opioids on the upper airway: a systematic review. Laryngoscope. 2016;126:270–84.
52. Boriosi JP, Eickhoff JC, Klein KB, Hollman GA. A retrospective comparison of propofol alone to propofol in combination with dexmedetomidine for pediatric 3T MRI sedation. Paediatr Anaesth. 2017;27:52–9.
53. Shin HJ, Kim EY, Hwang JW, Do SH, Na HS. Comparison of upper airway patency in patients with mild obstructive sleep apnea during dexmedetomidine or propofol sedation: a prospective, randomized, controlled trial. BMC Anesthesiol. 2018;18:120.
54. Butler MG, Hayes BG, Hathaway MM, Begleiter ML. Specific genetic diseases at risk for sedation/anesthesia complications. Anesth Analg. 2000;91:837–55.
55. Jones KL, Jones MC, del Campo M. Smith's recognizable patterns of human malformation. Philadelphia: Saunders; 2013.
56. Kurth CD, Spitzer AR, Broennle AM, Downes JJ. Postoperative apnea in preterm infants. Anesthesiology. 1987;66:483–8.
57. Miller MJ, Martin RJ. Apnea of prematurity. Clin Perinatol. 1992;19:789–808.
58. Poets CF, Stebbens VA, Richard D, Southall DP. Prolonged episodes of hypoxemia in preterm infants undetectable by cardiorespiratory monitors. Pediatrics. 1995;95:860–3.
59. Welborn LG, Rice LJ, Hannallah RS, Broadman LM, Ruttimann UE, Fink R. Postoperative apnea in former preterm infants: prospective comparison of spinal and general anesthesia. Anesthesiology. 1990;72:838–42.
60. Havidich JE, Beach M, Dierdorf SF, Onega T, Suresh G, Cravero JP. Preterm versus term children: analysis of sedation/anesthesia adverse events and longitudinal risk. Pediatrics. 2016;137:e20150463.
61. Abu-Shaweesh JM, Martin RJ. Neonatal apnea: what's new? Pediatr Pulmonol. 2008;43: 937–44.
62. Katz ES, Mitchell RB, D'Ambrosio CM. Obstructive sleep apnea in infants. Am J Respir Crit Care Med. 2012;185:805–16.
63. Martin RJ, Abu-Shaweesh JM. Control of breathing and neonatal apnea. Biol Neonate. 2005;87:288–95.
64. Praud JP. Larynx and neonatal apneas. Pediatr Pulmonol Suppl. 1999;18:190–3.
65. Scherrer PD, Mallory MD, Cravero JP, Lowrie L, Hertzog JH, Berkenbosch JW, Pediatric Sedation Research C. The impact of obesity on pediatric procedural sedation-related outcomes: results from the Pediatric Sedation Research Consortium. Paediatr Anaesth. 2015;25:689–97.
66. El-Metainy S, Ghoneim T, Aridae E, Abdel Wahab M. Incidence of perioperative adverse events in obese children undergoing elective general surgery. Br J Anaesth. 2011;106:359–63.
67. Nafiu OO, Green GE, Walton S, Morris M, Reddy S, Tremper KK. Obesity and risk of peri-operative complications in children presenting for adenotonsillectomy. Int J Pediatr Otorhinolaryngol. 2009;73:89–95.
68. Nafiu OO, Reynolds PI, Bamgbade OA, Tremper KK, Welch K, Kasa-Vubu JZ. Childhood body mass index and perioperative complications. Paediatr Anaesth. 2007;17:426–30.
69. Setzer N, Saade E. Childhood obesity and anesthetic morbidity. Paediatr Anaesth. 2007;17:321–6.
70. Hoffman AS, Matlow A, Shroff M, Cohen E. Factors impacting same-day cancellation of outpatient pediatric magnetic resonance imaging under anesthesia. Pediatr Radiol. 2015;45: 99–107.
71. Grunwell JR, Long LD, Bryan LN, Kelley T, Sabnis HS, Simon HK, Kamat PP. Factors affecting same-day cancelation of outpatient pediatric oncologic procedural sedation. Pediatr Hematol Oncol. 2018;35:309–15.

Chapter 26
Choosing a Sedation Regimen

Megan E. Peters and Gregory A. Hollman

Goals of Pediatric Procedural Sedation

Choosing the ideal sedation regimen achieves each of the central goals of pediatric procedural sedation. These goals are to maintain patient safety, promote procedural success, maximize patient comfort, and return the patient to their baseline clinical state [1–3]. First and foremost, the sedation regimen must preserve patient safety. It is essential to use the sedative regimen with the greatest safety profile that promotes both procedural success and patient comfort. Additionally, selecting the safest sedation agents requires a clear understanding of the sedative drug effects on the patient's upper airway and cardiorespiratory function. As a consequence, understanding the patient's underlying clinical condition and illness severity (e.g., American Society of Anesthesiologists (ASA) status) is necessary for choosing the safest sedation regimen. Titrating the sedative regimen to the desired clinical effect is another key factor in promoting patient safety during procedural sedation, particularly in critically ill patients. Successful completion of the procedure requires tailoring the sedative regimen to the characteristics and needs of the procedure. Procedural aspects that guide in choosing the best sedative regimen include the degree of invasiveness (pain), level of immobility required, and the urgency and length of the procedure. Consequently, the pharmacological properties of the sedation regimen should match the conditions needed for successful completion of the procedure. Ensuring patient comfort and pain control is a third priority of high-quality procedural sedation. Sedatives should be tailored to meet the needs of the patient and include reducing fear and anxiety, alleviating pain, and in many cases diminishing recall of the procedure and surrounding events. The final goal of the procedural sedation encounter is to return the patient to their baseline clinical state once the procedure has been completed.

M. E. Peters · G. A. Hollman (✉)
Department of Pediatrics, University of Wisconsin School of Medicine and Public Health, Madison, WI, USA
e-mail: mpeters@pediatrics.wisc.edu; ghollman@pediatrics.wisc.edu

P. P. Kamat, J. W. Berkenbosch (eds.), *Sedation and Analgesia for the Pediatric Intensivist*, https://doi.org/10.1007/978-3-030-52555-2_26

This chapter discusses the principles in choosing a sedative drug regimen that promotes safe and effective procedural sedation. The importance of understanding the basic pharmacological principles of sedative drugs and aligning them with the characteristics and requirements of the procedure will be considered in the next two sections. Lastly, a summary and practical approach to systematically choosing an appropriate procedural sedation regimen will be discussed.

Pharmacological Considerations and the Therapeutic Window

The key to successful pediatric procedural sedation is to achieve sedative drug concentrations that result in the therapeutic effects while remaining below concentrations associated with adverse events. The therapeutic window describes the drug concentration range that results in the desired clinical effect, beginning at concentrations just above subtherapeutic levels and just below that for adverse effects (Fig. 26.1).

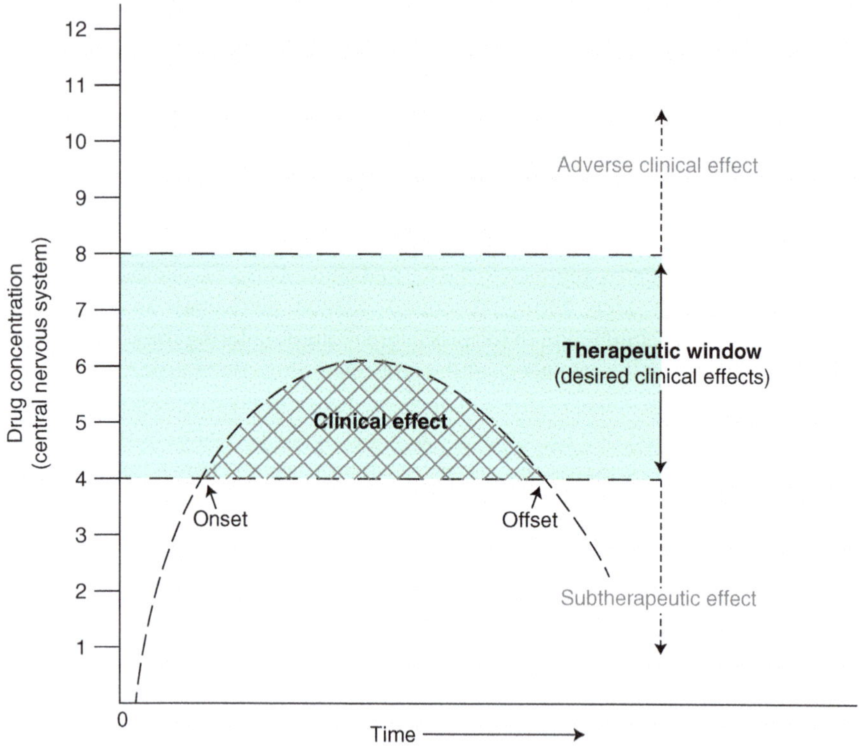

Fig. 26.1 The therapeutic window is the drug concentration range associated with the desired clinical effect. Concentrations below and above the therapeutic window are associated with subtherapeutic and adverse events, respectively. In this example, drug administration at time 0 results in the desired clinical effect (hatched lines) in the span of time between onset and offset of action

Describing the therapeutic window in terms of desired clinical effects facilitates matching the characteristics of the procedure to the clinical actions of the drug (e.g., painful procedures with a sedative analgesic). Adding the dimension of *time* to the therapeutic window based on the onset and duration of the procedure clarifies how fast and for how long the drug effects are required. As such, the desired clinical effects, largely determined by the nature of the procedure, facilitate the choice of a drug's pharmacodynamic properties, while the timing and length of the procedure clarify the selection of the drug's pharmacokinetic profile. Choosing the best sedative regimen begins with an in-depth understanding of the drug's pharmacodynamic and pharmacokinetic properties.

Pharmacodynamic Principles

The drugs pharmacodynamic action relates to the *drug concentration-target organ relationship*, "what the drug does to the body," and includes both the drug's desired and undesired clinical effects. A drug and its dose are typically chosen for their clinical action on a target organ, *effect site*, that results in the anticipated clinical effect. A sedative drug's clinical actions are usually described as quantitative in nature and subsequently dependent on the concentration of drug at the effect site. Consequently, greater clinical effect is associated with higher drug concentrations in the target organ. Electroencephalogram (EEG) analysis is a common surrogate monitor used to quantitate effect-site concentrations in the central nervous system and the resulting clinical effects of sedative drugs [4, 5]. In general, pharmacodynamic properties within a given class of sedative drugs (e.g., opioids) are similar and correspond with a specific receptor system (e.g., mu receptor). The common clinical effect among all sedative agents is their ability to simultaneously produce sedation (i.e., to calm and moderate excitement) and respiratory depression, although the degree of each will vary according to dose and drug. Pharmacodynamic features that distinguish sedative drugs from one another are their other clinical actions either directly or indirectly related to their ability to promote sedation. Other clinical properties used to select one sedative drug over another include the following.

Anxiolysis Sedative drugs with anxiolytic properties relieve apprehension and fear related to anticipation of an event. Sedatives with primary anxiolytic properties include nitrous oxide, benzodiazepines, and low-dose ketamine.

Amnesia (Anterograde) Anterograde amnesia is characterized by the partial or complete inability to recall information and events after the onset of sedation. Sedative drugs with anterograde amnestic effects include the benzodiazepines, propofol, and ketamine.

Analgesia Drugs with analgesic properties relieve pain and alter the perception of nociceptive stimuli. Opioids and ketamine are commonly used sedative drugs with analgesic properties.

Hypnosis A drug with hypnotic properties induces drowsiness and promotes the onset of sleep. Sedative drugs commonly used to promote sleep include dexmedetomidine, the barbiturates, and propofol.

Synergism Combining agents (e.g., an opioid with a benzodiazepine) can result in synergy in which the combined effects exceed the sum of individual effects, allowing smaller doses of individual drugs to achieve the desired clinical effect [6].

Pharmacokinetic Principles

The drug's pharmacokinetic properties relate to the *dose-concentration relationship* of the drug, "what the body does to the drug," and accounts for the relevant clinical consequences that result in onset of action, duration of effect, and elimination half-life. The pharmacokinetics of a drug distinguishes it within a given class and is often the principle factor in choosing one medication over another (e.g., fentanyl vs morphine). For most rapidly acting intravenous sedatives used for procedural sedation, onset of action and duration of effect can be described by a parallel three-compartment model, composed of a central compartment (plasma), a rapidly equilibrating, vessel-rich compartment, and a slowly equilibrating compartment, in addition to an "effect"-site component of negligible volume [7–9] (Fig. 26.2).

Following intravenous bolus administration, the simultaneous competing processes of distribution (reversible drug loss to and from the plasma) and elimination (irreversible drug loss from the body) occur. Peak plasma concentrations (central compartment) occur in approximately 30–45 seconds as drug is distributed to various compartments in the body. Immediately following intravenous drug delivery, the distribution phase of drug clearance from the plasma predominates and vessel-rich organs such as the central nervous system receive a relatively greater fraction

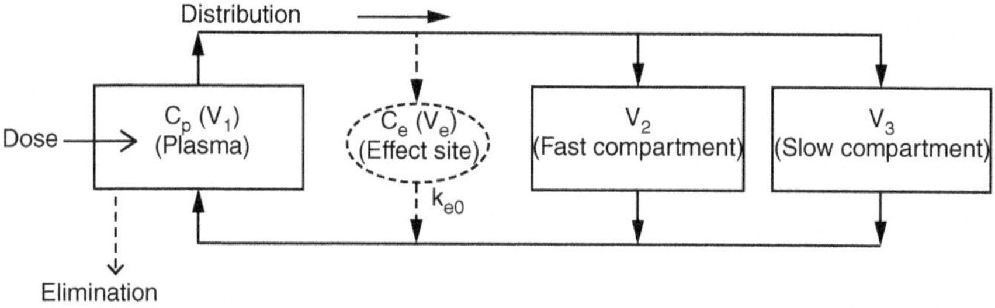

Fig. 26.2 Three-compartment parallel circuit model of intravenous drug administration, distribution, and elimination. Following drug delivery to plasma (V_1, central compartment), simultaneous distribution and elimination to and from the body occurs. K_{e0} is a measure of the rate of drug movement in and out of the effect-site compartment (V_e). The size of each arrow indicates the relative speed and fraction of drug to areas. C_P, plasma drug concentration; V_1, central (plasma) compartment; C_e, effect-site concentration; V_2, fast compartment; V_3, slow compartment

of the drug. The rate of drug movement from plasma to the effect site can be described as a first-order rate constant (k_{e0}). For rapidly acting sedative drugs, k_{e0} is small, and the drug rapidly enters the target organ (effect site) from the plasma during the early phases of distribution. Consequently, onset of clinical action is fast. Clinical effect is terminated during this phase as well, as drug concentrations rapidly decline in the central nervous system and gradually increase in slower compartments. Speed of action and duration of effect following a single dose of a fast-acting sedative agent is secondary to distribution in and out of the central nervous system, respectively [10, 11]. The fraction of drug irreversibly cleared from the body during elimination is initially small following a bolus and increases significantly following distribution equilibrium during the elimination phase (terminal half-life) of drug clearance [11].

Shortly following peak clinical action, effect-site drug concentrations of rapidly acting sedative agents will drop relatively quickly as drug is distributed to other compartments. In order to maintain a concentration range within the therapeutic window, additional drug must be administered during this time either as repeated boluses or as an infusion to overcome drug loss due to distribution and ongoing elimination. For short procedural sedations with rapidly acting sedative drugs, the distribution phase is unlikely to reach a steady state, and distribution remains the primary process terminating clinical action. For longer procedures where repeated drug dosing or a continuous infusion is used to maintain adequate drug concentrations, compartments become "saturated," and distribution approaches an equilibrium. Under these circumstances duration of effect becomes more dependent on drug clearance from the body during terminal elimination. The specifics of these processes will depend upon the individual drug pharmacokinetics and differences in patient physiology (e.g., cardiac output) [12, 13].

Pharmacodynamic-Pharmacokinetic Interactions

Applying both the sedative drug's pharmacodynamic and pharmacokinetic profiles helps appreciate a drug's clinical effect and onset and offset of action (see Fig. 26.3).

Drug dosing is based on achieving a concentration of drug in the central nervous system that results in the therapeutic end point and timed with performance of the procedure. The resulting plasma concentration following bolus administration at any one time is determined by the dose of drug and apparent volume of distribution. A *lag time* exists between peak drug plasma concentrations and peak effect-site (C_e) concentrations and is described by the linear time constant, k_{e0} (Fig. 26.3). The pharmacokinetic relationship between plasma and effect-site concentrations is the primary factor in categorizing how fast a drug works. Fast-acting sedative drugs such as propofol, midazolam, and ketamine have a short lag time (small k_{e0}) between plasma concentrations and effect-site concentrations [14]. While it is the unionized, nonprotein-bound portion of the drug that crosses the blood-brain barrier, the drug's degree of lipid solubility is the most important physicochemical property that

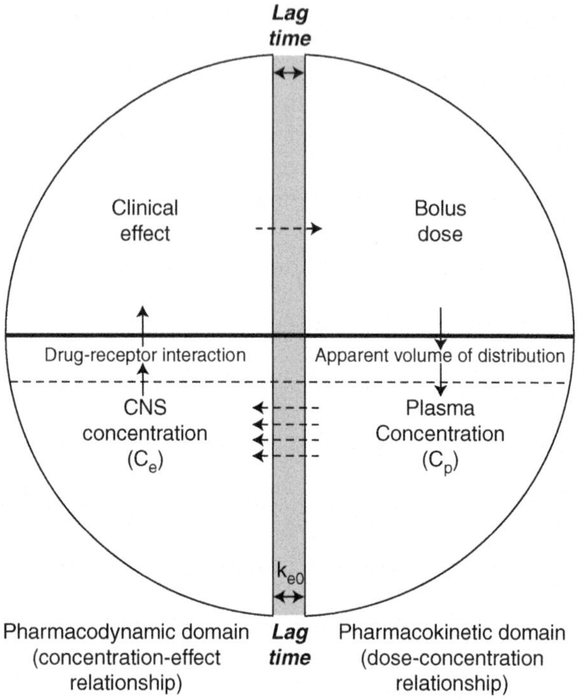

Fig. 26.3 Integration of a sedative drug's pharmacodynamic and pharmacokinetic domains. Plasma concentration (C_p) of a drug following bolus dosing is determined by the size of the bolus dose and the apparent volume of distribution (dose-concentration relationship). Clinical effect is determined by the effect-site (CNS) drug concentration (C_e) (concentration-effect relationship)

influences the speed of action and duration of effect. Following bolus dose intravenous administration, highly lipid-soluble drugs (e.g., ketamine, midazolam, or propofol) penetrate the CNS bio-phase quickly and bind to specific target receptors to result in clinical effect. A decline in effect-site concentration and receptor occupancy results in a diminution of the clinical activity. A second lag time exists between subtherapeutic clinical effects and administration of additional sedation and returns to the therapeutic drug concentration (Fig. 26.3). The duration of this time will be based on the timeliness of feedback-loop mechanisms (e.g., provider vigilance and monitoring).

Procedural Considerations

Diagnostic and therapeutic procedures conducted on children in the PICU are a part of routine daily practice [15, 16]. A recent prospective study found that a median of 11 painful and stressful procedures are performed daily on children in the PICU [15]. Successful selection of the procedural sedation regimen must take into consideration a number of procedural factors that include the anticipated physical and emotional consequences of the procedure (e.g., pain or anxiety) and the requirements for successful completion (e.g., degree of immobility or positioning).

Given their education, training, and experience in airway management and sedative administration, pediatric critical care medicine (PCCM) physicians are frequently tasked with facilitating an array of procedures for children, both inside and outside the PICU [15, 17, 18]. As the field of pediatric procedural sedation grows, the number of procedural sedations conducted by PCCM physicians outside the PICU will undoubtedly continue to increase [19]. Indeed, PCCM physicians comprise the single largest group of sedation providers belonging to the Pediatric Sedation Research Consortium (PSRC), a group of over 30 institutions that prospectively collects data on pediatric sedation encounters [20, 21]. Reports from the PSRC indicate that PCCM sedation providers most commonly provide procedural sedation for radiology procedures (e.g., magnetic resonance imaging (MRI) scans, nuclear medicine procedures, and computerized tomography (CT) scans) and hematology/oncology procedures (e.g., bone marrow biopsies and lumbar punctures). These two groups of procedures comprise nearly two-thirds of the cases sedated by PCCM physicians with the overall majority of procedures being conducted outside the PICU in radiology or sedation units [17, 20, 21]. However, PCCM physicians provide sedation for a host of other procedures as well both within and outside the PICU including upper and lower gastrointestinal endoscopy, laryngoscopy, bronchoscopy, dental restoration, fracture reduction, joint injection, foreign body removal, and cardiac catheterization [17, 22]. The range of sedative agents used for procedural sedation is also diverse. In a report from the PSRC regarding propofol use for procedural sedation by PCCM physicians, the addition of an opioid, benzodiazepine, or ketamine to the sedation regimen was common [17]. Arriving at the safest and most effective sedation regimen must consider a number of procedure variables such as positioning during the procedure (e.g., prone vs supine), direct access to the airway, and patient distance from the provider. Nevertheless, the most important aspects that guide selection of the sedation regimen include the procedure's level of invasiveness (intensity of pain), degree of immobility required, and timing.

Degrees of Invasiveness (Invasive vs Noninvasive) Procedures that require sedation can be categorized along a continuum of level of invasiveness. An illustration of this range and examples of the types of procedures along this continuum is shown in Fig. 26.4.

Invasive procedures are characterized by insertion of a device through the skin or body orifice and are accompanied by various intensities of pain and discomfort. Examples of highly invasive procedures conducted in the PICU include lumbar puncture, central venous catheter placement, arterial catheter placement, and chest tube placement. Stressful, less invasive procedures are probably the most frequent type of procedure conducted in the PICU and are frequently part of routine nursing cares [15, 18]. Procedures such as endotracheal tube suctioning, chest physiotherapy, urinary catheter placement, and nasogastric tube placement are examples of less invasive procedures that may result in significant physical and mental suffering [15]. These invasive and stressful procedures are a routine part of PCCM practice and are necessary to adequately deliver effective and safe critical care [15, 18, 23].

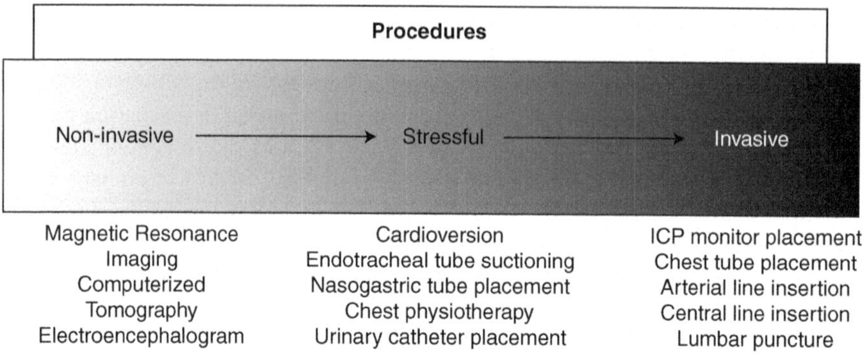

Fig. 26.4 Continuum of procedures based on level of invasiveness conducted within and outside the PICU. General examples of procedures falling along this continuum are listed

Recent studies have found a median of 10–12 invasive and/or stressful procedures conducted on PICU patients each day [15, 18]. While it would not be prudent to sedate for every instance of a stressful or invasive procedure, the emotional toll of repeated procedures must be acknowledged. In one prospective cohort study, children in the intensive care unit were exposed to almost 90 invasive procedures over the course of a 13-day PICU stay [16]. Follow-up analysis of this patient population demonstrated that the number of invasive procedures was the single most important predictor of posttraumatic stress up to 6 months after hospital discharge [24]. According to one recent retrospective study, a small percentage of patients receive procedural sedation or pain control when undergoing even the most invasive procedures (e.g., arterial line placement) [15]. While the quality of sedation and pain control in these studies has not been assessed, the negative consequences of poor procedural sedation and pain control in other pediatric populations are known. Most notably, pediatric oncology patients receiving inadequate pain relief during painful oncologic procedures report heightened pain and anxiety with repeated procedures, even after receiving analgesic agents [25–27]. These studies and others highlight the importance of adequate sedation and analgesia in vulnerable pediatric patients in the intensive care unit.

The amount of analgesia and depth of sedation a patient requires depend on the degree of invasiveness and pain associated with the procedure. Anticipation of pain associated with an invasive procedure by the patient and family is frequently a source of significant anxiety [25, 26]. Consequently, preparation of the patient prior to the procedure if possible and provision of adequate procedural pain control may significantly reduce the need for additional agents aimed solely at anxiolysis [25]. Ketamine and opioids such as remifentanil and fentanyl have pharmacokinetic profiles that render them highly useful in providing analgesia for procedures of brief duration. Additionally, when administered intravenously, opioids can induce a convenient, mild sedative effect, which is more pronounced when they are combined with agents such as benzodiazepines. The synergism of drug combinations is particularly beneficial, as the use of an analgesic agent alongside a sedative-hypnotic in painful procedures may decrease the cumulative need for both agents.

Noninvasive procedures conducted in the PICU consist of diagnostic imaging studies such as ultrasounds, echocardiograms, or electroencephalograms (EEG). Other relevant non-invasive procedures that take place outside the PICU include radiologic procedures such as CT, MRI, or nuclear medicine imaging studies. Despite the lack of pain or physical discomfort, procedures such as MRI often require deep sedation to be successfully performed due to their duration, requirement for immobility, and the intensity of audible stimulation during the scan [28].

Level of Immobility The requisite level of immobility needed to successfully complete a procedure varies by procedure type. On one end of the extreme, need for complete immobility are procedures such as MRI, CT, or nuclear medicine studies, while ultrasound imaging can frequently be performed with some movement and still reasonable images of diagnostic quality can be obtained. In addition, a number of invasive procedures requiring high levels of immobility previously done in the operating room may be performed in the PICU. For example, a motionless patient is needed for many high-risk invasive procedures, not only for successful completion but also for minimizing injury during the procedure. Examples of high-risk procedures requiring a motionless patient include intracranial pressure (ICP) monitor placement and chest tube placement. The degree of stillness required for a procedure to be successful will often determine whether deep sedation is required with a hypnotic agent like propofol or dexmedetomidine.

Timing and Duration The immediacy of performing the procedure and its anticipated duration are critical elements in choosing a sedation regimen. Some procedures simply must be completed expediently for the welfare of the patient (e.g., fracture reduction in the setting of vascular compromise). Intravenous administration is the fastest and most practical route of sedative drug delivery available to the PCCM provider. Fast-acting lipid-soluble intravenous sedative agents such as propofol, ketamine, and midazolam have an onset of action within 1–2 minutes following administration. These are ideal agents for procedures needed to be performed in an expeditious manner. For procedures exceeding 15–20 minutes, maintaining a relatively constant clinical effect requires frequent titration and/or continuous infusion of short-acting agents or administration of medications with a more prolonged clinical effect. In situations where the duration of the procedure is uncertain, continuous intravenous infusions of sedatives such as propofol and dexmedetomidine are useful to maintain control of a drug's clinical properties.

When IV access is not available or not otherwise necessary for the procedure, other routes of administration can lead to relatively fast absorption and onset of action. Alternative routes include buccal, oral, rectal, intranasal, and intramuscular routes. One major drawback of administering drugs via these routes is their clinical unpredictability. For example, orally and rectally administered medications have varying degrees of bioavailability and are also subject to first-pass hepatic metabolism. Consequently, administration via these routes may result in a variable degree of clinical effect and an inconsistent onset and cessation of action.

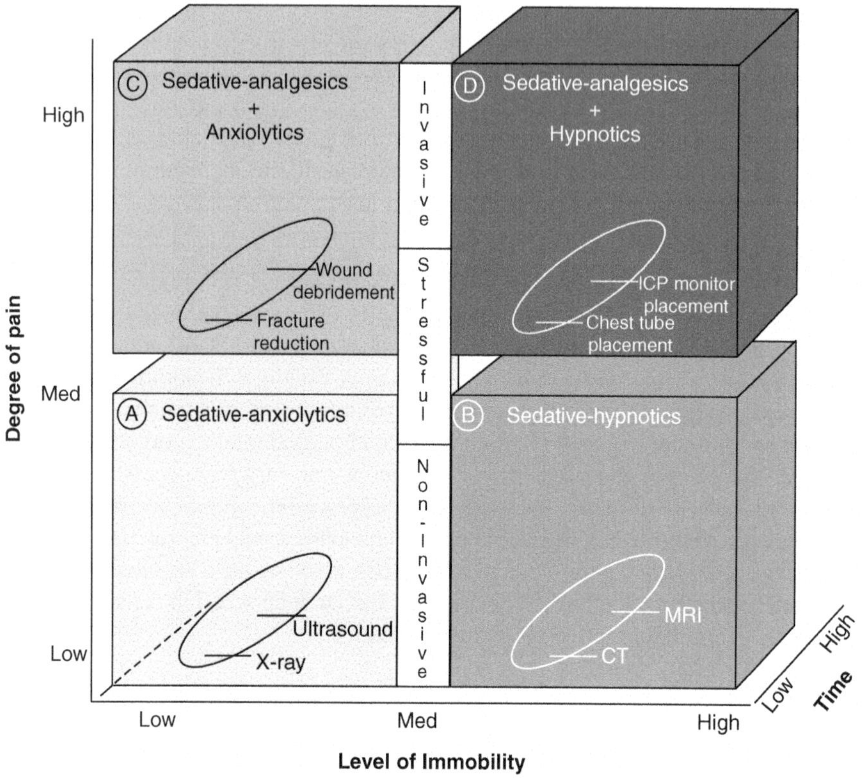

Fig. 26.5 Characteristics and requirements (degree of pain, level of immobility, and time) of procedures that determine the desired clinical actions of a sedative drug. US ultrasound, MRI magnetic resonance imaging, CT computed tomography, ICP intracranial pressure monitor

Summarizing Procedure Characteristics and Timing The three factors highlighted in the previous section, level of invasiveness, need for immobility, and timing (onset and duration) make up the three most important procedural factors when planning sedation. A useful way to depict these features is by displaying them on a three-dimensional Cartesian plane illustrating the procedure's level of immobility (x-axis), degree of pain (y-axis), and duration (z-axis) (see Fig. 26.5).

Procedures in Category A consist of low-intensity procedures requiring low levels of immobility and frequently no or minimal sedation. The primary variable in defining need for sedation and anxiolysis is often how long the procedure takes. Examples of Category A procedures include simple X-rays and ultrasonography. Category B procedures are noninvasive procedures requiring high levels of immobility for which a hypnotic agent for sleep may be indicated. Examples of relatively short vs long procedures in this category include CT and MRI, respectively. Category C procedures, which are of high intensity and where some degree of motion is acceptable, include fracture reduction and wound care-debridement. In all cases, an analgesic agent is the primary sedative drug and often combined with an anxiolytic. Category D procedures are the most complicated procedures to provide safe and effective sedation outside the operating room. Both levels of immobility and invasiveness are high, typically requiring a combination of a hypnotic agent and analgesic. Examples include chest tube placement and intracranial pressure monitor placement.

Approaches to Choosing a Sedative Regimen

Ultimately the most fundamental goal of procedural sedation is to choose the *right drug* at the *right dose* at the *right time*. In doing so the sedation provider must be mindful of the pharmacokinetic and pharmacodynamic profiles of the chosen sedation regimen. Answers to the following four questions facilitate a systematic approach to choosing the safest and most effective sedation regimen (see Fig. 26.6):

1. What are the desired clinical effects? This question is the central question and specifically relates to the therapeutic window. It is the sedation provider's most basic pharmacodynamic question in addressing what clinical actions are necessary for successful completion of the procedure and patient comfort.
2. How fast are the effects desired? The second question addresses how soon the procedure will be started. This question often focuses on the urgency of the

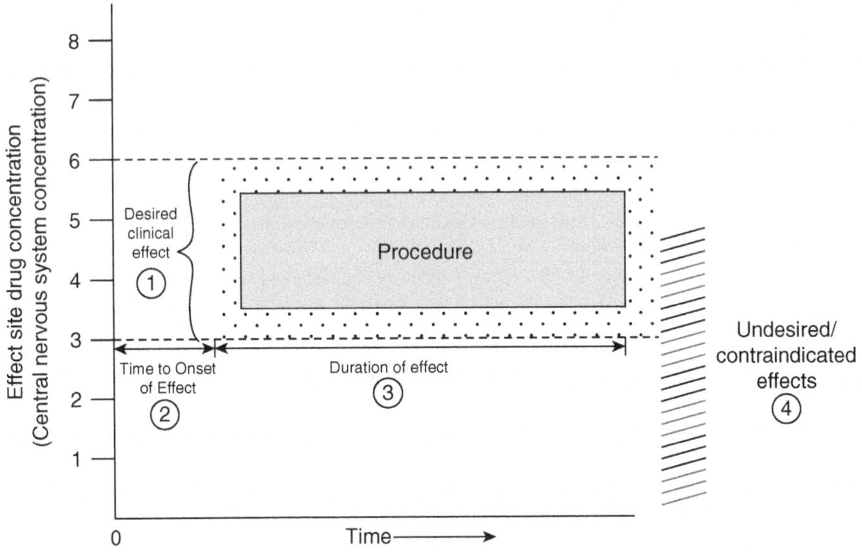

Fig. 26.6 A practical approach to choosing a safe and effective sedation regimen includes determining the (1) desired clinical effect, (2) time to onset of drug effect, (3) duration of drug effect, (4) undesired/contraindicated clinical effects

procedure, that is, how quickly are the sedative drug's pharmacological effects are needed.
3. How long are the effects desired? The third question addresses the duration of the procedure and whether frequent sedative drug titration or an infusion is required.
4. What drug effects are undesirable or contraindicated? The final question is frequently the question that directs the final decision in choosing the sedative regimen. Does the drug have properties that are either absolutely contraindicated (e.g., allergic reaction) or simply undesired (e.g., narrow therapeutic window)? These would create a situation in which patient safety is compromised.

At its core, the overall goals of procedural sedation are to maintain patient safety, successfully complete the procedure, and maintain patient comfort. To achieve these goals requires an in-depth understanding of the sedative drug's pharmacology and knowledge of the requirements and characteristics of the procedure. Given their expertise in cardiopulmonary physiology and airway management, pediatric critical care physicians are well suited to provide high-quality procedural sedation for children. As the variety of procedures in need of procedural sedation widens and intensivists are in need of selecting the most suitable sedation agents, these tenets for choosing sedation will continue to apply.

References

1. American Society of Anesthesiologists Task Force on Sedation and Analgesia by Non-Anesthesiologists. Practice guidelines for sedation and analgesia by non-anesthesiologists. Anesthesiology. 2002;96(4):1004–17.
2. Sury M, Bullock I, Rabar S, Demott K, Guideline Development G. Sedation for diagnostic and therapeutic procedures in children and young people: summary of NICE guidance. BMJ. 2010;341:c6819.
3. Zielinska M, Bartkowska-Sniatkowska A, Becke K, Hohne C, Najafi N, Schaffrath E, et al. Safe pediatric procedural sedation and analgesia by anesthesiologists for elective procedures: a clinical practice statement from the European Society for Paediatric Anaesthesiology. Paediatr Anaesth. 2019;29(6):583–90.
4. Gin T. Clinical pharmacology on display. Anesth Analg. 2010;111(2):256–8.
5. Kern SE, Stanski DR. Pharmacokinetics and pharmacodynamics of intravenously administered anesthetic drugs: concepts and lessons for drug development. Clin Pharmacol Ther. 2008;84(1):153–7.
6. Hendrickx JF, Eger EI 2nd, Sonner JM, Shafer SL. Is synergy the rule? A review of anesthetic interactions producing hypnosis and immobility. Anesth Analg. 2008;107(2):494–506.
7. Billard V. Pharmacokinetic-pharmacodynamic relationship of anesthetic drugs: from modeling to clinical use. F1000Res. 2015;4:F1000.
8. Hull CJ, McLeod K. Pharmacokinetic analysis using an electrical analogue. Br J Anaesth. 1976;48(7):677–86.
9. Mani V, Morton NS. Overview of total intravenous anesthesia in children. Paediatr Anaesth. 2010;20(3):211–22.
10. Fisher DM. (Almost) everything you learned about pharmacokinetics was (somewhat) wrong! Anesth Analg. 1996;83(5):901–3.

11. Henthorn TK, Krejcie TC, Avram MJ. Early drug distribution: a generally neglected aspect of pharmacokinetics of particular relevance to intravenously administered anesthetic agents. Clin Pharmacol Ther. 2008;84(1):18–22.
12. Kuipers JA, Boer F, Olofsen E, Olieman W, Vletter AA, Burm AG, et al. Recirculatory and compartmental pharmacokinetic modeling of alfentanil in pigs: the influence of cardiac output. Anesthesiology. 1999;90(4):1146–57.
13. Rigby-Jones AE, Sneyd JR. Pharmacokinetics and pharmacodynamics--is there anything new? Anaesthesia. 2012;67(1):5–11.
14. Cortinez LI. What is the ke0 and what does it tell me about propofol? Anaesthesia. 2014;69(5):399–402.
15. Baarslag MA, Jhingoer S, Ista E, Allegaert K, Tibboel D, van Dijk M. How often do we perform painful and stressful procedures in the paediatric intensive care unit? A prospective observational study. Aust Crit Care. 2019;32(1):4–10.
16. Rennick JE, Johnston CC, Dougherty G, Platt R, Ritchie JA. Children's psychological responses after critical illness and exposure to invasive technology. J Dev Behav Pediatr. 2002;23(3):133–44.
17. Kamat PP, McCracken CE, Gillespie SE, Fortenberry JD, Stockwell JA, Cravero JP, et al. Pediatric critical care physician-administered procedural sedation using propofol: a report from the Pediatric Sedation Research Consortium Database. Pediatr Crit Care Med. 2015;16(1):11–20.
18. Stevens BJ, Abbott LK, Yamada J, Harrison D, Stinson J, Taddio A, et al. Epidemiology and management of painful procedures in children in Canadian hospitals. CMAJ. 2011;183(7):E403–10.
19. Kudchadkar SR. Pediatric intensivists and elective procedural sedation: paradox or perfect pair? Pediatr Crit Care Med. 2015;16(1):77–8.
20. Cravero JP, Beach ML, Blike GT, Gallagher SM, Hertzog JH, Pediatric Sedation Research C. The incidence and nature of adverse events during pediatric sedation/anesthesia with propofol for procedures outside the operating room: a report from the Pediatric Sedation Research Consortium. Anesth Analg. 2009;108(3):795–804.
21. Cravero JP, Blike GT, Beach M, Gallagher SM, Hertzog JH, Havidich JE, et al. Incidence and nature of adverse events during pediatric sedation/anesthesia for procedures outside the operating room: report from the Pediatric Sedation Research Consortium. Pediatrics. 2006;118(3):1087–96.
22. Vespasiano M, Finkelstein M, Kurachek S. Propofol sedation: intensivists' experience with 7304 cases in a children's hospital. Pediatrics. 2007;120(6):e1411–7.
23. Southall DP, Cronin BC, Hartmann H, Harrison-Sewell C, Samuels MP. Invasive procedures in children receiving intensive care. BMJ. 1993;306(6891):1512–3.
24. Rennick JE, Morin I, Kim D, Johnston CC, Dougherty G, Platt R. Identifying children at high risk for psychological sequelae after pediatric intensive care unit hospitalization. Pediatr Crit Care Med. 2004;5(4):358–63.
25. Barbi E, Badina L, Marchetti F, Vecchi R, Giuseppin I, Bruno I, et al. Attitudes of children with leukemia toward repeated deep sedations with propofol. J Pediatr Hematol Oncol. 2005;27(12):639–43.
26. Dufresne A, Dugas MA, Samson Y, Barre P, Turcot L, Marc I. Do children undergoing cancer procedures under pharmacological sedation still report pain and anxiety? A preliminary study. Pain Med. 2010;11(2):215–23.
27. Weisman SJ, Bernstein B, Schechter NL. Consequences of inadequate analgesia during painful procedures in children. Arch Pediatr Adolesc Med. 1998;152(2):147–9.
28. Boriosi JP, Eickhoff JC, Klein KB, Hollman GA. A retrospective comparison of propofol alone to propofol in combination with dexmedetomidine for pediatric 3T MRI sedation. Paediatr Anaesth. 2017;27(1):52–9.

Part VII
Sedative and Analgesic Agents Available

Chapter 27
Analgesic Agents

Cheri D. Landers and Erin R. Powell

Pain is a subjective, complex, and multifactorial experience encompassing physical, psychological, emotional, and developmental components [1–3]. As a result, a multimodal strategy that targets each of these factors is most effective to manage pain in all settings [1, 2, 4]. Non-pharmacologic measures, which are discusseed elsewhere, are an important adjunct to pharmacologic agents in achieving adequate pain management. Additionally, mounting evidence suggests that painful procedures in neonates and children can have lifelong effects. Younger children who experience inadequate analgesia during a painful procedure may perceive poorly controlled pain in subsequent procedures [3]. Therefore, it is crucially important that neonates and children undergoing painful procedures receive adequate pain management, even for procedures that may be considered minor by many healthcare professionals such as peripheral intravenous cannulation, dressing changes, urinary catheter placement, and surgical drain removal. Adequate analgesia may also obviate the need for or decrease the amount of sedative required during procedures and increase the chance of a successful procedure [4]. For invasive procedures, such as lumbar puncture, bone marrow aspiration, fracture reduction, or burn debridement among others, analgesics are necessary in addition to sedatives or anxiolytics that do not provide pain management.

Assessment of pain relies on self-report and monitoring of behavioral and physiologic changes. There are many validated scoring tools to assess self-reported pain in the pediatric population, which are discussed elsewhere. Close observation of behavioral and physiologic changes are required for younger patients, older patients without the ability to effectively communicate, and patients who have received sedatives or anesthetics [2, 4]. Assessment and documentation of pain

C. D. Landers (✉) · E. R. Powell
Division of Pediatric Critical Care, University of Kentucky, Kentucky Children's Hospital, Lexington, KY, USA
e-mail: cdland2@uky.edu

P. P. Kamat, J. W. Berkenbosch (eds.), *Sedation and Analgesia for the Pediatric Intensivist*, https://doi.org/10.1007/978-3-030-52555-2_27

should occur before, during, and after the procedure to guide ongoing pain management.

In general, the American Academy of Pediatrics and the American Pain Society recommend that providers:

1. Provide a calm environment for procedures that reduces distress-producing stimulation.
2. Use appropriate pain assessment tools and techniques.
3. Anticipate predictable painful experiences, intervene, and monitor accordingly.
4. Use a multimodal (pharmacologic, cognitive, behavioral, and physical) approach to pain management, and use a multidisciplinary approach when possible.
5. Involve families and tailor interventions to the individual child [1].

When selecting any analgesic, providers should consider the actual and developmental age of the patient, underlying medical conditions, procedure(s) to take place, and prior adverse reactions to medications. In general, neonates have lower plasma protein concentrations, causing a higher proportion of free drug for highly protein-bound drugs. Neonates also have reduced clearance of many drugs due to incomplete maturation of hepatic enzymes and decreased renal filtration. On the contrary, young children (aged 2–6 years) have increased clearance of many drugs due to a larger liver-to-body-mass ratio. As a result, many drugs have a narrower therapeutic index in neonates, while young children may require more frequent dosing [2, 5]. The remainder of this chapter will discuss indications, pharmacology, dosing, and precautions for various analgesics.

Local Analgesics

Local analgesics can be effective as a single agent for minor procedures such as IV cannulation and laceration repair or used as an adjunct for invasive procedures such as lumbar puncture and renal or bone marrow biopsy. Local anesthetics are injected or administered topically [2, 6]. Local anesthetics block nerve conduction via reversible inhibition of sodium channels. Ester local anesthetics (tetracaine) are metabolized by plasma esterases, whereas amide local anesthetics (lidocaine, bupivacaine, prilocaine) are metabolized by the liver. Potency and time to onset of local anesthetics are related to lipid solubility; high lipid solubility confers higher potency and a longer duration of onset. Duration of action of local anesthetics is prolonged by protein binding and local sequestration by the addition of vasoconstrictors such as epinephrine [7]. Bupivacaine is an amide local anesthetic with high potency and long duration of action; however, it also has a low threshold for toxicity. The characteristics of local anesthetics are often compared to that of bupivacaine. Toxicity from local anesthetics generally occurs from improper use or overdose. Symptoms include somnolence, dizziness, paresthesias, coma, seizures, arrhythmia, and cardiac arrest [7–9]. Methemoglobinemia is associated with the use of local analgesics, especially benzocaine. Treatment of local anesthetic systemic toxicity includes supportive care for cardiopulmonary depression, benzodiazepines for the treatment of seizures, and lipid emulsion therapy.

Injectable Local Anesthetics

Lidocaine is the most commonly used local anesthetic in pediatrics. Lidocaine is an amide local anesthetic with a rapid onset of action (45–90 seconds), an intermediate duration of action (10–20 minutes), and a low likelihood of toxicity [8, 10]. Formulations are available that contain epinephrine to increase duration of action and decrease systemic uptake. The maximum single recommended dose of lidocaine without epinephrine is 4 mg/kg in neonates and 5 mg/kg in children, not to exceed the maximum adult dose of 300 mg [10]. The maximum single dose for formulations containing epinephrine is 7 mg/kg with a maximum adult dose of 500 mg [2, 8, 10].

Pain from the injection of local anesthetics can be a barrier to their use in pediatrics. Use of a j-tip device, which delivers 2–2.5 mg of 1% lidocaine solution via highly pressurized carbon dioxide into subcutaneous tissue, is an effective and pain-free route of administration [11]. The j-tip device produces an audible "pop" that can be distressing if patients are not adequately prepared. Other techniques "to decrease pain and distress from injection of local anesthetics include keeping needles out of sight of the child, buffering lidocaine with sodium bicarbonate in a 9:1 ratio, warming the local anesthetic, using a small-gauge needle (27 to 30 gauge), injecting slowly, injecting from wound edges rather than through intact skin when possible, and counterirritating surrounding skin during the injection" [12].

Regional analgesia may be beneficial for reduction of dislocated joints or fractures, but it is otherwise not commonly used during procedural sedation in pediatrics and is beyond the scope of this chapter. Regional analgesia for postoperative analgesia is discussed elsewhere.

Topical Local Anesthetics

A variety of topical anesthetic preparations are also available. Local hypersensitivity reactions are the most common adverse effects from topical anesthetics [9, 11, 13]. Agents for intact skin include lidocaine-prilocaine and liposomal lidocaine. Lidocaine-prilocaine is formulated as a cream containing equal parts 2.5% lidocaine and 2.5% prilocaine. Prilocaine is another amide local anesthetic with an intermediate onset and duration of action, similar potency to lidocaine, and the lowest toxicity of the amides. Prilocaine may cause methemoglobinemia in susceptible patients such as neonates [8]. The recommended dose is 1–2 g per 10 cm^2 area in infants and children 3 months of age or older and who weigh at least 5 kg [10]. Some clinicians recommend no more than 1 g/5 kg. The long duration of onset of

60 minutes limits its use in the acute setting. Despite its prilocaine component, several investigators have documented safe use of lidocaine-prilocaine in neonates [8]. Liposomal lidocaine is most commonly used as a 4% preparation, but it is also available as a 5% formulation. The recommended dose of liposomal lidocaine 4% is 1–2.5 g per 6.25 cm^2 of skin in infants and children older than 1 month of age [10]. The duration of onset is 30 minutes [14].

Topical agents available for use on open skin include TAC and LET. TAC is a solution or gel containing tetracaine, epinephrine, and cocaine. It was one of the first topical anesthetics manufactured, but due to its cocaine component, its use has largely been replaced by other formulations [9]. LET is a solution or gel containing 4% lidocaine, 0.1% epinephrine, and 0.5% tetracaine. Tetracaine is an ester local anesthetic with a relatively slow onset of action (low toxicity) and a potency and duration of action comparable to bupivacaine [8]. The recommended dose is 1–3 mL. The duration of onset is 20–40 minutes [10]. Use of LET is contraindicated on mucus membranes, end-arteriolar sites, and genitalia due to the risk of ischemia from epinephrine-induced vasoconstriction [14].

Vapocoolant sprays containing ethyl chloride or fluoromethane are also available for topical local analgesia on intact skin. These sprays work by producing a noxious cold stimulus via evaporation-induced skin cooling that may interfere with transmission of pain impulses. Blanching at the site should prompt discontinuation to avoid frostbite [9, 12, 13, 15].

Systemic Analgesics

For most invasive procedures, topical analgesia alone is inadequate and necessitates transition to or adjunctive use of systemic analgesics.

Non-opioid Systemic Analgesics

Acetaminophen (paracetamol) is the most commonly used systemic analgesic in children. Acetaminophen inhibits central prostaglandin synthesis. Dosing of acetaminophen is dependent on the formulation, but the total daily dose should not exceed 100 mg/kg for children, 75 mg/kg for infants, 60 mg/kg for term and preterm neonates older than 32 weeks post-conceptual age, and 40 mg/kg for preterm neonates younger than 32 weeks post-conceptual age [2, 16]. Hepatic toxicity, including progression to development of overt hepatic failure, can result from excessive doses of acetaminophen either when administered as a single overdose or with prolonged use of appropriate doses. Nonsteroidal anti-inflammatory drugs (NSAIDs), particularly ibuprofen, naproxen, or ketorolac, are also widely used in the pediatric population. NSAIDs inhibit cyclooxygenase enzymes, which decrease local prostaglandin synthesis. NSAIDs are contraindicated in patients with renal impairment, gastrointestinal bleeding, and platelet dysfunction. Alone, acetaminophen and NSAIDs are used to treat mild pain and are often inadequate as sole agents in procedural analgesia. However, both acetaminophen and NSAIDs are synergistic when coadministered with opioids and can be an useful adjunct to limit opioid doses. While all agents are available for enteral use, acetaminophen, ketorolac, and, more recently, ibuprofen are also available in IV formulations, decreasing the onset of action compared to oral dosing [2, 16]. However, inadequate data exist to allow specific recommendations for use of these agents, especially alone, for specific procedural analgesia applications.

Additionally, nonnutritive sucking of high-concentration sucrose solutions provides analgesia in infants up to 6 months of age and may be effective up to 1 year of age as an adjunct for procedural sedation. The mechanism of action for analgesia is likely through the endogenous release of endorphins. The onset of action is 2 minutes [4, 11].

Opioids

Opioids are the most common systemic analgesics used in pediatric procedural sedation. Numerous opioids exist for the management of acute pain with morphine and fentanyl being the most commonly used for procedural analgesia. Opioids exert their therapeutic effect by binding to central and peripheral μ receptors, which decreases the release of excitatory neurotransmitters. The agonism of μ_1 receptors is responsible for analgesia, while binding of μ_2 receptors causes both analgesia and respiratory depression. In addition to the differences in pharmacodynamic properties discussed earlier among different age groups, neonates and young infants are more susceptible to the adverse effects from opioids due to a larger proportion of μ_2 receptors and immature blood-brain barrier [16, 17]. Other adverse effects of opioids include nausea, emesis, and urinary retention [2]. There is no maximum recommended dose of opioid with the primary factor limiting use being the development adverse effects, especially hypotension or respiratory depression. Therefore, it is recommended that analgesia be initiated with low doses of opioids, which are then titrated by readministration to achieve effective pain relief while limiting the occurrence of adverse effects [6, 18]. When combined with other respiratory depressants, the opioid doses may need to be reduced to avoid respiratory depression. The effect of opioids can be reversed by the opioid receptor antagonist naloxone. The recommended dose of naloxone is 0.001–0.1 mg/kg, depending on the amount of reversal desired with dosing repeated every 2–3 minutes [10]. Repeat doses are often necessary since the duration of action of naloxone is shorter than that of most opioids. To avoid acute withdrawal responses or completely negate the analgesia achieved, it is recommended to start with lower doses of naloxone and repeat at 2–3-minute intervals to achieve adequate clinical effect.

Morphine is the prototypical opioid. The onset of action of intravenous morphine occurs at 5–10 minutes with the peak effect occurring at about 20 minutes with a duration of action of 2–4 hours. The recommended dose of morphine is 0.025 mg/kg/dose in infants <6 months and 0.05–1 mg/kg/dose in infants and children >6 months with a maximum of 2–5 mg/dose [10]. Children with previous opioid exposure may require higher doses. There are no dose adjustments provided in the manufacturer's labeling for intravenous dosing of morphine in renal or hepatic impairment; however, morphine and its metabolites are renally excreted, so caution should be used in those with renal impairment [10]. Histamine release with morphine administration can result in pruritis, nausea and vomiting, and may require caution for use in asthmatics and those with significant atopic history. Except for use in procedures of a longer duration, morphine use has mostly been supplanted by fentanyl.

Fentanyl is a synthetic opioid and is more potent than morphine with a shorter onset and duration of action, making it ideal for procedural sedation. The onset of action of intravenous fentanyl is <30 seconds with peak effect at 2–3 minutes and a duration of 20–40 minutes [6]. The recommended dose of intravenous fentanyl is 1–2 mcg/kg/dose up to 50 mcg/dose [10]. Children with previous opioid exposure may require higher doses. The recommended dose of fentanyl for analgesia is typically not associated with sedation. The same dose of intravenous fentanyl can be administered intranasally via an atomizer for needle-free dosing with an onset of action of ~10 minutes [11]. There are no dose adjustments provided in the manufacturer's labeling for intravenous dosing of fentanyl in renal or hepatic impairment; however, some clinicians recommend decreased dosing in renal impairment [10]. Oral transmucosal fentanyl is associated with a high incidence of emesis, limiting its use. Fentanyl is not associated with histamine release, resulting in less systemic pruritis, nausea and vomiting than morphine; however, it can produce nasal pruritus [6]. Hypotension in the hemodynamically stable patient is uncommon at doses required to achieve analgesia. Rapid administration and high doses of fentanyl are associated with chest wall rigidity and subsequent respiratory failure. Chest wall rigidity can sometimes be reversed with naloxone and in other cases requires administration of a paralytic.

Remifentanil is an ultrashort-acting synthetic opioid available for IV use only. It has a very short duration of action (8–10 minutes) with no active metabolites. It is broken down by plasma and other nonspecific esterases, so there are no concerns regarding use in the setting of hepatic or renal dysfunction. Similar to other opioids, its most concerning adverse effects include respiratory depression and hypotension. Its use has been described in combination with various other sedatives including benzodiazepines and propofol for invasive oncology procedures [19, 20], flexible bronchoscopy [21, 22], upper and lower GI endoscopy [23, 24], and dental procedures [25, 26]. While the rapid dissipation of action is appealing in the procedural sedation setting, it has a much narrower therapeutic window with regard to the development of significant respiratory depression and apnea. Consequently, its use remains relatively limited compared to other opioids for procedural sedation.

Dexmedetomidine

Dexmedetomidine is a selective alpha-2 receptor agonist with analgesic, anxiolytic, and sedative properties [11, 17]. Dexmedetomidine may be used to achieve procedural sedation and analgesia for mildly invasive procedures such as peripherally inserted central catheter (PICC) placement. Sedation with intravenous dexmedetomidine can be induced with doses of 0.5–2 mcg/kg/dose over 10 minutes and maintained with infusions of 0.5–2 mcg/kg/hour [10]. More rapid bolus administration is not recommended due to reports of the development of severe bradycardia or sinus pause. Infants and children younger than 2 years old may require a large bolus dose and a lower dose for continuous infusion due to their greater volume of distribution and longer half-life [17]. Intranasal formulations are also available with doses of 1.5 mg/kg [11]. There are no dose adjustments provided in the manufacturer's labeling for intravenous dosing of dexmedetomidine in renal or hepatic impairment; however, caution should be used in those with hepatic impairment, and some clinicians recommend dose reductions [10, 12]. Dexmedetomidine has less respiratory depressive effects as compared to opioids, but it is associated with increased incidence of bradycardia. Some patients receiving dexmedetomidine experience hypotension, while others experience hypertension [11, 17]. Due to relatively mild analgesia, use of dexmedetomidine as a sole analgesic agent has limited utility.

Ketamine

Ketamine is a dissociative anesthetic providing potent analgesia in addition to its sedative and amnestic properties. It therefore can be an ideal agent for painful procedures without requiring additional systemic analgesics unlike other sedatives or anesthetics. A thorough review of ketamine is provided elsewhere.

References

1. American Academy of Pediatrics. Committee on Psychosocial Aspects of Child and Family Health; Task Force on Pain in Infants, Children, and Adolescents. The assessment and management of acute pain in infants, children, and adolescents. Pediatrics. 2001;108(3):793–7.
2. Berde CB, Sethna NF. Analgesics for the treatment of pain in children. N Engl J Med. 2002;347(14):1094–103.
3. Weisman SJ, Bernstein B, Schechter NL. Consequences of inadequate analgesia during painful procedures in children. Arch Pediatr Adolesc Med. 1998;152(2):147–9.
4. Cramton RE, Gruchala NE. Managing procedural pain in pediatric patients. Curr Opin Pediatr. 2012;24(4):530–8.
5. Playfor S, Jenkins I, Boyles C, Choonara I, Davies G, Haywood T, Hinson G, Mayer A, Morton N, Ralph T, Wolf A, United Kingdom Paediatric Intensive Care Society Sedation; Analgesia and Neuromuscular Blockade Working Group. Consensus guidelines on sedation and analgesia in critically ill children. Intensive Care Med. 2006;32(8):1125–36.
6. Meyer S, Grundmann U, Gottschling S, Kleinschmidt S, Gortner L. Sedation and analgesia for brief diagnostic and therapeutic procedures in children. Eur J Pediatr. 2007;166(4):291–302.
7. Becker DE, Reed KL. Local anesthetics: review of pharmacological considerations. Anesth Prog. 2012;59(2):90–101.
8. Gunter JB. Benefit and risks of local anesthetics in infants and children. Paediatr Drugs. 2002;4(10):649–72.

9. Stewart GM, Simpson P, Rosenberg NM. Use of topical lidocaine in pediatric laceration repair: a review of topical anesthetics. Pediatr Emerg Care. 1998;14(6):419–23.
10. Lexi-Drugs. Lexicomp. Riverwoods: Wolters Kluwer Health, Inc. Available at: http://online.lexi.com.
11. Pacheco GS, Ferayorni A. Pediatric procedural sedation and analgesia. Emerg Med Clin North Am. 2013;31(3):831–52.
12. Young KD. Pediatric procedural pain. Ann Emerg Med. 2005;45(2):160–71.
13. Krauss B, Green SM. Sedation and analgesia for procedures in children. N Engl J Med. 2000;342(13):938–45.
14. Kundu S, Achar S. Principles of office anesthesia: Part II. Topical anesthesia. Am Fam Physician. 2002;66(1):99–102.
15. Farion KJ, Splinter KL, Newhook K, Gaboury I, Splinter WM. The effect of vapocoolant spray on pain due to intravenous cannulation in children: a randomized controlled trial. CMAJ. 2008;179(1):31–6.
16. Verghese ST, Hannallah RS. Acute pain management in children. J Pain Res. 2010;3:105–23.
17. Lucas SS, Nasr VG, Ng AJ, Joe C, Bond M, DiNardo JA. Pediatric Cardiac Intensive Care Society 2014 consensus statement: pharmacotherapies in cardiac critical care: sedation, analgesia and muscle relaxant. Pediatr Crit Care Med. 2016;17(3 Suppl 1):S3–S15.
18. Krauss B, Green SM. Procedural sedation and analgesia in children. Lancet. 2006;367(9512):766–80.
19. Litmans RS. Conscious sedation with remifentanil and midazolam during brief painful procedures in children. Arch Pediatr Adolesc Med. 1999;153:1085–8.
20. Ince IE, Iyilikci L, Yilmaz S, Güneş D, Akkuş M, Isguven D. Sedation for short hemato-oncologic invasive procedures in children: comparison of propofol-remifentanil and propofol-fentanyl. J Pediatr Hematol Oncol. 2013;35:112–7.
21. Reyle-Hahn M, Niggemann B, Max M, Streich R, Rossaint R. Remifentanil and propofol for sedation in children and young adolescents undergoing diagnostic flexible bronchoscopy. Paediatr Anaesth. 2000;10:59–63.
22. Berkenbosch JW, Graff GR, Stark JM, Ner Z, Tobias JD. Use of a remifentanil-propofol mixture for pediatric flexible fiberoptic bronchoscopy sedation. Paediatr Anaesth. 2004;14:941–6.
23. Abu-Shahwan I, Mack D. Propofol and remifentanil for deep sedation in children undergoing gastrointestinal endoscopy. Paediatr Anaesth. 2007;17:460–3.
24. Hirsh I, Lerner A, Shnaider I, Reuveni A, Pacht A, Segol O, Pizov R. Remifentanil versus fentanyl for esophagogastroduodenoscopy in children. J Pediatr Gastroenterol Nutr. 2010;51(5):618–21.
25. Lacombe GF, Leake JL, Clokie CM, Haas DA. Comparison of remifentanil with fentanyl for deep sedation in oral surgery. J Oral Maxillofac Surg. 2006;64:215–22.
26. Torun AC, Yilmaz MZ, Ozkan N, Ustun B, Koksal E, Kaya C. Sedative-analgesic activity of remifentanil and effects of preoperative anxiety on perceived pain in outpatient mandibular third molar surgery. Int J Oral Maxillofac Surg. 2017;46:379–84.

Chapter 28
Benzodiazepines and Barbiturates

Mudit Mathur and Mohammad Tariq Malik

Benzodiazepines

Mechanism of Action

Benzodiazepines are synthetic compounds whose core chemical structure consists of the fusion of a benzene ring and a diazepine ring. Benzodiazepines bind to the γ-aminobutyric acid type A receptor (GABA-A) shown in Fig. 28.1 at the alpha-subunit and potentiate GABA activity, thereby increasing conductance of the chloride channel and inhibiting neuronal excitability, which corresponds to their sedative, anticonvulsant, and muscle-relaxing effects. Antianxiety properties are related to increasing the inhibitory neurotransmitter glycine.

Because they have a lower tendency to cause a potentially fatal CNS depression when compared to barbiturates, benzodiazepines are widely used for procedural sedation, treatment of anxiety (anxiolytics) and insomnia (sedative/hypnotics), as well as other psychological conditions such as panic attacks and panic disorders.

M. Mathur (✉)
Pediatric Critical Care, Southern California Permanente Medical Group, Fontana, CA, USA

Kaiser Permanente School of Medicine, Pasadena, CA, USA
e-mail: mudit.mathur@kp.org

M. T. Malik
Pediatric Critical Care, Southern California Permanente Medical Group, Fontana, CA, USA

P. P. Kamat, J. W. Berkenbosch (eds.), *Sedation and Analgesia for the Pediatric Intensivist*, https://doi.org/10.1007/978-3-030-52555-2_28

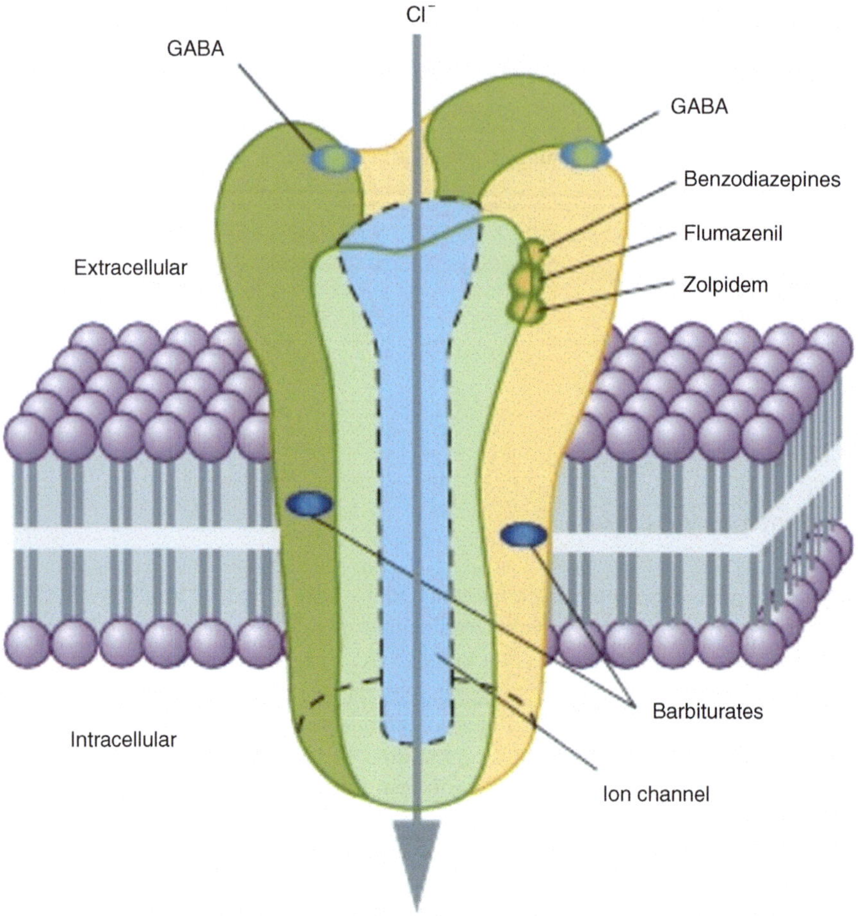

Fig. 28.1 Target receptor for benzodiazepines (Source: Katzung and Trevor [18]. www.accesspharmacy.com. Copyright © McGraw-Hill Education. All rights reserved)

Pharmacokinetics

Benzodiazepines are usually well absorbed by the gastrointestinal tract after oral administration. After intravenous administration, benzodiazepines quickly distribute to the brain and central nervous system. Benzodiazepine activity is terminated by redistribution like that of the lipid-soluble barbiturates. Following intramuscular injection, absorption of diazepam or chlordiazepoxide is slow and erratic, whereas absorption of intramuscular administration of lorazepam or midazolam appears to be rapid and complete. Lorazepam is also well absorbed after sublingual administration, reaching peak levels in 60 min.

Benzodiazepines and their metabolites are highly protein bound. They are widely distributed in the body and accumulate in lipid-rich areas preferentially such as the central nervous system and adipose tissue. The more lipophilic agents generally have the highest rates of absorption and fastest onset of clinical effects. Most benzodiazepines are oxidatively metabolized by the cytochrome P450 enzymes (phase I), conjugated with glucuronide (phase II), and excreted almost entirely in the urine. Some benzodiazepines exert additional actions via the production of active metabolites. Lorazepam does not have active metabolites and only undergoes conjugation. Diazepam and midazolam have active metabolites and require both oxidation and conjugation. Midazolam, one of the short-acting benzodiazepines, produces α-hydroxymidazolam, an active metabolite. Diazepam, a long-acting benzodiazepine, produces the active metabolites oxazepam, desmethyldiazepam, and temazepam; these metabolites further increase the duration of drug action especially in patients with extensive hepatic disease.

Benzodiazepines are classified in terms of their elimination half-life or relative potency. Short-acting benzodiazepines have a median elimination half-life of 1–12 h (temazepam, oxazepam), intermediate-acting benzodiazepines have an average elimination half-life of 12–40 h (alprazolam, clonazepam, lorazepam), and long-acting benzodiazepines have an average elimination half-life of 40–250 h (chlordiazepoxide, diazepam).

Dosing and Clinical Effects: Shown in Table 28.1

Midazolam

Midazolam is the benzodiazepine used most often for procedural sedation. It is a short-acting benzodiazepine with a rapid onset of action. Midazolam has good pre-procedural sedative, anxiolytic, amnestic, and muscle relaxant properties and is frequently used to provide mild sedation in children for diagnostic or radiographic procedures. Benzodiazepines are not reliable hypnotic agents but are useful as adjuncts with analgesics for painful procedures. Midazolam can be used alone for anxiolysis or in combination with synergistic agents such as short-acting opioids (e.g., fentanyl) for deeper levels of sedation and analgesia. Anterograde amnesia is one of the most important clinical effects of benzodiazepines, particularly in children undergoing invasive procedures. Midazolam can be administered through various routes, which makes it a very useful agent in children without vascular access.

Midazolam can be administered enterally using the intranasal, oral, or rectal route. Intranasal midazolam can be given as atomized midazolam at 0.3 mg/kg and is safe

Table 28.1 Intravenous benzodiazepines-typical dosing regimen

Benzodiazepine	Dose	Repeat dose as needed	Onset	Duration
Diazepam	0.1–0.15 mg/kg	0.05–0.1 mg/kg q 3–5 min	<60 s	60–120 min
Midazolam	0.05–0.1 mg/kg	0.05 mg/kg q 3–5 min	<60 s	15–60 min
Lorazepam	0.05 mg/kg	0.025–0.05 mg/kg q 10–15 min	2–3 min	1–2 h

and achieves faster sedation and better sedation scores as compared to 0.2 mg/kg [1]. Onset is in 10–15 min. It has been suggested to premedicate with intranasal lidocaine to decrease irritation and subsequent agitation [2, 3]. Oral dose is 0.3–0.5 mg/kg with onset in 20–30 min but may have variable onset and poor tolerability due to a bad taste. Rectal midazolam dose is 0.2–0.5 mg/kg to 1 milligram/kg once with onset in 15–20 min but may be associated with post-procedural agitation. Clinical trials have utilized the parenteral midazolam formulation for rectal administration.

Midazolam can be given parenterally via the intravenous or intramuscular route. The intravenous dose should be administered slowly over 1–2 min especially in neonates and young children undergoing procedural sedation. Intra-arterial administration is contraindicated. If given intramuscularly, it should be administered undiluted deep IM into a large muscle, generally into anterior-lateral aspect of thigh (vastus lateralis) in pediatric patients [4].

Caution is required if there is hepatic or renal impairment as half-life of midazolam and metabolites may be prolonged (no dosage adjustments needed).

Lorazepam

Lorazepam can be administered orally, intravenously, intramuscularly, or intranasally. It is metabolized through hepatic glucuronidation to lorazepam glucuronide and undergoes renal excretion. Lorazepam has poor lipid solubility and a high degree of protein binding (85–90%). Lorazepam has roughly double the potency of midazolam but no active metabolites. Because of its lack of water solubility, lorazepam may produce a burning sensation at the site of IV administration like that seen with diazepam. Lorazepam is not frequently used in procedural sedation because of its prolonged clinical action, its extreme amnestic properties, and primarily the difficulty in titrating the drug to clinical effect. Propylene glycol (1,2-propanediol) is the solvent used to deliver lorazepam IV. In neonates, large amounts of propylene glycol delivered orally, intravenously, or topically have been associated with potentially fatal toxicity, which manifests as metabolic acidosis, seizures, renal failure, and CNS depression. Toxicity has also been reported in children and adults after longer intravenous infusion with the development of hyperosmolality, lactic acidosis, seizures, and respiratory depression [5].

Diazepam

Diazepam is not an ideal sedative due to its erratic absorption, delayed onset, long half-life, active metabolites, and risk of phlebitis with intravenous administration. Additionally, it causes pain with injection. Duration of action after a single dose is determined by redistribution rather than metabolism. Rapid injection may cause respiratory depression or hypotension. Continuous infusion is not recommended because of precipitation in IV fluids and absorption of drug into infusion bags and tubing. Some dosage forms may contain benzyl alcohol or benzoate, which has been associated with a potentially fatal toxicity ("gasping syndrome") in neonates: metabolic acidosis, respiratory distress, gasping respirations, CNS dysfunction (including convulsions, intracranial hemorrhage), hypotension, and cardiovascular collapse [6]. Some dosage forms may contain propylene glycol as solvent; as with lorazepam, large amounts are potentially toxic and have been associated with hyperosmolality, lactic acidosis, seizures, and respiratory depression.

Adverse Effects

Midazolam can cause pain and reaction at injection site (severity less than diazepam). Benzodiazepines cause respiratory depression and apnea in high doses or when given concomitantly with other sedatives or narcotics. Benzodiazepines can cause hypotension as they have a mild negative inotropic effect especially with underlying myocardial depression. Benzodiazepines may cause myoclonus (preterm infants), seizure-like activity, and nystagmus. Neonates are more vulnerable to profound and/or prolonged respiratory depressant effects of midazolam. Midazolam exposure has been associated with abnormal hippocampal growth and neurodevelopmental outcome in preterm infants [7].

Paradoxical Reactions

Benzodiazepines mostly have a calming effect, but in a minority of patients, midazolam can cause paradoxical reactions characterized by acute excitement and an altered mental state with increased anxiety, hyperactivity, hostility, and rage. Agitation occurred in 20% of children undergoing sedation using midazolam in the ED [8]. The mechanism is thought to be due to the inhibition of the cortical restraint centers and decreased serotonin that may precipitate aggressive behavior [9]. Genetic factors and learning disabilities may contribute to paradoxical reactions. Flumazenil can reverse both respiratory depression and paradoxical reactions resulting from midazolam [10].

Conclusion

Benzodiazepines are commonly used sedatives with good sedative, anxiolytic, amnestic, and muscle relaxant properties but do not provide analgesia. Benzodiazepines have many desirable properties: a good safety profile, multiple options for routes of administration, and quick onset and short duration of action with relatively minimal side effects.

Barbiturates

Mechanism of Action

Barbiturates are derivatives of barbituric acid, a cyclic molecule. Different pharmacological properties result from substitutions at the 2 and 5 carbon positions. Barbiturates bind to the gamma-aminobutyric acid (GABA) receptors (A-subunit) in the central nervous system (CNS), causing synaptic inhibition and resulting in sedation. By depressing the reticular activating system in the CNS, they produce sedation in a dose-dependent manner. Barbiturates provide sedation but lack analgesic properties. The antianxiety properties are inferior to those exerted by benzodiazepines. Barbiturates can be useful as sole sedative agents for short noninvasive procedures, such as computed tomography scan or magnetic resonance imaging, and in conjunction with analgesics for painful invasive procedures in spontaneously breathing patients. An overdose of barbiturates can produce general anesthesia, necessitating support of respiratory and cardiovascular function.

Pharmacokinetics

Barbiturates are highly lipid soluble, thereby producing their effects on the CNS rapidly. They are initially redistributed from the brain to other tissues and ultimately metabolized in the liver by the cytochrome enzyme system through oxidation. Methohexital also undergoes demethylation and pentobarbital hydroxylation and glucuronidation. Essentially no unchanged drug is excreted in the urine; thus, the hepatic metabolism determines the elimination of the drug. Children less than 6 months of age may experience delayed metabolism or elimination of pentobarbital.

Barbiturates can be classified into ultrashort-acting (e.g., thiopental, methohexital), medium-acting (e.g., pentobarbital, secobarbital), and long-acting (phenobarbital) agents based on their pharmacokinetic and pharmacodynamic profiles. Long-acting agents such as phenobarbital have a slow onset time and a long half-life of 24–96 h, thus making them unsuitable for use as procedural sedation agents. Medium- and ultrashort-acting agents typically produce sedation lasting only 10–30 min, despite much longer elimination half-lives due to redistribution of the drug from the brain to other body tissues. Their more rapid onset and offset contribute to methohexital and pentobarbital being the barbiturates preferred for use in procedural sedation. However, when given as an infusion (e.g., pentobarbital to induce coma in patients with refractory seizures), metabolism and elimination, not redistribution, determines drug clearance. Therefore, as a prolonged infusion, pentobarbital clearance is extremely delayed (t½ 20–45 h). Dosing and clinical effects are shown in Table 28.2.

Table 28.2 Barbiturate dosing and clinical effects

Agent	Type	Dosing	Onset	Duration of action	Usual recovery time to discharge	Common adverse events	Special properties	Uses
Methohexital	Ultrashort-acting barbiturate	1–2 mg/kg initial IV or IM dose, may repeat 0.5 mg/kg at 5 min intervals x 3	IM: 2–10 min IV: 1–2 min	IM: 1–1.5 h IV: 7–10 min	<1 h, though pharmacological t½ 4–24 h	Hiccups, cough, secretions, airway obstruction (especially with increased patient weight)	Rapid onset and offset similar to propofol	Alternative to propofol for patients with egg/soy allergy or mitochondrial disorder
		25 mg/kg rectal	Rectal: 5–15 min	Rectal: 1–5 h	90 min, though pharmacological t ½ 4–24 h			
Pentobarbital	Medium-acting barbiturate	5 mg/kg oral/rectal, may repeat 2.5 mg/kg in 30 min × 2	Oral/rectal: 15–60 min	1–4 h	60–120 min but may be several hours Terminal half-life 26 ± 16 h	Emesis (smaller children), O_2 desaturation, prolonged sedation, paradoxical agitation	Suspension taste can be masked using a 3:1 ratio of pentobarbital to cherry syrup	
		2 mg/kg IV or IM, may repeat 2 mg/kg at 5 min intervals × 2	IM: 10–15 min IV: 3–5 min	15–45 min	60–120 min but may be several hours. Terminal half-life 26 ± 16 h	O_2 desaturation, agitation, airway obstruction, prolonged sedation		

A direct comparison of pentobarbital and methohexital as sedative agents in the emergency department for CT scans showed that patients receiving methohexital completed their scans quicker. They also had significantly shorter sedation and post-procedure recovery times [11]. More patients receiving pentobarbital (55%) required redosing compared to those receiving methohexital (33%). These results suggest that methohexital should be preferred over pentobarbital when rapid turnover in a busy sedation unit is a consideration. A study by Kamat et al. reported that methohexital can be used for radiological imaging in high-volume centers when propofol is not a preferred option in patients with propofol allergy, egg allergy with anaphylaxis, and mitochondrial diseases [12].

A study comparing oral and intravenous pentobarbital reported that while the time to sedation was longer when the oral route was used, the sedation effectiveness and time to discharge were comparable, as was the procedure success rate. Patients receiving IV pentobarbital experienced significantly higher oxygen desaturation events [13]. Thus, oral pentobarbital may be useful in infants who do not have IV access and are undergoing a study that does not need an IV catheter placed for administration of radiological contrast material.

Pentobarbital has been shown to be inferior to propofol in a large study reviewing the Pediatric Sedation Research Consortium database where pentobarbital was used in 2007 patients and propofol in 5072 patients 6 months to 6 years of age [14]. Pentobarbital use was more likely to result in procedure cancellation due to poor sedation level achieved, as well as prolonged recovery, unplanned admission, vomiting, and allergic complications. Though the procedure success rate was similar (around 95%) in both groups, the median recovery time with pentobarbital was also longer (75 min vs. 30 min with propofol). However, 75% of patients who received pentobarbital also received midazolam as an adjuvant, compared to only 5% of those receiving propofol, calling into question whether midazolam played a part in the prolonged recovery time seen in the pentobarbital group.

Pentobarbital has also been shown to be inferior to etomidate when used in the emergency department for CT scans [15]. Patients receiving pentobarbital had longer sedation times, longer time to discharge, and suffered an adverse event more commonly than those receiving etomidate.

Barbiturates enhance the binding of benzodiazepines to the benzodiazepine receptor. It may be hypothesized that using midazolam as an adjunct may reduce the total pentobarbital dose used due to synergistic actions. However, based on a study of over 1000 patients, there appears to be no advantage to using midazolam for this indication, as it had no effect on the pentobarbital dose required for sedation. Even after controlling for weight and age, the addition of midazolam prolonged the time to reach the desired sedation level as well as the time to discharge without affecting the rate of adverse events [16].

Adverse Effects

During procedural sedation, barbiturates may result in several major and minor adverse effects including respiratory depression, airway obstruction, apnea, hypersalivation, hiccups, oxygen desaturation, vomiting, allergic reaction, hypotension, reflex tachycardia, prolonged sedation, and sometimes paradoxical agitation. Extravasation or intra-arterial injection can cause tissue necrosis. Hypotension occurs due to direct myocardial depression and loss of arterial vascular tone. Therefore, barbiturates must be used with extreme caution if myocardial dysfunction or hypotension preexists as profound hypotension or cardiac arrest can occur. Some children may experience a paradoxical hyperkinetic reaction when given a barbiturate for sedation. This is an idiosyncratic reaction characterized by agitation, temper tantrums, incoherent speech, and disorientation. Barbiturate use as a sedative agent is contraindicated in the presence of hypersensitivity to barbiturates and underlying porphyria or any patient whose physical status would preclude elective procedural sedation. Barbiturates should be used with caution in patients with liver dysfunction, extreme obesity, or renal dysfunction.

Pentobarbital has also been associated with post-discharge adverse events. In a study with detailed telephone follow-up of 253 patients, almost 65% of patients experience some adverse events after discharge [17]. The most common events reported were incoordination of movements (54%), dizziness (31%), agitation (20%), and vomiting (15%). Since these adverse events were classified as minor, the authors recommended that parents of patients receiving pentobarbital be given detailed and standardized discharge instructions on what to expect.

Conclusion

Barbiturates are useful sedatives for brief noninvasive procedures, especially in patients where propofol is contraindicated (e.g., patients with egg/soy allergy or a mitochondrial disorder) or intravenous access is either not indicated or difficult to attain. Due to its quick onset, predictable physiological effects, good safety profile, and short duration of action, methohexital is the ultrashort-acting barbiturate preferred by many providers for producing and maintaining the desired level of sedation.

References

1. Baldwa NM, Padvi AV, Dave NM, Garasia MB. Atomised intranasal midazolam spray as premedication in pediatric patients: comparison between two doses of 0.2 and 0.3 mg/kg. J Anesth. 2012;26(3):346–50.
2. Calligaris L, Davide Z, Alessandra M, De Bortoli R, Chiaretti A, Barbi E. Concentrated midazolam for intranasal administration: a pilot study. Pediatr Emerg Care. 2011;27(3):245–7.
3. Lugo RA, Fishbein M, Nahata MC, Lininger B. Complication of intranasal midazolam. Pediatrics. 1993;92(4):638.
4. Lam C, Udin RD, Malamed SF, Good DL, Forrest JL. Midazolam premedication in children: a pilot study comparing intramuscular and intranasal administration. Anesth Prog. 2005;52(2):56–61.

5. Shehab N, Lewis CL, Streetman DD, Donn SM. Exposure to the pharmaceutical excipients benzyl alcohol and propylene glycol among critically ill neonates. Pediatr Crit Care Med. 2009;10(2):256–9.
6. Gershanik J, Boecler B, Ensley H, McCloskey S, George W. The gasping syndrome and benzyl alcohol poisoning. N Engl J Med. 1982;307(22):1384–8.
7. Duerden EG, Guo T, Dodbiba L, et al. Midazolam dose correlates with abnormal hippocampal growth and neurodevelopmental outcome in preterm infants. Ann Neurol. 2016;79(4):548–59.
8. Bellolio MF, Puls HA, Anderson JL, et al. Incidence of adverse events in paediatric procedural sedation in the emergency department: a systematic review and meta-analysis. BMJ Open. 2016;6(6):e011384.
9. Mancuso CE, Tanzi MG, Gabay M et al. Paradoxical reactions to benzodiazepines: literature review and treatment options. Pharmacotherapy. 2004;24(9):1177–85. https://doi.org/10.1592/phco.24.13.1177.38089.
10. Sharbaf Shoar N, Saadabadi A. Flumazenil. Treasure Island: StatPearls; 2019.
11. Chun TH, Amanullah S, Karishma-Bahl D, Machan JT, Andrada ER, Lewander WJ. Comparison of methohexital and pentobarbital as sedative agents for pediatric emergency department patients for computed tomography. Pediatr Emerg Care. 2009;25(10):648–50.
12. Jones NE, Kelleman MS, Simon HK, et al. Evaluation of methohexital as an alternative to propofol in a high volume outpatient pediatric sedation service. Am J Emerg Med. 2017;35(8):1101–5.
13. Mason KP, Zurakowski D, Connor L, et al. Infant sedation for MR imaging and CT: oral versus intravenous pentobarbital. Radiology. 2004;233(3):723–8.
14. Mallory MD, Baxter AL, Kost SI, Pediatric Sedation Research C. Propofol vs pentobarbital for sedation of children undergoing magnetic resonance imaging: results from the Pediatric Sedation Research Consortium. Paediatr Anaesth. 2009;19(6):601–11.
15. Baxter AL, Mallory MD, Spandorfer PR, et al. Etomidate versus pentobarbital for computed tomography sedations: report from the Pediatric Sedation Research Consortium. Pediatr Emerg Care. 2007;23(10):690–5.
16. Mason KP, Zurakowski D, Karian VE, Connor L, Fontaine PJ, Burrows PE. Sedatives used in pediatric imaging: comparison of IV pentobarbital with IV pentobarbital with midazolam added. AJR Am J Roentgenol. 2001;177(2):427–30.
17. Kaila R, Chen X, Kannikeswaran N. Postdischarge adverse events related to sedation for diagnostic imaging in children. Pediatr Emerg Care. 2012;28(8):796–801.
18. Katzung BG, Trevor AJ. Basic & clinical pharmacology. 13th ed. New York: McGraw-Hill; 2015.

Chapter 29
Alpha-agonists in Pediatric Procedural Sedation

Pradip P. Kamat

Mechanism of Action

Dexmedetomidine is a selective central alpha-2-agonist, which is an inhibitory pathway leading to decreased sympathetic output with multiple effects. Dexmedetomidine selectivity for alpha-2 vs. alpha-1 is 1620:1 compared to clonidine, which has a selectivity (alpha-2:alpha-1) of 220:1. Dexmedetomidine primarily binds to imidazoline receptors, which are not G-protein-coupled receptors. The imidazoline receptors play a central role in neuroprotection, memory, and blood pressure control [1].

Most of the action of DEX is at the level of the locus coeruleus in the brainstem (primarily sedation) and in the spinal cord (primarily analgesia). The vagomimetic effect on the heart as well as its effect through the alpha-2 receptors on blocking the cardioaccelerator nerve of the heart results in bradycardia [2].

Dexmedetomidine is a hypnotic, sedative, and amnestic agent with mild analgesic effects. Its action on peripheral vasculature (sympatholysis) results in hypotension [3]. Rapid intravenous administration of DEX can cause transient hypertension due to weak peripheral alpha-1 receptor agonist activity. Dexmedetomidine also has antishivering and mild diuretic effect [4]. An attractive property of DEX in procedural sedation is its ability to maintain airway reflexes and respiratory function [5]. However, a recent study, using pharyngeal critical pressures in adult volunteers not exposed to painful stimuli, reported that airway collapsibility with DEX is similar to propofol at similar levels of sedation. The applicability of the above study in infants and children is unclear at this time [6]. Other effects of DEX include decreased emergence delirium and neuroprotection [7, 8].

P. P. Kamat (✉)
Department of Pediatrics, Emory University School of Medicine, Atlanta, GA, USA
e-mail: Pradip.kamat@choa.org

P. P. Kamat, J. W. Berkenbosch (eds.), *Sedation and Analgesia for the Pediatric Intensivist*, https://doi.org/10.1007/978-3-030-52555-2_29

Pharmacokinetics and Pharmacodynamics

Dexmedetomidine is primarily used IV, but the same formulation can be used by intranasal or buccal routes. Following an IV dose, DEX works in 5–10 minutes with a peak effect noted in 15–30 minutes. Intranasal onset of action is in 45–60 minutes with a peak effect between 90 and 105 minutes. It is 93% protein bound [9]. Dexmedetomidine has an intranasal bioavailability of 65% (35–93%), and the intramuscular bioavailability is 104% [10]. The buccal bioavailability of DEX is 82%, whereas oral (subject to first-pass metabolism) is only 15%. Dexmedetomidine is primarily metabolized in the liver and excreted in the urine [11].

Dexmedetomidine is available as 200 mcg/2 ml, which is mixed with 48 cc NS to make a solution that delivers 4 mcg/ml. As opposed to benzodiazepines, patient is easily arousable from DEX sedation, which is called cooperative sedation.

Adverse Events

Adverse events include sedation, a dose-dependent decrease in heart rate and blood pressure, although <15% can manifest with hypertension due to stimulation of peripheral alpha-2 receptors, some of which are vasoconstrictive [12, 13]. Usually the drop in heart rate and blood pressure is <30% without a change in in the end-organ perfusion [14].

Withdrawal can be seen after prolonged infusion (>3–4 days) in terms of nervousness, agitation, tachycardia, headaches, and tachycardia. Atropine is not recommended in DEX-induced bradycardia as it causes sustained hypertension. The usual approach to DEX-induced bradycardia is to stop the infusion [15]. The sedation with DEX resembles natural non-rapid eye movement sleep with no interference with electroencephalogram [16]. Another benefit of the sedation with DEX resembling natural sleep is the absence of recovery-related agitation even in children with behavioral issues [17]. In fact DEX has been used for emergence reactions in anesthesiology. In a large report from the Pediatric Sedation Research Consortium (PSRC), Sulton et al. studied adverse events on 13, 072 children sedated using DEX [14]. The overall adverse event (AE) rate in that study was 466/13072 (3.6%, 95% CI 3.3–3.9%). The overall serious adverse event (SAE) rate was 45/13072 (0.34%, 95% CI 0.19–0.037%). Airway obstruction was the most common SAE: 35/13072 (0.27%, 95% CI 0.19–0.37%) [14]. In contrast PSRC study on propofol reported an AE rate of 5% and SAE rate of 2.5% [18].

Uses in Sedation

The main use of DEX is for radiological imaging and other procedures requiring patient to be motionless such as auditory brainstem responses (ABR), echocardiography, ultrasound, electroencephalogram, etc. [19]. Patients needing radiological imaging such as computed tomography, PET scan, short magnetic resonance imaging, and nuclear medicine imaging are perfect candidates for sedation with DEX [20, 21]. A combination of intravenous ketamine (1–2 mg/kg) with DEX can be used for short painful procedures including during cardiac catheterization [22].

Dosing

Different doses are suggested by various studies for radiological imaging but in general a slow loading dose over 10 minutes followed by an infusion for duration of the imaging procedure.

Intravenous DEX: Use 1–3 mcg/kg over 10 minutes followed by an infusion of 1–2 mcg/kg/h. Time to onset is 10–15 minutes, providing sedation for 30–45 minutes. Success rate is 84% and may require a second agent such as midazolam or ketamine.

In a large study published by Mason et al., a higher loading dose of DEX (3 mcg/kg over 10 minutes) followed by a 2 mcg/kg/h infusion was used in 747 consecutive patients receiving MRI sedation. Authors reported a high success rate (97.6%), lack of a need for adjuvant medications, and deviation of blood pressure and heart rate within 20% of the established awake norms [23].

The use of DEX in nuclear medicine was studied by Mason et al. [20]. In the largest retrospective study, 669 patients (age: 0.1–22.5 years) undergoing nuclear medicine imaging received DEX for sedation. A bolus of 2 mcg/kg was administered over 10 minutes; this dose could be repeated up to 2 additional times if the predefined sedation score was not achieved. In addition, patients also received a maintenance infusion of 1 mcg/kg/h. Authors reported a success rate of 99.7%. Hypotension (58.7%) and bradycardia (4.3%) were reported without the need for pharmacological therapy.

Intramuscular DEX dose is 1–4 mcg/kg. In a study of 65 children, Mason et al. used about 2.9 mcg/kg (MRI group) and 2.5 mcg/kg (CT group) with a mean time to sedation (13.1–13.4 minutes) and a time to discharge (17.1–21.9 minutes), and hypotension (defined as blood pressure <20%) was seen in 9 patients (14%). No bradycardia or hypertension or hypoxia was reported. The dose of DEX was not a predictor of hypotension [24].

In 315 patients with autism spectrum disorders and developmental disorders undergoing MRI, CT, EEG, or other imaging, Berkenbosch et al. used premedication with midazolam (IN or oral) or DEX, followed by an induction dose of 12 mcg/kg/h over 60 minutes [17]. No maintenance was used for short studies such as EEG, but a maintenance infusion of DEX was used for longer studies: the mean IV induction DEX dose of 1.4 ± 0.6 and a total dose of 2.6 ± 1.6 mcg/kg. About 90% of patients required concomitant midazolam and 7 patients required intervention for hypotension, bradycardia, or both, and two patients had recovery agitation. Overall success rate was 98.7%.

Intranasal DEX dose is 2–4 mcg/kg (use a mucosal atomizer device and split dose between the nostrils). Time of onset is 30–45 minutes, and duration of sedation is 45–60 minutes. A second intranasal agent such as midazolam can be added if DEX by itself is not proving the depth need for radiological imaging [25]. Sulton et al. reported on 224 children undergoing MRI using IN DEX [26]. The median dose in that study was 3/kg (IQR 2.5–3). Adjunctive midazolam was used in 219/224 (98%) of the patients.

Intranasal DEX is a great option for short imaging procedures, which do not require IV access for contrast (for eg. non-contrast brain MRI) [27]. Intranasal DEX can also be used in lieu of PO midazolam for anxiety prior to IV access. Studies have reported use of DEX prior to PIV placement in children with developmental delay or mild autism spectrum disorder (either buccal or intranasal) [28, 29]. Sedation providers need to be aware that mean time to achieve sedation in all patients is about 8.6 ± 4.6 minutes (range: 1–40 minutes). Additionally, duration to recovery post procedure is also prolonged with DEX [30]. This could affect the workflow at high-volume sedation programs.

A recent retrospective study by Boriosi et al. reported induction DEX (1–2 mcg/kg over 10 minutes) followed by the usual propofol infusion of 5–6 mg/kg/h for maintenance [31]. Propofol boluses of 0.5–1 mg/kg were allowed at the discretion of the physician. The DEX + propofol group had fewer adverse events (upper airway obstruction) compared to propofol alone. This is an interesting combination approach to infants and children who are premature, having history of obstructive sleep apnea and a recent upper respiratory tract infection, or any child with higher risk of upper airway obstruction.

For interventional procedures such as bronchoscopy, central venous line placement, and chest tubes, DEX was used in a dose of 1.5 mcg/k (range 1–3 mcg/kg) IV, but 50% required supplemental ketamine (0.7 mg/kg) [32]. There is an expanding role for DEX in pediatric dentistry in combination with an opioid or a benzodiazepine [33, 34]. The combination of DEX with either fentanyl or propofol has been used successfully for upper and lower GI endoscopy. However, use of DEX alone compared to propofol + fentanyl combination for ERCP was less effective in terms of analgesia provided as well as with agitation seen [35].

Summary

Dexmedetomidine could be the drug that has an evolving role in procedural sedation due to the nonavailability of chloral hydrate. Oral formulation of chloral hydrate is unavailable since 2012, leading to a few institutions compounding their own using raw ingredients for use in sedation of infants and young children. Chloral hydrate has a variable half-life and no antidote for toxicity and can result in clinical re-sedation, and there are concerns about genotoxicity as well as teratogenicity. Dexmedetomidine also has the advantage of being neuroprotective compared to chloral hydrate, which has been associated with neuronal apoptosis.

References

1. Zhang H, Yan X, Wang DG, et al. Dexmedetomidine relieves formaldehyde-induced pain in rats through both alpha2 adrenoceptor and imidazoline receptor. Biomed Pharmacother. 2017;90:914–20. https://doi.org/10.1016/j.biopha.2017.04.047.
2. Bloor BC, Ward DS, Belleville JP, Maze M. Effects of intravenous dexmedetomidine in humans. II. Hemodynamic changes. Anesthesiology. 1992;77(6):1134–42. https://doi.org/10.1097/00000542-199212000-00014.
3. Belleville JP, Ward DS, Bloor BC, Maze M. Effects of intravenous dexmedetomidine in humans. I. Sedation, ventilation, and metabolic rate. Anesthesiology. 1992;77(6):1125–33. https://doi.org/10.1097/00000542-199212000-00013.
4. Blaine Easley R, Brady KM, Tobias JD. Dexmedetomidine for the treatment of post-anesthesia shivering in children. Paediatr Anaesth. 2007;17(4):341–6. https://doi.org/10.1111/j.1460-9592.2006.02100.x.
5. Mahmoud M, Radhakrishman R, Gunter J, et al. Effect of increasing depth of dexmedetomidine anesthesia on upper airway morphology in children. Paediatr Anaesth. 2010;20(6):506–15. https://doi.org/10.1111/j.1460-9592.2010.03311.x.
6. Lodenius A, Maddison KJ, Lawther BK, et al. Upper airway collapsibility during dexmedetomidine and propofol sedation in healthy volunteers: a nonblinded randomized crossover study. Anesthesiology. 2019;131(5):962–73. https://doi.org/10.1097/ALN.0000000000002883.
7. Perez-Zoghbi JF, Zhu W, Grafe MR, Brambrink AM. Dexmedetomidine-mediated neuroprotection against sevoflurane-induced neurotoxicity extends to several brain regions in neonatal rats. Br J Anaesth. 2017;119(3):506–16. https://doi.org/10.1093/bja/aex222.
8. Sato M, Shirakami G, Tazuke-Nishimura M, Matsuura S, Tanimoto K, Fukuda K. Effect of single-dose dexmedetomidine on emergence agitation and recovery profiles after sevoflurane anesthesia in pediatric ambulatory surgery. J Anesth. 2010;24(5):675–82. https://doi.org/10.1007/s00540-010-0976-4.
9. Petroz GC, Sikich N, James M, et al. A phase I, two-center study of the pharmacokinetics and pharmacodynamics of dexmedetomidine in children. Anesthesiology. 2006;105(6):1098–110. https://doi.org/10.1097/00000542-200612000-00009.
10. Anttila M, Penttila J, Helminen A, Vuorilehto L, Scheinin H. Bioavailability of dexmedetomidine after extravascular doses in healthy subjects. Br J Clin Pharmacol. 2003;56(6):691–3. https://doi.org/10.1046/j.1365-2125.2003.01944.x.
11. Bhana N, Goa KL, McClellan KJ. Dexmedetomidine. Drugs. 2000;59(2):263–8. https://doi.org/10.2165/00003495-200059020-00012; discussion 269–270.
12. Mahmoud M, Mason KP. Dexmedetomidine: review, update, and future considerations of paediatric perioperative and periprocedural applications and limitations. Br J Anaesth. 2015;115(2):171–82. https://doi.org/10.1093/bja/aev226.
13. Mason KP, Zurakowski D, Zgleszewski S, Prescilla R, Fontaine PJ, Dinardo JA. Incidence and predictors of hypertension during high-dose dexmedetomidine sedation for pediatric MRI. Paediatr Anaesth. 2010;20(6):516–23. https://doi.org/10.1111/j.1460-9592.2010.03299.x.
14. Sulton C, McCracken C, Simon HK, et al. Pediatric procedural sedation using dexmedetomidine: a report from the Pediatric Sedation Research Consortium. Hosp Pediatr. 2016;6(9):536–44. https://doi.org/10.1542/hpeds.2015-0280.
15. Mason KP, Zgleszewski S, Forman RE, Stark C, DiNardo JA. An exaggerated hypertensive response to glycopyrrolate therapy for bradycardia associated with high-dose dexmedetomidine. Anesth Analg. 2009;108(3):906–8. https://doi.org/10.1213/ane.0b013e3181948a6f.
16. Mason KP, O'Mahony E, Zurakowski D, Libenson MH. Effects of dexmedetomidine sedation on the EEG in children. Paediatr Anaesth. 2009;19(12):1175–83. https://doi.org/10.1111/j.1460-9592.2009.03160.x.

17. Lubisch N, Roskos R, Berkenbosch JW. Dexmedetomidine for procedural sedation in children with autism and other behavior disorders. Pediatr Neurol. 2009;41(2):88–94. https://doi.org/10.1016/j.pediatrneurol.2009.02.006.
18. Kamat PP, McCracken CE, Gillespie SE, et al. Pediatric critical care physician-administered procedural sedation using propofol: a report from the Pediatric Sedation Research Consortium Database. Pediatr Crit Care Med. 2015;16(1):11–20. https://doi.org/10.1097/PCC.0000000000000273.
19. Berkenbosch JW, Wankum PC, Tobias JD. Prospective evaluation of dexmedetomidine for noninvasive procedural sedation in children. Pediatr Crit Care Med. 2005;6(4):435–9. https://doi.org/10.1097/01.PCC.0000163680.50087.93; quiz 440.
20. Mason KP, Robinson F, Fontaine P, Prescilla R. Dexmedetomidine offers an option for safe and effective sedation for nuclear medicine imaging in children. Radiology. 2013;267(3):911–7. https://doi.org/10.1148/radiol.13121232.
21. Mason KP. Sedation trends in the 21st century: the transition to dexmedetomidine for radiological imaging studies. Paediatr Anaesth. 2010;20(3):265–72. https://doi.org/10.1111/j.1460-9592.2009.03224.x.
22. Tobias JD. Dexmedetomidine and ketamine: an effective alternative for procedural sedation? Pediatr Crit Care Med. 2012;13(4):423–7. https://doi.org/10.1097/PCC.0b013e318238b81c.
23. Mason KP, Zurakowski D, Zgleszewski SE, et al. High dose dexmedetomidine as the sole sedative for pediatric MRI. Paediatr Anaesth. 2008;18(5):403–11. https://doi.org/10.1111/j.1460-9592.2008.02468.x.
24. Mason KP, Lubisch NB, Robinson F, Roskos R. Intramuscular dexmedetomidine sedation for pediatric MRI and CT. AJR Am J Roentgenol. 2011;197(3):720–5. https://doi.org/10.2214/AJR.10.6134.
25. Cozzi G, Norbedo S, Barbi E. Intranasal dexmedetomidine for procedural sedation in children, a suitable alternative to chloral hydrate. Paediatr Drugs. 2017;19(2):107–11. https://doi.org/10.1007/s40272-017-0217-5.
26. Sulton C, Kamat P, Mallory M, Reynolds J. The use of intranasal dexmedetomidine and midazolam for sedated magnetic resonance imaging in children: a report from the Pediatric Sedation Research Consortium. Pediatr Emerg Care. 2017. https://doi.org/10.1097/PEC.0000000000001199.
27. Lewis J, Bailey CR. Intranasal dexmedetomidine for sedation in children; a review. J Perioper Pract. 2019:1750458919854885. https://doi.org/10.1177/1750458919854885.
28. Jun JH, Kim KN, Kim JY, Song SM. The effects of intranasal dexmedetomidine premedication in children: a systematic review and meta-analysis. Can J Anaesth. 2017;64(9):947–61. https://doi.org/10.1007/s12630-017-0917-x.
29. Mondardini MC, Amigoni A, Cortellazzi P, et al. Intranasal dexmedetomidine in pediatrics: update of current knowledge. Minerva Anestesiol. 2019. https://doi.org/10.23736/S0375-9393.19.13820-5.
30. Olgun G, Ali MH. Use of intranasal dexmedetomidine as a solo sedative for MRI of infants. Hosp Pediatr. 2018. https://doi.org/10.1542/hpeds.2017-0120.
31. Boriosi JP, Eickhoff JC, Klein KB, Hollman GA. A retrospective comparison of propofol alone to propofol in combination with dexmedetomidine for pediatric 3T MRI sedation. Paediatr Anaesth. 2017;27(1):52–9. https://doi.org/10.1111/pan.13041.
32. Barton KP, Munoz R, Morell VO, Chrysostomou C. Dexmedetomidine as the primary sedative during invasive procedures in infants and toddlers with congenital heart disease. Pediatr Crit Care Med. 2008;9(6):612–5. https://doi.org/10.1097/PCC.0b013e31818d320d.
33. Mohite V, Baliga S, Thosar N, Rathi N. Role of dexmedetomidine in pediatric dental sedation. J Dent Anesth Pain Med. 2019;19(2):83–90. https://doi.org/10.17245/jdapm.2019.19.2.83.
34. Sago T, Shiiba S, Ando E, et al. Sedation with a combination of dexmedetomidine and midazolam for pediatric dental surgery. Anesth Prog. 2018;65(2):124–6. https://doi.org/10.2344/anpr-65-03-14.
35. Muller S, Borowics SM, Fortis EA, et al. Clinical efficacy of dexmedetomidine alone is less than propofol for conscious sedation during ERCP. Gastrointest Endosc. 2008;67(4):651–9. https://doi.org/10.1016/j.gie.2007.09.041.

Part VIII
Anesthetics

Chapter 30
Procedural Sedation in Children: Ketamine

Anuradha Menon and Yoke Hwee Chan

Introduction

Ketamine is a unique dissociative anesthetic capable of providing potent analgesia, anxiolysis, sedation, and amnesia while maintaining hemodynamic stability, spontaneous respiration, and retention of protective airway reflexes [1]. Stable hemodynamics and lack of respiratory depression make ketamine a safe and highly effective drug and one of the most frequently utilized in pediatric procedural sedation worldwide [2].

A structural analog of phencyclidine, ketamine was first developed in 1962 to reduce the troubling emergence of delirium that precluded its parent drug's widespread clinical use [3, 4]. Following US Food and Drug Administration (FDA) approval in 1970 as an anesthetic agent, its use has expanded far beyond the operating room and is now well established in the fields of emergency medicine, critical care, and pain management. New and emerging uses include its role in treating burns patients, chronic and neuropathic pain, refractory status epilepticus, and depression, among others [5–7].

The last two decades have seen its use in pediatric emergency departments (ED) increase worldwide for procedural sedation, generating a wealth of data that has demonstrated an excellent safety profile [8, 9]. An essential tool in the pediatric intensivist's arsenal for procedural sedation both in and outside the ICU, ketamine is used for both routine and complex procedures. In the developing world, particularly in resource-limited settings, ketamine is often the drug of choice where reliable ventilator equipment may not be readily available [10, 11], earning its place in the World Health Organization's (WHO) list of essential medications. However, it has not proven universally popular due to concerns regarding emergence phenomena, delirium, and potential for abuse due to its psychotropic properties and remains a controlled substance in some parts of the world.

A. Menon · Y. H. Chan (✉)
Department of Paediatric Subspecialties, Children's Intensive Care Unit, KK Women's and Children's Hospital, Singapore, Singapore
e-mail: Anuradha.Menon@singhealth.com.sg; Chan.Yoke.Hwee@singhealth.com.sg

P. P. Kamat, J. W. Berkenbosch (eds.), *Sedation and Analgesia for the Pediatric Intensivist*, https://doi.org/10.1007/978-3-030-52555-2_30

Pharmacology

A derivative of the cyclo-hexamine anesthetic agent phencyclidine, ketamine is a noncompetitive *N*-methyl-d-aspartate (NMDA) receptor antagonist. It blocks the phencyclidine binding site on the NMDA receptor located at spinal, thalamic, limbic, and cortical levels, thereby arresting neuronal depolarization, and interferes with sensory inputs to higher centers of the central nervous system (CNS) affecting pain, emotional response, and memory. The disconnection of the thalamocortical system from the limbic system gives rise to its unique dissociative properties, characterized by a lack of response to external stimuli. It resembles a cataleptic state in which the patient is non-communicative but appears awake, distinguishing ketamine from other agents used in procedural sedation [1, 12].

A multitude of secondary interactions with opioid receptors, monoaminergic receptors, muscarinic receptors, voltage-sensitive calcium, and sodium channels, as well as catecholamine receptors, are responsible for its various properties and systemic effects [1].

Most commercial preparations of ketamine for use in clinical settings exist as a racemic mixture of the two S(+) and R(−) isomers. Isolated S(+) ketamine is known to have a higher affinity to the NMDA receptor binding site, with 3–4 times greater potency. Besides, less cardiac stimulation, less motor activity, better analgesia, more rapid recovery, and a decreased incidence of emergence delirium have been described with its use [13, 14] and may be available for use in some countries.

Ketamine is highly lipophilic with low protein binding properties. Thus it is transferred rapidly across the blood-brain barrier, with a distribution half-life of only 10–15 min, and has a large volume of distribution. Ketamine undergoes metabolism primarily in the liver (80%) through the cytochrome systems to several metabolites, of which the active metabolite norketamine retains its anesthetic activity at one-third the potency of ketamine and contributes to its analgesic effects [15]. Inactive ketamine conjugates and metabolites are renally excreted, and elimination half-life is between 2 and 3 h [16–18]. Concomitant use with drugs that inhibit cytochrome P450 metabolism may therefore lead to inhibited ketamine metabolism and result in supra-therapeutic dosing.

Systemic Effects

Ketamine, via its sympathomimetic properties, increases arterial pressures and heart rate through direct CNS stimulation [19]. Consequently, myocardial oxygen demands and cardiac work are increased. Ketamine also causes direct relaxation of vascular smooth muscle, though due to its sympathetically mediated vasoconstriction, it has a relatively net stable effect on systemic vascular resistance. At higher doses, ketamine acts as a direct myocardial depressant and is cautioned for use in critical illness states where its negative inotropy may predominate [2, 20]. While earlier studies had shown an increase in pulmonary pressures with ketamine and cautioned its use in children with pulmonary hypertension and limited right ventricular function [21], recent studies have shown that ketamine does not affect pulmonary vascular resistance in children with pulmonary hypertension [21, 22].

Ketamine does not produce any significant respiratory depression. However, when administered intravenously, ketamine must be given slowly (over 1 min) to prevent apnea and transient respiratory depression [9, 23]. In addition to the maintenance of upper airway skeletal muscle tone and airway reflexes, ketamine is a bronchodilator. These effects on the airways are thought to be due to modulation of the inflammatory cascade, and a recent review has shown that there may be a role for ketamine in refractory asthma unresponsive to conventional treatment [24, 25]. An important consideration is its potential to increase salivary and tracheobronchial secretions, though unless clinically indicated, routine co-administration of antisialagogues has generally fallen out of favor [23, 26]. Due to its diverse molecular targets and neurophysiological properties, ketamine's precise effect on the CNS remains incompletely understood, but is an emerging area of research. Early data showed induction doses of ketamine increased cerebral blood flow, cerebral metabolism, and intracranial pressure (ICP) [27]. However, recent studies suggest ketamine does not cause clinically significant increases in ICP and has little impact on cerebral hemodynamics compared to other anesthetics [28–30]. Ketamine's action in inhibiting information transfer in cortical networks may confer potential neuroprotective benefits such as the attenuation of ischemic injury in traumatic brain injury, the management of refractory seizures, and the modulation of pathological states such as depression [31, 32].

Emergence phenomena include recovery agitation, "psychedelic" dreams, hallucinations, and depersonalization. These are generally uncommon in children and teenagers and if present are typically mild (1–2% in children vs. 10–20% in adults) [33]. Current evidence does not suggest any benefit from the prophylactic administration of concurrent benzodiazepines in children and recommends their role should be confined to treating unpleasant reactions should they arise [23, 33, 34].

Perturbations of the vestibular system are known to occur with ketamine use and include dizziness, nausea, and vomiting. Horizontal nystagmus is typical and frequently seen following administration. To allay undue anxiety, caregivers present should be told that this is an expected effect. Rates of emesis (6–28%) are higher with intramuscular administration, older age, and higher cumulative dosage [35–38] and may be ameliorated with the concomitant use of an antiemetic [39, 40]. Finally, ketamine produces an increase in muscle tone and occasionally muscle spasms, although it has been safely used in myopathies and malignant hyperthermia.

Indications

Ketamine is highly suited for a myriad of pediatric procedural sedation encounters both in and outside the ICU, both as an induction agent and in lower doses as a reliable sedative or analgesic drug.

In pediatric procedural sedation, ketamine is most often used for painful procedures in patients with a stable respiratory status and where complete immobility is not a prerequisite since ketamine causes transient hypertonicity or clonus. Examples include simple surgical procedures like incision and drainage, laceration repair, orthopedic procedures (e.g., fracture reduction), dental procedures, dressing changes in burns patients, bone marrow aspiration, and intrathecal chemotherapy administration in oncology patients.

Its sympathomimetic effects make it an ideal agent for rapid sequence induction (RSI) in patients who are hemodynamically unstable such as in sepsis, in cardiac disease, and in multi-trauma. For emergent procedures when fasting is not assured, ketamine may also be preferred due to its preservation of airway tone and reflexes. Its airway-preserving properties and bronchodilator properties make it an excellent choice for sedation and as a first-line agent for RSI in asthmatic patients.

Finally, at lower doses, ketamine is known to desensitize central pain pathways and modulate opioid receptors, making it suitable for use in patients with prolonged hospitalizations or ICU stays who may be developing a tolerance to opioids [41].

Dosing and Routes of Administration

Ketamine has a wide therapeutic range. It can be safely administered through multiple routes: intravenous, intramuscular, intranasal, intraosseous, oral, rectal, subcutaneous, and epidural.

Intravenous (IV) administration is 100% bioavailable and considered the ideal route of administration for procedural sedation if vascular access is easily established. Onset of action is rapid, approximately one-arm brain circulation time (30–45 s), with onset of dissociation noted within 1 min and effective procedural conditions lasting for about 5–10 min. A single loading dose of 0.5–2 mg/kg administered over 30–60 s is recommended (to prevent apnea and transient respiratory depression) and is often adequate for short procedures, although higher initial doses of 1.5–2 mg/kg compared to 1 mg/kg resulted in less re-dosing requirement and better physician satisfaction with the same sedation scores [42]. Longer procedures require the dissociative state to be maintained with intermittent boluses of 0.25–0.5 mg/kg or with a low-dose ketamine infusion depending on the provider's comfort. Cumulative IV dosing in excess of 5 mg/kg or an initial dose of ≥2.5 mg/kg has been associated with a higher incidence of adverse events [23]. Providers should consider maintenance of sedation and analgesia with other agents in these circumstances. Subanesthetic doses of 0.25–0.5 mg/kg IV (bolus) or 0.1–0.2 mg/kg/h IV continuous infusion are commonly used as adjuncts for post-operative pain or for sedation for tube tolerance following use in RSI or other routine ICU care.

In emergent settings or with uncooperative patients where obtaining vascular access is challenging, intramuscular (IM) ketamine is a good alternative. With only a slightly lower bioavailability of 93%, it is generally well tolerated though a higher incidence of nausea and vomiting has been described, particularly in adolescents

[35, 38]. When given IM at a dose of 4–5 mg/kg once, the same effect is achieved within 3–5 min, with effective procedural conditions lasting 10–30 min [43, 44]. Variations in dosing regimens exist with a recent population pharmacokinetics study of IM and IV ketamine in children recommending procedural sedation dose for IV ketamine at 2 mg/kg and IM ketamine at 6–8 mg/kg to provide adequate sedation for up to 20 min [45].

The availability and use of intranasal (IN) ketamine in pediatric procedural sedation are garnering more attention, though, at present, large and high-quality clinical trials are lacking [46]. Rapid systemic absorption combined with ease of access makes this route an appealing choice, especially in children. Onset of action is 10–15 min, consistent with IN ketamine's time to peak plasma concentration of 18–21 min [47, 48], and is described to be effective for up to 60 min following a single dose. Delivery via local instillation and use of mucosal atomizer devices has been described with good effect. However, significant heterogeneity exists between dosing and frequency, with reported ranges between 0.5 and 10 mg/kg [46]. Initial dosing in children older than 2 years is suggested at 0.5–0.8 mg/kg/dose; a second dose may be repeated in 10–15 min if required at 0.5 mg/kg/dose.

Transmucosal (oral and rectal) routes of administration are not commonly used for pediatric procedural sedation and analgesia owing to ketamine's extensive first-pass hepatic metabolism and variations in vascularity and gastrointestinal absorption resulting in reduced bioavailability, less predictable effectiveness, and delayed onset and recovery [47, 49]. Efforts are being made to develop suitable oral and sublingual formulations given the recent move toward using low-dose ketamine for pain and depression in adults [50].

It is important to note that ketamine does not exhibit the characteristic dose-response continuum to progressive titration. Below a certain threshold (1–1.5 mg/kg IV or 3–4 mg/kg IM), ketamine produces potent analgesia and sedation. Onset of the dissociative state is seen usually above a dose of about 1–1.5 mg/kg IV (range 0.25–1.5 mg/kg), and once this state is achieved, higher doses do not result in deeper levels of sedation as the dissociation has no observable levels of depth [8, 12]. The main goal of ketamine titration is to maintain the presence of this state over time required for completion of the procedure. There is some degree of tachyphylaxis reported with repeat use of ketamine [23].

Typical time from dosing until dischargeable recovery is 50–110 min when given IV and 60–140 min when given IM [23, 43, 51]. Minimum monitoring should include continuous electrocardiogram, non-invasive blood pressure, pulse oximetry, and end-tidal CO2 monitoring where available.

Adjuncts to Use/Co-administration with Other Drugs

Not infrequently, ketamine is used to achieve procedural sedation along with the other medications. Adjuncts include anticholinergics and antiemetics to mitigate systemic effects and co-administration of benzodiazepines, other anesthetic agents (propofol), and analgesics (e.g., opioids) for maintenance of sedation and analgesia in longer procedures. The choice of agent and exact timing of administration of these adjuncts – before, during, or after the procedure – also need to be carefully considered in the sedation plan and will depend upon procedure type, length, and patient factors. An individualized, tailor-made approach is recommended with the following guidelines in mind.

Anticholinergics

Anticholinergics (e.g., atropine or glycopyrrolate) have traditionally been administered with ketamine to decrease secretions, which may in turn predispose to increased cough, airway obstruction, and laryngospasm. This practice is no longer routinely advocated due to evidence from large pediatric studies which have demonstrated adjunctive anticholinergic use is associated with more adverse events, unless clinically indicated [9, 23, 52].

Antiemetics

Prophylactic ondansetron has been shown to decrease emesis rates in children by 8% in a randomized controlled trial in children undergoing procedural sedation in an ED setting and should therefore be considered in children at highest risk, namely, early adolescence, and those receiving IM route of administration [37, 39, 40].

Benzodiazepines

Benzodiazepine (most commonly midazolam) administration with ketamine is well known and primarily for the treatment and/or prevention of emergence reactions [53]. Emergence phenomena in children are rare and typically mild. Studies in children have yielded mixed results, and balancing this with potential respiratory complications and decreased hepatic clearance associated with benzodiazepine use, no strong recommendations can be made to strongly advocate its routine use [23, 33, 34, 54]. Emphasis on non-pharmacologic maneuvers where possible, such as recovering patients in a quiet and controlled environment with ample reassurance, may be effective in reducing the incidence and severity of emergence symptoms following ketamine sedation and where possible should be employed.

Ketamine and Propofol ("Ketofol")

Ketamine has been used safely in combination with propofol for induction and maintenance of sedation. This combination, "ketofol," has proven popular in both pediatric and adult procedural sedation [55]. Propofol, a sedative-hypnotic with a rapid onset of action and a quick recovery time, in addition has good antiemetic effects; however, it lacks analgesic properties. Its use is limited in practice by dose-dependent cardiorespiratory depression. The combination with ketamine, a dissociative agent that reliably produces analgesia and amnesia, results in lower doses of both drugs being used than typically required when each agent is used individually [56, 57]. In addition, ketofol also has the ability to counteract the emergence agitation and nausea associated with ketamine.

Studies in children suggest that ketofol use could have a slightly better time to sedation, and length of sedation and recovery time, compared to ketamine alone [58–61]. It does also appear that ketofol produces a more steady sedation depth not requiring as many repeat doses compared to propofol alone [60]. Better caregiver and provider satisfaction has also been reported with ketofol compared to ketamine or propofol use in isolation [59, 60] . Rates of severe adverse events and adverse events were higher when propofol was co-administered with ketamine compared with ketamine use alone in a large cohort of procedural sedation encounters in children performed outside of the OR within the pediatric sedation research consortium [52]. This is in contrast to smaller ED-based, single-center, prospective randomized controlled studies which did not show a significant difference in adverse respiratory events and a lower rate of nausea and vomiting in the ketofol group [59]. Though no standard dosing regimens are established, most studies and authors recommend a 1:1 ratio to provide ease of administration with good effects and safety profile [61, 62]. However, little data exists on the pharmacologic stability of mixing these two agents when combined, and future studies are needed in order to determine the best dose and method for delivery of ketofol [62, 63].

Ketamine and Dexmedetomidine ("Ketadex")

The moniker "ketadex" refers to the combination of ketamine with dexmedetomidine, a newer practice since the widespread use of dexmedetomidine in ICUs worldwide from the early 2000s. The rationale for this combination therapy lies in the potential synergistic effects of these agents [64]. Dexmedetomidine, a selective alpha-2-agonist, may decrease the tachycardia, hypertension, sialorrhea, and dissociative side effects associated with ketamine. Conversely, ketamine's rapid onset of action and sympathomimetic properties prevent the bradycardia and hypotension that is sometimes seen with dexmedetomidine. Literature on the use of ketadex for procedural sedation in children is limited. One prospective study comparing ketadex to ketofol showed similar efficacy in sedation and safety profile, but the ketofol group required less supplemental doses and had faster recovery time [65]. Another study comparing ketadex to ketamine/midazolam combination demonstrated faster recovery and less vomiting in the former group [66]. There were also retrospective case series and case reports describing the effectiveness of ketadex for pediatric procedural sedation [67]. Optimal dosing and adverse events in children however remain to be validated [67]. Most pediatric regimens described involve initial bolus doses of 1 ug/kg of dexmedetomidine and 1–2 mg/kg of ketamine followed by dexmedetomidine infusion at 0.7–2 ug/kg/h and ketamine as an infusion of 1 mg/kg/h or as top-up bolus doses of 0.5–1 mg/kg [67].

The abovementioned list of combination sedation regimen with ketamine is by no means exhaustive. The use of opioids, local anesthesia, chloral hydrate, etomidate, etc. has all been described but is beyond the scope of this chapter.

Contraindications and Special Precautions

Ketamine is not recommended for use in neonates and infants less than 3 months of age, due to the increased incidence of observed respiratory complications (apnea, laryngospasm, obstruction) and concerns regarding potential adverse effects on the developing brain [23]. Animal and retrospective human research implicate NMDA antagonists as a cause of apoptosis and neurodegeneration in developing brains, as seen with other drugs that share the same mechanism of action [68–70].

While patency of the airway is usually maintained during exposure to ketamine, attention to airway protection remains an essential aspect of procedural sedation, as partial obstruction and aspiration are possible especially in infants, where airway reflexes are more variable and unpredictable. A higher risk of airway complications with ketamine in infants less than 3 months of age has been described [9, 23] though this is more likely due to infant-specific differences in airway reactivity and anatomy rather than due to ketamine's properties itself.

The psychoactive properties associated with ketamine continue to limit its widespread clinical use and have led to its exploitation as a drug of abuse. Ketamine has been shown to exacerbate schizophrenia, and evidence suggests that alternative agents be used in such individuals [71].

In the setting of critical illness and compromised autonomic control where there are depletion of endogenous catecholamines and exhaustion of sympathetic compensatory mechanisms, ketamine's direct negative inotropic effects may become clinically significant [20, 72]. Data from adults suggest a reduced dose of ketamine for induction be considered in patients with shock and those with ischemic heart disease [73, 74].

Ketamine's use in traumatic brain injury and intracranial hypertension remains contentious but is no longer an absolute contraindication [23]. More recent studies in animals and ICU patients have undermined the belief that ketamine causes clinically significant increases in either intracranial or intra-ocular pressures and in fact suggest it may lower ICP without lowering blood pressure, therefore maintaining cerebral perfusion pressure [28–30].

Other relative contraindications include use in thyroid disease and porphyria due to concerns of enhanced sympathomimetic responses in these patients [23, 75]. Ketamine's potential to increase oral and tracheobronchial secretions must also be considered particularly in patients undergoing oral procedures and possible laryngeal stimulation for potential laryngospasm and adverse respiratory events [9, 52].

Conclusion

The ideal agent in procedural sedation is one that allows successful completion of the planned procedure in the least distressful means possible, while cardiopulmonary stability is maintained with minimal side effects. Ketamine's versatility and unique profile with flexible routes of administration make it a strong contender. The renewed and growing interest in ketamine for pediatric procedural sedation reflects its impressive risk-benefit ratio. It has successfully been used for a multitude of sedation encounters worldwide and has a vital role in the pre-hospital setting, in emergency medicine, and in critical care for pediatric procedural sedation. With its low cost and its wide therapeutic index, ketamine is an attractive choice for procedural sedation in the developing world where safety monitoring may be challenging due to resource limitations. Clinicians using ketamine must be knowledgeable with its effects and be adequately prepared to deal with complications should they arise.

However, ketamine is still associated with a certain stigma owing to concerns about its psychomimetic side effects, limiting its expanded clinical use. These adverse psychological effects are often transient and minor in children, offering increased opportunities for its use in this population, and moreover may be mitigated and managed well with the combined use with other agents. The increased availability of pure optical isomers of ketamine may help reduce unwanted side effects [76] and pave the way to its increased utilization worldwide.

References

1. Bergman SA. Ketamine: review of its pharmacology and its use in pediatric anesthesia. Anesth Prog. 1999;46(1):10–20.
2. Roback MG, Carlson DW, Babl FE, Kennedy RM. Update on pharmacological management of procedural sedation for children. Curr Opin Anaesthesiol. 2016;29(Suppl 1):S21–35.
3. Domino EF, Chodoff P, Corssen G. Pharmacologic effects of CI-581, a new dissociative anesthetic, in man. Clin Pharmacol Ther. 1965;6:279–91.
4. Corssen G, Domino EF. Dissociative anesthesia: further pharmacologic studies and first clinical experience with the phencyclidine derivative CI-581. Anesth Analg. 1966;45(1):29–40.
5. Zanos P, Moaddel R, Morris PJ, Georgiou P, Fischell J, Elmer GI, et al. NMDAR inhibition-independent antidepressant actions of ketamine metabolites. Nature. 2016;533(7604):481–6.

6. Gao M, Rejaei D, Liu H. Ketamine use in current clinical practice. Acta Pharmacol Sin. 2016;37(7):865–72.
7. Kurdi MS, Theerth KA, Deva RS. Ketamine: current applications in anesthesia, pain, and critical care. Anesth Essays Res. 2014;8(3):283–90.
8. Krauss B, Green SM. Sedation and analgesia for procedures in children. N Engl J Med. 2000;342(13):938–45.
9. Green SM, Roback MG, Krauss B, Brown L, McGlone RG, Agrawal D, et al. Predictors of airway and respiratory adverse events with ketamine sedation in the emergency department: an individual-patient data meta-analysis of 8,282 children. Ann Emerg Med. 2009;54(2):158–68.e1–4.
10. Green SM, Clem KJ, Rothrock SG. Ketamine safety profile in the developing world: survey of practitioners. Acad Emerg Med Off J Soc Acad Emerg Med. 1996;3(6):598–604.
11. Dong TT, Mellin-Olsen J, Gelb AW. Ketamine: a growing global health-care need. Br J Anaesth. 2015;115(4):491–3.
12. Green SM, Krauss B. The semantics of ketamine. Ann Emerg Med. 2000;36(5):480–2.
13. White PF, Ham J, Way WL, Trevor AJ. Pharmacology of ketamine isomers in surgical patients. Anesthesiology. 1980;52(3):231–9.
14. White PF, Schuttler J, Shafer A, Stanski DR, Horai Y, Trevor AJ. Comparative pharmacology of the ketamine isomers. Studies in volunteers. Br J Anaesth. 1985;57(2):197–203.
15. Herd DW, Anderson BJ, Holford NH. Modeling the norketamine metabolite in children and the implications for analgesia. Paediatr Anaesth. 2007;17(9):831–40.
16. Wieber J, Gugler R, Hengstmann JH, Dengler HJ. Pharmacokinetics of ketamine in man. Anaesthesist. 1975;24(6):260–3.
17. Clements JA, Nimmo WS, Grant IS. Bioavailability, pharmacokinetics, and analgesic activity of ketamine in humans. J Pharm Sci. 1982;71(5):539–42.
18. Mion G, Villevieille T. Ketamine pharmacology: an update (pharmacodynamics and molecular aspects, recent findings). CNS Neurosci Ther. 2013;19(6):370–80.
19. White PF, Way WL, Trevor AJ. Ketamine--its pharmacology and therapeutic uses. Anesthesiology. 1982;56(2):119–36.
20. Traber DL, Wilson RD, Priano LL. Differentiation of the cardiovascular effects of CI-581. Anesth Analg. 1968;47(6):769–78.
21. Williams GD, Friesen RH. Administration of ketamine to children with pulmonary hypertension is safe: pro-con debate: pro argument. Paediatr Anaesth. 2012;22(11):1042–52.
22. Friesen RH, Twite MD, Nichols CS, Cardwell KA, Pan Z, Darst JR, et al. Hemodynamic response to ketamine in children with pulmonary hypertension. Paediatr Anaesth. 2016;26(1):102–8.
23. Green SM, Roback MG, Kennedy RM, Krauss B. Clinical practice guideline for emergency department ketamine dissociative sedation: 2011 update. Ann Emerg Med. 2011;57(5):449–61.
24. Goyal S, Agrawal A. Ketamine in status asthmaticus: a review. Indian J Crit Care Med. 2013;17(3):154–61.
25. Kawasaki T, Ogata M, Kawasaki C, Ogata J, Inoue Y, Shigematsu A. Ketamine suppresses proinflammatory cytokine production in human whole blood in vitro. Anesth Analg. 1999;89(3):665–9.
26. Heinz P, Geelhoed GC, Wee C, Pascoe EM. Is atropine needed with ketamine sedation? A prospective, randomised, double blind study. Emerg Med J. 2006;23(3):206–9.
27. Wyte SR, Shapiro HM, Turner P, Harris AB. Ketamine-induced intracranial hypertension. Anesthesiology. 1972;36(2):174–6.
28. Bourgoin A, Albanese J, Wereszczynski N, Charbit M, Vialet R, Martin C. Safety of sedation with ketamine in severe head injury patients: comparison with sufentanil. Crit Care Med. 2003;31(3):711–7.
29. Bar-Joseph G, Guilburd Y, Tamir A, Guilburd JN. Effectiveness of ketamine in decreasing intracranial pressure in children with intracranial hypertension. J Neurosurg Pediatr. 2009;4(1):40–6.

30. Zeiler FA, Teitelbaum J, West M, Gillman LM. The ketamine effect on ICP in traumatic brain injury. Neurocrit Care. 2014;21(1):163–73.
31. Schroeder KE, Irwin ZT, Gaidica M, Nicole Bentley J, Patil PG, Mashour GA, et al. Disruption of corticocortical information transfer during ketamine anesthesia in the primate brain. NeuroImage. 2016;134:459–65.
32. Mashour GA. Network-level mechanisms of ketamine anesthesia. Anesthesiology. 2016;125(5):830–1.
33. Strayer RJ, Nelson LS. Adverse events associated with ketamine for procedural sedation in adults. Am J Emerg Med. 2008;26(9):985–1028.
34. Sherwin TS, Green SM, Khan A, Chapman DS, Dannenberg B. Does adjunctive midazolam reduce recovery agitation after ketamine sedation for pediatric procedures? A randomized, double-blind, placebo-controlled trial. Ann Emerg Med. 2000;35(3):229–38.
35. Green SM, Roback MG, Krauss B, Brown L, McGlone RG, Agrawal D, et al. Predictors of emesis and recovery agitation with emergency department ketamine sedation: an individual-patient data meta-analysis of 8,282 children. Ann Emerg Med. 2009;54(2):171–80.e1–4.
36. Roback MG, Wathen JE, MacKenzie T, Bajaj L. A randomized, controlled trial of i.v. versus i.m. ketamine for sedation of pediatric patients receiving emergency department orthopedic procedures. Ann Emerg Med. 2006;48(5):605–12.
37. Thorp AW, Brown L, Green SM. Ketamine-associated vomiting: is it dose-related? Pediatr Emerg Care. 2009;25(1):15–8.
38. Suryaprakash S, Tham LP. Predictors of emesis in children undergoing procedural sedation with intramuscular ketamine in a paediatric emergency department. Singap Med J. 2017;58(11):660–5.
39. Langston WT, Wathen JE, Roback MG, Bajaj L. Effect of ondansetron on the incidence of vomiting associated with ketamine sedation in children: a double-blind, randomized, placebo-controlled trial. Ann Emerg Med. 2008;52(1):30–4.
40. Lee JS, Jeon WC, Park EJ, Min YG, Kim GW, Jung YS, et al. Does ondansetron have an effect on intramuscular ketamine-associated vomiting in children? A prospective, randomised, open, controlled study. J Paediatr Child Health. 2014;50(7):557–61.
41. Sheehy KA, Lippold C, Rice AL, Nobrega R, Finkel JC, Quezado ZM. Subanesthetic ketamine for pain management in hospitalized children, adolescents, and young adults: a single-center cohort study. J Pain Res. 2017;10:787–95.
42. Kannikeswaran N, Lieh-Lai M, Malian M, Wang B, Farooqi A, Roback MG. Optimal dosing of intravenous ketamine for procedural sedation in children in the ED-a randomized controlled trial. Am J Emerg Med. 2016;34(8):1347–53.
43. Green SM, Rothrock SG, Lynch EL, Ho M, Harris T, Hestdalen R, et al. Intramuscular ketamine for pediatric sedation in the emergency department: safety profile in 1,022 cases. Ann Emerg Med. 1998;31(6):688–97.
44. Green SM, Hummel CB, Wittlake WA, Rothrock SG, Hopkins GA, Garrett W. What is the optimal dose of intramuscular ketamine for pediatric sedation? Acad Emerg Med. 1999;6(1):21–6.
45. Hornik CP, Gonzalez D, van den Anker J, Atz AM, Yogev R, Poindexter BB, et al. Population pharmacokinetics of intramuscular and intravenous ketamine in children. J Clin Pharmacol. 2018;58(8):1092–104.
46. Poonai N, Canton K, Ali S, Hendrikx S, Shah A, Miller M, et al. Intranasal ketamine for procedural sedation and analgesia in children: a systematic review. PLoS One. 2017;12(3):e0173253.
47. Malinovsky JM, Servin F, Cozian A, Lepage JY, Pinaud M. Ketamine and norketamine plasma concentrations after i.v., nasal and rectal administration in children. Br J Anaesth. 1996;77(2):203–7.
48. Weber F, Wulf H, Gruber M, Biallas R. S-ketamine and s-norketamine plasma concentrations after nasal and i.v. administration in anesthetized children. Paediatr Anaesth. 2004;14(12):983–8.
49. Qureshi FA, Mellis PT, McFadden MA. Efficacy of oral ketamine for providing sedation and analgesia to children requiring laceration repair. Pediatr Emerg Care. 1995;11(2):93–7.

50. Rolan P, Lim S, Sunderland V, Liu Y, Molnar V. The absolute bioavailability of racemic ketamine from a novel sublingual formulation. Br J Clin Pharmacol. 2014;77(6):1011–6.
51. Green SM, Rothrock SG, Harris T, Hopkins GA, Garrett W, Sherwin T. Intravenous ketamine for pediatric sedation in the emergency department: safety profile with 156 cases. Acad Emerg Med. 1998;5(10):971–6.
52. Grunwell JR, Travers C, McCracken CE, Scherrer PD, Stormorken AG, Chumpitazi CE, et al. Procedural sedation outside of the operating room using ketamine in 22,645 children: a report from the Pediatric Sedation Research Consortium. Pediatr Crit Care Med. 2016;17(12):1109–16.
53. Sener S, Eken C, Schultz CH, Serinken M, Ozsarac M. Ketamine with and without midazolam for emergency department sedation in adults: a randomized controlled trial. Ann Emerg Med. 2011;57(2):109–14.e2.
54. Wathen JE, Roback MG, Mackenzie T, Bothner JP. Does midazolam alter the clinical effects of intravenous ketamine sedation in children? A double-blind, randomized, controlled, emergency department trial. Ann Emerg Med. 2000;36(6):579–88.
55. Arora S. Combining ketamine and propofol ("ketofol") for emergency department procedural sedation and analgesia: a review. West J Emerg Med. 2008;9(1):20–3.
56. Green SM, Andolfatto G, Krauss B. Ketofol for procedural sedation? Pro and con. Ann Emerg Med. 2011;57(5):444–8.
57. Green SM, Andolfatto G, Krauss BS. Ketofol for procedural sedation revisited: pro and con. Ann Emerg Med. 2015;65(5):489–91.
58. Alletag MJ, Auerbach MA, Baum CR. Ketamine, propofol, and ketofol use for pediatric sedation. Pediatr Emerg Care. 2012;28(12):1391–5; quiz 6–8.
59. Shah A, Mosdossy G, McLeod S, Lehnhardt K, Peddle M, Rieder M. A blinded, randomized controlled trial to evaluate ketamine/propofol versus ketamine alone for procedural sedation in children. Ann Emerg Med. 2011;57(5):425–33.e2.
60. David H, Shipp J. A randomized controlled trial of ketamine/propofol versus propofol alone for emergency department procedural sedation. Ann Emerg Med. 2011;57(5):435–41.
61. Andolfatto G, Willman E. A prospective case series of pediatric procedural sedation and analgesia in the emergency department using single-syringe ketamine-propofol combination (ketofol). Acad Emerg Med. 2010;17(2):194–201.
62. Andolfatto G, Abu-Laban RB, Zed PJ, Staniforth SM, Stackhouse S, Moadebi S, et al. Ketamine-propofol combination (ketofol) versus propofol alone for emergency department procedural sedation and analgesia: a randomized double-blind trial. Ann Emerg Med. 2012;59(6):504–12.e1–2.
63. Izgi M, Basaran B, Muderrisoglu A, Ankay Yilbas A, Uluer MS, Celebioglu B. Evaluation of the stability and stratification of propofol and ketamine mixtures for pediatric anesthesia. Paediatr Anaesth. 2018;28(3):275–80.
64. Levanen J, Makela ML, Scheinin H. Dexmedetomidine premedication attenuates ketamine-induced cardiostimulatory effects and postanesthetic delirium. Anesthesiology. 1995;82(5):1117–25.
65. Tosun Z, Akin A, Guler G, Esmaoglu A, Boyaci A. Dexmedetomidine-ketamine and propofol-ketamine combinations for anesthesia in spontaneously breathing pediatric patients undergoing cardiac catheterization. J Cardiothorac Vasc Anesth. 2006;20(4):515–9.
66. Koruk S, Mizrak A, Gul R, Kilic E, Yendi F, Oner U. Dexmedetomidine-ketamine and midazolam-ketamine combinations for sedation in pediatric patients undergoing extracorporeal shock wave lithotripsy: a randomized prospective study. J Anesth. 2010;24(6):858–63.
67. Tobias JD. Dexmedetomidine and ketamine: an effective alternative for procedural sedation? Pediatr Crit Care Med. 2012;13(4):423–7.
68. Yan J, Li YR, Zhang Y, Lu Y, Jiang H. Repeated exposure to anesthetic ketamine can negatively impact neurodevelopment in infants: a prospective preliminary clinical study. J Child Neurol. 2014;29(10):1333–8.

69. Dong C, Anand KJ. Developmental neurotoxicity of ketamine in pediatric clinical use. Toxicol Lett. 2013;220(1):53–60.
70. Zou X, Patterson TA, Divine RL, Sadovova N, Zhang X, Hanig JP, et al. Prolonged exposure to ketamine increases neurodegeneration in the developing monkey brain. Int J Dev Neurosci. 2009;27(7):727–31.
71. Lahti AC, Koffel B, LaPorte D, Tamminga CA. Subanesthetic doses of ketamine stimulate psychosis in schizophrenia. Neuropsychopharmacology. 1995;13(1):9–19.
72. Sprung J, Schuetz SM, Stewart RW, Moravec CS. Effects of ketamine on the contractility of failing and nonfailing human heart muscles in vitro. Anesthesiology. 1998;88(5):1202–10.
73. Bovill JG. Intravenous anesthesia for the patient with left ventricular dysfunction. Semin Cardiothorac Vasc Anesth. 2006;10(1):43–8.
74. Page RL 2nd, O'Bryant CL, Cheng D, Dow TJ, Ky B, Stein CM, et al. Drugs that may cause or exacerbate heart failure: a scientific statement from the American Heart Association. Circulation. 2016;134(6):e32–69.
75. Kostrzewska E, Gregor A, Lipinska D. Ketamine in acute intermittent porphyria--dangerous or safe? Anesthesiology. 1978;49(5):376–7.
76. Harvey M, Sleigh J, Voss L, Jose J, Gamage S, Pruijn F, et al. Development of rapidly metabolized and ultra-short-acting ketamine analogs. Anesth Analg. 2015;121(4):925–33.

Chapter 31
Propofol

Kevin G. Couloures and Michael Hooper

Background

Propofol (2,6-diisopropylphenol) was originally discovered in 1977 by veterinarian John B. Glen, who was searching for alternatives to inhaled agents. The initial studies showed such a rapid recovery of coordination in mouse models compared to other intravenous induction agents used at that time (primarily sodium thiopental and other barbiturates) that it was thought to be ineffective. However, further investigation revealed that propofol actually produced a rapid induction of deep sedation or general anesthesia, which was short lived, void of undesired excitatory side effects, and from which recovery was rapid [1]. These attributes made it ideal for the newly evolving field of nonoperating room anesthesia (NORA), which further facilitated use in pediatric procedural sedation. The ability to have rapid induction of sedation with rapid recovery has led to it becoming the agent of choice during pediatric MRI and CT sedations and a common adjunct sedative in many other applications.

The quick onset of action for propofol is a result of its lipophilicity, which allows the drug to quickly cross the blood-brain barrier, with a blood-brain equilibration halftime of approximately 1 to 3 minutes. The mechanism of action for induction of sedation is believed to be agonist activation of gamma-aminobutyric acid $(GABA)_A$ receptors via ligand-gated chloride channels and antagonism of glutamatergic N-methyl-D-aspartate (NMDA) receptors [2]. The sum effect of these actions is to prolong the GABA receptor binding. In addition, propofol has potent antiemetic

K. G. Couloures (✉)
Stanford Medicine, Stanford, CA, USA
e-mail: kcouloures@stanford.edu

M. Hooper
Yale Medicine, New Haven, CT, USA
e-mail: michael.hooper@yale.edu

P. P. Kamat, J. W. Berkenbosch (eds.), *Sedation and Analgesia for the Pediatric Intensivist*, https://doi.org/10.1007/978-3-030-52555-2_31

properties, possibly due to serotonin antagonism, which can be used to advantage in children with a history of persistent postoperative vomiting after anesthesia.

The poor water solubility of propofol requires emulsion in lipids. While a 2% (20 mg/mL) formulation exists, by far the most commonly used formulation is a 1% solution (10mg/ml). The lipid component of the propofol emulsion has resulted in concerns for potential microbial contamination. As a result, different antimicrobials are added such as benzyl alcohol, ethylenediaminetetraacetic acid (EDTA), and sodium metabisulfite, depending on the manufacturer. The different formulations have negligible effects on propofol pharmacodynamics, but there is some concern that they may affect pain on injection. The concern for bacterial contamination results in the recommendation that unused propofol should be discarded after the vial has been open more than 6 hours. Additionally, unopened vials should be stored at 22 degrees Celsius and with no special light precautions.

The various components in the lipid emulsion include purified egg phospholipid (to solubilize the drug), soybean oil, and glycerol. Initial concerns that the egg-derived lecithin could potentiate anaphylaxis in egg-allergic patients have subsequently been shown to be unfounded. The American Academy of Allergy, Asthma, and Immunology reviewed the available data and published guidelines in which they report that it is safe to administer propofol to patients with soy allergy and egg allergy without any specific precautions [3]. The likely explanation for the low incidence of anaphylaxis is that the protein responsible for egg allergies is ovolecithin, which is found in egg whites and not the fat component in lecithin, which is in the egg yolk. Furthermore, the amount of lecithin contained in the lipid emulsion is very low (50ppm) and unlikely to cause a reaction [4]. A recent large retrospective study by Assehoi et al. failed to show correlation between food allergy and propofol on provocation testing that examined patients with allergies to egg, soy, and peanuts [5]. Only in those patients with documented anaphylaxis to eggs should consideration of alternative anesthetics be used.

Propofol has little to no oral bioavailability, a finding demonstrated in both animals and humans, which has been ascribed to the effects of first-pass metabolism of an 80% lipid emulsion [6–9]. It is also ineffective when administered by intramuscular or subcutaneous routes. Most likely the poor systemic uptake in these routes is due to its hydrophobic nature and its proclivity to cause inflammation and cellular necrosis [10]. Consequently, propofol is only administered as an intravenous administration. Efforts to formulate a version of propofol that does not require a lipid emulsion may change the potential routes of administration in the future.

A recently published review article by Dinis-Oliveira et al. [2] described the distribution of propofol as a three-compartment linear model: (a) a plasma compartment that rapidly equilibrates; (b) a compartment between the plasma and organs, which are highly perfused (e.g., the liver, lung, kidneys, and brain), that also rapidly equilibrates (distribution half-life of 1–8 minutes); and (c) a deep compartment, which lies between the CNS and less well-perfused tissues (e.g., adipose and skeletal muscle), that slowly equilibrates. The third compartment has a distribution half-life between 30 and 70 minutes, but that is followed by a rapid redistribution and rapid metabolism, which is responsible for the rapid offset of propofol's clinical effects as well as its limited residual post-sedation effects.

Increased adipose tissue concentration has a greater effect on propofol pharmacokinetics than other factors. The larger the amount of body fat one has seems to cause single IV dose effects to be short lived with greater volume of distribution. Higher plasma drug concentrations are seen in obese patients than other patients with less adipose tissue [2]. This is due to the fact that blood flow has greater distribution to non-adipose tissue than to adipose tissue. Eventually, however, adipose tissue may become drug saturated, which leads to prolonged drug action, although this is typically not an issue unless there has been exposure to prolonged continuous infusions. Propofol clearance is also enhanced by the associated increase in the liver volume and liver blood flow seen with increasing obesity [2].

The elimination of propofol is mainly through glomerular filtration (renal clearance of 120ml/min) mostly as water-soluble products and/or bile. Seventy-three percent of the dose is excreted in the first 24h and 88% by 120h. It appears that less than 1% is excreted unchanged in the urine with about 2% excreted in feces up to 48 hours after initial injection [2].

Use as an Anesthetic/Sedative Agent

Propofol was first used as an induction agent for anesthesia when initially introduced. As its favorable properties (rapid onset/offset, ability to maintain spontaneous respiration, generally well tolerated hemodynamically, and minimal emergence reactions) became better appreciated and practitioners found that anesthesia could be sustained without the use of inhaled anesthetics, it began to be used outside of the operating room. The move out of the operating room coincided with Cote's paper describing significant inherent risks with agents commonly used in the late 1990s [11]. As a result of the quest to find safer and more effective agents, pediatric intensive care and emergency room physicians were increasingly utilizing propofol for PPS. Cravero and Beach recognized this trend and utilized the large database accrued via the Pediatric Sedation Research Consortium as a way to track the use of propofol and its overall safety profile during PPS. From this, two reviews of over 50,000 procedural sedation encounters utilizing propofol have been published [12, 13]. In their analysis, there were no deaths recorded, two encounters requiring cardio-pulmonary resuscitations, and four pulmonary aspiration events. Of those 50,000 sedation encounters, >99% were completed without serious sequelae. The authors did report that airway events (stridor, laryngospasm, airway obstruction, wheezing, and central apnea) occurred at a rate of one in 65 sedation encounters and that one in 70 sedation encounters required advance airway and ventilation procedures.

Although propofol has an excellent safety profile in the hands of well-trained practitioners, it has significant effects on the pharyngeal musculature and should be used only by personnel proficient in advanced airway skills. The authors found it was the ability of the sedation provider to support the airway through maneuvers (e.g., effective jaw thrust, repositioning of the airway/head, and recognition for the need to place an oral or nasal airway) that prevented serious adverse events.

The impact of the use of these types of intervention by skilled providers (pediatric intensivist and emergency medicine physicians) has specifically been studied. Emrath et al. [14] analyzed data from an outpatient sedation service for which no code response team was available. They found that, in 655 procedures, no serious events occurred and there were no events that could not be handled by the providers. When they adjusted the overall adverse event rate for expected physiological changes that occur with sedation administration, the overall event rate was just over 10% with no serious adverse events recorded. This was in line with previous results by Cravero et al. [12, 13] (5.92%) for adverse events and Couloures et al. [15] (0.093%) for major complications. The caveat is that all the programs in the PSRC are highly motivated and organized systems. The reported incidence of serious events is low, but the events that could potentially cause harm are still not uncommon (1/89 PPS cases) [16]. Providers need to be skilled with airway management to quickly recognize and take action to prevent these minor events from becoming serious events. It is this benchmark, set by the PSRC, for skilled PPS providers of various clinical backgrounds that allow these sedations to be performed safely.

Recommendation Propofol is an effective and safe sedative agent when used by a practitioner skilled in airway management. The practitioner should be well versed in jaw thrust, placement of airway adjuncts, and bag valve mask ventilation in addition to invasive techniques such as endotracheal intubation.

The finding that propofol was safe and effective lead to studies comparing its effectiveness to other agents. Mallory et al. [17] used the PSRC database with over 7000 sedations for MRI using either propofol or pentobarbital. Both agents had completion rates over 96%, but pentobarbital was found to have additional risks associated with its use, which included prolonged recovery, unplanned admissions, more physiological changes, allergic complications, and inadequate sedation, resulting in cancellation of the procedure. The incidence of airway associated adverse events and complications were not significantly different between the two agents. However, the recovery time for pentobarbital was more than twice as long as that of propofol. Mallory et al. [16] also used the PSRC database to review emergency medicine physician provided sedations. When looking at over 25,000 procedures, a majority of which were for MRI, the safety of propofol for sedation was consistent with the benchmarks at the PSRC. Laryngospasm was seen at a rate of 0.11% vs. 1.2% in the APRICOT trial out of 31,127 patients, and they encountered one code event matching the PSRC's code rate of 0.4 code events/10,000 sedations. These data continue to confirm earlier reports [18] that propofol continues to be used increasingly outside the O.R. by emergency medicine trained physicians and was deemed to be safe with similar adverse event rates to those experienced by other providers. The risk factors for serious events are also consistent with other research, which included ASA physical status score >2, weight <5 kg, and young age. Despite the increased risk with young age, propofol continues to be utilized by the NICU prior to intubation, but there has been rare serious hypotension and one case report of subsequent cardiac arrest. Therefore, it should be used with caution in this population.

Recommendation Use of propofol in patients under 5 kg has a narrow therapeutic index since these patients are at higher risk for both central apnea due to incomplete development of respiratory drive centers and obstructive apnea due to small airway caliber. Hence, studies or procedures that are prolonged and during which the airway may not be readily accessible should be deferred until the patient is greater than 3 months or corrected gestational age of 60 weeks has been reached or be planned to be performed with a protected airway. Similarly, if there are additional comorbid conditions, then anesthesia with a protected airway may be a more prudent choice. Differentiation between ASA physical status 2 and 3 has low inter-rater reliability and hence less utility in determining risk.

Dosing depends on the procedure required, whether adjunct medications were given, and the length of the procedure. For most patients an initial IV bolus dose to achieve deep sedation is 1.5 to 3 mg/kg (usually as 1 mg/kg increments). However, lower doses are typically needed if adjunct medications are given or the patient is already receiving opioids for pain. Additional induction doses of 0.5 mg to 1 mg/kg may be given until the desired level of sedation is achieved. Slower administration generally leads to less apnea and desaturations. Infants and children often require higher weight-adjusted doses than adults (3–5 mg/kg). Sedation onset usually occurs within 1 minute and continuous infusions of 2 to 5 mg/kg/hour (or 120–300 mcg/kg/min) and may be adjusted as needed [19, 20].

Known adverse effects of propofol include dose-dependent respiratory depression/apnea, hypotension, and pain on injection. Apnea depends on the rapidity with which the initial dose is administered and the total dose administered. This is usually transient and patients recover quickly. Proper positioning of the airway and the use of supplemental oxygen via nasal cannula is usually enough to keep oxygen saturation at an acceptable level, and the supplemental oxygen can be titrated down quickly to maintain adequate oxygenation. Occasionally Bag Valve Mask (BVM) ventilation or jaw thrust will be required to alleviate the upper airway obstruction, but this can usually be anticipated by ascertaining information from the parents about recent congestion or history of snoring. The provider can then determine whether airway adjuncts are needed to safely continue the procedure. To avoid hypotension with a propofol infusion, administration of intravenous fluids concomitantly will help prevent severe hypotension. Pain at the induction site has also been well described. The incidence of pain at the injection site is decreased as larger veins are used or if it is injected into a free-flowing infusion. Additional strategies for relief include slower administration rate, pre-propofol administration of low-dose lidocaine, or, if planned, opioid and/or ketamine analgesia. The pain could be related to the propofol found on the outer membrane of the emulsion droplets, which stimulate pain receptors in the vein. One additional known side effect is extraneous limb movement on induction consistent with myoclonic movements. While benign, it can cause parents to become concerned if they are at the bedside during induction. The parents should be advised of this potential side effect pre-administration to avoid undue concern.

Recommendation

An infusion rate of isotonic fluid begun prior to induction of sedation may be efficacious in relieving propofol-induced hypotension or pain with injection. Patients undergoing treatment for childhood cancers will require fluid boluses before sedation to prevent hypotension despite echocardiographic evidence of normal cardiac function. The use of midazolam as an adjunct for IV placement or to decrease anxiety will increase the likelihood of hypotension.

Successful strategies for reduction of injection site pain have included small doses of lidocaine (0.2–0.5 mg/kg) or 2 mg/2 ml in a solution of per 180 mg of propofol or as a Bier's block with a tourniquet. Others have used fentanyl (0.5–1 microgram/kg) or ketamine (0.25–0.5 mg/kg) [21, 22].

The decision to use propofol as a sole agent or to be used with adjunct medications will depend on several factors, including the duration of the procedure, degree of anxiety, behavioral issues, and the nature of the procedure (painful vs. non-painful). For non-painful procedures such as CT or MRI scans, propofol is typically useful by itself, although concomitant use of other medications such as fentanyl or midazolam increases the potential for apnea, hypotension, and respiratory depression. Fentanyl is useful for those procedures that could be painful (e.g., lumbar puncture, bone marrow aspirate, joint injection). Dexmedetomidine has been used as an adjuvant for non-painful to mildly painful procedures. Dexmedetomidine has some analgesic properties and may also reduce propofol requirements, which may decrease the risk of clinically significant respiratory depression or airway obstruction [23, 24]. As with fentanyl, dexmedetomidine could potentiate side effects such as hypotension. Ketamine can be used in conjunction with propofol for mild-moderately painful procedures or for cases when the patient has questionable hemodynamic stability, a combination which has gained significant popularity and has been shown to better preserve blood cardiovascular stability vs. propofol alone [25–27]. Midazolam can be used prior to the placement of IVs and may decrease preinduction anxiety. Midazolam can help reduce the amount of propofol needed for induction of sedation and make the transition from a state of wakefulness to sedation smoother. However, as with the other adjuvants, it could potentiate airway obstruction, apnea, and hypotension.

Recommendation

CT or MRI – propofol at 100 to 150 mcg/kg/min is often effective. It can be titrated upward to a maximum of 250 mcg/kg/min in children, but this is typically only necessary for sedations lasting more than 90 minutes.

Bone marrow aspiration/biopsy – propofol in doses of 1.5–3 mg/kg with analgesia via fentanyl at 1 to 2 mcg/kg up to a maximum single dose of 50 mcg or ketamine at 1–2 mg/kg. Ketamine may be the preferred adjunct in those patients prone to hypotension.

Lumbar puncture – propofol at 1–3 mg/kg with or without adjunct analgesia via fentanyl at 1–2 mcg/kg given at least 3 minutes prior to procedure or ketamine 1–2 mg/kg. If topical analgesia has been utilized, adjunct analgesia may not be required.

IV placement – midazolam at 0.3 mg/kg up to 5 mg as an intranasal agent or 0.5 mg/kg up to 10 mg as an enteral agent.

Anxiolysis – intravenous midazolam at 0.05 mg/kg may be effective prior to propofol induction.

Another potential risk factor with propofol is in those patients with known mitochondrial disorders. Propofol can disrupt the function of the electron transport chain (ETC) [28, 29]. Propofol results in a decrease of ETC associated complexes I, II, and III, disruption of the transition pore, and reduction of the membrane potential [29, 30]. In addition the uptake of free fatty acids into mitochondria is inhibited. The ability of propofol to disrupt the mitochondrial electron transport chain leads to what has been described as propofol infusion syndrome (PRIS). PRIS is defined by metabolic acidosis, with a base deficit >10 mmol/l on at least one occasion, with heart and kidney effects and rhabdomyolysis following an infusion of propofol [31]. Risk seems to increase in children with inborn errors of mitochondrial fatty acid oxidation and is seen with high doses and prolonged infusions (>4–5 mg/kg/h and infusions >48 h: critical illness, concomitant use of catecholamine infusions, concomitant steroids, and young age) [32]. The common end point for PRIS is cardiovascular collapse. Treatment for PRIS has been largely supportive and included plasmapheresis, hemodialysis, partial exchange transfusion, and extracorporeal membrane oxygenation (ECMO). ECMO has been shown to be an effective strategy in case reports [33]. Given the short duration of most procedural sedation encounters, the likelihood of PRIS development during procedural sedation should be low, although some authors still suggest caution with propofol use in children with mitochondrial disorders [34].

Recommendation

Avoid the use of propofol in patients undergoing genetic evaluation or who appear syndromic, except for trisomy 21.

References

1. Glen JB. Animal studies of the anaesthetic activity of ICI 35 868. Br J Anaesth. 1980;52(8):731–42.
2. Dinis-Oliveira RJ. Metabolic profiles of propofol and fospropofol: clinical and forensic interpretative aspects %. J BioMed Res Int. 2018, 2018;16 https://doi.org/10.1155/2018/6852857.
3. https://www.aaaai.org/conditions-and-treatments/library/allergy-library/soy-egg-anesthesia - accessed 8/16/20
4. Martin-Hernandez C, Benet S, Marvin-Guy LF. Characterization and quantification of proteins in lecithins. J Agric Food Chem. 2005;53:8607–13.
5. Asserhoj LL, Mosbech H, Kroigaard M, Garvey LH. No evidence for contraindications to the use of propofol in adults allergic to egg, soy or peanutdagger. Br J Anaesth. 2016;116(1):77–82. https://doi.org/10.1093/bja/aev360.
6. Raoof AA, Augustijns PF, Verbeeck RK. In vivo assessment of intestinal, hepatic, and pulmonary first pass metabolism of propofol in the rat. Pharm Res. 1996;13(6):891–5.
7. Ceriana R, Braschi A, De Ponti F, Crema A, De Amici D. Is rectal administration of propofol effective? Anaesthesia. 1996;51(5):504.

8. Hiraoka H, Yamamoto K, Miyoshi S, et al. Kidneys contribute to the extrahepatic clearance of propofol in humans, but not lungs and brain. Br J Clin Pharmacol. 2005;60(2):176–82.
9. Hiraoka H, Yamamoto K, Okano N, Morita T, Goto F, Horiuchi R. Changes in drug plasma concentrations of an extensively bound and highly extracted drug, propofol, in response to altered plasma binding. Clin Pharmacol Therap. 2004;75(4):324–30.
10. McKune CM, Brosnan RJ, Dark MJ, Haldorson GJ. Safety and efficacy of intramuscular propofol administration in rats. Vet Anaesth Analg. 2008;35(6):495–500. https://doi.org/10.1111/j.1467-2995.2008.00418.x.
11. Coté CJ, Karl HW, Notterman DA, Weinberg JM, Closkey C. Adverse sedation events in pediatrics: analysis of medications used for sedation. Pediatrics. 2000;106:633–44. https://doi.org/10.1542/peds.106.4.633.
12. Cravero JP, Blike GT, Beach M, Gallagher SM, Hertzog JH, Havidich JE, Gelman B. Incidence and nature of adverse events during pediatric sedation/anesthesia for procedures outside the operating room: report from the Pediatric Sedation Research Consortium. Pediatrics. 2006;118(3):1087–96. https://doi.org/10.1542/peds.2006-0313.
13. Cravero JP, Beach ML, Blike GT, Gallagher SM, Hertzog JH. The incidence and nature of adverse events during pediatric sedation/anesthesia with propofol for procedures outside the operating room: a report from the pediatric sedation research consortium. Anesth Analg. 2009;108(3):795–804. https://doi.org/10.1213/ane.0b013e31818fc334.
14. Emrath ET, Stockwell JA, McCracken CE, Simon HK, Kamat PP. Provision of deep procedural sedation by a pediatric sedation team at a freestanding imaging center. Pediatr Radiol. 2014;44(8):1020–5. https://doi.org/10.1007/s00247-014-2942-z.
15. Couloures KG, Beach M, Cravero JP, Monroe KK, Hertzog JH. Impact of provider specialty on pediatric procedural sedation complication rates. Pediatrics. 2011;127(5):e1154–60. https://doi.org/10.1542/peds.2010-2960.
16. Mallory MD, Baxter AL, Yanosky DJ, Cravero JP. Emergency physician–administered propofol sedation: a report on 25,433 sedations from the Pediatric Sedation Research Consortium. Ann Emerg Med. 2011;57(5):462–468.e461. https://doi.org/10.1016/j.annemergmed.2011.03.008.
17. Mallory MD, Baxter AL, Kost SI. Propofol vs pentobarbital for sedation of children undergoing magnetic resonance imaging: results from the Pediatric Sedation Research Consortium. Pediatr Anesth. 2009;19(6):601–11. https://doi.org/10.1111/j.1460-9592.2009.03023.x.
18. Bassett KE, Anderson JL, Pribble CG, Guenther E. Propofol for procedural sedation in children in the emergency department. Annals of Emergency Medicine. 2003;42(6):773–82. https://doi.org/10.1016/s0196-0644(03)00619-x.
19. Barbi E, Petaros P, Badina L, Pahor T, Giuseppin I, Biasotto E, Ventura A. Deep sedation with propofol for upper gastrointestinal endoscopy in children, administered by specially trained pediatricians: a prospective case series with emphasis on side effects. Endoscopy. 2006;38(4):368–75. https://doi.org/10.1055/s-2005-921194.
20. Srinivasan M, Turmelle M, Depalma LM, Mao J, Carlson DW. Procedural sedation for diagnostic imaging in children by pediatric hospitalists using propofol: analysis of the nature, frequency, and predictors of adverse events and interventions. J Pediatr. 2012;160(5):801–806.e801. https://doi.org/10.1016/j.jpeds.2011.11.003.
21. Barbi E, Marchetti F, Gerarduzzi T, Neri E, Gagliardo A, Sarti A, Ventura A. Pretreatment with intravenous ketamine reduces propofol injection pain. Paediatr Anaesthes. 2003;13(9):764–8. https://doi.org/10.1046/j.1460-9592.2003.01150.x.
22. Picard P, Tramèr MR. Prevention of pain on injection with propofol: a quantitative systematic review. Anesth Analg. 2000;90(4):963–9. https://doi.org/10.1213/00000539-200004000-00035.
23. Nagoshi M, Reddy S, Bell M, Cresencia A, Margolis R, Wetzel R, Ross P. Low-dose dexmedetomidine as an adjuvant to propofol infusion for children in MRI: a double-cohort study. Paediatr Anaesth. 2018;28:639–46. https://doi.org/10.1111/pan.13400.
24. Boriosi JP, Eickhoff JC, Klein KB, Hollman GA. A retrospective comparison of propofol alone to propofol in combination with dexmedetomidine for pediatric 3T MRI sedation. Paediatr Anaesth. 2017;27:52–9. https://doi.org/10.1111/pan.13041.
25. Grunwell JR, Travers C, Stormorken AG, Scherrer PD, Chumpitazi CE, Stockwell JA, Roback MG, Cravero J, Kamat PP. Pediatric procedural sedation using the combination of

ketamine and propofol outside of the emergency department: a report from the pediatric sedation research consortium. Pediatr Crit Care Med. 2017;18:e356–e36. https://doi.org/10.1097/PCC.0000000000001246.
26. Chiaretti A, Ruggiero A, Barbi E, Pierri F, Maurizi P, Fantacci C, Bersani G, Riccardi R. Comparison of propofol versus propofol-ketamine combination in pediatric oncologic procedures performed by non-anesthesiologists. Pediatr Blood Cancer. 2011;57:1163–7. https://doi.org/10.1002/pbc.23170.
27. Phillips W, Anderson A, Rosengreen M, Johnson J, Halpin J. Propofol versus propofol/ketamine for brief painful procedures in the emergency department: clinical and bispectral index scale comparison. J Pain Palliat Care Pharmacother. 2010;24:349–55. https://doi.org/10.3109/15360288.2010.506503.
28. Savard M, Dupre N, Turgeon AF, Desbiens R, Langevin S, Brunet D. Propofol-related infusion syndrome heralding a mitochondrial disease: case report. Neurology. 2013;81(8):770–1. https://doi.org/10.1212/wnl.0b013e3182a1aa78.
29. Ramaiah R, Lollo L, Brannan D, Bhananker SM. Propofol infusion syndrome in a super morbidly obese patient (BMI = 75). Int J Crit Illn Inj Sci. 2011;1(1):84–6. https://doi.org/10.4103/2229-5151.79290.
30. Halestrap AP, Clarke SJ, Javadov SA. Mitochondrial permeability transition pore opening during myocardial reperfusion–a target for cardioprotection. Cardiovasc Res. 2004;61(3):372–85. https://doi.org/10.1016/s0008-6363(03)00533-9.
31. Finsterer J, Frank M. Propofol is mitochondrion-toxic and may unmask a mitochondrial disorder. J Child Neurol. 2016;31(13):1489–94. https://doi.org/10.1177/0883073816661458.
32. Diedrich DA, Brown DR. Analytic reviews: propofol infusion syndrome in the ICU. J Intensive Care Med. 2011;26(2):59–72. https://doi.org/10.1177/0885066610384195.
33. Culp KE, Augoustides JG, Ochroch AE, Milas BL. Clinical Management of Cardiogenic Shock Associated with prolonged propofol infusion. Anesth Analg. 2004;99(1):221–6. https://doi.org/10.1213/01.ane.0000117285.12600.c1.
34. Chidambaran V, Costandi A, D'Mello A. Propofol: a review of its role in pediatric anesthesia and sedation. CNS Drugs. 2015;29:543–63. https://doi.org/10.1007/s40263-015-0259-6.

Chapter 32
Nitrous Oxide

Robert Pettignano

Introduction

Nitrous oxide (N_2O) in combination with oxygen is being utilized more frequently to provide anxiolysis, amnesia, and analgesia during pediatric procedural sedation. Its advantages are relative noninvasive administration (face mask, nasal prongs), rapid onset, and rapid offset once discontinued, making it an appealing choice for brief procedures. Nitrous oxide also has a low incidence of adverse events with the most common events being nausea and emesis [1–5].

History

The chemical nitrous oxide was first discovered by the chemist Joseph Priestley in 1772. In the 1800s the pain-erasing effects of N_2O were identified by Humphry Davy, who began his experiments with the chemical at England's Pneumatic Institute [6]. Most of the experiments were performed on himself, and he became preoccupied with the euphoria he felt when inhaling the gas. After observing the effects of nitrous oxide on people who inhaled it, he coined the term "laughing gas." Although Davy recognized N_2O's ability to reduce or stop the sensation of pain, he did not identify it as an anesthetic for surgery. Instead in the 1830s N_2O was used as a recreational drug at "laughing gas" parties [7]. In 1844 during one of these parties, Horace Wells, a dentist, realized the potential of N_2O to prevent pain. In the morning after the party, Wells convinced a colleague to extract his tooth after inhaling N_2O, and he was astonished to realize that his tooth was removed without him feeling any pain. Subsequently he went to the Harvard Medical School in Boston to share his

R. Pettignano (✉)
Emory University School of Medicine, Atlanta, GA, USA
e-mail: Robert.Pettignano@choa.org

P. P. Kamat, J. W. Berkenbosch (eds.), *Sedation and Analgesia for the Pediatric Intensivist*, https://doi.org/10.1007/978-3-030-52555-2_32

discovery and prepared a demonstration to remove a tooth under the influence of N_2O. The demonstration did not go as planned. The person he selected to have his tooth removed screamed in pain. As it turned out, the man whose tooth was to be removed later admitted that he felt no pain; however, Wells had been labeled a fraud. Ironically, it took over 150 years before dental practices began using N_2O on a regular basis during dental procedures.

Nitrous Oxide: The Basics

Nitrous oxide is a colorless and relatively odorless gas that some have described as having a sweet taste and odor. It continues to be an integral part of a balanced anesthesia plan worldwide. Nitrous oxide is delivered either from a central gas supply in the hospital or from E-cylinders where it is stored under pressure as a liquid. Onset and offset of effects is in approximately 4–5 minutes. These changes in anesthesia depth and short recovery are related to the low solubility of N_2O in the blood. The primary mechanism of action of N_2O while not well defined appears to be its antagonism of N-methyl-D-aspartate (NMDA). Other mechanisms may involve dopaminergic and/or alpha-2-adrenergic receptors. The potency of inhaled anesthetics is described by and can be compared using the minimal alveolar concentration (MAC). MAC is the concentration of gas at 1 atmosphere that suppresses movement in 50% of patients in response to a surgical incision [8]. Factors that increase anesthetic concentration and therefore decrease induction time are increased concentration of the gas, high flow within the circuit, and increased minute ventilation (i.e., crying). N_2O is eliminated via the lungs. Its metabolism is independent of hepatic or renal function.

Nitrous Oxide Delivery: Nuts and Bolts

N_2O can be delivered via nasal cannula, nasal prongs (dental procedures), or face mask. Systems for delivery are either continuous flow or demand. The demand system requires the patient to generate a negative pressure of 3–5 cm H_2O in order for the demand valve to be opened and flow to be achieved.

In our institution N_2O is administered using a Porter/Matrx Tall 4 Cylinder E Stand equipped with a Porter MXR 3000 flowmeter® (Porter Instrument, Hatfield PA; a division of Parker Hannifin). The system is a continuous flow system that mixes oxygen and N_2O from separate E-cylinders. The system can provide 0% to a maximum of 70% N_2O. There are two important safety features in this system. The first ensures that at least 30% oxygen is provided to the patient, and the second is a fail-safe so that if the oxygen supply is exhausted, N_2O cannot be delivered. All expired gas is scavenged via the system to an external ventilation system.

At the start of the procedure, an appropriately sized mask with circuit is selected for the child. The child (patient) is then allowed to choose a scented lip balm, which is rubbed on the inside of the mask. The patient is monitored by direct observation and with pulse oximetry throughout N_2O delivery. The process of delivering N_2O is begun by flushing the circuit with O_2 and then delivering oxygen (FiO_2 1.0) via the mask to the patient. The mask can be held by a parent or caregiver to facilitate acceptance or by the physician if the patient allows. Oxygen is delivered for a minimum of 1–2 minutes followed by N_2O delivery to a maximum concentration of 70% for 4–5 minutes before beginning any procedure. Once the procedure is complete, oxygen (FiO_2 1.0) is once again administered for 3–5 minutes to prevent diffusion hypoxia (see below). An alternative method for administration is to give 100% oxygen for 1–2 min, followed by titration of N_2O in 10% intervals, increasing amounts of N_2O until the desired effect is achieved. The utilization of the former technique is reported to have an increase in nausea and emesis, while the latter takes longer in addition to an increased incidence of a dysphoric transition to the needed anxiolytic and analgesic state.

Safety Features for Delivery of Nitrous Oxide

In the United States a color-coding system is used for safety. The tanks, hoses, and outlets are color-coded to prevent administering the wrong gas. Air is yellow, oxygen is green, and N_2O is blue. Additionally, there is a pin-indexing system that allows only the correct tank be attached to the corresponding part on the delivery apparatus. Individual delivery devices may have some or all of the following safety features:

1. Mechanism to prevent delivery of a hypoxic mixture
2. In-line oxygen monitor
3. A mechanism to stop N_2O flow if the oxygen supply fails
4. A system to regulate the ratio of O_2 to N_2O so that an FiO_2 of 0.30 is the minimum concentration of oxygen that can be delivered and 70% is the maximum concentration of N_2O that can be delivered

To prevent staff exposure to N_2O, an active scavenging system connected to the hospital's vacuum system is needed, although there are no specific exposure limits to N_2O set by the Occupational Safety and Health Administration (OSHA).Studies have identified evidence of genomic alterations and cytotoxicity in situations of occupational exposure; however, it is debatable whether or not this exposure would translate to clinical disease [9]. Some studies have found an increased risk of spontaneous abortion in dental professionals with N_2O exposure, while others could not find a link [10, 11]. According to the American Society of Anesthesiologists, there are no data suggesting that waste anesthetic gases are a danger to women who are pregnant or considering becoming pregnant [12].

Nitrous Oxide: From Theory to Practice

Although the scope of this chapter is not meant to be a comprehensive review of nitrous oxide use in pediatrics, it is worthwhile reviewing a few common scenarios where usage appears to be safe and effective.

Dental Procedures

Nitrous oxide was first used as a dental anesthetic in the nineteenth century and has become the most commonly used inhalational anesthetic in dentistry [13]. Multiple studies have evaluated the use of N_2O for dental procedures and have found it safe and efficacious either alone or in combination with other sedatives and analgesics [14–16]. A survey by the ADA in 2007 estimated that 70% of dental practices using any form of sedation employed nitrous oxide-oxygen sedation [17].

Cannulation for Peripheral Intravenous Placement or Blood Draw

In a study by Furuya et al., 73 children were randomized into 4 groups to get N_2O at different concentrations (50 vs. 70%) and different durations of time (3 vs. 5 minutes). The results of their study showed that N_2O at concentration of 70% was more effective in reducing pain as evidenced by pain scores than at concentration of 50% N_2O. The difference in duration of administration did not significantly reduce the pain score. There was no difference in the number or severity of adverse events [18].

In a study of 70 patients randomized to receive either ELA or EMLA plus N_2O prior to venous cannulation, the pediatric patients who received EMLA plus N_2O had a statistically significant lower pain score as assessed by visual analogue scales [19]. A subsequent study by the same group of 90 patients randomized to receive either midazolam or N_2O at a concentration of 50% to measure time and IV placement efficiency revealed that the use of N_2O at this concentration reduced total procedure time and positively facilitated IV access [20].

In an open-label study that assessed patient satisfaction with a post-procedural survey, nurses, parents, and patients were asked to rate their satisfaction with the use of N_2O to reduce anxiety and provide analgesia. For patients who could not verbally respond to questioning, the physician administering N_2O determined the level of satisfaction based on markers of satisfaction such as ease of patient cooperation, lack of crying, or lack of withdrawal from IV placement when initiated. The authors found that N_2O for peripheral IV cannulation was very effective and had a high degree of patient/stakeholder satisfaction [21].

Lumbar Puncture

While lumbar puncture is probably one of the most common painful procedures carried out in pediatrics, there are a paucity of studies identifying its effectiveness in this procedure. In a letter to the editor, German described a study where children needing lumbar puncture received either N_2O at a fixed 50% nitrous-oxygen mixture or N_2O at a fixed 50% nitrous-oxygen mixture plus EMLA for lumbar puncture in the emergency department. Expected pain (pre) and experienced pain were evaluated in 19 patients. Seventy-nine percent of patients experienced less pain than expected, 10% an equivalent amount of pain, and 10% more pain than expected [22].

Livingston reported on the use of nitrous oxide (40–70%) in 78 oncology patients who underwent 350 lumbar punctures over time [23]. For 266 of the procedures, either topical or injected lidocaine was added for analgesia. Using nitrous oxide for anxiolysis and analgesia resulted in the successful completion of 344 procedures. No major complications were noted, and only 2% had minor adverse events (nausea, emesis, etc.). Although this is the only large study substantiating the use of nitrous oxide in lumbar puncture, it appears to be an effective sedative/analgesic to facilitate successful lumbar puncture in this patient population.

Voiding Cystourethrography

A prospective, randomized trial comparing the efficacy and safety of oral midazolam with 50% N_2O showed the two regimens to be equally safe and effective in reducing anxiety and distress for voiding cystourethrography; however, N_2O was more rapid in onset and had a shorter recovery time. The time to urination was increased with N_2O but not to statistical significance [24]. Of note, no topical anesthetic was used during this study as it was crafted to encourage the use of sedation. The addition of topical anesthetic would certainly add to the reduction of the pain associated with the procedure.

In a study comparing N_2O (70% nitrous/30% oxygen) to no sedation, pain and distress scores were significantly higher in the non-sedation group compared to those who received the N_2O mixture. There was no reference to the utilization of topical anesthetic use in either group [25].

Other Considerations

At the end of nitrous oxide administration, it rapidly diffuses from the blood back into the alveoli. The rapid diffusion from the blood to the alveolus reduces the oxygen tension in the lung that can cause hypoxia known as diffusion hypoxia [26].

During recovery from nitrous oxide anesthesia, supplemental oxygen at a FiO_2 of 1.0 can reduce or alleviate the above mentioned effect.

N_2O is contraindicated in patients with disease processes that may have air-filled cavities. Air-filled cavities such as pneumothorax, pneumocephalus, air embolism, intraocular air, and/or bowel obstruction contain nitrogen. N_2O displaces nitrogen approximately 30 times faster than the nitrogen can escape the closed space before entering the blood, therefore increasing the volume and pressure within the cavity to dangerous levels. In an animal model, inhalation of between 68 and 78% N_2O results in an increase in volume and pressure within the cavities of gas during bowel obstruction and pneumothorax. The rate at which pleural gas expanded was 15 times more rapid than that of the bowel gas space. The volume of a pneumothorax increased by 50% in 10 minutes and to about 80% in an hour [27].

Respiratory side effects include a decrease in the ventilator response to hypoxia in a dose-dependent manner, tachypnea, and reduced tidal volume [28]. N_2O also increases pulmonary venous tone that can exaggerate pulmonary hypertension. Monitoring by visual inspection and continuous oxygen saturation monitor is therefore required.

N_2O is known to increase cerebral blood flow, cerebral metabolic rate of oxygen consumption, and increased intracranial pressure; therefore, it should be avoided in patients with traumatic brain injury. The increases are mostly due to cerebral vasodilation; some of the effects may be attributed to sympathoadrenal stimulation [29, 30].

N_2O can trigger megaloblastic anemia and peripheral neuropathy in patients with vitamin B_{12} deficiency by inactivating methionine synthase, the enzyme required for vitamin B_{12} and folate metabolism. Patients with critical illness or an underlying vitamin B_{12} deficiency can suffer neurologic or hematologic effects [31].

Conclusion

Nitrous oxide has been found to be a very effective anxyolitic, amnestic and analgesic with very few side effects attributed to its use. Nitrous oxide should therefore be considered as a routine part of the armamentarium for physicians providing sedation for routine and repetitive minor procedures as described above.

References

1. Gall O, Annequin D, Benoit G, Glabeke E, Vrancea F, Murat I. Adverse events of premixed nitrous oxide and oxygen for procedural sedation in children. Lancet. 2001;358(9292):1514–5.
2. Kanagasundaram SA, Lane LJ, Cavalletto BP, Keneally JP, Cooper MG. Efficacy and safety of nitrous oxide in alleviating pain and anxiety during painful procedures. Arch Dis Child. 2001;84(6):492–5.
3. Brislin RP, Stayer SA, Schwartz RE, Pasquariello CA. Analgesia for venepuncture in a paediatric surgery centre. J Paediatr Child Health. 1995;31(6):542–4.

4. Tobias JD. Applications of nitrous oxide for procedural sedation in the pediatric population. Pediatr Emerg Care. 2013;29(2):245–65.
5. Tsze DS, Mallory MD, Cravero JP. Practice patterns and adverse events of nitrous oxide sedation and analgesia: a report from the pediatric sedation research consortium. J Pediatr. 2016;169:260–5 e2.
6. Goerig M, Schulte J, AM EJ. History of nitrous oxide—with special reference to its early use in Germany. Best Prac Res Clin Anaesthesiol. 2001;15:313–38.
7. Rutkow IM. American surgery: an illustrated history. Philadelphia: Lippincott-Raven; 1998.
8. Quasha AL, Eger EI, et al. Determination and application of MAC. Anesthesiology. 1980;5:315–44.
9. Wronska-Nofer T, Nofer JR, Jajte J, et al. Oxidatie DNA damage and oxidative stress in subjects occupationally exposed to nitrous oxide. Mutat Res. 2012;713:58–63.
10. Boivin JF. Risk of spontaneous abortion in women occupationally exposed to anaesthetic gases: a meta-analysis. Occup Environ Med. 1997;54(8):541–8.
11. Rowland AS, Baird DD, Shore DL, Weinberg CR, Savitz DA, Wilcox AJ. Nitrous oxide and spontaneous abortion in female dental assistants. Am J Epidemiol. 1995;141(6):531–8.
12. Miller RD, Pardo M. Basics of anesthesia, vol. 832. 6th ed. Philadelphia: Elsevier Saunders; 2011.
13. Mohan R, Asir VD, Shanmugapriyan, Ebenezr V, Dakir A, Balakrishnan, Jacob J. Nitrous oxide as a conscious sedative in minor oral surgical procedure. J Pharm Bioallied Sci. 2015;7(Suppl 1):S248–50. https://doi.org/10.4103/0975-7406.155939.
14. Berge TI. Acceptance and side effects of nitrous oxide oxygen sedation for oral surgical procedures. J Acta Odontologica Scandinavica. 1999;57:201–6.
15. Wilson KE, Welbury RR, Girldler NM. A randomised, controlled, crossover trial of oral midazolam and nitrous oxide for paediatric dental sedation. Anesthesia. 2002;57:860–7.
16. Hulland SA, Freilich MM, Sàndor GKB. Nitrous oxide–oxygen or oral midazolam for pediatric outpatient sedation. Oral Surg Oral Med Oral Pathol Oral Radiol Endod. 2002;93:643–6.
17. American Dental Association. Guidelines for the use of sedation and general anesthesia by dentists. October 2016. Accessed September 21, 2019.
18. Furuya A, Ito M, Fukao T, et al. The effective time and concentration of nitrous oxide to reduce venipuncture pain in children. J Clin Anesth. 2009;21(3):190–3.
19. Ekbom K, Jakobsson J, Marcus C. Nitrous oxide inhalation is a safe and effective way to facilitate procedures in paediatric outpatient departments. Arch Dis Child. 2005;90(10):1073–6.
20. Ekbom K, Kalman S, Jakobsson J, Marcus C. Efficient intravenous access without distress: a double-blind randomized study of midazolam and nitrous oxide in children and adolescents. Arch Pediatr Adolesc Med. 2011;165(9):785–91.
21. McCollum NL, Kamat PP, Stockwell JA, Travers C, McCracken CE, Thompson B, Pettignano R. Improving stakeholder satisfaction: nitrous oxide for peripheral intravenous cannulation for pediatric procedural sedation. J Radiol Nurs. 2017;36:238–41.
22. Germán M, Pavo MR, Palacios A, Ordoñez O. Use of fixed 50% nitrous oxide-oxygen mixture for lumbar punctures in pediatric patients. Pediatr Emerg Care. 2011;27(3):244–5.
23. Livingston M, Lawell M, McAllister N. Successful use of nitrous oxide during lumbar punctures: A call for nitrous oxide in pediatric oncology clinics. Pediatr Blood Cancer. 2017:64:e26610. https://doi.org/10.1002/pbc.26610
24. Keidan I, Zaslansky R, Weinberg M, Ben-Shlush A, Jacobson JM, Augarten A, Mor Y. Sedation during voiding cystourethrography: comparison of the efficacy and safety of using oral midazolam and continuous flow nitrous oxide. J Urol. 2005;174(4 Pt 2):1598–600. discussion 1601
25. Zier JL, Kvam KA, Kurachek SC, Finkelstein M. Sedation with nitrous oxide compared with no sedation during catheterization for urologic imaging in children. Pediatr Radiol. 2007;37(7):678–84.
26. Peyton PJ, Chao I, Weinberg L, Robinson GJ, Thompson BR. Nitrous oxide diffusion and the second gas effect on emergence from anesthesia. Anesthesiology. 2011;114(3):596–602. https://doi.org/10.1097/ALN.0b013e318209367b.

27. Eger EI, Saidman LJ. Hazards of nitrous oxide anesthesia in bowel obstruction and pneumothorax. Anesthesiology. 1965;26:61–6.
28. Yacoub O, Doell D, Kryger MH, et al. Depression of hypoxic ventilatory response by nitrous oxide. Anesthesiology. 1976;45:385–9.
29. Kaisti KK, Långsjö JW, Aalto S, et al. Effects of sevoflurane, propofol, and adjunct nitrous oxide on regional cerebral blood flow, oxygen consumption, and blood volume in humans. Anesthesiology. 2003;99(3):603–13.
30. Field LM, Dorrance DE, Krzeminska EK, Barsoum LZ. Effect of nitrous oxide on cerebral blood flow in normal humans. Br J Anaesth. 1993;70(2):154–9.
31. Berger JJ, Model JH, Sypert GW. Megaloblastic anemia and brief exposure to nitrous oxide: a causal relationship. Anesth Analg. 1988;67(2):197–8.

Part IX
Special Circumstances

Chapter 33
Child Life for Procedural Sedation

Jessica Brown

Overview and Child Life Background

Every year, children are hospitalized or visit the hospital for a variety of reasons. These visits can be a seemingly simple outpatient X-ray or as critical as an inpatient ICU admission. Within any visit to the hospital, the reality is that many children are ripped from the normal and carefree routine of childhood and trapped in an upended world where doctors, physician assistants, nurse practitioners, dietitians, nurses, and child life specialists come streaming in and out of their small rooms, poking, prodding, and talking to them in foreign medial language [10]. Within these stressful situations, many children and their families are able to receive support from child life specialists, who are trained pediatric health-care professionals with expertise in helping children and their families in hospitals and other settings overcome life's most challenging events related to health care, hospitalization, illness, and disability.

Child life specialists have a strong background in child development and ways to help support the family system as a whole. The educational background typically includes an emphasis on human growth and development, education, psychology, and a related field of study. They also have experience in how children respond to the many aspects of hospitalization [10]. Child life specialists strive to assist children in addressing their fears, clearing up misconceptions about the hospital, diagnosis, and procedures along with preparing the child for procedures using developmentally appropriate explanations.

Along with previous medical experiences, every child has other variables that are currently impacting how they are interpreting and coping with the environment around them. Hospitalizations in general have been referred to as a "landmark even in a child's life" [17] and can impact every child differently. It has been shown that

J. Brown (✉)
Children's Healthcare of Atlanta, Atlanta, GA, USA
e-mail: jessica.brown@choa.org

P. P. Kamat, J. W. Berkenbosch (eds.), *Sedation and Analgesia for the Pediatric Intensivist*, https://doi.org/10.1007/978-3-030-52555-2_33

after hospitalization, children's responses to the experience are continually refined by concurrent and future developmental processes, social and ecological encounters, and the interactions among them. Therefore, children's early experiences with hospitalization have enduring consequences, affecting individual's responses to hospitalization throughout their lifetimes [6]. Since a child can be so greatly impacted through a hospitalization, care is most effective when it is based on the unique situations, responses, needs, and resources of the specific child and family. Assessment and planning for psychosocial care need to consider the dynamic interactions between the strengths and vulnerabilities of each child and family and the changing nature of the child's health-care situation [8]. With the need to meet patients and families where they are, child life specialist are trained to utilize the stress potential assessment (Appendix A), taking into consideration different components of the child and family's life that might be impacting how they are coping within a current situation.

So, what does this mean for you? Although child life specialists are specially trained professionals on ways to prepare and support children through hospitalizations and medical procedures, there are many techniques the medical team can utilize to support the children they encounter during their day-to-day interactions.

Where to Begin

Going back to the basics, taking time to build rapport, and understanding the child and family help to build trust, leading to increased reporting of the actual reason for the visit [2, 20]. Medical providers who start by building rapport open the door to building strong relationships with patients. Rapport is built on mutual confidence, respect, and acceptance. As health-care providers the main responsibility is to establish oneself as a trusting, useful individual. Taking this time to build rapport builds trust, which can lead to improved communication with patients and families and increases overall satisfaction with their health-care experience. In addition to the improved health-care experience, children are more likely to be compliant and cooperative with care when they trust their medical provider.

Children are typically scared or confused about why they need to be in the hospital or have a procedure completed or why a health-care provider needs to talk to them. In every interaction a child experiences, they need to see adults as neutral and empathetic. Along with this approach, communication must be tailored to the child's developmental level, need, previous experience, and general interest. The medical team can utilize nonintimidating, empathic styles including getting down on the child's level, referring to the child and parents by name, showing interest in the child as a person, matching tone and affect to the child and family, and always leading with a smile. Remembering body position is important including avoiding body positioning of power and keep your arms and legs uncrossed. Reinforcing a trusting relationship will go a long way within everyday interactions.

Be thoughtful of language used as children are concrete and can misinterpret or read into what is said to them. If you ask a child "may I" or end with "ok," you open the door for the child to say "no," which then violates trust when a procedure needs to be completed anyway. If you are providing information/preparation to a child on a procedure, medication, or any other item within the hospital that might be new to them, keep in mind that they might very well take you literally when you say something, for example, "CAT scan," they might be looking for the cats and "we are going to put you to sleep," afraid they might die since their dog was "put to sleep" and he never came home (Appendix B). You want to make sure to be honest with avoiding making statements that sound like promises as most times they cannot be kept. Always remember you do not have to know everything, and that is okay. It is okay to say "I do not know" and just listen to the child or parent talk.

Before the Procedure/Preparation

Once rapport and trust is established, it is important to continue this vital relationship through possible procedures as communication is the most common "procedure" in medicine [12]. Making sure all members of the medical team engage in open and honest communication with the patient and family is instrumental in supporting patient's coping. The goal of psychological preparation is to increase children and family members' sense of predictability and control over potentially overwhelming life experiences, allowing them to proceed in these situations with a sense of mastery and with the lowest possible level of distress. This, in turn, may contribute to the optimal emotional adjustment of children and families to hospitalization, health care, illness, or other potentially stressful events [9]. Continued and consistent communication assists patients and families not only in understanding of procedures and diagnosis but also in keeping a clear and consistent message among health-care providers. If patients feel like they cannot trust the health-care providers who are caring for them, they are less likely to be cooperative throughout their stay. Although child life specialists are specially trained in order to provide developmentally appropriate preparation and support for procedure, it is everyone's responsibility on the medical team to make sure they are providing the children they are interacting with accurate information.

During a Procedure/Support

Every child reacts differently to the situations they are placed into. It does not matter whether that same child had the procedure previously or whether it is the first time, coping can vary day to day and situation to situation. Since these experiences are so individualized, a child's understanding and plan for coping should be reassessed prior to every procedure experience. In the following sections we will discuss different strategies to support patients during procedures along with ways to assist patients in creating a coping plan prior to beginning a procedure.

One Voice

During a procedure many things are happening at once. There might be one or more nurses needed in the room, a physician, a child life specialist, and maybe even a parent. With all of those people, one cannot forget the patient who might be crying or fighting, depending on their age or how scared they are. In the heat of the moment, it is easy for everyone to want to "fix" or "calm" the situation/child and begin to talk at once. Everyone might be trying to reassure or encourage the child that they are doing a "great job," although it all turns into a jumbled mess and the child no longer knows who to listen to and can become overstimulated. During a procedure, one voice methodology should be utilized as a way to support the coping needs of the child.

One Voice Methodology

- **O**ne voice should be heard during procedure.
- **N**eed parental involvement.
- **E**ducate patient before the procedure about what is going to happen.
- **V**alidate child with words.
- **O**ffer the most comfortable, nonthreatening position.
- **I**ndividualize your game plan.
- **C**hoose appropriate distraction to be used.
- **E**liminate unnecessary people not actively involved with the procedure.

When using One Voice, only one person should be talking to the child during a procedure. This person should be designated to be the supportive voice to the child and should have a trusting relationship with the patient and family. Not only is this person someone the child can look to as a trusting safe person, but they also can help to set the tone for the room with a quiet, soothing voice. Throughout the procedure any additional conversation that needs to take place should be kept at a very low volume or happen outside the room.

Positioning for Comfort

Once a child enters the hospital, they have the potential to experience many different situations including a variety of sensory input during a possible procedure they might be having. Unfortunately within these experiences, many children become fearful and end up needing to be held or "restrained" in order for the procedure to be completed. Challenges may be experienced when the need to safely complete a procedure ends up leaving a longer-term impact on a child's ability to cope with medical procedures. The use of restraint to accomplish the medical procedure may worsen the child's experiences [3, 15] and is potentially harmful and traumatizing. When looking at the potential long-term effects of medical restraint during procedures, it is always good to know there are other ways to safety. One of these is to utilize positioning for comfort during a procedure. Positioning for comfort additionally gives the parents the chance to be involved during a procedure in a safe and directed way, which has been shown to reduce the stress and anxiety of children when their parents are close by and involved. Since many parents are equally if not more stressed when their child needs to undergo a procedure of any kind, being able to assist during the procedure allows the parent to have an alternative focus and assist in keeping their child calm. If a child needs to be restrained during a procedure, control is also taken away from the parent, which can raise their anxiety, in turn raising the anxiety of their child. In certain situations health-care providers have felt that the parent's strong emotions, such as tears, anger, insecurity, or doubts during a procedure, affected the child in such a way that the child's tears, anger, and resistance increased [14]. Along with involving parents in positioning for comfort, parents have to also be given the choice or option if they do not feel comfortable being the one "holding" their child. Parents need to know it is okay if they do not want to be the one providing comfort through those holds but standing back and being there to provide support and comfort to their child when the procedure is complete. This is especially true when it comes to parents of young infants and younger children. In these situations it is appropriate for other health-care providers to utilize positioning for comfort with them, being the ones either holding or positioning the child in a position where they are not being only "restrained" to the bed. If this situation does arise where a parent cannot safely assist during a procedure, health-care professionals need to make sure they are providing preparation and explanations throughout the procedure.

When a child is restrained, they are typically laid flat on their back and either held by multiple staff members or wrapped in a blanket or sheet, which puts the child into one of the most vulnerable positions and takes away all sense of control they might have over the situation. Some medical providers are fearful of attempting positioning for comfort as they are afraid that either the child will not be able to be held still enough or they will not have enough control. This technique can and will provide security and comfort for a child during a potential stressful and painful procedure. There are a variety of positions (Appendix C) that can be utilized during a variety of procedures including blood draws, IV placements, NG tube placements, and injections to name a few. Utilizing these positions allows the child to feel safe and secure while gaining a sense of control over in an environment where they have very little. Once a child is in a comforting position, it allows the caregiver to another health-care provider to engage the child in distraction, which we will talk more about in a later section.

Coping Plans/Strategies

Another step in assisting a child in coping while they are in the hospital and undergoing a procedure is to make sure and create a coping plan or strategy prior to the start of a procedure. A coping plan can be utilized for a variety of situations including having a general plan to assist a patient through a procedure, if a patient has a developmental delay or autism, and also to create a plan with parents to support younger patients. Within these plans the medical team learns from not only the patient but also the parents on ways to best support their child throughout an upcoming procedure. A coping plan can range from simple to more complex. Being as simple as whether a child likes to watch during a procedure or look away or more complex in a parent being able to provide strategies and ideas on the best way to support their child. For older children a coping plan allows a child a chance to regain a sense of control in allowing them to choose how they would like their procedure to play out. With younger children staff needs to look to the parents for assistance in the creation of this plan as they are the experts on their child and how they have reacted previously within the same or similar situation. If the coping preferences of children are not known or cannot be determined, it is probably best to attempt to distract the child. Clinically, we have found that toddlers and most young children do better with distraction techniques. If a young child then directs his or her attention back to the procedure, clinical judgment must be used to assess how effectively the child is coping, and adjustments in the intervention may be made if needed. Older children and adolescents may need to be provided a choice of whether it is more helpful to attend or distract from a procedure [7].

Coping Plans and Children with Autism

When a child has any additional needs, for example, a diagnosis of autistic spectrum disorder (ASD), it adds to the possible complexity of meeting their needs and providing support. Children with autism can range from having decreased interest in social interactions to having marked deficits in verbal and nonverbal social communication, limited initiation of social interactions, and reduced or abnormal responses to social overtures from others to severe deficits in verbal and nonverbal social communication skills, causing severe impairments in functioning, very limited initiation of social interactions and minimal response to social overtures from others [5]. Autism may affect as many as one in 59 children and affects all racial, ethnic, and socioeconomic groups [4]. With the increase in the number of children seen within the health-care setting with a diagnosis of autism, special care needs to be taken to ensure their needs are appropriately met and there is not a significant long-term impact. Children with ASD can have difficulties with new environments and changes in their normal routine. Components of a health-care visit can be very stressful to the child, parent, and health-care professional, and painful procedures can leave lasting negative memories. These memories can have a significant impact on future visits, resulting in behaviors such as tantrums and aggressions toward health-care personnel [13]. Since there is the opportunity for the health-care environment to greatly impact children with ASD, it is important for preplanning prior to a procedure. Child life specialists can be utilized to help with this process, but if a child life specialist is not available, then other members of the health-care team can be a part of asking parents questions as a way to learn more about their child and ways to help them cope (Appendix D). Asking questions to get to know the patient prior to or in the beginning of the patient's visit will give the health-care providers invaluable insight into ways to support patients and families throughout any given procedure.

Since each child with ASD manifests a range of characteristics of this disorder including mild to severe symptoms of autism [13], the outpatient setting brings its own unique set of challenges. Remembering that the parents of children with ASD are often extremely knowledgeable and are an excellent resource [13], it means they should be the first line of defense before a child's initial visit. Since these visits are typically procedure based and quicker, many times a child with ASD does not have as much time to adjust to the environment, staff, and unfamiliar materials. Care should be taken to items needed in the room and the environment should be uncluttered, with supplies and equipment set up ahead of time and screened from view prior to the patient entering the exam or procedure room [13]. With having limited time to adjust to a change in their routine and a new environment, some children with ASD may become anxious upon arrival for a medical visit due to the unfamiliar surrounding or memories of past experiences [13]. In knowing that anxiety could be a part of their visit, make sure to circle back around to the first steps in involving the parents in creating the most supportive plan possible.

Distraction

The child has been prepared, they are in a position of comfort, and the procedure is set to begin, now what? This is when distraction comes into play. Many children who come in the hospital environment have had previous medical experience or have heard stories of someone else who has. Children are at risk of developing anticipatory fears of painful procedures and perhaps exposed to traumatic experiences if they are not provided with a supportive and understanding environment [11]. Distraction is hypothesized to be an effective strategy for decreasing procedural pain, fear, and distress by reducing the sensory and affective components of pain and the diversion capacity left to process the pain [18]. Characteristics of effective distraction are interventions that are interesting to the child, consistent with the child's energy level, stimulate at least one of the major senses, and can change with the pain [16]. Distraction techniques and items can vary, depending on the age and interest of the child. They can vary from rattles, bubbles, I-spy books, magic wands, singing songs, video games, virtual reality, iPad games, and videos on the Internet. Along with using items for distraction, controlled breathing, guided imagery, and positive self-talk can also be used. Guided imagery can be led by a parent or health-care provider and is used to provide additional relaxation and a sense of security, using the ability to imagine and incorporate as many scenes as possible. With positive self-talk, you encourage the child to replace negative thoughts with positive ones, replacing "I can't do this" or "this is going to hurt real bad" with "this might hurt, but I will feel better soon." All caregivers and health-care staff need to remember that all distraction techniques are individualized to meet the child's developmental and individualized needs [1]. Utilizing these individualized plans for distraction, knowing that they can change and also that some children do not want to be distracted in the moment, but rather leading up to the procedure and immediately following the procedure. Reinforce to the child it is "okay" if they would like to watch during the procedure while giving them a job to help, which might be to make sure their arm stays still. This is also the time to remind a child it is okay to cry, as crying is not necessarily a sign of poor coping rather a coping mechanism. Crying cannot always be classified as a symptom of ineffective coping [19]. The important part to evaluate is how the patient is acting post procedure to see if they return to pre-procedure baseline. Are they able to return to interacting with their parents and staff? Do they calm when held by parents? If they are able to do these things, this will let you know they are coping with the procedure that just took place. If not, they will need follow-up to assist in coping especially for future hospital visits. If they are able to calm, remind the parents we can never ask a child to like a procedure that needs to take place, but it is the after picture that truly lets us know how they are doing.

Conclusion

When painful procedures are an everyday part of the pediatric health care, a "bad" experience during one of these procedures can lead to the development of considerable anxiety in children during subsequent medical treatments [7]. Health-care providers have the opportunity to influence children every day both positively and negatively, depending on the interactions that take place. Children and parents cannot learn effective coping skills to manage a procedure if none are modeled or taught [7]. When a child and family comes into the hospital environment, whether they have been there 100 times or it is their first, each and every one is different and holds new challenges. They look to the medical team for support and guidance as they navigate this foreign and ever-changing environment. Remember that every action, word, and gesture has the chance to impact some of the most vulnerable children and make a possible lifelong impact.

Appendix A

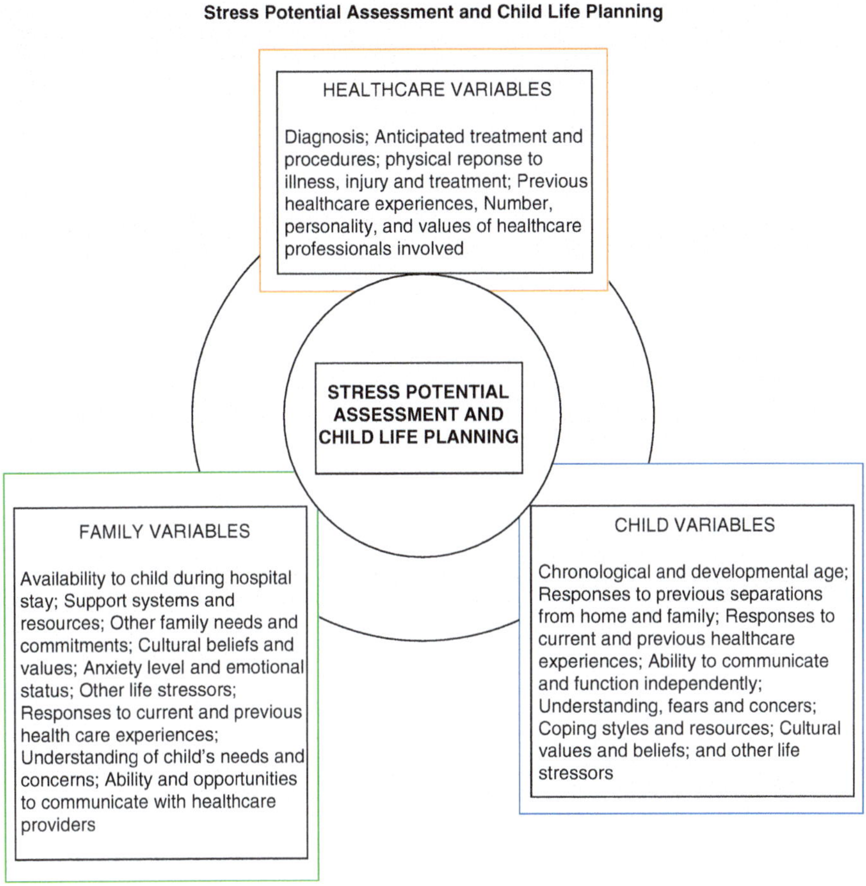
Stress Potential Assessment and Child Life Planning
HEALTHCARE VARIABLES
Diagnosis; Anticipated treatment and procedures; physical reponse to illness, injury and treatment; Previous healthcare experiences, Number, personality, and values of healthcare professionals involved
STRESS POTENTIAL ASSESSMENT AND CHILD LIFE PLANNING
FAMILY VARIABLES
Availability to child during hospital stay; Support systems and resources; Other family needs and commitments; Cultural beliefs and values; Anxiety level and emotional status; Other life stressors; Responses to current and previous health care experiences; Understanding of child's needs and concerns; Ability and opportunities to communicate with healthcare providers
CHILD VARIABLES
Chronological and developmental age; Responses to previous separations from home and family; Responses to current and previous healthcare experiences; Ability to communicate and function independently; Understanding, fears and concers; Coping styles and resources; Cultural values and beliefs; and other life stressors

Appendix B: Misconceptions in Health-Care Language for Children

Commonly used language	What kids might think	Suggested language
Shot Intravenous (or IV)	You're going to hurt me? Are you mad at me? Poison ivy	A "poke" or "medicine through a small needle" First explain what a vein is, then explain that "medicine works best when it goes into the vein through a small straw or tube" or "quickest way to get medicine."
Take your vitals	Stealing something from me; unknown medical term	"Measure your temperature," "check how fast and strong your heart is working" "Listen to your lungs breathe"
Put you to sleep (anesthesia)	Like my pet was put to sleep and never came back?	"Give you medicine that will make you sleep during the whole (test, surgery), so you don't feel anything that hurts"
Dressing change	Why are they going to undress me? Do I have to change my clothes? Will I be naked?	"Put on a new, clean bandage"
Take a picture (X-ray, CT, or MRI)	This camera does not look like our camera at home! That is really big. Should I say "cheese"?	"We're going to take a picture of the inside of your body using this big camera" (describe appearance, sounds, and movement of the equipment, as well as expectations from the child [i.e., hold still])

Adapted from Gaynard et al. [8]

Abbreviations: CT computed tomography, *MRI* magnetic resonance imaging

Appendix C: Positioning for Comfort

Positioning for Comfort:

Chest to chest for IM injections

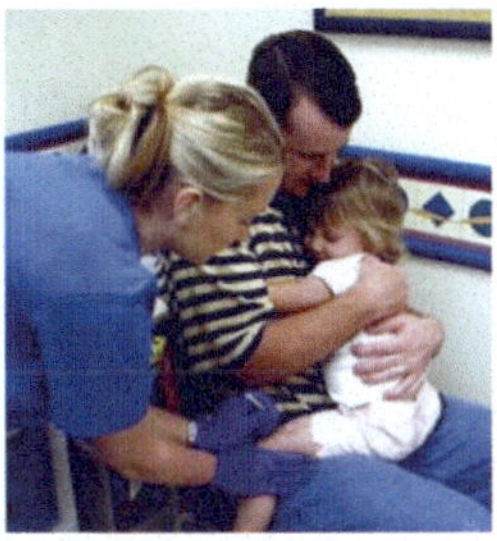

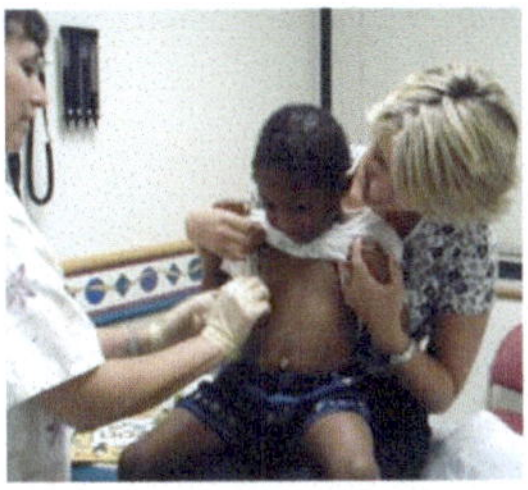

Forward facing of parents lap (port access, IV placement)

Chest to chest

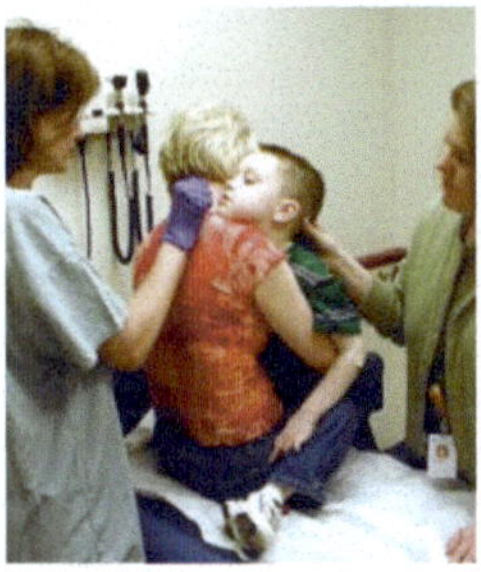

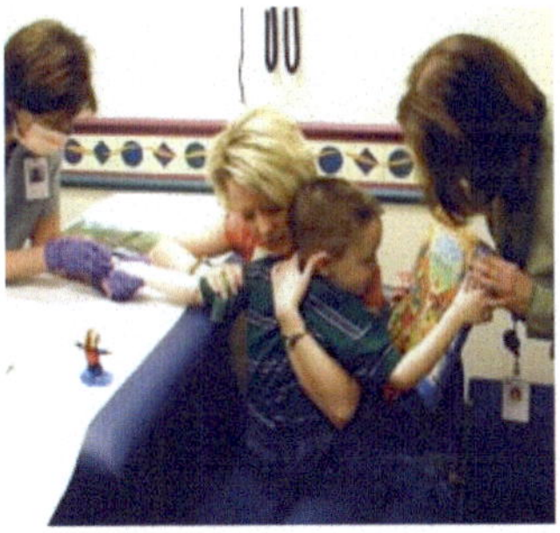

Straddling lap of caregiver

Side-sitting

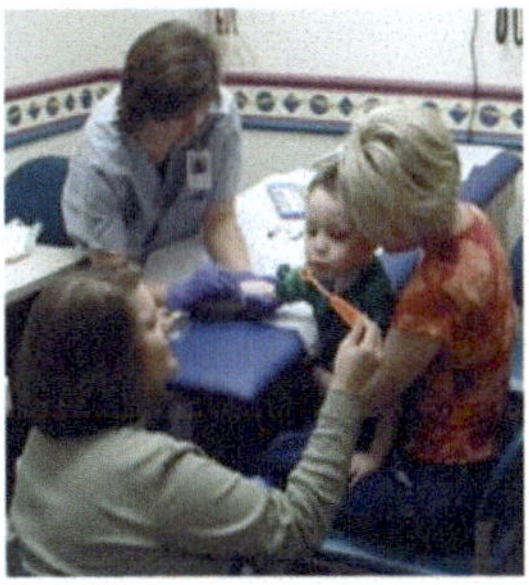

Appendix D: Ideas on Questions to Ask in Creating a Coping Plan

- What are the stress triggers for your child?
- How does your child show you he/she is stressed?
- What items help your child calm when they are stressed or remain calm?
- Has your child had previous experiences within the medical environment? If so, how have they coped, and has anything made it better or worse?
- How does your child communicate?
- Is there anything else that would be good for us to know about your child?

References

1. Bandstra NF, Skinner L, LeBlanc C, et al. The role of child life in pediatric pain management: a survey of child life specialists. J Pain. 2008;9(4):320–9. https://doi.org/10.1016/j.jpain.2007.11.004.
2. Bernzweig J, Takayama JL, Phibbs C, Lewis C, Pantell RH. Gender differences in physician-patient communication. Evidence from pediatric visits. Arch Pediatr Adolesc Med. 1997;151(6):586–91.
3. Brenner M. Child restraint in the acute setting of pediatric nursing: an extraordinarily stressful event. Issues Compr Pediatr Nurs. 2007;30(1-2):29–37. https://doi.org/10.1080/01460860701366658.
4. Center for Disease Control (2017). Facts about autism spectrum disorders. Retrieved from https://www.cdc.gov/ncbddd/autism/data.html.
5. Diagnostic and statistical manual of mental disorders (2013). DSM-5. Arlington, VA; American Psychiatric Association.
6. Elder GH. The life course as development theory. Child Dev. 1998;69:1–12.
7. Fanurik D, Koh J, Schmitz M, Brown R. Pharmacobehavioral intervention: integrating pharmacologic and behavioral techniques for pediatric medical procedures. Child Health Care. 1997;26(1):31–46.
8. Gaynard L, Wolfer J, Goldberger J, Thompson R, Redburn L, Laidley L. Psychosocial care of children in hospitals: a clinical practice manual. Rockville: Child Life Council; 1998.
9. Goldberger J, Mohl AL, Thompson R. Psychological preparation and coping. In: Thompson RH, editor. The handbook of child life: a guide for pediatric psychosocial care. Springfield: Charles C. Thomas; 2009. p. 160–98.
10. Kaddoura M, Cormier K, Leduc J. Resource collaboration: the benefits of utilizing child life specialists when dealing with pediatric stress. Educ Res Q. 2013;37(2):3–21.
11. Kuttner L. A child in pain: What health professionals can do to help. Bethel: Crown House Publishing Company; 2010.
12. Levetown M. Communicating with children and families: from everyday interactions to skill in conveying distressing information. Pediatrics. 2008;121(5):e1441–60. https://doi.org/10.1542/peds.2008-0565.
13. Souders MC, Freeman KG, DePaul D, Levy SE. Caring for children and adolescents with autism who require challenging procedures. Pediatr Nurs. 2002;28(6):555–83.
14. Svendsen EJ, Pedersen R, Moen A, Bjørk IT. Exploring perspectives on restraint during medical procedures in paediatric care: a qualitative interview study with nurses and physicians. Int

J Qual Stud Health Well Being. 2017;12(1):1363623. https://doi.org/10.1080/17482631.2017.1363623.
15. Synder BS. Preventing treatment interference: nurses' and parents' intervention strategies. Pediatr Nurs. 2004;30(1):31–40.
16. Twycross A, Dowden S, Stinson J. Managing pain in children: a clinical guide for nurses and healthcare professionals. 2nd ed. Wiley-Blackwell: Chichester; 2014.
17. Vessey JA. Children's psychological responses to hospitalization. Annu Rev Nurs Res. 2003;21:173–201.
18. Vessey JA, Carlson KL, McGill J. Use of distraction with children during an acute pain experience. Nurs Res. 1994;43(6):369–72.
19. Vingerhoets A, et al. Is there a relationship between depression and crying? A review. Acta Psychiatr Scandinavac. 2007;115:340–51.
20. Wertlieb D. Converging trends in family research and pediatrics, recent findings for the task force on the family. Pediatrics. 2003;111(6 pt 2):1572–87.

Chapter 34
Risk Stratification for Procedural Sedation

Eitan Neeman and Kevin G. Couloures

Overview

Sedation, the process of decreasing one's level of consciousness so they can tolerate an uncomfortable or painful procedure, should be done in a setting prepared for the possible adverse events associated with decreased consciousness. The decline in awareness and possible loss of protective reflexes carries an inherent risk, and the healthcare provider must continuously assess the risks versus benefits of sedation. When the patient is being evaluated for a nonurgent procedure, then we must consider if sedating the patient electively is in their best interest.

The three main aspects to consider are the type of procedure, chronic conditions affecting the patient, and any acute change in their usual state of health. While the optimal situation would be a short and non-painful procedure in a previously healthy patient, with no current illness, pediatric patients in need of sedation often present with an acute or chronic illness, and procedures in this population are more technically challenging and hence prolonged, compared to the same procedures in the adult population.

Older agents such as pentobarbital and chloral hydrate not had only a lower safety profile but also diminished patient satisfaction [1–4] due to the need for a longer recovery period and irritability after the procedure. This is partially due to

E. Neeman
Yale School of Medicine, New Haven, CT, USA

Pediatric Intensive Care Unit, Soroka University Medical Center and Faculty of Health Sciences, Ben-Gurion University of the Negev, Beer-Sheva, Israel
e-mail: eitanne@bgu.ac.il

K. G. Couloures (✉)
Stanford School of Medicine, Palo Alto, CA, USA

Pediatric Intensive Care Unit, California Pacific Medical Center, San Francisco, CA, USA
e-mail: kcouloures@stanford.edu

P. P. Kamat, J. W. Berkenbosch (eds.), *Sedation and Analgesia for the Pediatric Intensivist*, https://doi.org/10.1007/978-3-030-52555-2_34

their extended half-life as well as the potential for delayed apneic episodes [5]. As the field of sedation has progressed, newer drugs with enhanced safety and satisfaction profiles have appeared, thus allowing the sedation practitioner to provide safe sedation for an expanded patient population and improved patient/family satisfaction due to better recovery profiles.

Location of Procedure

The optimal setting for a planned procedural sedation is an area where all supplies and equipment are available, such as the operating room or the pediatric ICU. Guidelines and minimal required equipment lists have been previously published [6]. However, many sedations occur outside of these setting, such as the radiology suite or a dedicated treatment room, with excellent safety records. This has been demonstrated with both propofol [7] and ketamine [8]. In the study utilizing propofol, serious side effects such as aspiration or CPR were exceedingly rare (four and two episodes, respectively, out of 49,836 sedations – 0.8 aspiration episodes per 10,000 sedation events and 0.4 CPR episodes per 10,000 sedation events). These rates are lower than those observed in patients undergoing general anesthesia (GA): Zgleszewski et al., in a single-center retrospective review, found a rate of 5.1 cardiac arrests per 10,000 GA events [9]; Kelly and Walker reported an aspiration rate of two per 10,000 elective procedures undergoing GA [10]. Less serious side effects such as desaturation or central apnea were more common (154 and 575 per 10,000 sedations, respectively), and while the rate of post-extubation stridor in GA is low [11], it has not been reported in the sedation literature. Other side effects such as laryngospasm were below 100 per 10,000 sedations. In a similar retrospective series, ketamine had an overall adverse event rate of 7.26% or 726 per 10,000 sedation encounters, with a severe adverse event (AE) frequency of 1.77% or 177 per 10,000 sedation encounters. The sedation team must be well aware of all the possible complications and be prepared to manage these events, should they occur. These very rare events must be anticipated, and a system to rehearse and practice for these low-frequency/high-acuity events must be in place, since simulation has been shown to improve tasks related to patient safety during sedation [12].

Procedure Type

Data regarding the procedure type show that even renal biopsies can be performed outside of the OR with sedation [13]. In the study by Kamat et al., which included 174 renal biopsies, 30% required blowby oxygen and 12% required CPAP. The use of fentanyl with propofol had a significantly higher success rate in comparison with other drug combinations. In children undergoing esophagogastroduodenoscopy, colonoscopy, or both, a retrospective study has shown a low overall adverse events prevalence, less than 5%. One of the independent predictors was the type of procedure, namely, esophagogastroduodenoscopy, hinting that procedures adjacent to the airway involve a higher risk for adverse events when compared to a procedure that did not manipulate the airway [14]. In comparison, a recent retrospective review for pediatric patients undergoing sedation for MRI demonstrated a 2% risk of unplanned intubation [15]. Another review, looking at the AE rate in a freestanding imaging center, demonstrated that desaturations occurred in 11.5% of cases but were handled by the sedation team successfully [16]; it can be assumed that painful procedures are protective for adverse events such as desaturation and apnea because of the stimulation involved, causing increase in motor tone during the procedure.

Chronic Conditions

First, we must consider the child's age and whether they were born at full-term or premature. Infants under the gestational age of 60 weeks are at risk for apnea several hours after the sedation/anesthetic event and hence require prolonged monitoring or overnight admission. Prematurity also confers increased risk that persists throughout childhood and up until early adulthood [17]. It is still unclear if the risk arises from early birth itself and its effects on organ development or the comorbidities and interventions that come with it such as prolonged respiratory support and recurrent airway manipulations.

Research varies regarding the minimal age for undergoing elective sedation outside the OR. In a retrospective study, age below 5 years almost doubled the rate of any AE (7.8% vs. 4% in older than 5). However, the majority of these adverse events were desaturations and airway obstruction, which in the hands of the experienced provider are readily recognized and managed. The authors mention several factors, including the relatively smaller airway and decreased respiratory reserves in small children [14]; other contributing factors to this increased risk are higher basal metabolic rate and larger head size that is more likely to flex forward and obstruct the airway during sedation. Several studies using newer agents such as dexmedetomidine demonstrated excellent safety profiles in younger babies and post-prematurity infants, as summarized by Scherrer [18]. Najafi et al. [19] used IV dexmedetomidine to sedate children with respiratory comorbidities and required smaller doses for children under 1 year of age. Olgun [20] used the intranasal route to administer dexmedetomidine as a single agent to patients 12 months and under, who underwent MRI, with an overall success rate higher than 96% and without any significant AEs. In a retrospective chart review by Jenkins [21], patients under 6 months of age sedated with propofol had a 99% success rate (defined as completion of study using sedation with satisfactory image quality and no motion artifact) but with a 12.7 AE rate, and 4.3% had a serious AE, with airway obstruction being the most common. The authors tie the higher dose required during the sedation of this young population to the relatively high frequency of airway AEs. A recent retrospective study that compared babies undergoing sedation and general anesthesia showed no apneic events in either preterm or term population post procedure in the sedation group, which used propofol almost exclusively [22]. This implies a possible change in the post-sedation management of this population: the historical "late effects" of sedation such as apnea might not be applicable when IV/IN agents are used compared to prior agents such as chloral hydrate and pentobarbital, which were given via the enteral route.

We recommend that sedation of the premature and former premature infants requires heightened awareness and proficient airway management skills, since airway and respiratory adverse events were most commonly reported in this cohort.

The American Society of Anesthesiologists physical status (ASA-PS) score has also been used to differentiate those children at increased risk for adverse events, but the score was not designed to be used in this manner, and there is a considerable inter-rater variation for the same patient's score between different providers and between different specialties and experience [23] [24]. Newer scores with better predictive ability have been proposed [25] but are not widely used. High Mallampati score was not in itself associated with a higher rate of AEs, including desaturations, apnea, or bag mask ventilation. There was, however, an increased need for patient repositioning [26]. Special consideration should be given to patients with underlying airway anomalies and deviation from normal in any other organ system, such as chronic heart disease, lung diseases [27], bleeding disorders, and neurologic changes such as baseline decreased level of consciousness or poorly controlled seizure disorders.

The child's weight also plays an important role in the pre-procedural assessment. Obese patients, defined as BMI ≥95th percentile for age and gender, are at increased risk for AEs, especially respiratory ones (airway obstruction, desaturation, secretions, and laryngospasm). In addition, they had a higher rate of inability to complete the associated procedure and a longer recovery period. In Scherrer's multivariate analysis of more than 5000 patients, obesity was shown to be independently associated with minor and moderate but not major adverse events [28]. Additionally, Hirsch [29] has shown that children with obesity are almost twice as likely to have a desaturation related to procedural sedation compared with children of other weight status. There is also a tendency to overestimate their sedative requirements, as measured by Chidambaran on 20 patients with BMI greater than the 97th percentile. The authors recommend titrating propofol according to bispectral index (BIS) levels, as the current weight-based dosing is inaccurate [30]. However, BIS monitoring is not a routine practice in pediatric procedural sedation practice. Underweight patients, defined as less than fifth percentile for age, pose a risk as well; a study in oncologic patients showed them to be at increased risk for AEs [31].

We recommend that sedation of the overweight and underweight child requires proficient airway management skills, since weight-based regimens may result in more frequent desaturation events. Use of the ideal body weight for initial dosing in the obese patient with upward titration as needed will help avoid airway-related events related to a deeper than intended level of sedation.

Many obese patients suffer from obstructive sleep apnea (OSA), which can create challenges in maintaining airway patency and excessive body motion due to snoring while the patient is supine. Enlarged tonsils or underlying disorders such as Down's syndrome can also result in airway obstruction during sleep, independent of the patient's weight. In patients with OSA, dexmedetomidine has been shown to be of benefit, as upper airway reflexes remained active during sedation and patients can compensate for airway obstruction, similar to natural sleep [32]. Of note, both OSA and obesity were found to be risk factors for failed sedation in a single-center study investigating root causes of failed procedural sedation [33].

We recommend that children who require positive pressure airway during sleep either be sedated solely with dexmedetomidine or a combination of dexmedetomidine (induction) and propofol (infusion for maintenance) or be referred to anesthesia. The use of agents other than dexmedetomidine will frequently require placement of an oral airway to maintain airway patency during deep sedation.

The sedation of a child with preexisting acyanotic cardiac disease presents unique challenges. The child with cyanotic disease would preferentially be seen by a cardiac anesthetist in large academic centers. However, in situation where access to cardiac anesthesia is limited or not available, the use of agents such as dexmedetomidine and propofol is preferred. Propofol, despite its negative effect on blood pressure, has not been shown to decrease cerebral tissue oxygenation in a 32 patients' series. The authors speculate this is caused by decreased oxygen consumption of the sedated brain with intact cerebral autoregulation [34]. Although the use of dexmedetomidine has been shown to be safe and effective both during heart surgery [35] and postoperative ICU sedation in patients with acyanotic heart disease [36], evidence is lacking regarding its use in procedural sedation in this patient population. Congenital heart disease could not be evaluated as a predictor of failed sedation in one study, since these patients had been classified as ASA 3 [33]. In addition, as dexmedetomidine depresses nodal function in the heart [37, 38], EKG testing prior to administration in the patients with known heart disease may be prudent. Additionally, dexmedetomidine should not be used for patients with heart block, prolonged QT interval, or ones using digoxin.

We recommend dexmedetomidine as a first-line agent, for its established safety profile for patients with acyanotic heart disease, except for those with preexisting heart block or prolonged QT interval. Propofol can be used in the hemodynamically stable patient, who has a good cardiac output. Patients with cyanotic heart disease should be referred to a cardiac anesthesia team regardless of function or palliation stage.

Autistic spectrum patients, despite their normal physiological responses, require special attention from the sedation team. These measures may include minimizing wait times, avoiding benzodiazepines, additional staff and preparation visits to familiarize the patient with the settings, and minimizing distractions throughout the visit. A practice survey of sedation for autistic spectrum patients undergoing MRI showed significant variation between institutions [39], but no increased frequency of AE, albeit additional personnel requirement before induction. In the series, 10% of patients required four or more providers to ensure patient and provider safety [40]. Regarding the preferred medication regimen in this population, a recent comparative study showed recovery and discharge times were significantly lower when using propofol, while the use of dexmedetomidine maintained more stable hemodynamics. Both propofol and dexmedetomidine proved to be adequate and safe for procedural sedation [41]. Dexmedetomidine doses were shown to be significantly lower in autistic patients than other patients undergoing MRI sedation, without increase in complications [42].

We recommend avoidance of benzodiazepine and prefer dexmedetomidine as the agent of choice in patients with autistic spectrum disorder. Policies should also be in place to minimize wait time and distractions and provide additional staff as needed.

Another high-risk patient group, who requires frequent sedation, is the oncologic patients. These patients often benefit from aggregation of several procedures during a single sedation, although a retrospective review has shown that these combined procedures require more propofol, and have a higher but manageable risk for AEs [43]. In this patient population, ketamine has been shown to be superior to pethidine (meperidine) in a randomized crossover trial [44], and the combination of propofol and ketamine was better than ketamine alone, as shown in another randomized trial [45]. Another RCT compared propofol to ketamine-midazolam combination; the authors conclude that ketamine-midazolam combination is safer and more effective. Propofol was faster in onset and recovery and had smoother emergence, albeit poor efficacy at recommended initial doses [46]. Of note, ketamine has been associated with laryngospasm [8] and should only be administered by those prepared to deal with this infrequent event.

We recommend ketamine-propofol combination or propofol-fentanyl combination for sedation of oncologic patients. The clinician should be aware of their side effects, namely, laryngospasm for the former and hypotension for the latter, and be ready to manage these, should they appear. A readily accessible record of prior sedative agents and their effect on the sedation event and recovery will also help guide future sedation encounters.

Acute Conditions

The most common illness in our population is upper respiratory infections (URI). These episodes are closely linked to an increase in anesthesia-related adverse events such as breath holding and desaturations but not to laryngospasm or bronchospasm [47]. A single-center evaluation of risk factors for sedation failures identified URI as having increased odds ratio for a failed sedation [33] . A recent observational study in patients undergoing procedural sedation has shown increased rate of airway AE, but overall the risk remained low; the rates of major airway AEs such as laryngospasm, aspiration, emergent airway interventions, unplanned admission, and emergent call for anesthesia all remained <1% regardless of URI status. Current URI and thick secretions (vs. clear) increased the frequency of airway AEs. No relationship between URI status and non-airway AEs was found [48]. We feel it is important to distinguish between increased secretions alone, which may require increased suctioning frequency, to the presence of cough; as the coughing child is sedated and loses the ability to generate a cough, one can assume the risk of aspiration and airway AE will increase. The presence of a URI in itself does not preclude a patient from undergoing sedation but requires a risk-benefit analysis regarding the length and urgency of the procedure.

We recommend that in the child with URI without cough and baseline saturation > 95%, suctioning be performed shortly after induction of sedation, as this will help decrease desaturation events and minimize the risk of laryngospasm triggered by secretions.

Fever is usually a sign of intercurrent illness, and thus, an assessment of its source should occur and whether this would influence his respiratory or cardiovascular status during the sedation. One review recommends postponing an elective procedure requiring anesthesia 1–3 weeks after vaccination [49]. There is currently not an accepted standard or guideline regarding this.

We recommend that elective sedation be delayed until 1–2 weeks after the illness. Sedation of patients, who cannot be deferred due to protocol adherence, should be evaluated on a case-by-case basis.

Current ASA guidelines dictate a fasting period of 8 hours (excluding human milk and clear liquids) without distinction between general anesthesia and procedural sedation. These guidelines have been used in procedural sedation since any sedation might need manipulation of the airway, but this is not an evidence-based practice; a retrospective review by Beach et al. did not find a significant difference of complications between patients with different NPO status [50]. Another retrospective study in an institution where children scheduled for elective procedures were allowed to drink clear fluids until called to the operating suite found a 0.03% chance of aspiration in more than 10,000 cases [51]. Furthermore, a growing body of evidence question this requirement: a single-center prospective study failed to find an association between a shortened fasting time and increased frequency of vomiting [52], and other studies showed no difference in complication rate [53] [54]. These studies suggest that using shorter fasting time may be a safe alternative for procedure cancellation and rescheduling. Of note, use of nitrous oxide is increasing in our practice. Although associated with a low rate of AEs, the odds of vomiting increased when concomitant opioids were administered and NPO clear fluids <2 hours [55].

We recommend that patients be NPO for 6 hours for light meals, cow's milk, and formula, 4 hours for breast milk, and 2 hours for apple juice, water, and Pedialyte®. Allowing clears up until 2 hours before the procedure helps decrease patient/family concern about prolonged NPO periods.

Pediatric Sedation Service teams are frequently asked to provide procedural sedation for hospitalized patients, but since the patient is hospitalized, a careful review of their respiratory and hemodynamic status along with a physical examination prior to determining sedation is appropriate; if the patient requires supplemental oxygen, has borderline hypotension or airway anomalies, deferring to anesthesia would also be appropriate. However, bedside placement of peripherally inserted central catheter (PICC) lines, short oncologic procedures, and liver or renal biopsies can be readily handled by a well-organized sedation service.

References

1. Teshome G, Belani K, Braun JL, Constantine DR, Gattu RK, Lichenstein R. Comparison of dexmedetomidine with pentobarbital for pediatric MRI sedation. Hosp Pediatr. 2014;4(6):360–5.
2. Fong CY, Tay CG, Ong LC, Lai NM. Chloral hydrate as a sedating agent for neurodiagnostic procedures in children. Cochrane Database Syst Rev. 2017;(11):CD011786.
3. Yuen VM, Li BL, Cheuk DK, Leung MKM, Hui TWC, Wong IC, et al. A randomised controlled trial of oral chloral hydrate vs. intranasal dexmedetomidine before computerised tomography in children. Anaesthesia. 2017;72(10):1191–5.
4. Cao Q, Lin Y, Xie Z, Shen W, Chen Y, Gan X, et al. Comparison of sedation by intranasal dexmedetomidine and oral chloral hydrate for pediatric ophthalmic examination. Paediatr Anaesth. 2017;27(6):629–36.
5. Cote CJ, Notterman DA, Karl HW, Weinberg JA, McCloskey C. Adverse sedation events in pediatrics: a critical incident analysis of contributing factors. Pediatrics. 2000;105(4 Pt 1):805–14.
6. Cote CJ, Wilson S, American Academy of P, American Academy of Pediatric D. Guidelines for monitoring and management of pediatric patients before, during, and after sedation for diagnostic and therapeutic procedures: update 2016. Pediatrics. 2016;138:1.
7. Cravero JP, Beach ML, Blike GT, Gallagher SM, Hertzog JH, Pediatric Sedation Research C. The incidence and nature of adverse events during pediatric sedation/anesthesia with propofol for procedures outside the operating room: a report from the Pediatric Sedation Research Consortium. Anesth Analg. 2009;108(3):795–804.
8. Grunwell JR, Travers C, McCracken CE, Scherrer PD, Stormorken AG, Chumpitazi CE, et al. Procedural sedation outside of the operating room using ketamine in 22,645 children: a report from the Pediatric Sedation Research consortium. Pediatr Crit Care Med. 2016;17(12):1109–16.
9. Zgleszewski SE, Graham DA, Hickey PR, Brustowicz RM, Odegard KC, Koka R, et al. Anesthesiologist- and system-related risk factors for risk-adjusted pediatric anesthesia-related cardiac arrest. Anesth Analg. 2016;122(2):482–9.
10. Kelly CJ, Walker RW. Perioperative pulmonary aspiration is infrequent and low risk in pediatric anesthetic practice. Paediatr Anaesth. 2015;25(1):36–43.
11. Litman RS, Keon TP. Postintubation croup in children. Anesthesiology. 1991;75(6):1122–3.
12. Ben-Ari M, Chayen G, Steiner IP, Schinasi DA, Feldman O, Shavit I. The effect of in situ simulation training on the performance of tasks related to patient safety during sedation. J Anesth. 2018;32(2):300–4.
13. Kamat PP, Ayestaran FW, Gillespie SE, Sanders RD, Greenbaum LA, Simon HK, et al. Deep procedural sedation by a sedationist team for outpatient pediatric renal biopsies. Pediatr Transplant. 2016;20(3):372–7.
14. Biber JL, Allareddy V, Allareddy V, Gallagher SM, Couloures KG, Speicher DG, et al. Prevalence and predictors of adverse events during procedural sedation anesthesia-outside the operating room for esophagogastroduodenoscopy and colonoscopy in children: age is an independent predictor of outcomes. Pediatr Crit Care Med. 2015;16(8):e251–9.
15. Kim D, Lee EK, Jeong JS, Gil NS, Hahm TS, Shin YH. Incidence and risk factors of unplanned intubation during pediatric sedation for MRI. J Magn Reson Imaging. 2019;49(4):1053–61.
16. Emrath ET, Stockwell JA, McCracken CE, Simon HK, Kamat PP. Provision of deep procedural sedation by a pediatric sedation team at a freestanding imaging center. Pediatr Radiol. 2014;44(8):1020–5.
17. Havidich JE, Beach M, Dierdorf SF, Onega T, Suresh G, Cravero JP. Preterm versus term children: analysis of sedation/anesthesia adverse events and longitudinal risk. Pediatrics. 2016;137(3):e20150463.
18. Scherrer PD, Rogers AP, Kamat PP. Shifting the paradigm: the quiet revolution of pediatric procedural sedation practice. Hosp Pediatr. 2018;8(6):372–4.
19. Najafi N, Veyckemans F, Van de Velde A, Poelaert J. Usability of dexmedetomidine for deep sedation in infants and small children with respiratory morbidities. Acta Anaesthesiol Scand. 2016;60(7):865–73.

20. Olgun G, Ali MH. Use of intranasal Dexmedetomidine as a solo sedative for MRI of infants. Hosp Pediatr. 2018;
21. Jenkins E, Hebbar KB, Karaga KK, Hirsh DA, Fortenberry JD, McCracken CE, et al. Experience with the use of propofol for radiologic imaging in infants younger than 6 months of age. Pediatr Radiol. 2017;47(8):974–83.
22. Rozema T, Westgate PM, Landers CD. Apnea in preterm and term infants after deep sedation and general anesthesia. Hosp Pediatr. 2018;8(6):314–20.
23. Tollinche LE, Yang G, Tan KS, Borchardt R. Interrater variability in ASA physical status assignment: an analysis in the pediatric cancer setting. J Anesth. 2018;32(2):211–8.
24. Bernard PA, Makin CE, Hongying D, Ballard HO. Variability of ASA physical status class assignment among pediatric sedation practitioners. Int J Adolesc Med Health. 2009;21(2):213–20.
25. Malviya S, Voepel-Lewis T, Chiravuri SD, Gibbons K, Chimbira WT, Nafiu OO, et al. Does an objective system-based approach improve assessment of perioperative risk in children? A preliminary evaluation of the 'NARCO'. Br J Anaesth. 2011;106(3):352–8.
26. Iyer MS, Pitetti RD, Vitale M. Higher Mallampati scores are not associated with more adverse events during Pediatric procedural sedation and analgesia. West J Emerg Med. 2018;19(2):430–6.
27. Della Rocca G. Anaesthesia in patients with cystic fibrosis. Curr Opin Anaesthesiol. 2002;15(1):95–101.
28. Scherrer PD, Mallory MD, Cravero JP, Lowrie L, Hertzog JH, Berkenbosch JW, et al. The impact of obesity on pediatric procedural sedation-related outcomes: results from the Pediatric Sedation Research Consortium. Paediatr Anaesth. 2015;25(7):689–97.
29. Hirsch DG, Tyo J, Wrotniak BH. Desaturation in procedural sedation for children with long bone fractures: does weight status matter? Am J Emerg Med. 2017;35(8):1060–3.
30. Chidambaran V, Sadhasivam S, Diepstraten J, Esslinger H, Cox S, Schnell BM, et al. Evaluation of propofol anesthesia in morbidly obese children and adolescents. BMC Anesthesiol. 2013;13:8.
31. Rogerson CM, Abulebda K, Hobson MJ. Association of BMI with propofol dosing and adverse events in children with cancer undergoing procedural sedation. Hosp Pediatr. 2017;7(9):542–6.
32. Mahmoud M, Ishman SL, McConnell K, Fleck R, Shott S, Mylavarapu G, et al. Upper airway reflexes are preserved during Dexmedetomidine sedation in children with down syndrome and obstructive sleep apnea. J Clin Sleep Med. 2017;13(5):721–7.
33. Grunwell JR, McCracken C, Fortenberry J, Stockwell J, Kamat P. Risk factors leading to failed procedural sedation in children outside the operating room. Pediatr Emerg Care. 2014;30(6):381–7.
34. Fleck T, Schubert S, Ewert P, Stiller B, Nagdyman N, Berger F. Propofol effect on cerebral oxygenation in children with congenital heart disease. Pediatr Cardiol. 2015;36(3):543–9.
35. Pan W, Wang Y, Lin L, Zhou G, Hua X, Mo L. Outcomes of dexmedetomidine treatment in pediatric patients undergoing congenital heart disease surgery: a meta-analysis. Paediatr Anaesth. 2016;26(3):239–48.
36. Gupta P, Whiteside W, Sabati A, Tesoro TM, Gossett JM, Tobias JD, et al. Safety and efficacy of prolonged dexmedetomidine use in critically ill children with heart disease*. Pediatr Crit Care Med. 2012;13(6):660–6.
37. Hammer GB, Drover DR, Cao H, Jackson E, Williams GD, Ramamoorthy C, et al. The effects of dexmedetomidine on cardiac electrophysiology in children. Anesth Analg. 2008;106(1):79–83. table of contents
38. Su F, Hammer GB. Dexmedetomidine: pediatric pharmacology, clinical uses and safety. Expert Opin Drug Saf. 2011;10(1):55–66.
39. Kamat PP, Bryan LN, McCracken CE, Simon HK, Berkenbosch JW, Grunwell JR. Procedural sedation in children with autism spectrum disorders: a survey of current practice patterns of the society for pediatric sedation members. Paediatr Anaesth. 2018;28(6):552–7.
40. Kamat PP, Karaga MK, Wisniewski BL, McCracken CE, Simon HK, Sidhu R, et al. Outpatient procedural sedation of patients with autism spectrum disorders for magnetic resonance imaging of the brain using propofol. J Child Neurol. 2018;33(5):313–9.

41. Abulebda K, Louer R, Lutfi R, Ahmed SS. A comparison of safety and efficacy of dexmedetomidine and propofol in children with autism and autism spectrum disorders undergoing magnetic resonance imaging. J Autism Dev Disord. 2018;48(9):3127–32.
42. Ahmed SS, Unland T, Slaven JE, Nitu ME, Rigby MR. Successful use of intravenous dexmedetomidine for magnetic resonance imaging sedation in autistic children. South Med J. 2014;107(9):559–64.
43. Patel MM, Kamat PP, McCracken CE, Simon HK. Complications of deep sedation for individual procedures (lumbar puncture alone) versus combined procedures (lumbar puncture and bone marrow aspirate) in pediatric oncology patients. Hosp Pediatr. 2016;6(2):95–102.
44. Abdolkarimi B, Zareifar S, Golestani Eraghi M, Saleh F. Comparison effect of intravenous ketamine with pethidine for analgesia and sedation during bone marrow procedures in oncologic children: a randomized, double-blinded, crossover trial. Int J Hematol Oncol Stem Cell Res. 2016;10(4):206–11.
45. Chiaretti A, Ruggiero A, Barbi E, Pierri F, Maurizi P, Fantacci C, et al. Comparison of propofol versus propofol-ketamine combination in pediatric oncologic procedures performed by non-anesthesiologists. Pediatr Blood Cancer. 2011;57(7):1163–7.
46. Chayapathi V, Kalra M, Bakshi AS, Mahajan A. A comparison of ketamine + midazolam to propofol for procedural sedation for lumbar puncture in pediatric oncology by nonanesthesiologists-a randomized comparative trial. Pediatr Blood Cancer. 2018;65(8):e27108.
47. Tait AR, Malviya S, Voepel-Lewis T, Munro HM, Seiwert M, Pandit UA. Risk factors for perioperative adverse respiratory events in children with upper respiratory tract infections. Anesthesiology. 2001;95(2):299–306.
48. Mallory MD, Travers C, McCracken CE, Hertzog J, Cravero JP. Upper respiratory infections and airway adverse events in pediatric procedural Sedation. Pediatrics. 2017;40(1):e20170009
49. Bertolizio G, Astuto M, Ingelmo P. The implications of immunization in the daily practice of pediatric anesthesia. Curr Opin Anaesthesiol. 2017;30(3):368–75.
50. Beach ML, Cohen DM, Gallagher SM, Cravero JP. Major adverse events and relationship to nil per Os status in pediatric sedation/anesthesia outside the operating room: a report of the Pediatric Sedation Research Consortium. Anesthesiology. 2016;124(1):80–8.
51. Andersson H, Zaren B, Frykholm P. Low incidence of pulmonary aspiration in children allowed intake of clear fluids until called to the operating suite. Paediatr Anaesth. 2015;25(8):770–7.
52. Chumpitazi CE, Camp EA, Bhamidipati DR, Montillo AM, Chantal Caviness A, Mayorquin L, et al. Shortened preprocedural fasting in the pediatric emergency department. Am J Emerg Med. 2018;36(9):1577–80.
53. Clark M, Birisci E, Anderson JE, Anliker CM, Bryant MA, Downs C, et al. The risk of shorter fasting time for pediatric deep sedation. Anesth Essays Res. 2016;10(3):607–12.
54. Malia L, Laurich VM, Sturm JJ. Adverse events and satisfaction with use of intranasal midazolam for emergency department procedures in children. Am J Emerg Med. 2018;
55. Tsze DS, Mallory MD, Cravero JP. Practice patterns and adverse events of nitrous oxide Sedation and analgesia: a report from the Pediatric Sedation Research Consortium. J Pediatr. 2016;169:260–5.e2.

Chapter 35
Nursing Considerations

Nancy Crego

Pre-procedure Nursing Considerations

Prior to starting any sedation procedure, it is important for nurses to be familiar with any state regulatory and organization level limitations to sedation practice. These may include limitations on the depth of sedation achieved and restrictions on the sedative medications that can be administered by nurses. However, state regulatory practices vary widely and continue to evolve [1].

State Regulations

Nursing regulatory bodies such as the National Council of State Boards of Nursing, protect the public's health and welfare by assuring that safe and competent care is provided by licensees [2]. Nursing practice is regulated through individual state nurse practice acts that are evidence based, responsive to the evolving needs of the public, and include collaboration with other organizations and agencies also interested in protection of the public, patient safety, and education [2]. One challenge of this regulatory system is that licensing procedures and nursing practices vary by state. Thus, licensees must be aware of the specific sedation regulations in their state. There is currently no up-to-date centralized list of nurse sedation regulations. However, the National Council of State Boards of Nursing maintains a complete list of contact information for each individual state board of nursing and can be accessed at https://www.ncsbn.org/contact-bon.htm.

N. Crego (✉)
Duke University School of Nursing, Durham, NC, USA
e-mail: Nancy.Crego@Duke.edu

P. P. Kamat, J. W. Berkenbosch (eds.), *Sedation and Analgesia for the Pediatric Intensivist*, https://doi.org/10.1007/978-3-030-52555-2_35

Organizational Policies and Procedures

Nurse sedation practice is also guided by individual organizational policies that consider state regulation, national standards set by the Joint Commission, and professional standards such as the American Association of Critical-Care Nurses. These policies provide much greater detail as to organizational practices related to sedation such as screening procedures, monitoring, equipment, and training/credentialing requirements. Additionally, organizational policies addressing emergency response procedures and quality improvement processes that are applicable to sedation may be addressed in separate policies. An in-depth understanding of all sedation-related organizational policies, procedures, and processes are needed to enable nurses to provide safe sedation care.

Sedation Competency

Nursing competence is defined as an "expected level of performance that integrates knowledge, skills, abilities and judgment" [3]. Sedation competency includes the ability to perform a pre-procedural assessment that incorporates sedation risk assessment, knowledge and experience with various sedative medications, appropriate implementation and analysis of monitoring data, identification and recognition of changes in sedation levels, and the ability to recognize and intervene appropriately when complications arise [4]. Table 35.1 provides a detailed list of the components of nurse sedation competency.

Assessment of sedation competency differs by institution but may include knowledge tests, simulation, and/or review of completed cases.

Setting

Sedation is provided in many locations and for many different types of procedures that require varying depth of sedation. Although there is a greater risk for complications associated with deeper sedation levels, these can arise at any point [5]. One important aspect of maintaining a safe sedation environment is assuring the appropriate equipment and systems are in place to respond to emergencies in any location in which sedation occurs [6–8].

Equipment

Ensuring a safe environment begins with assuring that all emergency equipment is available in working order and in the appropriate sizes. A systematic approach is needed to ensure that all necessary equipment is available prior to starting any

Table 35.1 Pediatric sedation nurse moderate sedation competencies

Pre-procedure	Intra-sedation	Post-sedation
Knowledge Institution-approved sedation providers, locations, and procedures [a]Pre-procedure health-related questions to determine appropriateness for sedation	Knowledge Medications approved for provider use Sedative medication dosing, side effects, administration rate, administration interval, and applicable reversal agents Use of emergency medications and equipment	Knowledge Sedative medication duration and side effects Specific post-procedural requirements (e.g., positioning) Institution-approved discharge criteria and procedures
Actions Pre-sedation health evaluation and physical assessment immediately prior to sedation Verify consent Consider age-appropriate comfort/distraction techniques Verify/obtain intravenous access Review/obtain applicable laboratory work Perform pre-procedure education Prepare medications Evaluate sedation environment and equipment Perform time-out procedures	Actions Consider safety, procedural requirements, and comfort when positioning infant/child/adolescent Monitor physiologic parameters and sedation level throughout procedure using institutional guidelines Support airway, breathing, and circulation using appropriate equipment Document intra-sedation physiologic parameters, sedation levels, interventions, medications administered, and patient response at set intervals per institutional policy	Actions Maintain fall prevention procedures Maintain continuous physiologic monitoring until achieving institution-approved discharge criteria Assess and manage oxygenation (e.g., clearing airway, discontinuing airway adjuncts) as directed Assess for changes in sedation level using institution-approved scoring tool Assess and maintain hydration status or discontinue as directed Provide oral and written post-sedation care instruction to caregiver/transfer information including procedure specific, medication, safety, dietary precautions, and contact information for post-sedation care

[a]Questions vary by institution

Society for Pediatric Sedation Nursing Committee. Sedation Nurse Competencies: Society for Pediatric Sedation 2019 [cited 2019 April]. Available from: https://www.pedsedation.org/sps-nursing/

procedure. Table 35.2 outlines emergency sedation equipment using the acronym SOAPME [6]. Emergency response plans should include a process to assure that emergency equipment is readily available at the location where the procedure is completed and when transferring sedated patients from one location to another.

Remote Locations

Many sedation procedures occur outside of the intensive care unit. The need for sedation care in remote locations, however, can increase the risk of sedation due to

Table 35.2 Sedation equipment

S – Suction	Functioning Appropriate sized: Yankauer suction catheters
O – Oxygen	Functioning flowmeter, adequate supply Appropriate sized: cannula/mask
A – Airway	Functioning and appropriate sized: nasopharyngeal, oropharyngeal, endotracheal, face mask, stylet, bag valve mask (self-inflating/anesthesia), laryngoscope blade and handle
P – Pharmacy	Sedatives, analgesics, reversal agents, and emergency resuscitation medications
M – Monitors	Functioning and appropriate sized: pulse oximeter, noninvasive blood pressure/heart rate, stethoscope, end-tidal CO2
E – Extra equipment	Alcohol wipes, pacifier, saline flush, code cart (etc.)

Leroy et al. [4]

environmental factors that can lead to substandard monitoring combined with subsequent respiratory depression [9]. For example, high levels of acoustic noise, a dark environment, limited equipment compatibility, and obstructed patient visualization during magnetic resonance imaging (MRI) may compromise continuous monitoring of the sedated patient [7]. Preparations for logistical challenges such as proximity to emergency equipment, location of outlets and oxygen sources, and communication systems needed in the event an emergency response is required are important factors in assuring a safe environment [10]. Trainings using techniques such as simulation and frequent communication between the sedation personnel and personnel in the remote location are needed in order to adapt existing sedation practices and develop processes to maintain patient safely.

Patient Preparation

Prescreening

Pre-sedation screening techniques vary depending on the institutional sedation delivery system. When outpatient sedation services are provided within the intensive care unit, screening procedures are the same as those used for outpatients. Patient parents/caregivers are called prior to the procedure and asked a series of questions to determine if the patient is in an appropriate condition to be sedated and are provided with instructions for pre-sedation preparation. Depending on institutional policy, additional screening techniques may include requests for digital pictures to assess for presence of jaw or facial abnormalities. Nurses frequently perform this pre-sedation screen. Common prescreening questions include the following [8, 11, 12]:

- Past medical history
- Presence of allergies
- Patient and biological family anesthesia/sedation history

- Current medications
- History of chronic pulmonary or cardiac disease
- Obesity
- Central or obstructive sleep apnea
  - Documentation from a sleep study
  - Chronic snoring
  - Any jaw or facial abnormality
- Post-gestational age of neonates
- Swallowing dysfunction
- Presence of fever or any current illness
- Presence and type of internal or external medical devices
- Previous surgical procedures and any adverse reactions
- Presence of any syndromes (e.g., Pierre Robin, trisomy 21) that could increase the potential for airway or other sedation complications

Pre-sedation preparation for critically ill patients may require additional coordination or consultation prior to the planned procedure. Assessment of current intravenous access and compatibility with procedural sedatives, coordination with respiratory therapy for ventilated patients having a procedure outside the critical care unit, and consideration of fluid maintenance needs if enteral feeding is discontinued for NPO status are examples of additional steps needed prior to sedation. Alterations in personnel staffing may also be necessary in order to assure an adequate number of staff are available to respond to non-sedation-related unit needs while sedation is in progress.

Developmental Concerns

Understanding differences in the developmental needs of children is an integral part of providing comprehensive pediatric intensive care nursing [13]. The strategies used to address developmental needs vary depending on the child's baseline developmental level and current physiologic condition. Bright Futures, a pocket guide published by the American Academy of Pediatrics, is a free online comprehensive guide to expected motor and social developmental milestones throughout childhood that clinicians and parents/caregivers can use to identify developmentally supportive activities (http://brightfutures.aap.org/3rd_Edition_Guidelines_and_Pocket_Guide.html) [14]. Some of these practices, such as reading to children, can be incorporated into the intensive care unit setting. Developmental care practices can include alterations in the environment or individual patient interventions. Examples of environmental alterations in intensive care that support developmental needs include reducing environmental noise and light during usual naptime or regular sleep hours. Individual patient developmentally supportive interventions can include clustering care to reduce sleep interruptions at night and providing age-appropriate toys, music, or videos at the bedside when patients are awake and interactive activities such as video games. Several of these interventions can be integrated into the care provided during a procedure (e.g., MRI video goggles) or immediately pre- or post-sedation. Parents/caregivers and child life specialists are important partners in providing the child with developmentally supportive care during sedation and in educating the patient about the procedure and sedation process.

Parent/Caregiver and Patient Education

Pre- and post-sedation parent/caregiver and patient education is an important aspect of holistic care. An assessment of parent/caregiver and patient understanding of sedation and the procedure to be completed is necessary in order to identify any misconceptions that may exist [15]. Teaching should be individualized to address specific language needs, be developmentally appropriate, include strategies for parents/caregivers to partner in the pre- and post-sedation care of the patient, provide accurate information, and assist parents in setting post-sedation expectations.

Parent presence during sedation procedures if permitted by institutional policy may require additional education regarding anticipated changes in patient level of consciousness and safety precautions in locations such as radiology. When parents are not at the bedside, information about the anticipated length of the procedure, waiting areas, and mechanisms to obtain updates on their child can assist in reducing parent/caregiver anxiety about sedation.

Intra-procedural Considerations

Medication Administration

There are numerous sedative medications and medication administration routes that nurses must be familiar with. A detailed description of sedative and analgesic medication side effects, indications, doses, and precautions can be found in prior chapters. Nurses must be familiar with their individual state regulations and any organizational policies delineating dosing limitations, monitoring, or other precautions prior to administering sedative drugs. Nursing competencies related to sedative medications include knowledge of contraindications, side effects, appropriate and maximum dosing, route options, onset and duration of effects, as well as reversal agents whether administered by the nurse or other providers [11].

In the intensive care setting, intravenous access may be complicated depending on the number of medication infusions that may not be compatible with sedative medications (e.g., vasoactives, lipids). It is important to consult medication compatibility charts, the pharmacist, and medical team to determine if medication infusions must be altered to accommodate sedative medication boluses or infusions. If additional intravenous access is necessary, procedural needs should be considered when deciding the anatomical placement of the catheter. If a sedative infusion is intended, procurement of equipment such as a syringe/infusion pump should be obtained. Appropriate labeling of medication syringes/bags and lines as well as verification of the concentration and correct programming of infusions should be completed per institutional policy.

Time-Out and Monitoring

Time-out procedures including verification of the correct patient, site-marking procedures, and verification of correct procedures should be completed and documented per institutional policy.

Monitoring equipment (e.g., pulse oximetry probes, blood pressure cuffs) should be selected considering the patients' size, and alarm parameters should be set using age parameters and consideration of baseline readings. Verification of the presence of monitor tracings and functioning of equipment (e.g., blood pressure) should be determined when obtaining pre-sedation vital sign readings. Continuous monitoring including oxygen saturation, heart rate, respiratory rate, and capnography (as required by institutional policy) should be maintained throughout the procedure. Assessment of sedation level, airway patency, respiratory status, color, pain/comfort score, blood pressure, and temperature should be obtained and documented as delineated by institutional policy [11].

Continuous evaluation and communication of changes in monitoring parameters indicating complications should be immediately noted and appropriate interventions initiated. Table 35.3 outlines common sedation complications encountered during procedures and the applicable interventions [5, 16, 17]. Documentation of intra-procedural assessments, patient responses, and interventions should be completed as per institutional policy.

Post-procedural Considerations

Recovery Phase

Post-procedure recovery is affected by the sedative medications used and depth of sedation and may vary depending on individual patient response to medications. The length of the recovery period depends upon the patient's return to baseline physiologic status including level of consciousness. Inclusion of the parent/caregiver during the recovery period can provide comfort to the child and reduce parental anxiety. The same equipment, monitoring, and documentation requirements during the intra procedural phase should be maintained until the patient meets the criteria for discontinuation of sedation monitoring as delineated by institutional policy.

Table 35.3 Common sedation complications and interventions

Airway/breathing	Circulation	Neurologic
Complications		
Apnea Obstruction Laryngospasm Bronchospasm Secretions Poor ventilation Shallow	Hypotension Infiltrated IV access Bradycardia Hyperemesis	Emergence delirium "Failed" sedation Prolonged sedation Oversedation Uncontrolled pain
Interventions		
Airway positioning Bag-valve-mask ventilation Oral/nasal/tracheostomy/endotracheal suctioning Airway adjuncts Blowby oxygen Nasal cannula/face mask Oral and nasal airway	Intravenous fluid bolus and continuous infusion Central line and peripheral line management Chest compressions Vasoactive/emergency medication administration	Administration of reversal agents Safety precautions (e.g., seat belts, magnetic field precautions) Administration of analgesic medications and initiation of developmentally appropriate comfort measures

Society for Pediatric Sedation Nursing Committee. Sedation Nurse Competencies: Society for Pediatric Sedation 2019 [cited 2019 April]. Available from: https://www.pedsedation.org/sps-nursing/

Monitoring for Complications

Continuous monitoring for the same complications and interventions described in the intra-procedural sedation phase should occur during sedation recovery, refer to Table 35.3. Additional safety precautions that should be put in place include positioning the patient to maintain airway patency using a neck/shoulder roll, maintaining procedure-related requirements (e.g., securing dressings, side-lying position), and removing airway adjuncts and oxygen delivery systems as patient returns to baseline oxygenation. Discontinuation of intravenous fluid such as removing the peripheral intravenous catheter or flushing lines that are no longer in use may also be required. The patient's developmental comfort needs such as adequate pain control and potential safety hazards including risk for falls should also be addressed.

Discharge/Transfer/Discontinuation of Recovery Monitoring

Once the patient's physiologic and neurologic status returns to baseline and/or institutional criteria to discontinue recovery monitoring are met, the patient may be prepared for discharge or transfer. Discharge criteria often include standard measurement tools to detect return to pre-sedation status including pain level and hydration status. Documentation of vital signs, sedation level, and recovery measures should be completed prior to discharge or transfer.

Discharge/Transfer Education

Discharge instructions provided to parent/caregiver/receiving provider may vary depending on the specific side effects and potential complications associated with the sedative agents used. Parents should receive information (verbal and written) about the signs and symptoms of common problems, such as potential airway complications, falls risk, appropriate diet advancement, timing to restart at home medications, and contact information for the sedation provider in the event questions arise. Prescriptions for at-home analgesics as well as recommendations for alternative pharmacologic and non-pharmacologic pain control should also be provided. Lastly, restrictions or requirements associated with the procedure and instructions for follow-up appointments/consultations should be provided at discharge.

Follow-Up

Evaluation of sedation outcomes including patient status after discharge/transfer is necessary in order to detect delayed complications. This if often accomplished through telephone calls to parents/caregivers or contact with the accepting patient care unit. Follow-up questions assess complications such as nausea/vomiting, pain level, and changes in respiratory or neurologic condition or the need to obtain a higher level of care (e.g., emergency department visit/increased inpatient monitoring). Follow-up data should be incorporated into existing quality improvement processes.

References

1. Crego N. Procedural sedation practice: a review of current nursing standards. J Nursing Regulat. 2015;6(1):50–6.
2. National Council of State Boards of Nursing. Guiding principles of nursing regulation: National Council of State Boards of Nursing; 2007. Available from: https://www.ncsbn.org/1325.htm
3. American Nurses Association. Position statement on professional role competence. American Nurses Association; 2014. https://www.nursingworld.org/practice-policy/nursing-excellence/official-position-statements/id/professional-role-competence/
4. Leroy PL, Schipper DM, Knape HJ. Professional skills and competence for safe and effective procedural sedation in children: recommendations based on a systematic review of the literature. Int J Pediatr. 2010;2010:934298.
5. Cravero JP, Blike GT, Beach M, Gallagher SM, Hertzog JH, Havidich JE, et al. Incidence and nature of adverse events during pediatric sedation/anesthesia for procedures outside the operating room: report from the Pediatric Sedation Research Consortium. Pediatrics. 2006;118(3):1087–96.
6. Cote CJ, Wilson S. American Academy of Pediatric Dentistry, American Academy of Pediatrics. Guidelines for monitoring and management of pediatric patients before, during,

and after sedation for diagnostic and therapeutic procedures: update 2016. Pediatr Dentist. 2016;38(4):E19c–E39.

7. Practice Guidelines for Moderate Procedural Sedation and Analgesia 2018: a report by the American Society of Anesthesiologists Task Force on Moderate Procedural Sedation and Analgesia, the American Association of Oral and Maxillofacial Surgeons, American College of Radiology, American Dental Association, American Society of Dentist Anesthesiologists, and Society of Interventional Radiology. Anesthesiology. 2018;128(3):437–79.
8. Mason KP. Pediatric sedation outside the operating room. New York: Springer; 2012.
9. Eichhorn V, Henzler D, Murphy MF. Standardizing care and monitoring for anesthesia or procedural sedation delivered outside the operating room. Curr Opin Anaesthesiol. 2010;23(4):494–9.
10. Lu AC, Wald SH, Sun EC. Into the wilderness?: The growing importance of Nonoperating Room Anesthesia Care in the United States. Anesth Analg. 2017;124(4):1044–6.
11. Society for Pediatric Sedation Nursing Committee. Sedation Nurse Competencies: Society for Pediatric Sedation 2019 [cited 2019 April]. Available from: https://www.pedsedation.org/sps-nursing/.
12. Gooden CK, Lowrie LH, Jackson BF. The pediatric procedural sedation handbook. New York: Oxford Press; 2018.
13. Curtis K, Foster K, Mitchell R, Van C. Models of care delivery for families of critically ill children: an integrative review of international literature. J Pediatr Nurs. 2016;31(3):330–41.
14. Hagan JF, Duncan PM. Bright futures guidelines for health supervision of infants, children and adolescents [pocket guide]. 4th ed. Elk Grove Village: American Academy of Pediatrics; 2017.
15. Panella JJ. Preoperative care of children: strategies from a child life perspective. AORN J. 2016;104(1):11–22.
16. Crego N, Baernholdt M, Merwin E. Differences in pediatric non-interventional radiology procedural sedation practices and adverse events by registered nurses and physicians. J Pediatr Nurs. 2017;35:129–33.
17. Mallory MD, Travers C, McCracken CE, Hertzog J, Cravero JP. Upper respiratory infections and airway adverse events in pediatric procedural sedation. Pediatrics. 2017;140(1):e20170009. https://doi.org/10.1542/peds.2017-0009

Part X
Sedation Training

Chapter 36
Simulation in Pediatric Procedural Sedation

Girish G. Deshpande, Gregory S. Podolej, and Nadia Shaikh

Introduction

Pediatric procedural sedation (PPS) is commonly employed to help minimize pain and anxiety during medical procedures as well as provide sedation for diagnostic imaging studies.

Infants and children represent a high-risk population due to their airway anatomy, cardiorespiratory physiology, and varying responses to sedation-analgesia medications [1]. Premature and young infants as well as high ASA (IV–V) class patients are more likely to experience adverse events related to sedation-analgesia administration [2].

Cote et al. in their 2000 landmark study described adverse events associated with pediatric sedation including respiratory depression (most common), oxygen desaturation, laryngospasm, cardiac arrest, and bradycardia, resulting from inadequate monitoring, inadequate pre-sedation evaluation, medication errors, and inadequate resuscitation by the providers [3].

The American Academy of Pediatrics revised the guidelines for pediatric procedural sedation by non-anesthesiologists in 2016 [4]. Adherence to such guidelines and performance of structured risk assessments have decreased the risk associated with PPS [5]. Furthermore, the Joint Commission on Accreditation of Healthcare

G. G. Deshpande (✉)
Critical Care Medicine, University of Illinois College of Medicine at Peoria, Children's Hospital of Illinois, Peoria, IL, USA
e-mail: girish@uic.edu

G. S. Podolej
Emergency Medicine, OSF St Francis Medical Center, Peoria, IL, USA

N. Shaikh
Pediatric Hospital Medicine, University of Illinois College of Medicine at Peoria, Children's Hospital of Illinois, Peoria, IL, USA
e-mail: nshaikh@uic.edu

P. P. Kamat, J. W. Berkenbosch (eds.), *Sedation and Analgesia for the Pediatric Intensivist*, https://doi.org/10.1007/978-3-030-52555-2_36

Organizations (JCAHO) guidelines require that a sedation practitioner be able to rescue a patient from a level of sedation deeper than intended [6].

Analysis of settled injury and liability claims found that, in addition to poor resuscitation, a delay in resuscitation (caused by a lack of vigilance and ignoring warnings from alarm systems) resulted in injury to patients. The authors of the article concluded that respiratory depression caused by over-sedation was a principal mechanism of injury which could be prevented by appropriate monitoring, vigilance by the provider, and early resuscitation [2].

The Role of Simulation in PPS

Simulation is a versatile tool within the realm of PPS. In the following paragraphs, we will discuss the utility of simulation within the context of clinical training, system and process improvement, as well as evaluation and assessment of patients. Simulation allows learners to experience realistic high-risk and high-acuity scenarios in a safe learning environment without exposing patients to risk [7]. High-fidelity simulators provide ideal opportunities for hands-on training with the use of real instruments and can demonstrate realistic adverse reactions such as laryngospasm or respiratory depression. Simulators can also be used to maintain rarely used critical skills such as cardiopulmonary resuscitation.

Simulation-based medical education (SBME) has become a cornerstone of medical education and has been shown to be superior to standard education with respect to skill acquisition and retention [8]. The concept of deliberate practice allows learners to repeat process to mastery learning [9] in order to assimilate key concepts (knowledge base and problem-solving) and learn the attitudes (team dynamics) and procedural skills (hands-on learning) required of successful PPS.

A PPS training curriculum must primarily meet the needs of the learners and implement the IOM quality framework with a focus on providing safe, effective, timely, patient-centered, efficient, and equitable clinical care [10]. These needs should be reflected in the learning objectives, course content, and learner assessments. The curricular development process requires rigorous planning in order to optimize resource allocation.

Debriefing

> If simulation is the body, then debriefing is its soul. – Girish Deshpande, MD

Debriefing is defined by Fanning and Gaba as a "facilitated or guided reflection in the cycle of experiential learning." This involves active participation of learners, guided by a trained facilitator or instructor whose primary goal is to help learners identify and close gaps in their knowledge and skills [11, 12]. Debriefing facilitates introspection by the learners of their performance during the simulation scenario. This self-reflection is a powerful learning experience which helps incorporate the learning objectives into future actions. Debriefing may be augmented by recorded video-playback as it provides an objective, time-coded record of trainee communication and actions and creates a powerful stimulus for learning.

Simulation with debriefing can be used for both training and assessment. For formative assessment, we recommend using structured debriefing after simulation with an emphasis on learner perspectives. For summative assessments, we recommend a rigorous standard setting procedure followed by a simulation-based assessment with a goal toward mastery learning. Table 36.1 provides several suggested critical actions that can be both taught and assessed using simulation. Instructors will find that simulation is helpful in providing comprehensive training including knowledge, procedural skills, as well as teamwork.

Types of Simulators (Table 36.2)

There are multiple simulation modalities that can be utilized to meet the needs of a PPS training curriculum. The use of simulation technology should be based on the learning objectives with consideration of available resources. High-fidelity simulation can be cost prohibitive and may not be required in every scenario. For example, if the educational objective is to practice bag-valve mask ventilation or intubation, this can be accomplished via a simple task trainer. If the learning objective is to monitor complex drug interactions or simulate nuances in airway management, then a high-fidelity mannequin would be best suited for this role. When possible, the use of high-fidelity simulation helps assimilate the multitude of competencies required of PPS as well as recreate the complexities of patient care.

Simulation modalities extend beyond silicone. In addition to computer-based simulation training, recent advances in technology have led to the development of widely available virtual reality (VR) modules that can completely immerse learners in their environments with extreme fidelity. The majority of this software is still proprietary and not available commercially at the time of this publication.

Institutional Application of Simulation in PPS (Clinical Training and Team Dynamics, System and Process Improvement, Quality and Safety Initiatives)

Many hospitals and medical institutions have accepted simulation as a modality for clinical training, building team dynamics, system and process improvement, as well as quality and safety initiatives. The following outline provides a structure to be considered when incorporating simulation in PPS at the institutional level and helps the instructor to decide which modality best suits the needs of the program.

Table 36.1 Using simulation for PPS critical actions

	Select critical actions during sedation	Benefit of simulation	Limitation of simulation
1	History and physical examination	Key portions of history and physical can be practiced to mastery learning standards, amenable to checklists	Mannequin may not accurately mimic certain anatomic abnormalities (e.g., Pierre Robin or difficult airway). Standardized participants are required for the history
2	Establishing intravenous (IV) access for moderate to deep sedation	Learners are able to practice all the steps of the procedure without harming patients	Mannequin IV sites may not adequately mimic difficulty of placing a pediatric IV where patients need to be restrained or held
3	Selection of appropriate sedation drugs	Learners can become familiar with the physiologic response to various sedative agents without risk to patients	Only high-fidelity mannequins can be programmed to respond to specific stimuli
4	Continuous monitoring during sedation	Learners recognize the importance of monitoring changes in vital signs including end-tidal CO2 and oxygen saturation in a variety of circumstances	Nuances in physiologic changes can only be recreated with high-fidelity mannequins or mimicked by programming the monitor
5	Airway skills: Jaw thrust, head positioning, oral, nasopharyngeal airway	Learners can practice these critical procedures with low-fidelity mannequins or task trainers in a safe environment without patient harm	Mannequins cannot fully recreate the realism of human patient anatomy
6	Bag-mask ventilation		
7	Endotracheal intubation		
8	Addressing sedation complications (e.g., laryngospasm, hypotension, adverse drug response)	Rarely encountered adverse reactions can be practiced on-demand and tailored to learner needs	Not all simulation modalities or simulation mannequins can realistically replicate these responses. May require high-fidelity or VR simulation
9	Teamwork	Principles of teamwork can be practiced until proficiency is achieved	None
10	Leadership skills	Leadership skill can be taught using simulation and can be reinforced until team achieves proficiency	None

Table 36.2 Selected List of Simulation Mannequins and their role in PPS simulation

Manufacturer	Mannequin model	Description	Application in PPS simulation
Gaumard	Premie™ Blue	High-fidelity 28-week premature infant	Establishing intravenous (IV) access for moderate to deep sedation Continuous monitoring during sedation Airway skills: Jaw thrust, head positioning, oral, nasopharyngeal airway Bag-mask ventilation Endotracheal intubation Addressing sedation complications (e.g., laryngospasm, hypotension, adverse drug response) Teamwork
	Premie HAL®	High-fidelity 30-week premature infant	
	Premie HAL® Skills Trainer	High-fidelity 24-week premature infant	
	Super Tory® Advanced Newborn Patient Simulator	Ultra-high-fidelity full-term newborn	
	Newborn Tory® Neonatal Care Patient Simulator	High-fidelity full-term newborn	
	Newborn HAL® Full-Term Newborn Patient Simulator	High-fidelity full-term newborn	
	Code Blue® III Newborn Advanced Life Support Training Simulator	High-fidelity full-term newborn	
	PEDI® Blue Newborn Patient Simulator	High-fidelity full-term newborn	
	Multipurpose Patient Newborn	High-fidelity full-term newborn	
	Pediatric HAL® – Pediatric Patient Simulator	Ultra-high-fidelity pediatric mannequin	
	Code Blue® III Pediatric Advanced Life Support Training Simulator	High-fidelity pediatric mannequin	
	Pediatric HAL® S3004	One-year-old pediatric patient high-fidelity simulator	
	Five-Year-Old Multipurpose Patient Simulator (S157)	High-fidelity 5-year-old pediatric simulator	
	Pediatric HAL® S3005	Five-year-old pediatric patient high-fidelity simulator	
	One-Year-Old Multipurpose Patient Simulator	One-year-old pediatric patient high-fidelity simulator	
Koken	Neonatal Resuscitation Model	High-fidelity mannequin with manual bulb for pulsation	
Nasco	Pediatric Simulator 3	Computer-based pediatric simulator	
Laerdal	Premature Anne™	High-fidelity portable wireless 25-week-old premature infant	
	Premature Anne™ Task Trainer	High-fidelity 25-week-old premature infant	
	SimNewB®	High-fidelity newborn infant, wireless	

(continued)

Table 36.2 (continued)

Manufacturer	Mannequin model	Description	Application in PPS simulation
Laerdal	Nursing Kid	Low-fidelity task training mannequin	Establishing intravenous (IV) access for moderate to deep sedation Continuous monitoring during sedation Airway skills: Jaw thrust, head positioning, oral, nasopharyngeal airway Bag-mask ventilation Endotracheal intubation Teamwork
	Nursing Baby	Low-fidelity task training mannequin	
CAE Healthcare	Luna	High-fidelity neonatal mannequin	
	BabySIM	High-fidelity infant mannequin	
	PediaSIM	High-fidelity 6-year-old pediatric mannequin	
Gaumard	One-Year-Old PEDI®	One-year-old pediatric patient high-fidelity simulator	
Gaumard	Newborn PEDI® Newborn Skills Trainer	Full-term newborn	
Gaumard	Susie® and Simon® Newborn Patient Simulator	High-fidelity full-term newborn	*Note-Features vary with model number Establishing intravenous (IV) access for moderate to deep sedation Airway skills: Jaw thrust, head positioning, oral, nasopharyngeal airway Bag-mask ventilation Teamwork
Simulaids	Pediatric Intubation Head	Airway training simulation head	Airway skills: Jaw thrust, head positioning, oral, nasopharyngeal airway Bag-mask ventilation Endotracheal intubation
TruCorp	Pediatric Intubation Head	Airway training simulation head	
Gaumard	One-Year-Old Pediatric Airway Trainer	Airway training mannequin	
	5-Year-Old Patient, PEDI® Airway Trainer	Airway training mannequin	
Laerdal	Pediatric Intubation Trainer	Low-fidelity airway training mannequin	
	Neonatal Intubation Trainer	Airway training simulation head	
Laerdal	Newborn Anne™	Low-fidelity full-term newborn	Airway skills: Jaw thrust, head positioning, oral, nasopharyngeal airway Bag-mask ventilation Endotracheal intubation Teamwork
Laerdal	NeoNatalie™	Low-fidelity inflatable neonatal mannequin, portable	Airway skills: Jaw thrust, head positioning, oral, nasopharyngeal airway Bag-mask ventilation Teamwork

Manufacturer	Mannequin model	Description	Application in PPS simulation
TruCorp	TruMonitor App	Patient monitor simulator	Continuous monitoring during sedation Addressing sedation complications (e.g., laryngospasm, hypotension, adverse drug response)
Gaumard	1-Year-Old Patient Injection Training Arm	Pediatric task trainer	Establishing intravenous (IV) access for moderate to deep sedation
	Newborn Injection Training Arm	Pediatric task trainer	
	5-Year-Old Patient Injection Training Arm	Pediatric task trainer	
Laerdal	Infant Virtual I.V. (Discontinued)	Virtual reality pediatric IV trainer with haptic feedback	
Gaumard	Mike® and Michelle® One-Year-Old Pediatric Care Simulator	Low-fidelity pediatric simulator	Teamwork

1. Scenario Development: learning objectives, learners, case content
2. Location: in situ vs simulation lab
3. Resource Allocation: time, faculty availability, standardized participants, equipment
4. Assessment: debriefing, formative vs summative

Curriculum Development for Sedation-Analgesia and Clinical Training

Exposure to procedural sedation and analgesia during residency training can be limited and occurs only during select pediatric critical care or emergency department rotations. Because of this, several academic programs have developed their own curricula for trainees based on the needs of the institution and core competencies as required by the Residency Review Committee [13].

The Society for Pediatric Sedation (SPS) is another source for multidisciplinary leadership in advancing the quality and safety of pediatric sedations. They offer a Sedation Provider Course – a 1-day course intended to provide sedation practitioners with the basic knowledge and core competencies that promote safe and effective procedural sedation practices for children. More importantly, the course is designed to meet the needs of the experienced sedation provider seeking both cognitive (didactic)- and psychomotor (simulation)-based education and training. It focuses on patient selection and risk assessment (safety), general approach to procedural sedation, monitoring, drug pharmacology, and the recognition and management of the more common sedation-related adverse events.

Simulations can be conducted both in the simulation centers and in situ. The benefits of in situ simulations are that they can be used for evaluation of team members and detecting latent errors in the system. In situ simulations are often unannounced and serve to familiarize learners with the actual setting and equipment utilized in patient care. They can be performed at any time of day or night. The drawbacks are that they only target the learners on shift and may interrupt the clinical workflow.

Simulations in a simulation center can be used for training or standardized testing. They are often scheduled so that learners can prepare for them mentally and they minimize interruption of clinical workflow. They are usually limited temporally to day time hours and also by the equipment available in the simulation center (which may not reflect that used in the clinical environment).

Though we provide a brief synopsis of benefits and limitations of simulation modalities, the benefits and limitations of both in situ and simulation center scenarios are described in detail in the 2008 AHRQ publication *Advances in Patient Safety: New Directions and Alternative Approaches; Vol 3: Performance and Tools* [14].

Sedation-Analgesia Team Dynamics

A team is defined as "Two or more individuals with specialized knowledge and skills who perform specific roles and complete interdependent tasks to achieve a common goal or outcome" [15].

In most settings, sedation team members have the benefit of familiarity with each other on both professional and personal levels and have previously established team roles. In pediatric code situations, the nearest responders who provide care often do not have the advantage of being familiar with their team members and must rely on their individual communication skills and knowledge of team dynamics to facilitate patient care. This area is ripe for a simulation-based approach which has shown improvement in education, patient safety, and team training [16, 17]. Team dynamics play a significant role in patient outcomes in acute situations which underscores the importance of practice and for coordinated efforts for optimal human resource management in order to deliver safe and effective care.

TeamSTEPPS (Team Strategies and Tools for Enhancing Performance and Patient Safety) is a program introduced by the Agency for Healthcare Research and Quality (AHRQ) and the Department of Defense (DoD) in collaboration with the American Institute for Research in 2002 to identify best practices and set the standard for medical team training. It identifies four essential components of effective team training: leadership, situation monitoring, mutual support, and communication. These can be used as the outcomes and evaluation parameters while training the sedation teams [18].

The main themes in crisis resource management have been identified by Cheng et al. (2012): leadership and followership, communication, teamwork, resource use, and situational awareness [19]. We utilize this framework to enumerate the critical elements of teamwork below:

Elements of Teamwork (Diagram 36.1)

a. *Leadership*: Usually rests on the shoulders of the sedation provider. Leader positions himself/herself to have an overall view of the patient and cardiorespiratory monitors, as well as the team members. The responsibility of the leader includes assigning the roles to all team members; analyzing, interpreting, and sharing the information received; and creating a shared mental model about the situation at hand. The leader also gives constructive feedback (performance monitoring) and provides support and interchanges the roles based on the skill needs (backup behavior) while being respectful of all team members.

b. *Team Members (Followership)*: Sedation nurses, advanced practice providers, residents, and clinical technicians are often members of the team. The team members need to be competent at their individual tasks while at the same time facilitating teamwork by sharing their observations, interpretations, and interventions with the leader. They need to feel safe and empowered to share their thoughts in critical settings (flattening of hierarchy). They need to be respectful of constructive feedback and correct their actions to make their interventions effective.

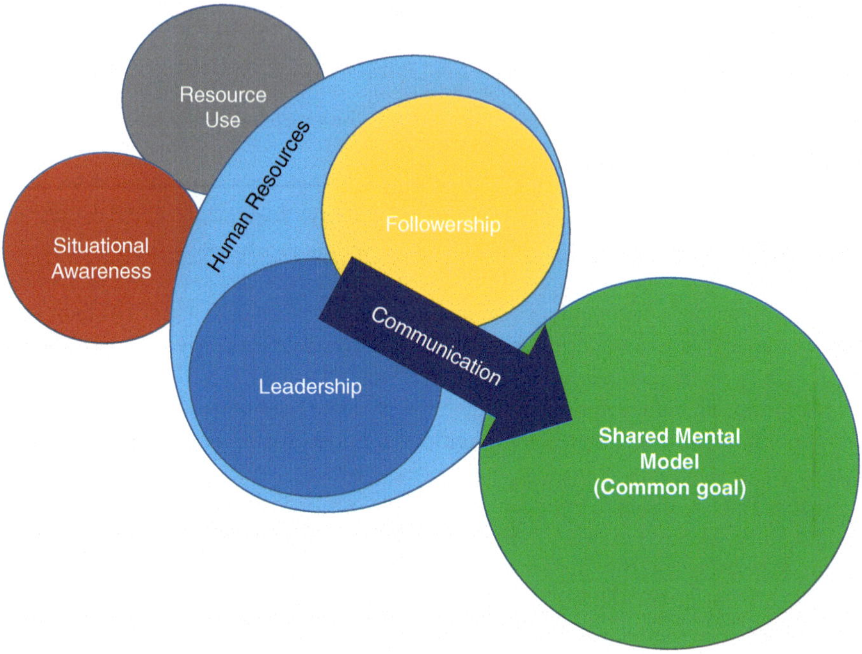

Diagram 36.1 Elements and interactions of team dynamics (Original contribution courtesy of Dr. Girish Deshpande)

c. *Communication*: Arguably this is the most important component of effective teamwork. Greater than two-thirds of errors in medical management are due to breakdown in communication. Components of communication are:

   i. *Assertive communication*: The "flattening of hierarchy" is achieved when all team members feel empowered to speak up if they have concern that something might be wrong. Team leaders can encourage this behavior by intermittently asking for the input of the team members.
   ii. *Closed-loop communication*: When the leader gives an instruction to a team member, the team member should verbally acknowledge the instruction, repeat the instruction back to the leader (check-back), and report to the leader once the instruction is completed or followed.
   iii. *Information sharing and inquiry*: This is the ongoing process of bidirectional (leader to team member and vice versa) knowledge-sharing and real-time corrections of errors. This helps prevent inappropriate actions and minimizes fixation errors.

d. *Human Resources*: The leader should constantly reassess the utilization of human resources (team members) to ensure that all the needed team roles are safely and effectively fulfilled such that tasks are carried out successfully.

e. *Material Resources*: All equipment necessary for resuscitation is in good working order and readily available for use by team members familiar with the location and operation of the supplies.
f. *Situational Awareness*: The team should be aware of the dynamic status of the patient during resuscitation and base their perceptions on the latest information available. It is a good practice to periodically have a team huddle (or "recap") to review the condition of the patient and response to interventions (shared mental model). The leader should also make sure to attend to the patient's family (if present) at the bedside and/or assign an alternative individual to do so.

System and Process Improvement
Simulation can be used for evaluating providers and team members for credentialing, for re-credentialing, and for detecting latent errors or system issues. It is also useful for process improvement or risk mitigation purposes when migrating into new clinical environments. Simulation-based assessment (SBA) has already been used in regulatory systems for healthcare professionals. For example, successful completion of the Fundamentals of Laparoscopic Surgery course is now required by the American Board of Surgery for initial certification in surgery. Several SBAs are being used for as part of the American Board of Medical Specialties maintenance of certification (MOC) program. The American Board of Anesthesiology requires completion of simulator training as a part of its MOC program, and the American Board of Internal Medicine provides a cardiac catheterization simulator formative assessment as an option for interventional cardiologists [20].

System's Issues
Problems surrounding the organizational, human, technical, and facility-related systems can be identified and rectified using simulation especially when a new facility is opened for patient care. Villamaria et al. in their study "Using simulation to orient code blue teams to a new hospital facility" concluded that clinical simulation can be effectively used to orient code blue teams and identify critical safety issues in a newly constructed healthcare facility [21].

The use of in situ simulation has become standard for not only education but also as a tool for prospective systems analysis for the identification and mitigation of latent safety threats [14]. A variety of follow-up interventions (both formal and informal) have been deployed to address outcomes of these events including bedside just-in-time education, the development or adaptation of formal educational curricula, policy changes, and various process improvement methods. In situ simulation also allows the ability to re-test the system of care following interventions. Integration of the program within the institutional quality and safety reporting structure allows the information to remain protected while providing a mechanism to utilize the error reporting system for simulated events and allow routine communication back to the administrative level where policy change often originates. To promote this culture of safety, information is always de-identified, and findings are never punitive or linked to individual participants. At this institution, findings have been categorized into three main areas: clinical care/education, equipment, and systems/process. Examples issues identified for each category are listed below

Table 36.3 Examples of system issues identified during in situ simulations

Category	Finding	Actions taken
Clinical care/education	Use of a pump for rapid fluid bolus was insufficient Medication dosing and location for benzodiazepines for acute seizure	Bedside education followed by integration of rapid infusion techniques for providers Bedside education and revision of medication storage area
Equipment	Broselow tape missing from code cart	Immediate notification of central supply, cross-check of all existing carts
Systems/process	Delayed response by rapid response team after change in unit location Lack of access for off-unit providers serving on rapid response team into med room where glucose monitoring devices were kept Differentiating the use of the rapid response team vs code blue team	Immediate addition of wayfinding signage, education within huddles and via email for to address Immediate change in badge access Policy clarification, education, and signage

Table 36.4 Examples of learner feedback. Question: Following the simulation, can you identify a change in your practice? If so, please provide an example

Clinical care	Communication/teamwork
Use of diazepam before lorazepam based on available and accessibility in unit Differentiating SVT perfusing vs SVT with poor perfusion Upper extremity access for adenosine	Ask questions when not sure why a medical decision was made – exp. ice to face; ask who leader is Make sure a PERT (rapid response) is called Make sure dose/route is right/better communication

(Table 36.3). Follow-up feedback is solicited from each participant and includes an opportunity to identify a change in practice (Table 36.4). Informal qualitative analysis of comments for in situ simulations between 2016 and 2018 revealed that errors were equally divided between clinical care and teamwork communication. Aggregate results were presented to unit managers and quality and safety leaders (unpublished data, courtesy of Trina Croland, MD).

Examples of Clinical Simulation Scenarios

Following are simulation case scenarios for learners to serve as a guide:

1. *Scenario*: learning objectives, learners, case content
2. *Location*: in situ vs simulation lab

3. *Resources*: time, faculty availability, standardized participants, equipment
4. *Assessment*: debriefing, formative vs summative

Location All the following scenarios can be conducted as in situ (mock code) or in simulation lab.

Resources To conduct these training sessions, you will require high-fidelity mannequins, standardized participants as a parent, a confederate nurse, a trained facilitator, and equipment including pediatric crash cart, etc.

Case Scenario 1

Learning Objectives:

- Identify chest wall rigidity as an adverse effect of fentanyl.
- Appropriate management of chest wall rigidity.
- Documentation and disclosure to the family.
- Team dynamics.

Case Content

A 6-month-old infant is undergoing sedation-analgesia for bone marrow aspiration in the Procedure room located on the Pediatric ICU. Infant has pancytopenia identified on a CBC performed for his pallor and tiredness. There is no other significant medical, birth, and perinatal history. There are no known allergies. Immunizations are up to date. He is currently on amoxicillin for otitis media. His vitals are as follows: temp., 36.9 °C; HR, 140/min; RR. 28/min; BP, 72/43 mm Hg; and SpO2, 100% on room air. The infant appears pale and has few bruises over his extremities; otherwise extremities are warm and well perfused with brisk capillary refill. Oropharynx is normal with pale mucous membranes. Lungs are clear to auscultation. Heart sounds are normal with soft ejection systolic murmur. His abdomen is soft with moderately enlarged liver and spleen. Infant is awake and has no focal motor deficits.

You choose combination of propofol and fentanyl for sedation and analgesia after obtaining informed consent from the parents. Patient is on the cardiorespiratory monitor and nasal end-tidal CO2. Timeout is observed. Upon administration of fentanyl by a new nurse, infant suddenly becomes cyanotic, with desaturations down to 60%, and his heart rate drops down to 80s with no visible respirations. End-tidal CO2 not picking up. You do not notice any chest rise spontaneously or with bagging that is requiring higher pressures. Patient continues to have desaturations.

Expected Actions:

1. Position the head and continue bag-mask ventilation.
2. Call for naloxone IV 0.01mg/kg and prepare for Rapid Sequence Intubation (with midazolam,vecuronium).

Debriefing Points:

1. Identification of adverse event and interpretation of end-tidal CO2.
2. Fentanyl-induced chest wall rigidity – needs naloxone or a paralytic.
3. Root cause of the adverse event – system issues identification.
4. Honest and complete disclosure and documentation.

Case Scenario 2

Learning Objectives:

- Recognition of medication interactions
- Documentation and disclosure to the family

Case Content

A 7-month-old infant with history of new-onset seizure is admitted for work-up. Patient has had low-grade fever for the past 2 days with URI symptoms. He has no other significant medical history. His immunizations are up to date. There are no known allergies. Patient has been obtunded and very agitated to be held still. Neurologist wants to measure the opening pressure while doing lumbar puncture (LP). Pediatric ICU fellow decides to perform LP under sedation-analgesia using midazolam and fentanyl.

His vitals prior to the procedure are as follows: T, 38.9 °C; HR, 148/min; RR, 38/min; BP, 81/42 mm Hg; and SpO2, 99% on room air. Lungs/heart/abdomen examination is normal. No focal motor deficits are identified; patient is extremely squirmy during positioning for LP. Sedation medications are pushed, and the patient goes into deep sedation with hypoventilation (RR: 12/min), hypotension (63/32 mm Hg), and desaturations (down to 80s) after 0.1 mg/kg of midazolam. Patient's airway is adjusted, and he continues to require bagging so the fellow decides to give him the reversal agent flumazenil. Patient develops generalized tonic-clonic seizures.

Expected Actions:

1. Airway opening by positioning, with bag-mask ventilation.
2. Administer IV midazolam 0.1 mg/kg for seizures.
3. IV fluid bolus of NS 20 ml/kg.
4. If no improvement: proceed with RSI.

Debriefing Points:

1. Drug interactions should be reviewed closely prior to case initiation. In this case flumazenil is contraindicated in patient with seizures and should have been avoided.
2. Supportive care with airway management and fluid boluses generally suffices to stabilize such events.
3. Honest and complete disclosure and documentation of the event.

Case Scenario 3

Learning Objectives:
- Common sedation complications and interventions

Case Content
A 6-year-old patient is undergoing a scheduled lumbar puncture for intrathecal chemotherapy and bone marrow aspiration for acute lymphoblastic leukemia. Patient is otherwise asymptomatic and has been afebrile. His vital signs are as follows: T, 37.8 °C; HR, 108/min; RR, 24/min; BP, 108/68 mm Hg; and SpO2, 98% on room air. His cardiovascular and pulmonary examination is normal. Liver is 3 cm below the right costal margin, and spleen is 2 cm below the left costal margin. He is awake and has no focal motor deficits.

You decide to use midazolam and ketamine for sedation-analgesia. You administer 0.1 mg/kg of midazolam intravenously followed by 1 mg/kg of ketamine. Patient develops nystagmus in eyes within a minute, immediately followed by severe respiratory distress with cough and desaturations down to 80s. HR is 158/min; BP is 147/85 mm Hg; and RR in 40s. Patient also develops high-pitched inspiratory sound.

Expected Actions:
1. Bag-mask ventilation.
2. Deepen the sedation with IV propofol 1 mg/kg.
3. Prepare for RSI, if no improvement: proceed with RSI.

Debriefing Points:
1. Ketamine can induce life-threatening laryngospasm requiring administering PPV or deepening of sedation.
2. If patient is dropping saturations and blood pressure quickly, he needs to be paralyzed and intubated immediately.

Case Scenario 4

Learning Objectives:
Common sedation complications and interventions

Case Content
A 5-year-old, previously healthy child is undergoing MRI of the brain for recurrent headaches for the past 3 weeks. He is immunized, has no allergies, and has no significant medical or surgical history. His initial vitals are as follows: T, 37.3 °C; HR, 108/min; RR, 26/min; BP, 96/58 mm Hg; and SpO2, 99% on room air. He weighs 20 kg. Physician orders 1/kg propofol and the new nurse hands over 1 ml/kg propofol. Physician administers the propofol that was handed to him. Right after the

initial bolus, the patient goes apneic, with SpO2 85% and falling with HR 80/min and rapidly falling and BP 68/44 mm Hg. When asked you tell the team that the patient was given 1 ml/kg (20 ml) of propofol instead of 1 mg/kg [20 mg which is 2 ml as the concentration is 10 mg/ml].

Expected Actions:

1. Bag-mask ventilation until patient recovers

Debriefing Points:

1. Identifying system errors ranging from medication order to medication administration and risk mitigation.
2. Always clarifying the units of the drugs by readback method.
3. Medicine administration errors are completely preventable if one uses appropriate precautions while ordering, writing, drawing in a syringe, or administering. While ordering, be clear about the unit of the drug, the route, and over how much duration it needs to be administered.

Case Scenario 5

Learning Objectives:

Cumulative effect of sedation-analgesia medications

Case Content

A 10-year-old boy is admitted to Pediatric Intermediate Care Unit a week ago, for partial amputation of right foot as a result of foot getting caught in an auger on the farm. He underwent wound debridement and surgical amputation of front half of right foot a day after admission. Currently he is receiving hydromorphone PCA at a basal rate with intermittent boluses with lockout for pain management.

You are scheduled to provide sedation-analgesia for dressing and wound vac. change in am. He is otherwise healthy and has no allergies. After talking to parents, you decide to use propofol and fentanyl for the procedural sedation. His initial vital signs are as follows: HR 100/min, RR 22/min, BP 118/68, and SpO2 100% on room air. He weighs 50 kgs. Oropharyngeal examination is Mallampati 3 with no loose teeth, and the rest of the systemic exam is normal except for the amputated right foot. You administer 1 mg/kg IV propofol. You repeat another dose of propofol, followed by 50 mcg of fentanyl as he is not completely asleep. Propofol infusion is started at 2 mg/kg/hour by RN. As they start with dressing change, you hear stertor, and SpO2 is 94% on room air.

Expected Actions:

1. Move to the head end of the bed and apply jaw thrust and have someone listen for air exchange.
2. Look at end-tidal CO2.

3. Stop/titrate down propofol infusion until stable.
4. Start supplemental oxygen via nasal cannula.
5. Be ready with bag-mask ventilation and consider if patient has continued desaturations or apnea.
6. Consider naloxone for apnea.

Debriefing Points:
1. Taking into account the cumulative effect of sedation regimen in patients on strong analgesia protocol.
2. Patient has just taken the dose of hydromorphone from PCA, and there is already a continuous infusion going through. A smaller dose of fentanyl could have been useful. One may consider naloxone if patient goes apneic.
3. Discontinue continuous infusion of propofol if already started.

Case Scenario 6

Learning Objectives:
Role of close monitoring until after the end of procedure

A 13-year-old boy diagnosed with ALL who is on induction therapy presented to the clinic for his scheduled LPIT with chemotherapy. He has gained weight due to steroid therapy over the last month, and his BMI is 31%. You have sedated him in the past, and you choose to use propofol and fentanyl for him as before. The induction goes smoothly requiring some airway adjustment and supplemental oxygen that you expected.

At the completion of chemotherapy infusion, when you have cleared his line with a saline push, you notice that his breathing pattern is paradoxical. His saturations suddenly drop down to 64% with the HR 110, and he loses his capnography waveform. The nurse tries to do jaw thrust which doesn't help. While turning up the oxygen, the nurse starts to suction his mouth with no improvement. While the bag mask is placed, you give 1 mg/kg of propofol bolus to reverse his laryngospasm, and the patient suddenly takes a deep breath and begins to recover.

Expected Actions:
1. Ask someone to listen to the lungs for air movement while jaw thrust is applied.
2. Start positive pressure ventilation.
3. Deepen the sedation with propofol bolus.
4. Prepare for RSI with paralytics.

Debriefing Points:
1. Laryngospasm can happen due to many risk factors including insufficient depth of sedation, obesity, gastroesophageal reflux, asthma, and URTI with children being at a higher risk.

2. Most complications occur during induction but it is important to be prepared for any sudden and emergence complications at the end of the procedure.
3. Suctioning can sometimes worsen the spasm.

References

1. Coté CJ, Notterman DA, Karl HW, Weinberg JA, McCloskey C. Adverse sedation events in pediatrics: a critical incident analysis of contributing factors. Pediatrics. 2000;105(4):805–14. https://doi.org/10.1542/peds.105.4.805.
2. Bhananker SM, Posner KL, Cheney FW, Caplan RA, Lee LA, Domino KB. Injury and liability associated with monitored anesthesia care: a closed claims analysis. Anesthesiology. 2006;104(2):228–34. https://doi.org/10.1097/00000542-200602000-00005.
3. Coté CJ, Notterman DA, Karl HW, Weinberg JA, McCloskey C. Adverse sedation events in pediatrics: a critical incident analysis of contributing factors. Pediatrics. 2000;105(4 Pt 1):805–14.
4. Cote CJ, Wilson S, American Academy of Pediatrics, American Academy of Pediatric Dentistry. Guidelines for monitoring and management of pediatric patients before, during, and after sedation for diagnostic and therapeutic procedures: Update 2016. Pediatrics (Evanston). 2016;138(1):e20161212.
5. Hoffman GM, Nowakowski R, Troshynski TJ, Berens RJ, Weisman SJ. Risk reduction in pediatric procedural sedation by application of an American Academy of Pediatrics/American Society of Anesthesiologists Process Model. Pediatrics. 2002;109(2):236–43. https://doi.org/10.1542/peds.109.2.236.
6. The Joint Commission releases Improving America's hospitals: The Joint Commission's annual report on quality and safety 2007. Jt Comm Perspect. 2007;27(12):1–3.
7. Shetty R, Thyagarajan S. Simulation in pediatrics: is it about time? Ann Card Anaesth. 19(3):505–10.
8. McGaghie WC, Issenberg SB, Cohen ER, Barsuk JH, Wayne DB. Does simulation-based medical education with deliberate practice yield better results than traditional clinical education? A meta-analytic comparative review of the evidence. Acad Med. 2011;86(6):706–11. https://doi.org/10.1097/ACM.0b013e318217e119.
9. Ericsson KA. Deliberate practice and acquisition of expert performance: a general overview. Acad Emerg Med. 2008;15(11):988–94. https://doi.org/10.1111/j.1553-2712.2008.00227.x.
10. Institute of Medicine (US) Committee on Quality of Health Care in America. Crossing the quality chasm: a new health system for the 21st century. 2001. https://doi.org/10.17226/10027.
11. Fanning RM, Gaba DM. The role of debriefing in simulation-based learning. Simul Healthc. 2007;2(2):115–25. https://doi.org/10.1097/SIH.0b013e3180315539.
12. Raemer D, Anderson M, Cheng A, Fanning R, Nadkarni V, Savoldelli G. Research regarding debriefing as part of the learning process. Simul Healthc. 2011;6 Suppl(7):S52–7. https://doi.org/10.1097/SIH.0b013e31822724d0.
13. Tripathi S, Raju V, Horack KA, Bronson DL, Deshpande GG. Successful development and implementation of pediatric sedation-analgesia curriculum for residents. J Pediatr Intensive Care. 2018;7(3):129–34. https://doi.org/10.1055/s-0038-1624570.
14. Patterson MD, Blike GT, Nadkarni VM. In situ simulation: challenges and results. In: Advances in patient safety: new directions and alternative approaches (Vol. 3: Performance and Tools). Agency for Healthcare Research and Quality (US); 2008.
15. Baker DP, Gustafson S, Beaubien J, Salas E, Barach P. Medical teamwork and patient safety: the evidence-based relation. AHRQ Public. 2005;5:53):1–64.

16. Pian-Smith MCM, Simon R, Minehart RD, et al. Teaching residents the two-challenge rule: a simulation-based approach to improve education and patient safety. Simul Healthc. 2009;4(2):84–91. https://doi.org/10.1097/SIH.0b013e31818cffd3.
17. Robertson B, Kaplan B, Atallah H, Higgins M, Lewitt MJ, Ander DS. The use of simulation and a modified TeamSTEPPS curriculum for medical and nursing student team training. Simul Healthc. 2010;5(6):332–7. https://doi.org/10.1097/SIH.0b013e3181f008ad.
18. American Institutes for Research. Training guide: using simulation in TeamSTEPPS® training. Rockville, MD: Agency for Healthcare Research and Quality. AHRQ Publication No. 11-0041 EF. February 2011
19. Cheng A, Donoghue A, Gilfoyle E, Eppich W. Simulation-based crisis resource management training for pediatric critical care medicine: a review for instructors. Pediatr Crit Care Med. 2012;13(2):197–203.
20. Holmboe E, Rizzolo MA, Sachdeva AK, Rosenberg M, Ziv A. Simulation-based assessment and the regulation of healthcare professionals. Simul Healthc. 2011;6(7):S58–62. https://doi.org/10.1097/SIH.0b013e3182283bd7.
21. Villamaria FJ, Pliego JF, Wehbe-Janek H, et al. Using simulation to orient code blue teams to a new hospital facility. Simul Healthc. 2008;3(4):209–16. https://doi.org/10.1097/SIH.0b013e31818187f3.

Index

P. P. Kamat, J. W. Berkenbosch (eds.), *Sedation and Analgesia for the Pediatric Intensivist*, https://doi.org/10.1007/978-3-030-52555-2

The manufacturer's authorised representative in the EU is Springer Nature Customer Service Centre GmbH, Europaplatz 3, 69115 Heidelberg, Germany. If you have any concerns regarding our products, please contact ProductSafety@springernature.com

Printed and bound by CPI Group (UK) Ltd, Croydon, CR0 4YY
30/09/2026
02225705-0006